COMPREHENSIVE
RADIOGRAPHIC
PATHOLOGY

Fourth Edition

COMPREHENSIVE RADIOGRAPHIC PATHOLOGY

Ronald L. Eisenberg, MD, JD, FACR
Chairman of Imaging, Department of Radiology
Highland General Hospital
Oakland, California;
Clinical Professor of Radiology
University of California at San Francisco and Davis
San Francisco, California

Nancy M. Johnson, BA, RT (R) (CV) (CT) (QM)
Faculty, Medical Radiography Program
GateWay Community College
Phoenix, Arizona

With 967 illustrations

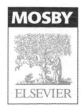

MOSBY
ELSEVIER

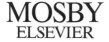

11830 Westline Industrial Drive
St. Louis, Missouri 63146

Comprehensive Radiographic Pathology

ISBN-13:   978-0-323-03624-5
ISBN-10:   0-323-03624-4

Notice

Previous editions copyrighted 2003, 1995, 1990.

ISBN-13: 978-0-323-03624-5
ISBN-10: 0-323-03624-4

Executive Editor: Jeanne Wilke
Managing Editor: Mindy Hutchinson
Senior Developmental Editor: Linda Woodard
Associate Developmental Editor: Christina Pryor
Publishing Services Manager: Pat Joiner
Senior Project Manager: Rachel E. Dowell
Design Direction: Andrea Lutes

Printed in the United States of America

Last digit is the print number: 9 8 7 6 5 4 3 2 1

To all students and radiographers
wishing to better understand the value
of the profession of radiologic technology

ACKNOWLEDGMENTS

I would like to acknowledge and thank the technologists who helped me in updating the text and images. Also, without the support and assistance of my editors (from the publishing side) and my family (from the home front) this endeavor would not have been successful. Thank you all!

Nancy Johnson

REVIEWERS

Donna J. Crum, MS, RT (R) (CT)
Program Director—Radiography
St. Catharine College
St. Catharine, Kentucky

Kelli Welch Haynes, MSRS, RT (R)
Assistant Professor/Clinical Coordinator
Northwestern State University
Shreveport, Louisiana

Jeannie Kilgore, RT (ARRT) (R), BS, MEd
Program Director/Instructor
Clovis Community College
Clovis, New Mexico

Mimi L. Polczynski, MS Ed, RT (R) (M) (CT)
Radiology Program Director
Kaskaskia College
Centralia, Illinois

PREFACE

Understanding the basic principles of pathology is an essential part of the radiologic technologist's training. Knowing how disease processes work and recognizing the radiographic appearance of specific diseases can aid the technologist in selecting proper modalities and determining the need for repeat radiographs in different situations. This kind of knowledge enables the radiologic technologist to become a more competent professional and a contributing member of the diagnostic team.

Organization

Fully illustrated and well organized, *Comprehensive Radiographic Pathology* meets the needs of today's student and practicing radiographers. The book opens with a preliminary chapter on disease processes that introduces the pathologic terms used throughout the text. Chapter 2 describes the advantages and limitations of seven widely used modalities: ultrasound, computed tomography (CT), magnetic resonance imaging (MRI), nuclear medicine, single-photon emission computed tomography (SPECT), positron emission tomography (PET), and fusion imaging.

Each of the remaining chapters is a systematic approach to the diseases involving a specific organ system. These chapters begin with an overview of physiology. For each of the most common pathologic conditions associated with the system, there is a brief description of the disease and its clinical manifestations, followed by imaging findings and treatment. Summary tables follow each major discussion, reiterating the location, radiographic appearance, and treatment of the diseases just presented.

Distinctive Features

- Comprehensive coverage provides the most thorough explanations of any radiographic pathology text of those pathologies that can be diagnosed with medical imaging.
- Navigating the chapters is easy with the standardized heading scheme and chapter outlines for the systems chapters.
- *Radiographers Notes* in every chapter instructs the students with ways to deal effectively with varying patient needs and provides perspective on why learning pathology is important for radiography practice.
- Systems approach makes it easy to locate information and to study one area at a time, assimilating details in a logical sequence. It provides the best framework for building understanding of pathology.
- Summary tables make it easy to locate information and to study one area at a time, assimilating details in a logical sequence. The tables summarize the radiographic appearance and treatment of each disease which have been updated for all pathology conditions included in the text.
- Coverage of the alternative imaging modalities that supplement plain film imaging for diagnosis of some pathology conditions orients readers to think about other imaging modalities that may be needed to ensure proper diagnosis of certain pathologies.
- Treatment sections provide useful background on some treatment and prognosis content even though radiographers are not involved beyond the diagnostic stage of patient care.
- Student workbook provides extra opportunities for review and self-assessment.

New to this Edition

- Discussions on fusion imaging—PET/CT—and updated discussions of common modalities that were previously included: ultrasound, CT, MRI, nuclear medicine, SPECT, and PET.
- Many new images using these modalities, as well as plain film radiography, have been added to update existing content and to illustrate new discussions.
- New discussions on hepatitis, anthrax, and severe acute respiratory syndrome (SARS).
- New student workbook reinforces information from the textbook.

Pedagogical Features

- Each chapter opens with a listing of prerequisite knowledge including goals and objectives. A list of key terms has been added with a chapter outline to aid the student in navigating the content.
- *Radiographers Notes* offer helpful suggestions for producing optimal radiographs of the organ system

featured in each chapter. Information especially relevant to radiologic technologists is included, such as technique adjustments for patients with specific conditions and special patient handling requirements. If multiple imaging modalities can be used, the most appropriate initial procedure is indicated, as well as the sequence in which various imaging studies should be performed.

- The body system chapters are organized as follows: physiology, identification of anatomic structures on radiographs, pathologic conditions, radiographic appearance, and treatment.
- Each section of related pathologies is summarized in a table at the end of the section. The tables name the disorder, and then list the location, radiographic appearance, and treatment for easy review and enhanced retention.
- Finally, each chapter ends with a series of review questions to help readers assess their comprehension of the material. An answer key is found at the back of the book, along with several appendixes, an extensive glossary, and a list of major prefixes, roots, and suffixes to help readers determine the meaning of unfamiliar words.

Ancillaries

For the Instructor

- **Instructor's Electronic Resource** available on CD-ROM includes an image collection of approximately 700 images available in jpeg and PowerPoint formats as well as a test bank in ExamView of approximately 500 questions.
- **Evolve Learning Resource** is an interactive learning environment designed to work in coordination with *Comprehensive Radiographic Pathology,* fourth edition. All of the material included in the Instructor's Electronic Resource is also available on Evolve. Instructors may use Evolve to provide an Internet-based course component that reinforces and expands the concepts presented in class. Evolve may be used to publish the class syllabus, outlines, and lecture notes; set up "virtual office hours" and e-mail communication; share important dates and information through the online class calendar; and encourage student participation through chat rooms and discussion boards. Evolve allows instructors to post exams and manage their grade books online. For more information, visit http://evolve.elsevier.com/Eisenberg/pathology or contact an Elsevier sales representative.

For the Student

- The new **Workbook** contains a variety of exercises for each of the 12 chapters in the book. Examples include matching terms with their definitions, labeling diagrams, fill-in-the-blanks, pathology case studies, short answer questions, multiple choice questions, and a posttest. Completing the workbook activities will ensure understanding of disease processes, their radiographic appearance, and their likely treatment. The addition of the student workbook creates a more complete learning package for students that will assist them in understanding the complex disease processes that will be diagnosed with the help of the medical images they will produce as imaging technologists. The answers for the exercises are located in the back of the workbook.

By understanding the disease processes, their radiographic appearance, and their treatment covered in this textbook and its ancillaries, the technologist will be prepared to contribute to the diagnostic team.

CONTENTS

COMPREHENSIVE
RADIOGRAPHIC
PATHOLOGY

CHAPTER **1**

INTRODUCTION TO
Pathology

Chapter Outline

Disease
    Inflammation
    Edema
    Ischemia and Infarction
    Hemorrhage
    Alterations of Cell Growth
    Neoplasia
Hereditary Diseases
    Disorders of Immunity
    Acquired Immunodeficiency Syndrome
    Hepatitis

Key Terms

abscess
acquired immunodeficiency syndrome (AIDS)
active immunity
anaphylactic
anaplastic
anasarca
antibodies
antigens
atrophy
autosomes
bacteremia
benign
cancers
carcinomas
community acquired
dominant
dysplasia
edema
elephantiasis
grading
granulation tissue
hematogenous spread
hematoma
hemorrhage
hepatitis
hereditary diseases
hyperplasia
iatrogenic
idiopathic

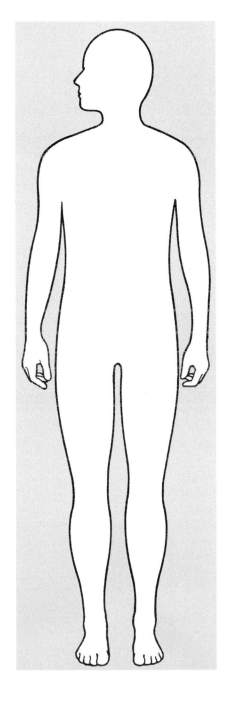

immune	mutations	sarcomas
infarct	neoplasia	signs
inflammation	nosocomial	staging
ischemia	oncology	symptoms
lymphatic spread	permeable	toxoid
malignant	pyogenic	undifferentiated
metastasize	recessive	vaccine

Prerequisite Knowledge

The student should have a basic knowledge of the normal anatomy and physiology of the human body. A good foundation in medical terminology, including word roots, prefixes, and suffixes (see Appendix A) will be most helpful for assimilating the somewhat difficult information presented in this and future chapters. In addition, proper learning and understanding of the material will be facilitated if the student has some clinical experience in all areas of radiography of the human body and in image evaluation, including a concept of the changes in technique required to compensate for density differences produced by underlying pathologic conditions.

Goals

To acquaint the student radiographer with basic medical terminology used to describe various pathologic conditions occurring in the human body (including hereditary diseases, immune reactions, and acquired immunodeficiency syndrome [AIDS]).

Objectives

After reading this chapter, the reader will be able to:
1. Classify the more common diseases in terms of their attenuation of x-rays
2. Explain the changes in technical factors required for obtaining optimal quality radiographs in patients with various underlying pathologic conditions
3. Define and describe all bold-faced terms in this chapter
4. Differentiate inflammation, edema, infarction, hemorrhage, and neoplasia
5. Characterize the various alterations of cell growth
6. Describe the various immune reactions of the body
7. Describe AIDS and the precautions necessary when taking a radiograph of patients with AIDS or any patient with whom contact with any body fluid is possible (Standard Precautions)

Disease

Pathology is the study of diseases that can cause abnormalities in the structure or function of various organ systems. In essence, a disease is the pattern of the body's response to some form of injury that causes a deviation from or variation of normal conditions. Diseases may be hereditary or may result from a broad spectrum of traumatic, infectious, vascular, or metabolic processes presenting by a set of characteristics known as **signs** and **symptoms**. Signs represent the measurable or objective manifestations of the disease process. The experience the patient feels and describes are the symptoms, those (subjective) manifestations that are not measurable or observable. They may reflect alterations of cell growth, as in neoplasia (tumors), or they may even be caused by physicians and their treatment **(iatrogenic).** Incidences of infections being developed at the acute care facility are called **nosocomial,** whereas those contracted outside the healthcare facility are known as **community acquired**. In some cases the underlying cause is unknown, and the disease is termed **idiopathic.**

This chapter discusses several basic reactions of the body that characterize the underlying mechanisms for the radiographic manifestations of most pathologic conditions. These processes include inflammation, edema, ischemia and infarction, hemorrhage, and alterations of cell growth leading to the development of neoplasms (tumors). In addition, this chapter deals with hereditary diseases and immune reactions, such as AIDS and hepatitis.

Inflammation

Acute **inflammation** is the initial response of body tissues to local injury. The various types of injury include those caused by blunt or penetrating trauma, infectious organisms, and irritating chemical substances. Regardless of the underlying cause, the inflammatory response consists of four overlapping events that occur sequentially:
1. Alterations in blood flow and vascular permeability

RADIOGRAPHER *Notes*

Radiography of patients with underlying pathologic conditions can present problems for even the most experienced radiographers. Adjustments in patient position may be necessary to prevent excessive pain caused by the body's response to trauma or certain disease processes. A change in routine projections may be indicated to visualize subtle alterations in the normal radiographic appearance. Many disease processes also alter the density of the structures being radiographed and therefore require changes in technique. For example, extensive edema may require an increased technique, whereas severe atrophy may require a decreased technique. Unless the radiographer has access to previous films with recorded exposure factors, a standard technique chart should be used to determine the initial exposures. Any necessary adjustments can then be made on subsequent films.

The box on p. 4 lists the relative attenuations of x-rays that can be expected in advanced stages of various disease processes. In chest radiography, 110 to 125 kilovolts peak (kVp) is optimal; therefore adjust milliampere-second (mAs) factors to control density. In skeletal radiography, when bone *quality* changes are expected, the best exposure factor to change is the kilovolt level (beam quality change for structural change). When bone *quantity* changes, the mAs value is the exposure factor to change to control density (beam quantity increases to ensure that enough radiation reaches the film without changing the contrast). For example, in osteoporosis there is a decrease in bone quantity and quality; however, a decrease in kilovolts produces a higher-quality image. The normal kilovolt level easily penetrates the diseased bone, producing a low-contrast image with loss of visibility of detail.

Certain diseases suppress the normal immune response. Immunocompromised patients (such as those with advanced leukemia) may require special care to prevent their acquiring a disease from the radiographer. Personal protective equipment (PPE) aids in preventing the spread of microorganisms to the patient and to the healthcare worker. The patient may have to be placed in protective isolation (or "reverse" isolation), and the radiographer may be required to wear mask, gown, and gloves before approaching the patient.

Diseases such as AIDS and hepatitis require that the radiographer wear rubber or latex gloves to be protected against exposure to blood and body fluids, which could contaminate any area near the patient. When examining a patient with AIDS who has a productive cough, the radiographer must wear a mask and possibly protective eye goggles if there is a need to be very close to a patient's face. It is important to remember that many patients having radiographic procedures have not been diagnosed and thus all patients should be treated as though they may have a communicable disease. Therefore whenever exposure to any type of body secretion or blood may occur, the healthcare worker should wear appropriate PPE.

---

2. Migration of circulating white blood cells to the interstitium of the injured tissue
3. Phagocytosis and enzymatic digestion of dead cells and tissue elements
4. Repair of injury by regeneration of normal parenchymal cells or proliferation of granulation tissue and eventual scar formation

The earliest bodily response to local injury is dilation of arterioles, capillaries, and venules, leading to a dramatic increase in blood flow in and around the injury site. This hyperemia produces the heat and redness associated with inflammation. As hyperemia develops, the venules and capillaries become abnormally **permeable,** allowing passage of protein-rich plasma across vessel walls into the interstitium. This inflammatory exudate in the tissues results in the swelling associated with inflammation, which produces pressure on sensitive nerve endings and causes pain. The protein-rich exudate of inflammation must be differentiated from a transudate, a low-protein fluid such as that seen in the pulmonary edema that develops in congestive heart failure.

Very early in the inflammatory response, leukocytes (white blood cells, especially neutrophils and macrophages) of the circulating blood migrate to the area of injury. These white blood cells cross the capillary walls into the injured tissues, where they engulf and enzymatically digest infecting organisms and cellular debris, a process called phagocytosis.

The removal of necrotic debris and any injurious agents, such as bacteria, makes possible the repair of the injury that triggered the inflammatory response. In many tissues, such as the lung after pneumococcal pneumonia, regeneration of parenchymal cells

Relative Attenuation of X-Rays in Advanced Stages of Diseases

Skeletal System
Additive (increased attenuation)
 Acromegaly
 Acute kyphosis
 Callus
 Charcot's joint
 Chronic osteomyelitis (healed)
 Exostosis
 Hydrocephalus
 Marble bone
 Metastasis (osteosclerotic)
 Osteochondroma
 Osteoma
 Paget's disease
 Proliferative arthritis
 Sclerosis
Destructive (decreased attenuation)
 Active osteomyelitis
 Active tuberculosis
 Aseptic necrosis
 Atrophy (disease or disuse)
 Blastomycosis
 Carcinoma
 Coccidioidomycosis
 Degenerative arthritis
 Ewing's tumor (in children)
 Fibrosarcoma
 Giant cell tumor
 Gout
 Hemangioma
 Hodgkin's disease
 Hyperparathyroidism
 Leprosy
 Metastasis (osteolytic)
 Multiple myeloma
 Neuroblastoma
 New bone (fibrosis)
 Osteitis fibrosa cystica
 Osteoporosis/osteomalacia
 Radiation necrosis
 Solitary myeloma

Respiratory System
Additive (increased attenuation)
 Actinomycosis
 Arrested tuberculosis (calcification)
 Atelectasis
 Bronchiectasis
 Edema
 Empyema
 Encapsulated abscess
 Hydropneumothorax
 Malignancy
 Miliary tuberculosis
 Pleural effusion
 Pneumoconiosis
  Anthracosis
  Asbestosis
  Calcinosis
  Siderosis
  Silicosis
 Pneumonia
 Syphilis
 Thoracoplasty
Destructive (decreased attenuation)
 Early lung abscess
 Emphysema
 Pneumothorax

Circulatory System
Additive (increased attenuation)
 Aortic aneurysm
 Ascites
 Cirrhosis of the liver
 Enlarged heart

Soft Tissue
Additive (increased attenuation)
 Edema
Destructive (decreased attenuation)
 Emaciation

From Thompson TT: *Cahoon's formulating x-ray techniques,* ed 9, Durham, NC, 1979, Duke University Press.

permits reconstitution of normal anatomic structure and function. However, some tissues, such as the heart after myocardial infarction, cannot heal by regeneration. A fibrous *scar* replaces the area of destroyed tissue with **granulation tissue.** Granulation tissue refers to a combination of young developing capillaries and actively proliferating fibroblasts, which produce connective tissue fibers (collagen) that replace the dead tissue. Eventually the strong connective tissue contracts to produce a fibrous scar. In the abdomen, such fibrous adhesions can narrow

loops of intestine and result in an obstruction. The accumulation of excessive amounts of collagen (more common in African Americans) may produce a protruding, tumorlike scar known as a keloid. Unfortunately, surgery to remove a keloid is usually ineffective because the subsequent incision tends to heal in the same way.

Many injuries heal by a combination of regeneration and scar tissue formation. An example is the response of the liver to repeated and persistent alcoholic injury; the result is cirrhosis, in which irregular lobules of regenerated liver cells are criss-crossed and surrounded by bands of scar tissue. Scar tissue formation consists of fibrous connective tissue, which can be divided into primary union (surgical incision) and secondary union (non-surgical; gun shot wound).

The five clinical signs of acute inflammation are rubor (redness), calor (heat), tumor (swelling), dolor (pain), and loss of function. The localized heat and redness result from increased blood flow in the microcirculation at the site of injury. The swelling occurs because the exudate increases the amount of interstitial fluid, resulting in pressure on nerve endings and thus pain, which results in a loss of function.

Acute inflammation can also lead to systemic manifestations. Fever is especially common in inflammatory conditions associated with the spread of organisms into the bloodstream. The number of circulating white blood cells also increases (leukocytosis).

Some bacterial organisms (such as staphylococci and streptococci) produce toxins that damage the tissues and incite an inflammatory response. The presence of **pyogenic** bacteria leads to the production of a thick, yellow fluid called pus, which contains dead white blood cells, inflammatory exudate, and bacteria. A suppurative inflammation is one that is associated with pus formation. When a pyogenic infection occurs beneath the skin or in a solid organ, it produces an **abscess,** a localized, usually encapsulated, collection of pus. All pyogens, wherever they become implanted, have the ability to invade blood vessels to produce **bacteremia,** with the potential involvement of other organs and tissues in the body.

A granulomatous inflammation manifests as a distinct pattern seen in relatively few diseases, including tuberculosis, syphilis, and sarcoidosis. A granuloma is a localized area of chronic inflammation, often with central necrosis. It is characterized by the accumulation of macrophages, some of which fuse to form multinucleated giant cells.

Edema

Edema is the accumulation of abnormal amounts of fluid in the intercellular tissue spaces or body cavities. Localized edema results from an inflammatory reaction, whereas generalized edema occurs with pronounced swelling of subcutaneous tissues throughout the body **(anasarca).** Localized edema may result from inflammation, with the escape of protein-rich intravascular fluid into the extravascular tissue. It may also result from a local obstruction to lymphatic drainage; for example, in filariasis, a parasitic worm causes lymphatic obstruction, and the resulting localized edema is termed **elephantiasis.** Generalized edema occurs most frequently in patients with congestive heart failure, cirrhosis of the liver, and certain forms of renal disease. Because of the effect of gravity, generalized edema is usually most prominent in dependent portions of the body. Thus ambulatory patients tend to accumulate fluid in tissues around the ankles and lower legs, whereas in hospitalized patients who are non-ambulatory or sedentary, the edema fluid collects most prominently in the lower back, sacral areas, and lung.

Extravascular fluid can also accumulate in serous cavities to produce pleural and pericardial effusions and peritoneal ascites. Edema may produce minimal clinical symptoms or be potentially fatal. If localized to the subcutaneous tissues, large amounts of edema may cause minimal functional impairment. In contrast, pulmonary edema, pericardial effusion, or edematous swelling of the brain may have dire consequences.

Ischemia and Infarction

Ischemia refers to an interference with the blood supply to an organ or part of an organ, depriving the organ's cells and tissues of oxygen and nutrients. Ischemia may be caused by a narrowing of arterial structures, as in atherosclerosis, or by thrombotic or embolic occlusion (Figure 1-1). Depending on several factors, occlusion of an artery or vein may have little or no effect on the involved tissue, or it may cause death of the tissue and even of the individual. A major determinant is the availability of an alternative or newly acquired route of blood supply (collateral vessels). Other factors include the rate of development of the occlusion, the vulnerability of the tissue to hypoxia, and the oxygen-carrying capacity of the blood. Slowly developing occlusions are less likely to cause tissue death (necrosis) because they provide an opportunity for the development of alternative pathways of flow. Ganglion cells of the nervous system and myocardial muscle cells undergo irreversible damage if deprived of their blood supply for 3 to 5 minutes. Anemic or cyanotic patients tolerate arterial insufficiency less well than normal individuals do, and thus occlusion of even a small vessel in such an individual may lead to death of tissue.

An **infarct** is a localized area of ischemic necrosis within a tissue or organ produced by occlusion of either its arterial supply or its venous drainage. The two most common clinical forms of infarction are myocardial and pulmonary. Almost all infarcts result from thrombotic or embolic occlusion. Infrequent causes include twisting of an organ (volvulus), compression of the blood supply of a loop of bowel in a hernia sac, or trapping of a viscus under a peritoneal adhesion.

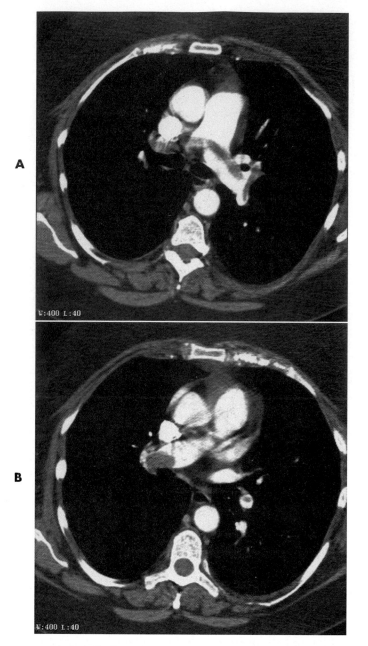

FIGURE 1-1 Pulmonary embolism (saddle type) **(A)** blocking both the right and left pulmonary arteries, and **(B)** a blockage nearly complete on the right.

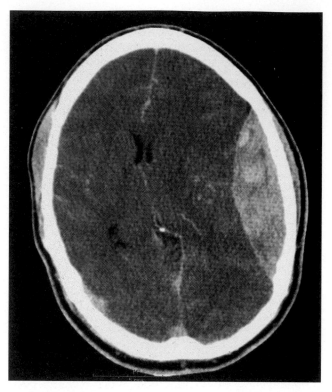

FIGURE 1-2 Subdural hematoma on the left causing midline shift of the ventricles.

In cases in which ischemia continues to progress, resulting in an infarction, necrosis may result due to lack of blood flow. This progressive situation can result in a condition called gangrene. Severe arterial disease of the lower extremities may result in necrosis of several toes or a large segment of the foot, causing gangrene. A frequent presenting symptom in diabetic patients is ischemia of the foot, which may progress to infarction and result in gangrene.

Infarctions tend to be especially severe because they occur more often in the patients least able to withstand them. Thus infarcts tend to occur in elderly individuals with advanced atherosclerosis or impaired cardiac function. The periods after surgery and delivery also have increased occurrence of infarctions.

Hemorrhage

The term **hemorrhage** implies rupture of a blood vessel. Rupture of a large artery or vein is almost always caused by some form of injury, such as trauma, atherosclerosis, or inflammatory or neoplastic erosion of the vessel wall. Hemorrhage may be external, or the blood may be trapped within body tissues, resulting in an accumulation termed a **hematoma** (Figure 1-2). The accumulation of blood in a body cavity results in hemothorax, hemopericardium, hemoperitoneum, or hemarthrosis (blood in a joint). Minimal hemorrhages into the skin, mucous membranes, or serosal surfaces are called petechiae; slightly larger hemorrhages are termed purpura. A large (greater than 1 to 2 cm) subcutaneous hematoma, or bruise, is called an ecchymosis.

The significance of hemorrhage depends on the volume of blood loss, the rate of loss, and the site of the hemorrhage. Sudden losses of up to 20% of the blood volume or slow losses of even larger amounts may have little clinical significance. The site of the hemorrhage is critical. For example, an amount of bleeding that would have little clinical significance in the subcutaneous tissues may cause death when located in a vital portion of the brain. Large amounts of external bleeding lead to the chronic loss of iron from the body and anemia. In contrast, internal hemorrhages into body cavities, joints, or tissues permit the iron to be recaptured for the synthesis of hemoglobin and the development of normal red blood cells.

Alterations of Cell Growth

Changes in the number and size of cells, their differentiation, and their arrangement may develop in response to physiologic stimuli. **Atrophy** refers to a reduction in the size or number of cells in an organ or tissue, with a corresponding decrease in function. It must be distinguished from hypoplasia and aplasia, in which failure of normal development accounts for small size.

An example is the disuse atrophy that occurs with immobilization of a limb by a plaster cast. The muscle mass of the encased limb reduces dramatically. Because the cast also removes the stress and strain from the enclosed bone that normally stimulates new bone formation, normal bone resorption continues unchecked and the loss of calcified bone can be detected on radiographs. In this situation, there is rapid recovery from the atrophic appearance when the cast is removed and normal function is resumed.

Pathologic, irreversible atrophy may be caused by loss of innervation, by hormonal stimulation, or by decreased blood supply. For example, stenosis of a renal artery may cause atrophy of the kidney with shrinkage of individual nephrons and loss of interstitial tissue.

Hypertrophy refers to an increase in the size of the cells of a tissue or organ in response to a demand for increased function. This must be distinguished from **hyperplasia,** an increase in the number of cells in a tissue or organ (Figure 1-3). Hypertrophy occurs most often in cells that cannot multiply, especially those in myocardial and peripheral striated muscle. Myocardial hypertrophy is necessary to maintain cardiac output despite increased peripheral resistance in patients with arterial hypertension or aortic valve disease. After the loss of a normal kidney, hypertrophy of the kidney on the opposite side occurs in an attempt to continue adequate renal function.

Examples of hyperplasia include (1) proliferation of granulation tissue in the repair of injury and (2) the increased cellularity of bone marrow in patients with hemolytic anemia or after hemorrhage. Hyperplasia of the adrenal cortex is a response to increased adrenocorticotropic hormone (ACTH) secretion; hyperplasia of the thyroid gland occurs with increased thyrotropic hormone secretion by the pituitary gland.

Dysplasia is a loss in the uniformity of individual cells and their architectural orientation; it is typically associated with prolonged chronic irritation or

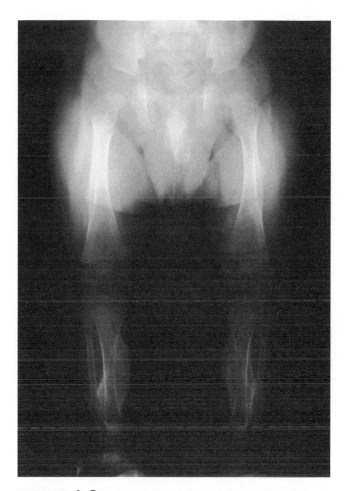

FIGURE 1-3 Infantile cortical hyperostosis (Caffey's disease). Affected bones demonstrate cortical thickening with new periosteal bone formation bilaterally on the femurs and tibias.

inflammation. Removal of the irritant may result in a return to normal, but often the tissue change persists, and it may evolve into a totally abnormal growth pattern. Thus dysplasia is generally considered at least potentially premalignant—a borderline lesion that may heal or progress to cancer.

Neoplasia

Neoplasia, from the Latin word for "new growth," refers to an abnormal proliferation of cells that are no longer controlled by the factors that govern the growth of normal cells. Neoplastic cells act as parasites, competing with normal cells and tissues for their metabolic needs. Thus tumor cells may flourish and the patient becomes weak and emaciated, a condition termed cachexia.

Neoplasms are commonly referred to as tumors; indeed the study of neoplasms is called **oncology,** derived from the Greek word *oncos,* meaning "tumor." Although the word *tumor* originally referred to any swelling, which could also be produced by edema or hemorrhage in tissue, the word now refers almost exclusively to a neoplasm.

Neoplasms are divided into benign and malignant categories on the basis of their potential clinical behavior. **Benign** tumors closely resemble their cells of origin in structure and function. They remain localized, without spreading to other sites, and thus can usually be surgically removed with resultant survival of the patient.

Nevertheless, some benign tumors can have severe consequences because of their position or hormonal secretion. For example, a benign pituitary tumor can cause pressure atrophy and destruction of the surrounding gland, and a benign tumor of the islets of Langerhans in the pancreas can produce excessive amounts of insulin, resulting in possibly fatal low levels of blood glucose. Other potentially dangerous benign tumors include those arising in the brain or spinal cord, which may influence central nervous system function. Tumors of the trachea or esophagus may occlude the air supply or make it impossible to swallow.

Malignant neoplasms invade and destroy adjacent structures and spread to distant sites **(metastasize),** causing death. Malignancies tend to be poorly differentiated so that it may be impossible to determine the organ from which they originate. Malignant tumors are collectively referred to as **cancers.** This term is derived from the Latin word for "crab," possibly because the fingerlike projections that extend into underlying tissue resemble crablike claws.

All tumors, both benign and malignant, have two basic components: (1) the parenchyma (organ tissue), made up of proliferating neoplastic cells, and (2) the supporting stroma (supporting tissue), made up of connective tissue, blood vessels, and possibly lymphatic vessels. The parenchyma of the neoplasm largely determines its biologic behavior and is the component that determines how the tumor is named.

Most benign tumors consist of parenchymal cells that closely resemble the tissue of origin. Their names come from adding the suffix -*oma* to the cell type from which the tumor arose. For example, benign tumors of fibrous tissue are termed fibromas, whereas benign cartilaginous tumors are chondromas (Figure 1-4). The term adenoma is applied to benign epithelial neoplasms that grow in glandlike patterns. Benign tumors that form large cystic masses are called cystadenomas. Lipomas consist of soft fatty tissue, myomas are tumors of muscle, and angiomas are tumors composed of blood vessels. An epithelial tumor that grows as a projecting mass on the skin or from an inner mucous membrane (such as the gastrointestinal tract) is termed a papilloma or a polyp.

Malignant neoplasms of epithelial cell origin are called **carcinomas,** from the Greek word *karkinos,* meaning "crab." Carcinomas affect epithelial tissues, skin, and mucous membranes lining body cavities. Adenocarcinoma refers to malignancies of glandular tissues, such as the breast, liver, and pancreas, and of the cells lining the gastrointestinal tract. Squamous cell carcinoma denotes a cancer in which the tumor cells resemble stratified squamous epithelium, as in the lung and head and neck regions. At times, the tumor grows in such a bizarre pattern that it is termed **undifferentiated** or **anaplastic** (without form).

Sarcomas are highly malignant tumors arising from connective tissues, such as bone, muscle, and

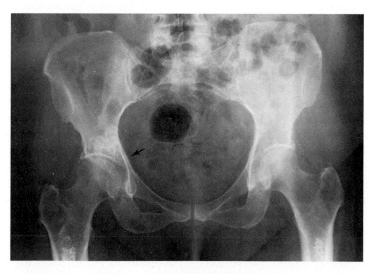

FIGURE 1-4 Enchondroma, a lobulated area with increased density in the supraacetabular region on the right side.

cartilage. Although they are less common than carcinomas, sarcomas tend to spread more rapidly.

Substantial evidence exists indicating that most tumors arise from a single cell (monoclonal origin). The rate of growth generally correlates inversely with the level of parenchymal differentiation. Thus well-differentiated tumors tend to grow slowly, whereas bizarre, undifferentiated neoplasms have a rapid growth rate.

Although the cause of cancer is still unknown, many possible causative factors (carcinogens) have been implicated. Chemical carcinogens may cause structural alteration of the deoxyribonucleic acid (DNA) molecule (mutation), which may lead to the development of a neoplasm. Examples of chemical carcinogens include air and water pollution, cigarette smoke, asbestos, and a variety of other substances used in industry, food, cosmetics, and plastics. The development of specific types of cancer in certain families suggests a possible genetic predisposition. Excessive exposure to ultraviolet radiation (sunshine) may lead to the development of skin cancer. Survivors of the atom bomb who received huge doses of radiation have demonstrated a high incidence of leukemia. A greater-than-expected rate of leukemia was also seen in persons working with x-radiation before the need for proper protection was appreciated.

The study of experimental animal tumors has offered convincing evidence that DNA and ribonucleic acid (RNA) viruses can induce neoplastic transformation. Viruses that invade normal cells may alter their genetic material, leading to the abnormal cell divisions and rapid growth observed in malignant tumors.

The clinical symptoms of cancer vary with the site of malignancy. A blood-tinged stool, a change in bowel activity (e.g., intermittent constipation and diarrhea), or intestinal obstruction is suggestive of gastrointestinal malignancy. Difficulty in swallowing (dysphagia) or loss of appetite (anorexia), especially if accompanied by rapid weight loss, suggests a neoplasm in the esophagus or stomach. Hematuria may indicate kidney or bladder cancer, whereas difficulties in urination (e.g., urgency, a burning sensation, or an inability to start the stream of urine) in an elderly man may be a sign of prostate tumor. Hemoptysis (coughing up blood), a persistent cough, or hoarseness may suggest a neoplasm in the respiratory tract. Severe anemia may develop from internal bleeding or from malfunction of the bone marrow caused by growth of a malignant lesion in the skeleton.

It should be stressed that these clinical symptoms may also be caused by benign disease. Nevertheless, because they may signal an underlying malignancy, they should be carefully investigated to exclude the presence of cancer.

Pain is frequently not an early sign of cancer. Unfortunately, pain may be appreciated only when the malignancy has spread too extensively to be curable. Secondary infections are common and an increasing cause of death. Most cancer patients are immunologically compromised, either because of their original disease or as a result of radiation or chemotherapy. In addition to having typical bacterial and viral infections, immunocompromised patients with malignancy are especially susceptible to unusual opportunistic infections, such as *Pneumocystis carinii* pneumonia and cytomegalovirus.

Some cancers that are still at a curable stage can be detected by screening procedures. Routine mammography may identify nonpalpable breast cancer; a Papanicolaou (Pap) smear may show otherwise unsuspected cancer of the cervix. Surgical removal of these small tumors without metastatic spread offers an excellent prognosis.

Malignant neoplasms disseminate to distant sites by one of three pathways: (1) seeding within body cavities, (2) lymphatic spread, and (3) hematogenous spread.

Seeding (diffuse spread) of cancers occurs when neoplasms invade a natural body cavity. For example, a tumor of the gastrointestinal tract may penetrate the wall of the gut (visceral peritoneum), permitting metastases to enter the peritoneal cavity and implant at distant sites. A similar sequence may occur with lung cancers in the pleural cavity. Neoplasms of the central nervous system (medulloblastoma, ependymoma) may spread from the cerebral ventricles by means of the cerebrospinal fluid to reimplant on the meningeal surfaces within the brain or in the spinal cord.

Lymphatic spread is the major metastatic route of carcinomas, especially those of the lung and breast. The pattern of lymph node involvement depends on the site of the primary neoplasm and the natural lymphatic pathways of drainage of that region. Carcinomas of the lung metastasize first to the regional bronchial lymph nodes and then to the tracheobronchial and hilar nodes. Carcinoma of the breast usually arises in the upper outer quadrant and first spreads to the axillary nodes. Medial breast lesions may drain through the chest wall to nodes along the internal mammary artery.

The **hematogenous spread** of cancer is a complex process involving several steps. Tumor cells invade and penetrate blood vessels, traveling as neoplastic emboli in the circulation. These emboli of tumor cells are trapped in small vascular channels of distant organs, where they invade the wall of the arresting vessel and infiltrate and multiply in the adjacent tissue. The localization of hematogenous metastases tends to be determined by the vascular connections and anatomic relationships between the primary neoplasm and the metastatic sites. For example, carcinomas arising in abdominal organs, such as the gastrointestinal tract, tend to metastasize to the liver because of the flow of portal vein blood to that organ. Cancers arising in midline organs close to the vertebral column (e.g., prostate, thyroid) tend to embolize through the paravertebral venous plexus to seed the vertebral column. Neoplasms in organs drained by the inferior and superior vena cava, such as the kidney, tend to metastasize to the lung. However, several well-defined patterns of metastatic spread cannot be easily explained by vascular-anatomic relationships. Some examples include the tendency for carcinoma of the lung to involve the adrenal glands, simultaneous metastatic deposits in the brain and adrenal glands, and pituitary metastases occurring from breast carcinomas.

The **grading** of a malignant tumor assesses aggressiveness, or degree of malignancy. The grade of a tumor usually indicates its biologic behavior and may allow prediction of its responsiveness to certain therapeutic agents. **Staging** refers to the extensiveness of a tumor at its primary site and the presence or absence of metastases to lymph nodes and distant organs, such as the liver, lungs, and skeleton. The staging of a tumor aids in determining the most appropriate therapy. Well-localized tumors without evidence of metastases may be surgically removed. Fast-growing, undifferentiated tumors, such as those found in patients with Hodgkin's disease, may respond best to radiation therapy. Cancer of the prostate responds to hormonal therapy, either by the removal of the sources of male gonadal hormones that stimulate tumor growth or by the administration of female gonadal hormone (estrogen) that inhibits it. Chemotherapy uses one or a combination of cytotoxic substances that kill neoplastic cells, but these drugs may injure many normal cells and result in significant complications.

Hereditary Diseases

Hereditary diseases pass from one generation to the next through the genetic information contained in the nucleus of each cell. They reflect an abnormality in the DNA, which provides the blueprint for protein synthesis in the cell. In many hereditary diseases, an error in a single protein molecule leads to enzyme defects; membrane receptor and transport system defects; alterations in the structure, function, or quantity of nonenzyme proteins; and unusual drug reactions.

The most common hereditary abnormality is an enzyme deficiency. This leads to a metabolic block that results in a decreased amount of a substance needed for normal function, or in an accumulation of a metabolic intermediate that may cause injury. An example of the first mechanism is albinism, the absence of pigmentation resulting from an enzymatic deficiency that prevents the synthesis of the pigment melanin. An example of the second mechanism is phenylketonuria, in which the absence of an enzyme leads to the accumulation of toxic levels of the amino acid phenylalanine.

A defect in the structure of the globin molecule leads to the development of the hemoglobinopathies, such as sickle cell disease and thalassemia. An example of a genetically determined adverse reaction to drugs is glucose 6-phosphate dehydrogenase deficiency, in which an insufficient amount of the enzyme results in a severe hemolytic anemia in patients receiving a common antimalarial drug.

Despite our extensive knowledge of the biochemical basis of many genetic disorders, there are a large number of conditions for which the underlying mechanism is still unknown. This list includes cystic fibrosis (Chapter 3), neurofibromatosis, retinoblastoma, familial colonic polyposis (Chapter 5), and Huntington's disease (Chapter 8).

Each human cell contains 46 chromosomes divided into 23 pairs. The chromosomes in turn contain thousands of genes, each of which is responsible for the synthesis of a single protein. Forty-four of the chromosomes are called **autosomes;** the other two are the X and Y chromosomes, which determine the sex of the person. A combination of XY chromosomes results in a male, whereas an XX configuration results in a female.

Each person inherits half of his or her chromosomes from each parent. If the genes inherited from each parent are the same for a particular trait, the person is *homozygous* for that trait. If the genes differ (e.g., one for brown eyes and one for blue eyes), the person is *heterozygous* for that trait. **Dominant** genes always produce an effect regardless of whether the person is homozygous or heterozygous; **recessive** genes manifest themselves only when the person is homozygous for the trait. In determining eye color, brown is dominant, whereas blue is recessive. It must be remembered that although a recessive trait must have been contributed by both parents, the possibility exists that neither parent demonstrates that trait. For example, two parents, each with one gene for brown eyes and one gene for blue eyes, would show the dominant brown coloration, although they could each contribute a blue-eye gene to their offspring, who would manifest the recessive blue-eye trait.

For some traits, the genes are codominant, so that both are expressed. An example is the AB blood type, in which the gene for factor A is inherited from one parent and that for factor B is inherited from the other.

Mutations are alterations in the DNA structure that may become permanent hereditary changes if they affect the gonadal cells. Mutations may result from radiation, chemicals, or viruses. They may have minimal effect and be virtually undetectable or be so serious that they are incompatible with life, causing the death of a fetus and spontaneous abortion.

Autosomal dominant disorders are transmitted from one generation to the next. These disorders affect females and males, and both can transmit the condition. When an affected person marries an unaffected person, half the children (on the average) will have the disease. The clinical manifestations of autosomal dominant disorders can be modified by reduced penetrance and variable expressivity. Reduced penetrance means that not everyone who has the gene will demonstrate the trait; variable expressivity refers to the fact that a dominant gene may manifest somewhat differently in different individuals (Figure 1-5) (e.g., polydactyly may be expressed in the toes or in the fingers as one or more extra digits). Examples of autosomal dominant disorders include achondroplasia (Chapter 4), neurofibromatosis, Marfan's syndrome (Chapter 12), and familial hypercholesterolemia.

Autosomal recessive disorders result only when a person is homozygous for the defective gene. The trait does not usually affect the parents, although siblings may show the disease. On average, siblings have a one-in-four chance of being affected; two out of four will be carriers of the gene, and one will be normal. Recessive genes appear more frequently in a family, and close intermarriage (as between first cousins) increases the risk of the particular disease. Unlike autosomal dominant diseases, the expression of the defect tends to be uniform in autosomal recessive diseases and the age of onset is frequently early in life. Examples of autosomal recessive disorders include phenylketonuria (Chapter 12), cystic fibrosis (Chapter 3), galactosemia, glycogen and lipid storage diseases (Chapter 12), Tay-Sachs disease, and sickle cell anemia (Chapter 9).

Sex-linked disorders generally result from defective genes on the X chromosome because the Y chromosome is small and carries very few genes. Most of these conditions are transmitted by heterozygous female carriers virtually only to sons, who have only the single, affected X chromosome. Sons of a heterozygous woman have a one-in-two chance of receiving the mutant gene. An affected man does not transmit the disorder to sons, but all his daughters carry the genetic trait. In rare cases a female may have the sex-linked disease if she is homozygous for the recessive gene. Virtually all sex-linked disorders are recessive. The most common example of a sex-linked disorder is color blindness. Other conditions include glucose 6-phosphate dehydrogenase deficiency, and some types of hemophilia (Chapter 9) and muscular dystrophy (Chapter 12).

Disorders of Immunity

The immune reaction of the body provides a powerful defense against invading organisms by allowing it to recognize foreign substances **(antigens),** such as bacteria, viruses, fungi, and toxins, and to produce **antibodies** to counteract them. The antibody binds together with the antigen to make the antigen harmless. Once antibodies have been produced, a person becomes **immune** to the antigen.

Antibodies, or immunoglobulins, form in lymphoid tissue, primarily in the lymph nodes, thymus gland, and spleen. Although an infant has some immunity at birth, most immunity is acquired either naturally by exposure to a disease or artificially by immunization. There are two types of artificial immunity: active and passive. In **active immunity,** a person forms

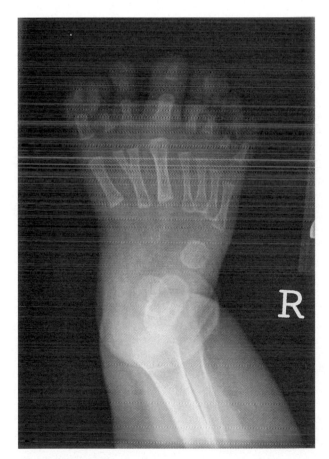

FIGURE 1-5 Right foot image with seven metatarsals and eight digits demonstrating polydactyly.

antibodies to counteract an antigen in the form of a vaccine or a toxoid. A **vaccine** consists of a low dose of dead or deactivated bacteria or viruses. Although these organisms cannot cause disease, they are foreign proteins containing antigens that stimulate the body to produce antibodies against them. A **toxoid** is a chemically altered toxin, the poisonous material produced by a pathogenic organism. As with a vaccine, the toxin cannot cause disease but does trigger the development of antibodies. Examples of active immunity are the vaccines given to prevent smallpox, polio, measles, tetanus, and diphtheria. Active immunity persists for a long time, although a relatively long time is required to build up immunity, and a booster shot frequently gives a stronger effect.

Passive immunity refers to the administration of a dose of preformed antibodies from the immune serum of an animal, usually a horse. This type of immunity acts immediately, but lasts for a relatively short time. It is used in situations in which a person is exposed to a serious disease (hepatitis, rabies, tetanus), but has no immunity against it and thus requires an immediate supply of antibodies to prevent a possibly fatal infection.

Several fundamental mechanisms of immunologic responses to antigens exist. The first type is a rapidly occurring reaction in which antigens are attacked by antibodies previously bound to the surface of mast cells. The mast cells release histamine, which causes a local increase in vascular permeability and smooth muscle contraction. Disorders resulting from localized reactions of this type (which probably have a genetically determined predisposition) include hay fever, asthma, and gastrointestinal allergies. Generalized, or systemic, **anaphylactic** reactions are characterized by hypotension and vascular collapse (shock) with urticaria (hives), bronchiolar spasm, and laryngeal edema. This reaction causes acute death in patients who are hypersensitive ("allergic") to the sting of bees, wasps, and other insects and to medications, such as penicillin and the iodinated contrast materials used in radiology.

In the second type of immune reaction, called a cytotoxic reaction, either the antigen is a component of a cell or it attaches to the wall of red blood cells, white blood cells, platelets, or vascular endothelial cells. The reaction with an antibody leads to cell destruction by lysis or phagocytosis. Examples of a cytotoxic immune reaction include the transfusion reaction occurring after the administration of ABO-incompatible blood, and erythroblastosis fetalis, the hemolytic anemia of the Rh-positive newborn whose Rh-negative mother has produced anti-Rh antibodies.

The third type of immune reaction, a delayed reaction, occurs in an individual previously sensitized to an antigen. As an example, the first time a person touches poison ivy no reaction occurs. However, on the next exposure to poison ivy, antibodies are present to attack the antigen, and the patient develops the typical rash and irritation. A similar process produces a reaction to tuberculosis, leprosy, many fungal diseases, and other infections. This process also represents the principal component of rejection in organ transplants.

Acquired Immunodeficiency Syndrome

Acquired immunodeficiency syndrome (AIDS), which most commonly affects young homosexual men and intravenous drug abusers, is characterized by a profound and sustained impairment of cellular immunity that results in recurrent or sequential opportunistic infections and a particularly aggressive form of Kaposi's sarcoma. AIDS has also been reported in a substantial number of hemophiliacs, in recipients of transfusions, and increasingly in heterosexual partners of affected individuals. AIDS is attributable to infection with retroviruses (RNA viruses) known as human immunodeficiency viruses (HIV). This immune deficiency predominantly involves the lungs, gastrointestinal tract, and central nervous system. Pulmonary infections are extremely common in patients with AIDS and are frequently caused by organisms that only rarely produce disease in individuals with normal immune systems. About 60% of AIDS victims develop one or more attacks of *Pneumocystis carinii* pneumonia, which is characterized by a sudden onset, a rapid progression to diffuse lung involvement, and a considerable delay in resolution. *Pneumocystis carinii* cannot be cultured, and the disease is usually fatal if untreated. An open-lung biopsy is often necessary to make the diagnosis if a sputum examination reveals no organisms in a patient suspected of having this disease.

Gastrointestinal manifestations of AIDS include a variety of sexually transmitted diseases involving the rectum and colon, infectious processes (such as shigellosis, amebiasis, candidiasis, and giardiasis), and alimentary tract dissemination (spread) of Kaposi's sarcoma. Kaposi's sarcoma, a systemic disease, characteristically affects the skin and causes an ulcerated hemorrhagic dermatitis. Metastases to the small bowel, which are relatively common, consist of multiple reddish or bluish red nodules that intrude into the lumen of the bowel (Figure 1-6). Similar lesions can develop throughout the gastrointestinal tract. Central ulceration of the metastases causes gastrointestinal bleeding and a characteristic radiographic appearance of multiple "bull's-eye" lesions simulating metastatic melanoma.

About 40% of all AIDS victims have neurologic symptoms, most commonly progressive dementia.

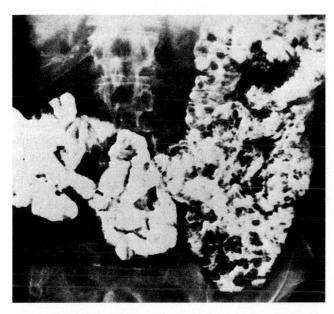

FIGURE 1-6 Kaposi's sarcoma. Small bowel study shows multiple intramural nodules (predominantly involving the jejunum) that distort the mucosal pattern and produce contour defects and intraluminal lucencies.

Patients who develop mass lesions of the brain commonly have focal neurologic symptoms and signs.

Radiographic Appearance

The typical early radiographic finding of *P. carinii* pneumonia is a hazy, perihilar, granular infiltrate that spreads to the periphery and appears predominantly interstitial. In later stages the pattern progresses to patchy areas of air-space consolidation with air bronchograms, indicating the alveolar nature of the process (Figure 1-7). The radiographic appearance may closely resemble pulmonary edema or bacterial pneumonia.

Magnetic resonance imaging (MRI) best demonstrates the multiple manifestations of AIDS in the central nervous system, where areas of increased signal intensity can be seen on T2-weighted images. Atypical brain abscesses and meningeal infection often occur, most commonly related to toxoplasmosis, cryptococcosis, cytomegalovirus, and herpesvirus (Figure 1-8). Increasing evidence indicates that cerebral infections may manifest from the HIV itself. Patients with AIDS also have a high incidence of lymphoma involving the central nervous system.

Treatment

Although much research has been initiated, no cure for AIDS has been found. Currently, treatment assists in maintaining quality of life and management of symptoms as they manifest. Antiviral drugs assist in suppressing the HIV infection. A healthy lifestyle free of stress, alcohol, and illegal drugs is recommended.

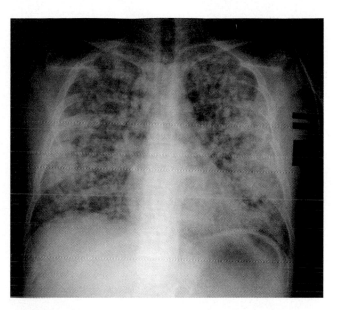

FIGURE 1-7 *Pneumocystis carinii* pneumonia. Diffuse bilateral air-space consolidation is suggestive of severe bacterial pneumonia or pulmonary edema.

HIV carriers should avoid infections if possible because they may accelerate the HIV process.

Hepatitis

Hepatitis is the most prevalent inflammatory disease of the liver. The most common causes are a viral infection or a reaction to drugs and toxins. The viral types of hepatitis include hepatitis A virus (HAV), hepatitis B virus (HBV), hepatitis C virus (HCV), and hepatitis E virus (HEV).

Hepatitis A virus, previously known as "infectious hepatitis," is transmitted in the digestive tract from oral or fecal contact. In most cases the disease is self-contained and has a favorable prognosis.

Hepatitis B virus, previously known as "serum hepatitis," is contracted by exposure to contaminated blood or blood products, or through sexual contact. Healthcare workers are more susceptible to this virus and are usually required to have been vaccinated or prove immunity. Ninety percent recover without incident; however, because of the high incidence (200,000 to 300,000 new cases/year), the vaccine has become required as part of the childhood immunization process.

Hepatitis C virus, formally known as "non-A, non-B hepatitis," is the common cause of chronic hepatitis, cirrhosis, and hepatocellular carcinoma. Because it is contracted by blood transfusion or sexual contact, some believe healthcare workers are more susceptible; however, 40% of cases are of an unknown source found in the general population. It is estimated that 50% with HVC related cirrhosis will

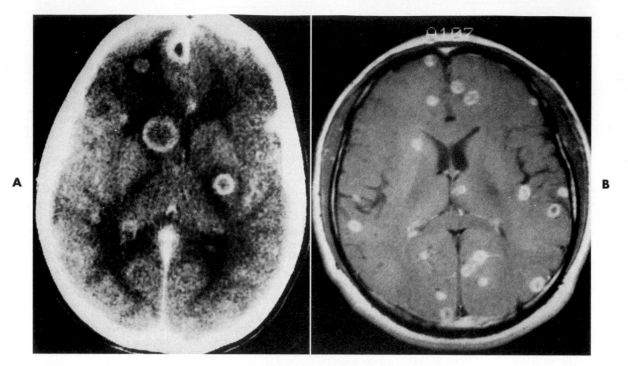

FIGURE 1-8 Neurologic manifestations of AIDS. **A,** Computed tomographic scan shows multiple ring-enhancing lesions caused by cryptococcal brain abscesses. **B,** MRI, after intravenous administration of contrast medium, demonstrates multiple enhancing abscesses caused by toxoplasmosis.

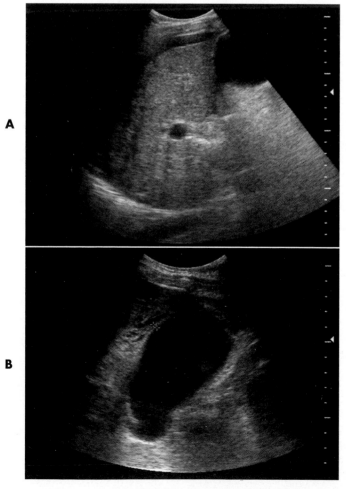

FIGURE 1-9 Autoimmune hepatitis: 18-year-old female with end-stage liver disease. On the ultrasound, the liver demonstrates an internal coarse texture **(A)** and a lobulated surface **(B),** which is consistent with severe cirrhosis.

develop cancer. In the United States and Western Europe, HCV cirrhosis is the principal cause leading to liver transplantation.

Hepatitis E virus is self-limited and acquired by the ingestion of food or water that has been contaminated with fecal material.

Radiographic Appearance

Viral hepatitis in the earliest stages is not visible on diagnostic images. The later stages resulting in cirrhosis or hepatocellular carcinoma can be demonstrated on ultrasound, computed tomography (CT), and MRI. On ultrasound, cirrhosis caused by viral hepatitis usually presents as macronodules, which may vary in size from 3 mm to 5 cm. The liver has an internal coarse texture with increased echogenicity, and the surface may have a nodular appearance representing fibrosis (Figure 1-9). Portal hypertension, due to enlargement or blockage of the portal system, can also be detected. CT demonstrates hepatocellular necrosis with scattered inflammatory cells and evidence of a fatty liver. Normally the density of the liver should be similar to that of the spleen. In fatty liver, infiltrates of fat appear as discrete or diffuse areas of low density within the liver. Contrast-enhanced CT in the portal venous phase is best for demonstrating a lobulated liver. Due to atrophy, the intrahepatic fissures become more visually prominent. T1-weighted contrast MR images show irregular diffuse enhancement with ill-defined surfaces; there may be rim enhancement in the venous phase. T2-weighted fat-suppressed images demonstrate a heterogeneous mass appearance with moderate elevation of the signal intensity. MRI enhancement with gadolinium is superior to that produced by iodinated contrast on CT for distinguishing abnormalities.

Treatment

At this time, prevention is the best method to control hepatitis. Standard Precautions for healthcare workers should include the use of PPE for all patients. Vaccines exist for hepatitis A virus and hepatitis B virus. For short-term immunization, immune globulin is used.

REVIEW QUESTIONS

1. The accumulation of abnormal amounts of fluid in the spaces between cells or in body cavities is termed _____.

2. _____ is the process by which white blood cells surround and digest infectious organisms.

3. A tumorlike scar is referred to as a(n) _____.

4. Inflammation with pus formation is termed _____.

5. An interruption in the blood supply to an organ or body part is referred to as _____.

6. A localized area of ischemic necrosis in an organ or tissue is termed a(n) _____.

7. A swelling caused by bleeding into an enclosed area is termed _____.

8. A decrease in function of an organ or tissue because of a reduction in the size or number of cells is termed _____.

9. The term _____ means new growth.

10. The term for benign epithelial neoplasms that have a glandlike pattern is _____.

BIBLIOGRAPHY

General Radiology

Beers MH, Berkow R: *The Merck manual of diagnosis and therapy*, New Jersey, 1999, Merck Publishing Group.

Eisenberg RL: *Diagnostic imaging in internal medicine*, New York, 1985, McGraw-Hill.

Eisenberg RL: *Diagnostic imaging in surgery*, New York, 1986, McGraw-Hill.

Juhl JH, Crummy AB: *Essentials of radiologic imaging*, Philadelphia, 1987, Lippincott.

Putman CE, Ravin CE: *Textbook of diagnostic imaging*, Philadelphia, 1988, Saunders.

Rumack CM, Wilson SR, Charborneau JW: *Diagnostic ultrasound*, St Louis, 2005, Mosby.

CHAPTER **2**

SPECIALIZED IMAGING
Techniques

Chapter Outline

Diagnostic Imaging Modalities
    Ultrasound
    Computed Tomography
    Magnetic Resonance Imaging
    Nuclear Medicine
    Single-Photon Emission Computed
     Tomography
    Positron Emission Tomography
    Fusion Imaging

Key Terms

anechoic
annihilation
collimator
computed tomography (CT)
CT number
diffusion imaging
direct fusion
echogenic
fat-suppressed images
functional MR (fMR)
gamma camera
helical
hyperechoic
integrated imaging
isoechoic
magnetic resonance imaging (MRI)
nuclear medicine
positron emission tomography (PET)
radiofrequency (RF) pulse
radiopharmaceutical
single-photon emission computed tomography
  (SPECT)
spin-echo (SE)
T1-weighted images
T2-weighted images
ultrasound
volume-rendered imaging

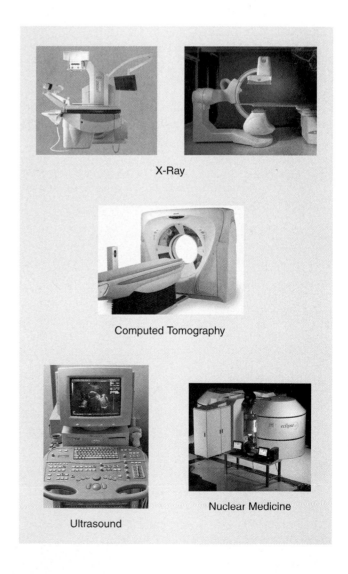

X-Ray

Computed Tomography

Ultrasound

Nuclear Medicine

Prerequisite Knowledge

The student should have a basic knowledge of diagnostic imaging modalities of the human body. A good foundation of basic imaging terms and physics will be most helpful to aid in understanding the somewhat difficult pathologic processes and their relationship to image appearance presented in future chapters. In addition, proper learning and understanding of the material will be facilitated if the student has some clinical experience in all areas of radiography of the human body and image evaluation, including a concept of the modality of choice to best demonstrate underlying pathologic conditions.

Goals

To introduce the student radiographer to some basic specialized imaging techniques used to demonstrate the pathologic conditions related to different disease processes.

Objectives

After reading this chapter, the reader will be able to:
1. Describe the theory of image production with ultrasound and why this modality becomes the optimal choice to demonstrate the pathologic conditions
2. Describe the theory of image production with computed tomography (CT) and the body structures best demonstrated
3. Briefly describe the theory of image production with magnetic resonance imaging (MRI) and the different sequences used to demonstrate specific tissue
4. Describe the theory of image production with nuclear medicine, single-photon emission computed tomography (SPECT), and positron emission tomography (PET)
5. Identify the fusion imaging techniques required to produce optimal quality images in patients with various underlying pathologic conditions

RADIOGRAPHER *Notes*

A medical radiographer is one of the patient's healthcare team for care, diagnosis, and treatment, especially in the diagnostic imaging department. As a team member, our role is to produce the best quality images for diagnosis. Not only radiologists and physicians view the images; technologists using other imaging modalities—such as ultrasound, CT, MRI, nuclear medicine, SPECT, and PET— view these images as a basis for producing studies in other modalities.

As a part of the team, communication is very important. To accomplish this task, the radiographer may need to gather information from the patient (patient history). Once the added information is recorded, the technologist may confer with the radiologist to ensure that the correct exam has been ordered. In some cases, even though the exam is correct, it would be beneficial if additional image projections were taken to provide supplementary information. The better radiographers understand their role in imaging, the more adept they will be at producing the correct images for the specific pathophysiologic condition of the patient.

To best demonstrate the pathology, all imaging technologists must do their part to provide added information. The imaging team is responsible for providing the best images to complement each other. The collection of images from all modalities aids the diagnostician in making an accurate diagnosis.

Diagnostic Imaging Modalities

As the world of technology advances, medical imaging modalities have become more technical. This requires the radiographer to have a broader and more specific skill set to produce quality images.

The first of these new modalities was ultrasound, which was capable of producing images without the use of ionizing radiation, providing a diagnostic tool to view soft tissues, especially in the fetus. In the early to mid-1970s, computed axial tomography (now known as CT) provided revolutionary new images of the brain that demonstrated the bone structure, white and gray matter, and the fluid-filled ventricles. Eventually, CT eliminated the need for pneumoencephalogy and replaced many cerebral angiograms. Scientists integrated the use of strong magnets and radiofrequencies to provide another mode of producing images without the use of ionizing radiation—nuclear magnetic resonance (now known as MRI). Magnetic resonance imaging offers clinicians images with high soft tissue resolution and the ability to visualize structural and functional tissue. CT and MRI now provide diagnosticians with three-dimensional (axial, sagittal, and coronal) images and offer a way to separate overlapping anatomic structures. With continuing research, nuclear medicine expanded its role by adding movement and a computer that allowed more than anterior and posterior projections, resulting in the development of SPECT. Additional research developments in radiopharmaceuticals led to the creation of a positron-emitting radionuclide, which resulted in the newest modality—PET. Now the concept of multiplanar imaging and gamma camera movement (tomography) has provided healthcare with two new perspectives in molecular imaging.

Computerized technology has become prevalent in imaging today. Imaging modalities with special software can now be integrated to create a fused image (superimposition of two different modalities). PET/CT is the most prominent hybrid equipment available today. As computed technology continues to become more complex, the modalities of today's imaging department will also become more complicated. However, these positive changes result in images that are more precise and have greater sensitivity. This offers the diagnostician a quicker, more accurate diagnosis to meet the patient's needs.

Ultrasound

Ultrasound is a widely accepted cross-sectional imaging technique because of its low cost, availability, and ability to differentiate cystic (gallbladder), solid (liver), and complex (liver tumor) tissue. Ultrasound (Figure 2-1) is a noninvasive imaging modality that uses high-frequency sound waves produced by electrical stimulation of a specialized crystal. When the high-frequency sound waves pass through the body, their intensity is reduced by different amounts, depending on the acoustic properties of the tissues through which they travel. The crystal mounted in a transducer sends the signal and also acts as a receiver to record echoes reflected back from the body whenever the sound wave strikes an interface between two tissues that have different acoustic properties. The transducer records the tiny changes of the signal's pitch and direction. A water-tissue interface can produce strong reflections (echoes), whereas a solid tissue mass that contains small differences in composition can cause weak reflections. The display of the ultrasound image on a television monitor shows both the intensity level of the echoes and the position in the body from which they were scanned. Ultrasound images may be displayed as static grayscale images or as multiple (video) images that permit movement to be viewed in real time. Depending on the equipment used, the interactions of the tissue with the sound wave determine how the tissue or organ is visualized and described.

In general, fluid-filled structures have intense echoes at their borders, no internal echoes, and good transmission of the sound waves. **Anechoic** tissue or structures (which are echo free or lacking a signal) transmit sound waves easily and appear as the dark region on the image; examples are the gallbladder and a distended urinary bladder. Solid structures (e.g., a gallbladder with gallstones) produce internal echoes of variable intensity. Because the solid

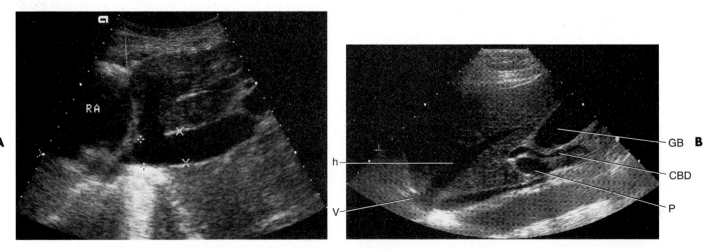

FIGURE 2-1 Ultrasound images of normal abdomens. **A,** Right atrium of the heart *(RA),* the inferior vena cava (marked for measurement), and the hepatic vein joining the inferior vena cava. **B,** Gallbladder *(GB),* common bile duct *(CBD),* portal vein *(P),* hepatic vein *(h),* and inferior vena cava *(V).*

structure tends to attenuate the sound waves, the posterior margin appears less sharply defined than the anterior margin, and only a portion of the beam is transmitted. The terms **hyperechoic** and **echogenic** indicate that the tissue structure exhibits a relatively strong reflection, a bright intensity appearing light gray to white on the image (e.g., stones and bone). Hypoechoic tissue exhibits relatively weak reflections that appear dark gray to gray on the image (e.g., the gastrointestinal tract). The term **isoechoic** is used to describe two structures that have the same echogenicity even though the tissue may not be the same; for example, liver tissue is isoechoic to renal cortex. Complex tissue types have both anechoic and echogenic areas (Figure 2-2).

The major advantage of ultrasound is its safety. There has been no evidence of any adverse effect on human tissues at the intensity level currently used for diagnostic procedures. Therefore ultrasound is the modality of choice for examinations of children and pregnant women in whom a potential danger exists from the radiation exposure of other imaging studies. Ultrasound is by far the best technique for evaluating fetal age and placenta placement, congenital anomalies, and complications of pregnancy (Figure 2-3). Abdominal ultrasound is used extensively to evaluate the intraperitoneal and retroperitoneal structures, to detect abdominal and pelvic abscesses, and to diagnose obstruction of the biliary and urinary tracts. Pelvic ultrasound images of the prostate gland aid in the detection and accurate staging of neoplasms. Pelvic imaging is performed by a transabdominal (organs), transvaginal (uterus), or transrectal (prostate gland) approach.

Vascular or color-flow Doppler studies assess the patency of major blood vessels, demonstrating obstructions (stenoses), blood clots, plaques, and emboli. The color-flow duplex system, in which conventional real-time imaging is integrated with Doppler imaging (to produce quantitative data) and with color, depicts motion and the direction and velocity of blood flow. The color and intensity represent the direction of flow and the velocity, respectively (e.g., in the carotid artery).

Other uses of ultrasound include breast imaging (to differentiate solid from cystic masses) (Figure 2-4), musculoskeletal imaging (to detect problems with tendons, muscles, and joints, and soft tissue fluid collections or masses) (Figure 2-5), and as an imaging guide for invasive procedures (biopsies, aspirations, and drain placement) (Figure 2-6).

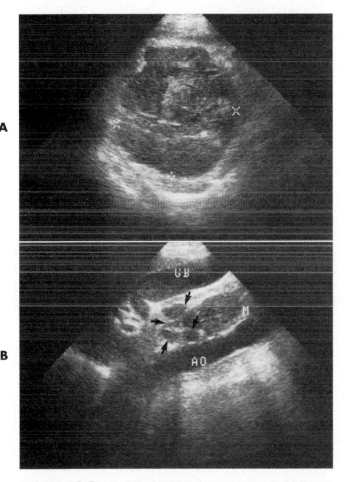

FIGURE 2-2 Ultrasound images of the abdomen. **A,** Transverse right kidney demonstrates a hyperechoic area *(white)* within the mass caused by renal cell carcinoma. **B,** Gallbladder *(GB)* and aorta *(AO)* are hypoechoic compared with the pancreas. Focal masses *(arrows)* within the pancreas are all isoechoic (i.e., similar in density).

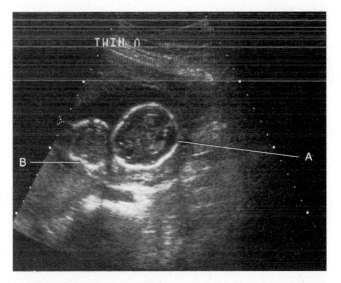

FIGURE 2-3 Sonogram of the abdomen of a woman with a multiple pregnancy. Cranial architecture is normal in fetus *A* and abnormal in fetus *B*, which documented fetal demise × 2 of fetuses *B* and *C* (not imaged).

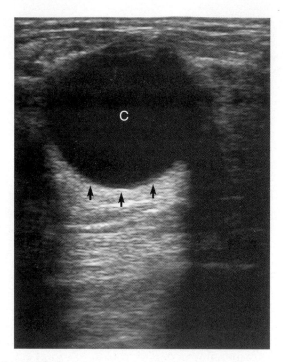

FIGURE 2-4 Ultrasound image of a breast. The sonogram shows an anechoic mass *(C)* with a well-defined back wall and distal enhancement *(arrows)*.

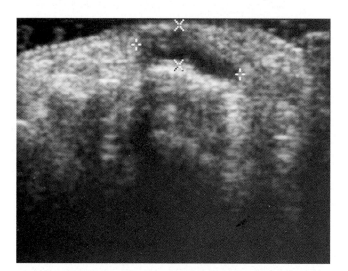

FIGURE 2-5 Ultrasound image of a wrist demonstrating the musculoskeletal architecture. A cystic structure (15 mm × 5 mm) can be seen near the dorsal aspect of base of the fourth and fifth metacarpals.

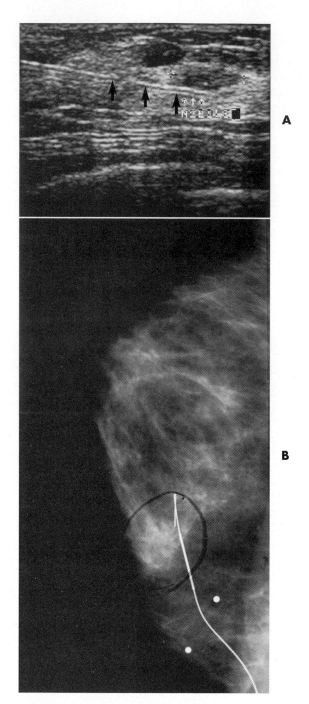

FIGURE 2-6 Ultrasound-guided localization. **A,** Ultrasound needle localization for surgical biopsy of the breast. **B,** Mammography image verifying needle localization.

Ultrasound is a quick, inexpensive procedure for evaluating postoperative complications, although it may be difficult to perform in some patients because of overlying dressings, retention sutures, drains, and open wounds, which may prevent the transducer from being in direct contact with the skin. In children with open fontanelles, ultrasound can image the intracranial structures. High-resolution, real-time ultrasound systems can assist surgeons during operative procedures. This technique has been applied to the neurosurgical localization of brain and spine neoplasms, to the evaluation of intraventricular shunt tube placement, to the localization of renal calculi, and to surgical procedures involving the hepatobiliary system and pancreas.

The role of ultrasound imaging has expanded as a result of the availability of multifrequency transducers (2 megahertz to 15 megahertz) and advances in software (signal-processing) technology. The resultant higher-resolution images are used in musculoskeletal, breast, and small-parts imaging. The latest technologies include harmonic imaging (which involves a broad band of low frequencies and can suppress reflection from surrounding tissue) to reduce image noise and artifact, sonoCT real-time compound imaging (a combination of multiple lines of sight that increases image clarity and provides more diagnostic information), and contrast agents (microbubble echo-enhancing agents) that increase vasculature definition. Harmonic imaging produces diminished noise images, increasing the resolution in a hypersthenic patient so that patient size does not prevent obtaining diagnostic images. SonoCT real-time compound imaging provides a wider field of view in real time, which allows visualization of an entire fetus in a single pass. Contrast agents, injectable low solubility gas bubbles (less than 5 μm) such as perfluorochemicals (inert dense fluids), increase the differentiation of tissues and enhance visibility of detail in tumors, small and stenotic vessels, heart studies, and ultrasound hysterosalpingography.

Ultrasound imaging requires an expanded knowledge of anatomy, physiology, and pathology to locate and demonstrate the specific region of interest. The quality of the scans is operator dependent, and extensive instruction and guidance are required to produce optimal images.

The major limitation of ultrasound is the presence of acoustic barriers, such as air, bone, and barium. For example, air reflects essentially the entire ultrasound beam, so that structures beneath cannot be imaged. This special problem interferes with imaging of the solid abdominal organs (e.g., the pancreas) in a patient with adynamic ileus, and it is the major factor precluding ultrasound examination of the thorax. For an ultrasound examination of the pelvis, the patient usually drinks a large amount of fluid to fill the bladder, thus displacing the air-filled bowel from the region of interest. More information on ultrasound imaging can be found on the following web sites: www.aium.org, www.sdms.org, and www.ardms.org.

Computed Tomography

Computed tomography (CT) produces cross-sectional tomographic images by first scanning a slice of tissue from multiple angles with a narrow x-ray beam, then calculating a relative linear attenuation coefficient (representing the amount of radiation absorbed in tissue for the various tissue elements in the section), and finally displaying the computed reconstruction as a gray-scale image on a television monitor. Unlike other imaging modalities (except for the more recent MRI), CT permits the radiographic differentiation of a variety of soft tissues from each other (Figure 2-7). CT is extremely sensitive to slight (1%) differences in tissue densities; for comparison, detection by conventional screen-film

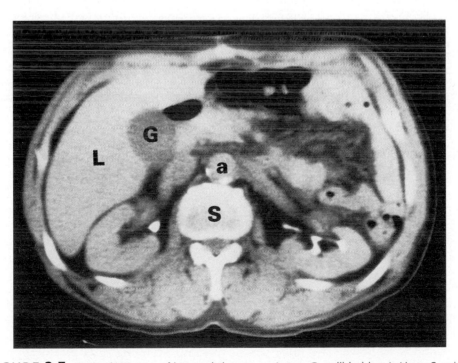

FIGURE 2-7 Normal CT scan of lower abdomen. *a*, Aorta; *G*, gallbladder; *L*, Liver; *S*, spine.

radiography requires differences in tissue density of at least 5%. Thus, in the head, CT can differentiate between blood clots, white matter and gray matter, cerebrospinal fluid, cerebral edema, and neoplastic processes.

The **CT number** reflects the attenuation of a specific tissue relative to that of water, which is arbitrarily assigned a CT number of 0 and appears gray on the image. The highest CT number (1000) represents bone, which appears white, and the lowest CT number (−1000) denotes air, which appears black. Fat has a CT number less than 0, whereas soft tissues have CT numbers higher than 0. The use of the computer allows the image to be manipulated by adjusting the window widths (gray scale—contrast scale) and window levels (density). From the radiographer's perspective, the window width determines the number of densities that can be visualized on the monitor. The window level is the midpoint or center of the total number of densities being viewed in a selected window width. Predetermined window widths and window levels are used to demonstrate specific parts of the anatomy (lung, liver, bone). Technical improvements in CT instrumentation and tube heat unit capacity have greatly reduced the time required to produce a single slice (1 to 2 seconds), and this permits the CT evaluation of virtually any portion of the body. In most instances, some type of preliminary film is obtained (either a radiograph or a CT-generated image) for localization, the detection of potentially interfering high-density material (metallic clips, barium, electrodes), and correlation with the CT images. An overlying grid with numeric markers permits close correlation between the subsequent CT scans and the initial scout film (Figure 2-8).

The intravenous injection of iodinated contrast material has become an integral part of many CT examinations. Scanning during or immediately after the administration of contrast material permits the differentiation of vascular from nonvascular solid structures. Differences in the degree and the time course of contrast enhancement may permit the detection of neoplastic or infectious processes within normal parenchymal structures. Because of its relatively low CT number, fat can serve as a natural contrast material and can outline parenchymal organs. In patients with malignant lesions, the loss of adjacent fat planes strongly suggests tumor extension. For abdominal studies, especially those of the pancreas and retroperitoneum, dilute oral contrast material is frequently given to demonstrate the lumen of the gastrointestinal tract, and it permits the distinction between loops of bowel and solid abdominal structures.

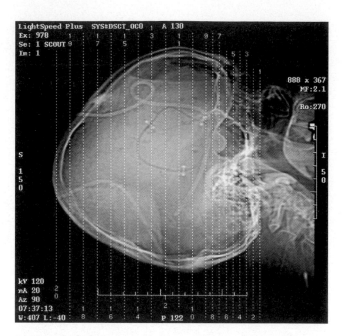

FIGURE 2-8 CT scout image with overlying grid representing scan slices.

Conventional CT produces images using a section thickness of 5 to 10 mm. In high-resolution CT, thin sections (1.5- to 2.0-mm slices) are used to produce a very detailed display of lung anatomy. High-resolution CT is far more sensitive and specific than plain chest radiographs (or conventional CT) for the diagnosis of parenchymal lung disease (Figure 2-9).

CT technology has moved to spiral (**helical**) scanning. In this technique, continual CT scanning is performed as the patient moves through the gantry (unlike the multiple single scans in conventional CT) (Figure 2-10). This permits much faster scanning without respiratory motion and provides data that can be easily reformatted in coronal and sagittal planes, and in the standard axial plane. The newest scanners with subsecond scanning abilities produce images of the chest (taking 20 to 30 seconds to complete the scan protocol) that demonstrate the pulmonary arteries without motion and can detect pulmonary emboli. CT imaging protocols for some procedures (e.g., obtaining images of the kidneys and liver) may require three-phase scanning (arterial, capillary, and venous phases, and an excretory phase) to demonstrate all anatomic (tissue) structures (Figure 2-11). The single-scan protocol changed with subsecond scanning because the intravenous bolus injection appears very dense on the image and may obscure the pathologic features. Subsecond scanning requires delayed scanning and second and third phases to demonstrate a higher sensitivity than single-slice scanning. Subsecond scanning also produces abdominal studies with much less peristaltic motion, which results in a

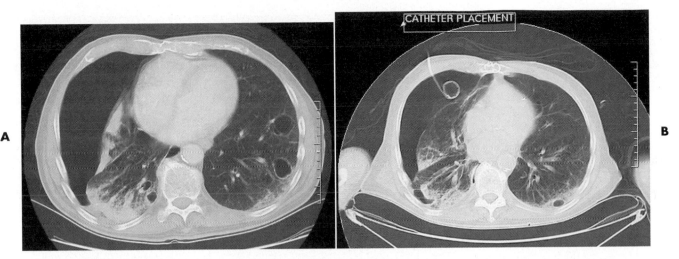

FIGURE 2-9 High-resolution CT scan of the lung. **A,** A pneumothorax can be seen in the right side of the lung of an emphysematous patient, and blebs (high-density areas) in the left lung. **B,** Visualization of catheter placement in the treatment for the pneumothorax.

higher-quality examination. Spiral CT allows reconstruction of images in three dimensions and can demonstrate vascular lesions without the need for arteriography (Figure 2-12). With the thin slices of spiral scanning and the addition of three-dimensional software, the reconstruction can produce virtual colonoscopy and bronchoscopy images.

The newest-generation scanner performs multiple slices (multidetectors producing 8 to 64 slices) per rotation, offers pitch variability (table movement), and variable rotation speed of the tube. It also contains software programming for instantaneous three-dimensional images (Figure 2-13). With the development of 16-slice scanners and beyond, CT angiography (CTA) became more precise and prevalent. Clinicians and radiologists are quickly accepting the use of CT for vascular imaging; however the complexity of the imaging protocol creates the need for extensive specialized education for the radiographer to produce the highest quality images. An understanding of vascular anatomy, blood flow rates related to blood pressure, and ejection fraction rates and possible pathophysiologic conditions that can influence protocol must be considered. Using **volume-rendered imaging** and 3-D volume rendering, the vascular system can be viewed from all perspectives (360 degrees). The faster scanning times and thinner slices have also made cardiac scanning a possibility, beyond electron-beam CT scanning. As technology continues to expand, the next-generation scanner will possibly have 128 to 256 channels; however, because of the amount of data that would be collected and our inability to view and use this much information, this appears to be years away.

Magnetic Resonance Imaging

Magnetic resonance imaging (MRI), once called nuclear magnetic resonance (NMR), has in a few short years become an important clinical tool for a variety of conditions (Figure 2-14). It has become the modality of choice for imaging the central nervous system and spine. It is also the first line of imaging for most conditions of the musculoskeletal system, and it is a problem solver in the abdomen and pelvis.

Although the physics of MRI is beyond the scope of this book, the basic technique consists of inducing hydrogen atoms (protons) to alternate between a high-energy state and a low-energy state by absorbing and then releasing, or transferring, energy. This absorption of energy is accomplished by placing the anatomic part to be imaged in a strong static magnetic field and directing a **radiofrequency (RF) pulse** of a specific frequency at the area. As protons absorb energy, they move into a high-energy state. After a predetermined time, the RF pulse is turned off and the protons begin to release, or transfer, their absorbed energy as they move back to a low-energy state. This process is called relaxation and it occurs over time. Two types of relaxation, T1 and T2, occur simultaneously. A listening device called a receiver coil, placed near the anatomic site, is able to detect and calculate the time it takes for both T1 and T2 relaxation types. A complex computer program named Fourier transform translates the information from the receiving coil into a computer-generated, gray-scale image.

To generate an MR image, the radiographer selects a group of scanning parameters referred to as a pulse

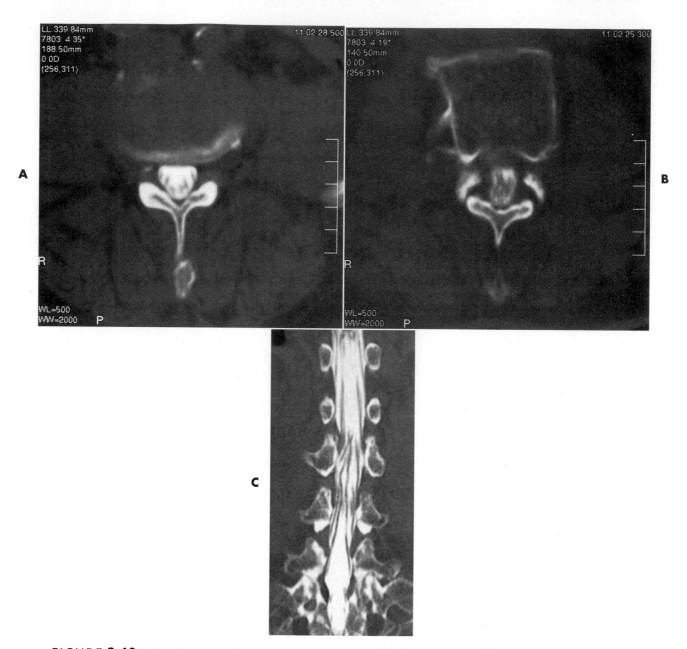

FIGURE 2-10 CT myelogram: 10 cc nonionic contrast agent was injected into the subarachnoid space. Following the myelogram, CT images using 3-mm slices were taken on a 16-slice scanner. On axial projections, **(A)** demonstrates subarachnoid (SA) space enhancement with the vertebral disk anteriorly, and **(B)** illustrates the SA shifted to the left. The coronal reconstruction **(C)** better demonstrates an impingement on the right at the level of L2-L3.

sequence. This pulse sequence contains a set of RF pulses and their timing, which is usually represented by a specific echo time (TE) and a repetition time (TR). The TE is the time between the end of the last RF pulse and the point when the receiving coil "listens" for the MR signal (known as an echo). The TR is the time it takes to play out the entire set of RF pulses before repeating. The most commonly used pulse sequences are termed **spin-echo (SE)** and fast, or turbo, spin-echo (FSE). By varying the TE and TR, the radiographer is able to produce an image that is weighted, demonstrating T1 relaxation or T2 relaxation, proton density, or a combination of all three, which allows a superb display of the differences between normal and abnormal tissues. In general, a pulse sequence using a short TR (500 to 700 msec) and a short TE (20 to 30 msec) provides a T1-weighted image. A pulse sequence using a long TR (2000 to 2500 msec) and a long TE (60 to 80 msec) provides a T2-weighted image. A pulse sequence using a short TE (15 to 30 msec) and an intermediate TR (2000 msec) provides a proton-density, or spin-density, image.

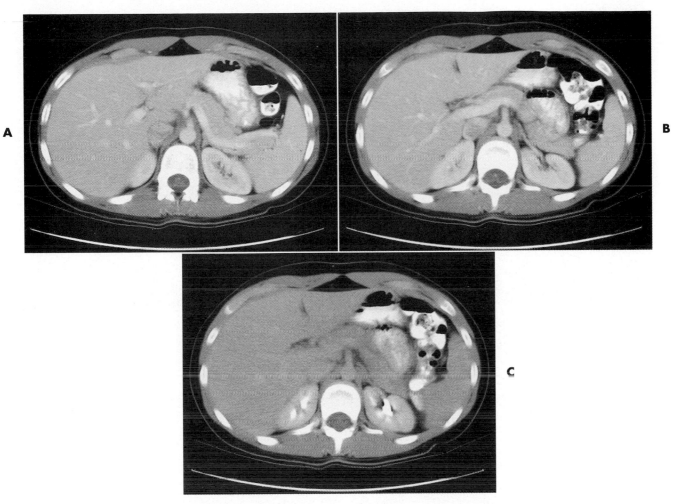

FIGURE 2-11 Three-phase CT scanning protocol for an abdomen. **A,** Arterial phase demonstrating the abdominal aorta and kidney. **B,** Portal venous phase seen in the liver. **C,** Excretory phase of the kidneys is visualized.

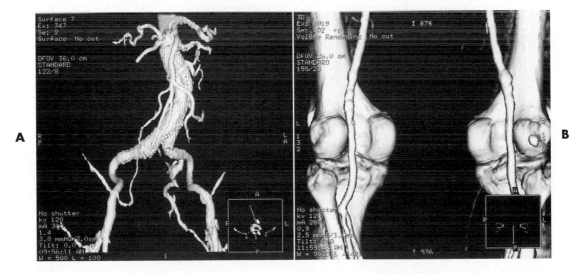

FIGURE 2-12 CTA. **A,** Special software is used to demonstrate the abdominal aorta, the renal arteries, the superior mesenteric artery, and the iliac arteries. **B,** Three-dimensional software in a femoral arterial run-off is used to demonstrate the popliteal arteries.

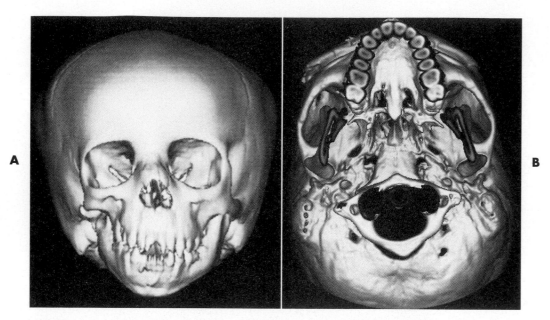

FIGURE 2-13 Three-dimensional CT images. **A,** Skull of 3-year-old girl with closed sutures (craniosynostosis) and shape deformity. **B,** Three-dimensional cut-away illustrating the base of a normal skull. The mandible has been removed from the image.

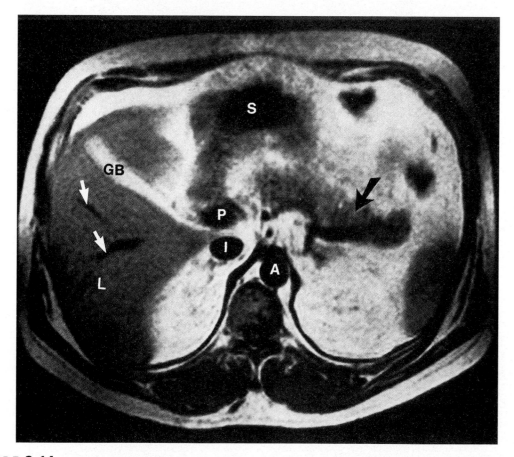

FIGURE 2-14 MRI of normal upper abdomen. Transverse scan shows liver *(L)* and branches of portal veins *(white arrows)*. Gallbladder *(GB)* has high intensity in this fasting person. Pancreas *(black arrow)* and stomach *(S)* are easily seen. Inferior vena cava *(I)*, aorta *(A)*, and main portal vein *(P)* are seen with signal void because they contain flowing blood.

Although the degree of signal intensity of various substances on MR scans is complex and depends on multiple factors, some generalizations can be made. On **T1-weighted images**, substances causing high signal intensity (i.e., appearing bright) include fat, subacute hemorrhage, highly proteinaceous material (e.g., mucus), slow-flowing blood, and intravenous contrast material (e.g., gadolinium). Water, as in cerebrospinal fluid or simple cysts, has a relatively low signal intensity and appears dark. Soft tissue has an intermediate level of signal intensity (Figure 2-15, *A*).

On **T2-weighted images,** water has a high signal intensity (it appears bright), whereas muscle and other soft tissues (including fat) tend to have lower signal intensity and appear intermediate to dark. Cortical bone, calcium, air, and fast-flowing blood appear very dark on most imaging sequences (see Figure 2-15, *B* and *C*).

MRI has many of the advantages offered by other imaging modalities, without the associated disadvantages, and it is complementary to other modalities. Like ultrasound, MRI produces images in multiple planes without the use of ionizing radiation. Unlike

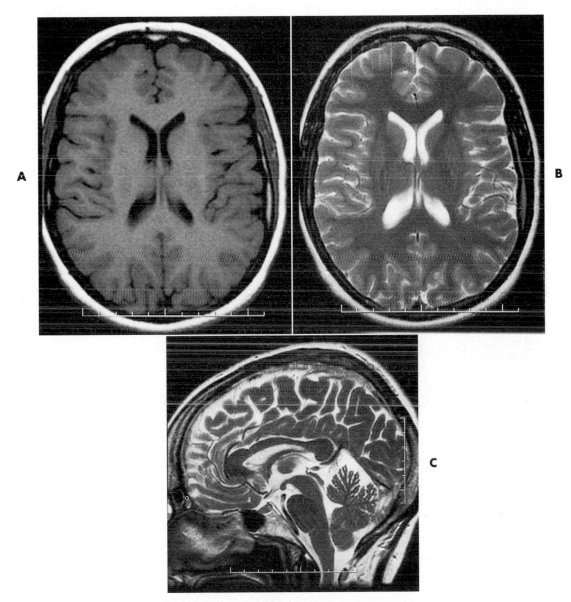

FIGURE 2-15 MRI of normal brain. **A,** T1-weighted spin-echo image (TE = 9 msec, TR = 466 msec). The ventricles and cerebrospinal fluid areas appear dark, and the white and gray matter are shades of gray. **B,** T2-weighted fast spin-echo image (TE = 101 msec, TR = 4500 msec). The cerebrospinal fluid produces a high signal intensity *(white area)* on the image. **C,** Sagittal T2-weighted fast spin-echo image (TE = 104 msec, TR = 4000 msec) demonstrates cerebral cortex, ventricles, pons, and cerebellum.

ultrasound, MRI depends less on the operator's skill and the habitus of the patient and can penetrate bone without significant decrease in intensity (i.e., without attenuation), so that the underlying tissue can be clearly imaged. The ability to image directly in any plane allows the best visualization of normal and abnormal anatomy.

Unlike other imaging modalities that depend on information from one parameter (such as CT, which depends on electron density), MRI derives information from multiple biologic parameters, such as proton density (Figure 2-16, *A*) and T1 and T2 relaxation times. MRI provides excellent spatial resolution, equal to that of CT, and far better contrast resolution of soft tissue. The intravenous injection of contrast material is unnecessary with MRI because flowing blood produces a signal void that contrasts sharply with adjacent structures.

Although MRI demonstrates improved sensitivity for detection of abnormal tissue, up to now it has not shown significantly improved specificity. In the head, for example, infarction, edema, tumor, infection, and demyelinating disease all produce identically high signal intensity on T2-weighted images. The introduction of intravenous contrast materials and different types of pulse sequences is helping increase specificity.

Disadvantages of MRI include a longer scanning time, leading to image degradation resulting from patient and physiologic motion. Patient claustrophobia is a possibility, and monitoring a patient in a somewhat closed environment may be difficult. Furthermore, imaging patients with pacemakers (which may not operate properly) or ferromagnetic intracranial aneurysm clips (which may slip and result in hemorrhage) is contraindicated.

MR angiography permits high-quality images of the arterial and venous systems without the need for contrast material (Figure 2-17, *A*). Recent advances using rapidly infused intravenous contrast (e.g., gadolinium chelates) coupled with subsecond scanning result in superb diagnostic images of the arterial and venous systems without the need for invasive catheter angiography (Figure 2-17, *B* and *C*). This modality and CTA have substantially supplanted contrast angiography for the diagnosis of vascular disease.

Spectroscopic examinations (MRSI) using high magnetic fields to assess various chemical elements permit the sophisticated biochemical analysis of tissues in vivo. Two major clinical applications include staging carcinoma of the prostate and follow-up of brain tumors after treatment. New technology and FDA-approved techniques allow MRI and MRSI to be completed simultaneously. Improved hardware and software and the development of specific magnetic contrast agents should improve the specificity of this modality to make MRI the imaging procedure of choice for a broad spectrum of clinical applications.

New and faster sequencing pulses and stronger gradients produce diffusion and perfusion images that have expanded the clinical applications of MRI. **Diffusion imaging** relies on the movement of molecules and random thermal motion. (In this instance, random movement of water is known as diffusion.) This application of diffusion gradients requires the use of pulses to cancel normal tissue random motion, recording a high signal in tissue with reduced diffusion because of edema. Using ultrafast echo-planar imaging techniques, this altered diffusion can be

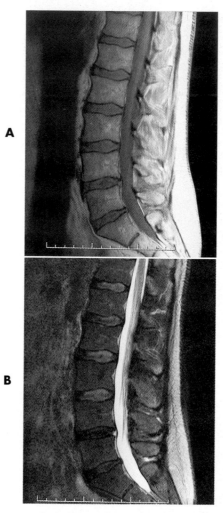

FIGURE 2-16 MRI of sagittal lumbar spine with small disk protrusion at L4-L5 and slightly desiccated disk spaces. **A,** Proton density fast spin-echo image demonstrating, disk protrusion. **B,** Fat-suppressed image. Spinal fluid has high intensity and spinal nerves have a lower intensity signal.

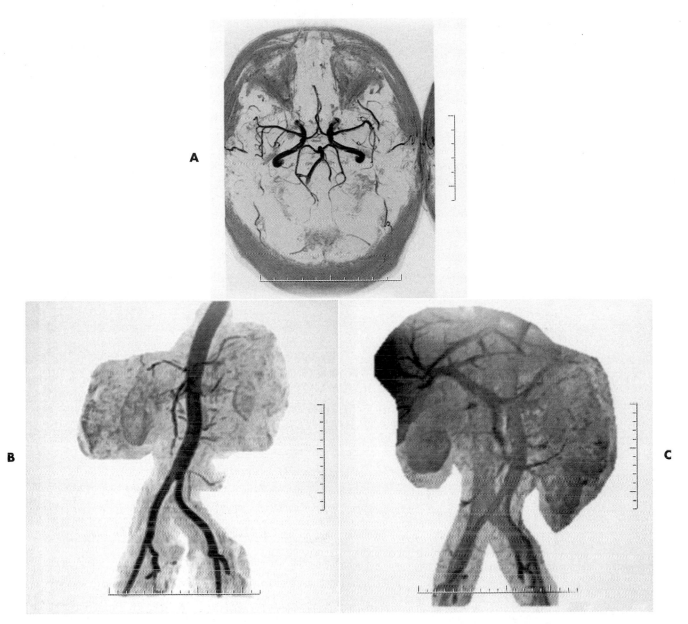

FIGURE 2-17 MR angiography. **A,** Collapsed view of the cerebrum showing a normal circle of Willis. **B,** Gadolinium enhancement of the abdomen demonstrates renal and mesenteric arteries. **C,** The venous phase demonstrates the portal circulation in the same patient.

imaged within minutes from the onset of symptoms. MR perfusion imaging illustrates microcirculation (demonstrating blood volume) with an increased signal intensity by using an enhancement agent (e.g., rapidly infused gadolinium) or motion-sensitive gradients (e.g., diffusion imaging uses RF inversion of saturation pulses). These images of the brain, visceral organs (e.g., the liver), and myocardium demonstrate circulation in viable tissue, which helps to distinguish old from new infarctions or ischemic regions. Minor tissue characteristics show morphologic changes: for example, diffusion-weighted images show how

much tissue has been affected by altered blood flow (e.g., as after an infarction), whereas perfusion images demonstrate the region of tissue that continues to be at risk. In brain or liver tissue, malignancies have increased tissue metabolism or perfusion and demonstrate an increased signal (i.e., a bright image). In cerebral blood volume, an area of stroke demonstrates a low perfusion and appears dark. Currently, diffusion and perfusion imaging assist in demonstrating stroke lesions early, increasing the possibility of revascularization with immediate treatment. Myocardial images acquired at rest or after exercise may demonstrate a decreased signal, indicating ischemic or infarcted tissue.

One of the unique advantages of MRI is its ability to acquire images with selective tissue suppression. The tissue most often suppressed in routine imaging is fat. **Fat-suppressed images** require heavy weighting (i.e., saturation or full magnetization) on the T1 sequence to ensure a large contrast difference between fat and water. Fat saturation techniques produce images in which fat gives off little or no signal (see Figure 2-16, *B*). This technique effectively demonstrates small lesions when there are only subtle differences with increasing lesion conspicuity in a normal T1-weighted image. Fat-suppression images are employed when imaging the skull base and the soft tissues of the neck, the abdomen, and the pelvis. When bone marrow is being imaged, fat suppression accentuates marrow edema, such as is found in stress fractures and bone bruises.

Functional MR (fMR) allows the localization of specific regions of the brain that correspond to various functions, such as the motor, sensory, memory, vision, and language functions. The technique used to create fMR images applies an ultrafast gradient to generate a functional map that is laid over a high-resolution anatomic image. The image maps brain activity because the increased blood flow to the activated cerebral cortex produces a signal change. The combined images allow the diagnostician to precisely plan interventions that will spare specific functional areas. Future uses of fMR will be in the evaluation of stroke, epilepsy, pain, and behavioral problems.

Current trends in MRI are moving to higher magnet strengths. 3-tesla magnets, previously used for brain research, are now finding their way into the mainstream. The lower strength magnets, 1 to 1.5 tesla, are being reconfigured—open or ultra–short-bore—to be more patient-friendly.

Nuclear Medicine

In radiography, ionizing radiation interacts with tissue to produce an image. In **nuclear medicine**, however, the patient ingests, or is injected with, a radiopharmaceutical that emits radiation, and an image is created from the signals radiating from the patient (Figure 2-18). The dose of **radiopharmaceutical** is calculated on the basis of the specific half-life and decay rate of its attached radionuclide. The amount of ionizing radiation to the patient in a nuclear medicine study is similar to that in a plain radiographic examination. The injected radionuclide does not produce the pharmacologic side effects or complications seen with radiographic iodinated contrast agents, making the study safer for all patients with an iodine allergy.

A **gamma camera** with a sodium iodide crystal detects the ionizing radiation emitted from the patient. Interaction of the gamma rays with the crystal produces light scintillation, which is converted to a digital signal on a computer monitor. The scintigraphic image, which defines the distribution of the radioactive nuclide, represents the physiologic map of the organ or system being imaged.

The physiologic map produced by some nuclear medicine procedures allows changes to be detected earlier than plain radiographic images because the functional perspective makes it more sensitive, which may lead to an earlier diagnosis and thus a better prognosis. Abnormal radionuclide images demonstrate hot spots (produced by an increase in uptake that is directly proportional to the emission of gamma radiation) or cold spots (which reflect a decreased uptake).

The images obtained using nuclear medicine techniques are excellent for documenting organ physiology, but they can be lacking in anatomic information. Plain radiographic images can therefore be useful for correlative purposes.

New technology has expanded the role of nuclear medicine to include tumor imaging. These studies help determine tumor size, location, and recurrence. Because radiopharmaceuticals differ in their ability to demonstrate various tumors, a choice is made on the basis of the suspected diagnosis (Figure 2-19). The scintigraphic images can be used to document diagnoses and for treatment management.

Single-Photon Emission Computed Tomography

Single-photon emission computed tomography (SPECT) represents another aspect of nuclear medicine imaging (Figure 2-20). The radiopharmaceuticals used in SPECT are the same as those used in planar nuclear medicine. The SPECT camera is a gamma camera with the ability to rotate independently around the patient. With the aid of a computer, it can create three-dimensional slices at any level in the body. The three-dimensional images are created by initially acquiring projections 180 to 360 degrees around the patient. The software then performs a reconstruction of the raw data to produce a three-dimensional image that is "sliced" up into transverse, sagittal, and coronal sections, very much like CT or MRI. To gather the tomographic information, a detector array rotates 360 degrees around the patient. This is similar to a CT scanner, but in SPECT, instead of the source (the x-ray tube) and the detector array moving simultaneously, the source (the patient) emits the signal while the detector array rotates. The signal, which the computer

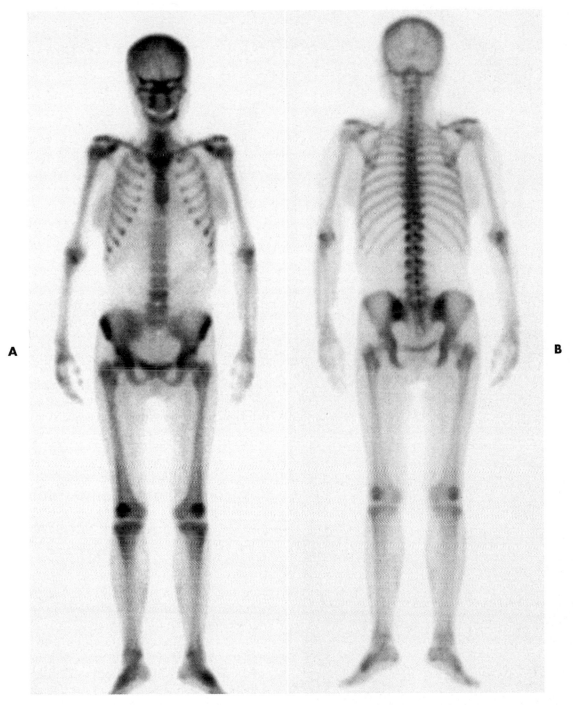

FIGURE 2-18 Nuclear medicine bone scan (technetium 99m–labeled bone scintigraphy). This normal scan demonstrates the anterior **(A)** and posterior **(B)** perspectives in a patient with hypercalcemia.

reconstruction algorithm analyzes, determines the position and strength of the data to create an image. Because the position and attenuation coefficients are unknown, the information must be inferred by the signal detector system, resulting in decreased resolution and sensitivity.

The gamma camera, which detects the gamma rays used in SPECT, has a **collimator** containing multiple parallel channels to allow the rays to pass. By placing the collimator in front of the camera and moving the camera, attenuation prevents many of the gamma rays from reaching the camera, decreasing the amount of data collected. Attenuation also occurs when gamma rays interact with the body. Compton scattering and photoelectric effect take place and lead to a loss of image contrast. To compensate for this

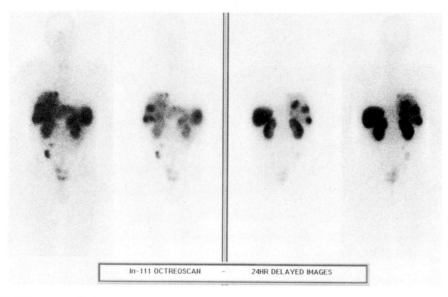

In-111 OCTREOSCAN - 24HR DELAYED IMAGES

FIGURE 2-19 This 24-hour indium-111 octreotide scan illustrates multiple hepatic carcinoma metastases.

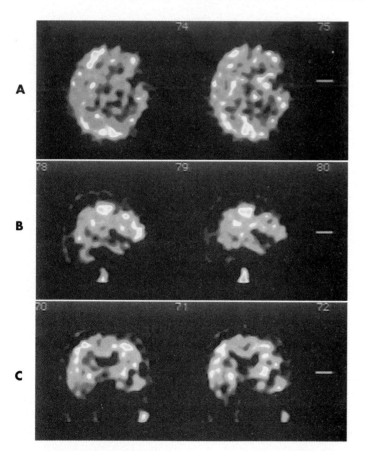

FIGURE 2-20 SPECT images of the brain reconstructed into three planes of view: **A,** Transverse. **B,** Sagittal. **C,** Coronal.

loss, the computer reconstruction software must correct for attenuation.

Today, a disadvantage of SPECT is the gamma camera, which allows imaging of a region of interest that is only the size of the camera. As technology improves, the resolution and sensitivity of this modality will increase. Currently the advantage of SPECT is that it costs half the price of PET imaging. SPECT imaging provides useful information in evaluating patients with many disease states: coronary artery disease, ventricular function disorders, ventricular wall motion abnormalities (Figure 2-21), infection, tumors (evaluation and staging), strokes, focal seizures, and traumatic brain injuries.

Positron Emission Tomography

In **positron emission tomography (PET)**, as in nuclear medicine procedures, a radionuclide tracer is used to produce images (Figure 2-22). However, here the radiopharmaceutical is different because it decays by positron emission. A positron emitted from the radionuclide tracer interacts with an electron. This **"annihilation"** interaction produces two high-energy photons (gamma rays) in opposite directions (separated by 180 degrees). If both gamma rays are detected simultaneously within the field, the computer can localize the interaction and add these signals to the image distribution. Detection of only one interaction will not be counted in the distribution because the computer must receive two signals simultaneously to satisfy the program. These simultaneous signals produce multiple lines of response, which determine the location of the signal and produce an image. The tracer in the radionuclide represents a naturally occurring substance in the body, such as carbon, oxygen, nitrogen, or glucose. The imaging distribution of these molecules creates a finely detailed metabolic representation of the area of interest. The body or organ metabolism illustrates the biochemistry of the tissue, distinguishing diseased

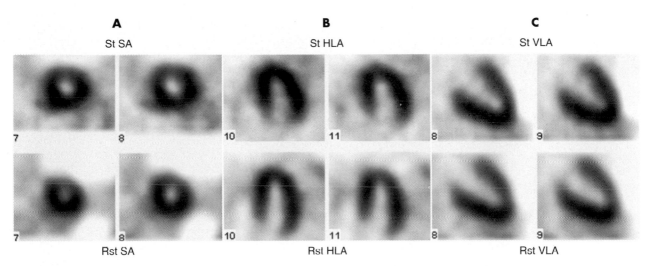

FIGURE 2-21 SPECT images of the normal heart in three planes of view, completed at rest *(Rst)* and stress *(St)* levels, with image reconstruction. **A,** Short axis *(SA)* shows the coronal heart plane. **B,** Horizontal long axis *(HLA)* shows the oblique transaxial plane. **C,** Vertical long axis *(VLA)* shows the oblique sagittal plane.

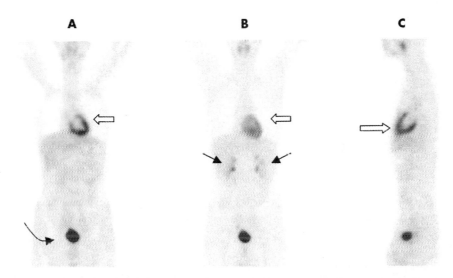

FIGURE 2-22 Normal PET scan with multiplanar body imaging. **A,** Coronal plane. **B,** Projection plane. **C,** Sagittal plane. Bladder *(curved arrow)*, heart *(open arrows)*, and kidney *(solid arrows)*.

or dead tissue from healthy or normal tissue, and demonstrating tissue viability. Thus PET images the distribution of the gamma rays in the specific organs of interest and provides diagnosticians with a biologic map.

With PET imaging, multiple detectors (sometimes in excess of 8000) receive the signal, and computerized software converts the raw data to a three-dimensional image in three planes: axial, coronal, and sagittal. In PET imaging, attenuation correction is resolved by performing a transmission scan on each patient. The computer reconstruction software then corrects for each patient's individual body contour and attenuation

factor. This attenuation correction to the image resolution and sensitivity of PET images produces higher-quality images compared with SPECT. Radiation exposure rates to the patient for PET imaging are similar to those in nuclear medicine studies; however, the technologist receives higher doses because of the energy level of the radionuclide.

PET is especially useful in three medical specialties: oncology, cardiology, and neurology. For oncology patients, this imaging modality can accurately image the whole body with one pass, permitting the detection of metastases in multiple organs and aiding in tumor staging. Because PET produces a metabolic image, follow-up scans can be used to demonstrate the effectiveness of radiation or chemotherapy treatment by documenting any changes (Figure 2-23). In cardiology patients, PET assists in screening for coronary artery disease by demonstrating myocardial perfusion (flow rates, flow reserves, and viable myocardium) (Figures 2-24 and 2-25).

In neurologic patients, PET can be used to evaluate for stroke and to identify epileptic foci for surgical intervention (Figure 2-26). The scanning environment (i.e., sound and light) may influence the scan results because these stimuli can affect the metabolism of the temporal and occipital regions of the brain; therefore the environment needs to be strictly controlled. Brain disorders that can be demonstrated by PET imaging include Parkinson's disease, schizophrenia, Huntington's disease, and Alzheimer's disease. Oxygen, carbon monoxide, and glucose (used most often) are tracers that are used in brain imaging to demonstrate different aspects of cerebral function. Unlike the anatomic map produced by CT and MRI, the physiologic map provided by PET may permit earlier detection of abnormalities by demonstrating pathology before morphologic changes and lead to prompt treatment interventions and a better prognosis.

Fusion Imaging

The future of imaging takes on a new look by combining anatomic images with metabolic function images. This new imaging integration provides a high degree of clarity to view the pathophysiologic changes without viewing each modality separately. By fusing the morphology and physiology, the diagnosis can be made much quicker and with increased accuracy.

Integrated imaging is accomplished using special software designed to overlay or fuse multidimensional computed data from MRI, CT, nuclear

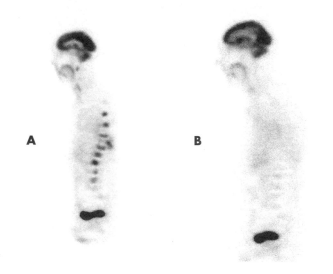

FIGURE 2-23 PET used to assess effectiveness of chemotherapy. **A,** Image before therapy. **B,** After chemotherapy, the image demonstrates decreased uptake of ^{18}F-fluorodeoxyglucose.

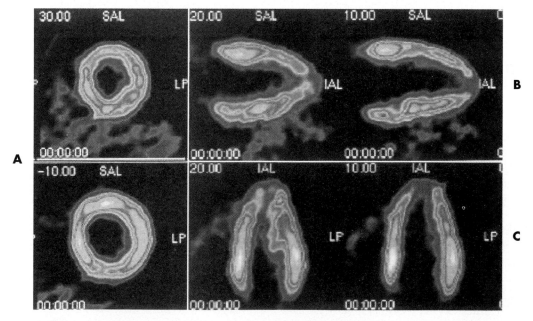

FIGURE 2-24 Normal PET images of the heart. Cardiology procedure demonstrating: **A,** Short axis. **B,** Long vertical axis using ^{18}F-fluorodeoxyglucose. **C,** Horizontal long axis (HLA) with normal perfusion.

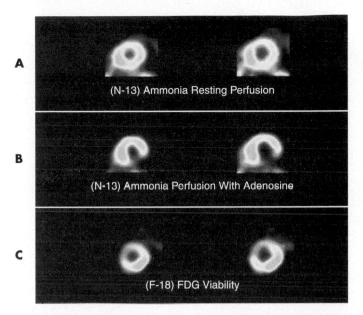

FIGURE 2-25 PET images demonstrating myocardial viability. Cardiac resting and artificial stress (adenosine) perfusion images of the short axis using $^{13}NH_3\{\Sigma Y\}–\{/\Sigma Y\}$ ammonia. **A,** At rest, perfusion is normal. **B,** After artificial stress, uptake in the inferolateral wall is decreased. **C,** Viability scan with ^{18}F-fluorodeoxyglucose suggests ischemia of the right coronary artery and the left circumflex coronary artery. Perfusion of the region indicates that the myocardium remains viable.

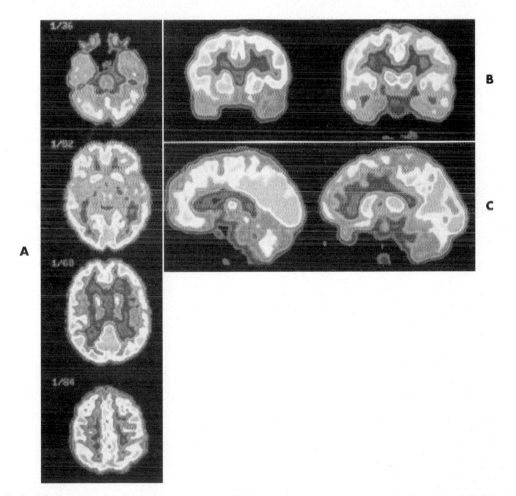

FIGURE 2-26 PET image of the brain. Normal ^{18}F-fluorodeoxyglucose uptake in the brain is indicated by the symmetric and consistent blood flow and metabolism in three planes. **A,** Axial or transverse. **B,** Coronal. **C,** Sagittal.

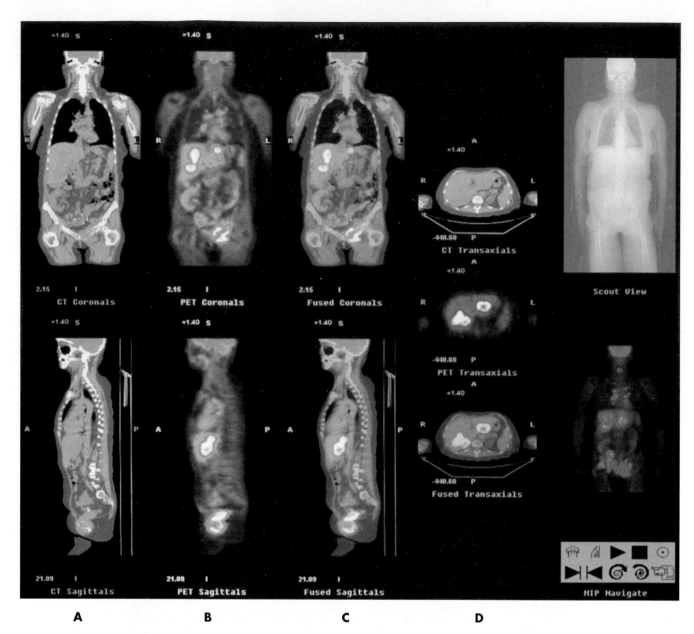

FIGURE 2-27 PET/CT of the body. **A,** Provides the anatomic landmarks in the coronal and sagittal planes using the CT images. PET coronal and sagittal images **(B)** demonstrate increased molecular uptake. The fused images **(C)** provide greater detail by locating the increased uptake in its anatomic position. **D,** Provides the axial projection through the liver.

medicine, SPECT, or PET into a single set of images. Many angles viewed in this manner provide improved visualization of the anatomic site of interest. Currently, **direct fusion** equipment (also known as hybrid technology) for PET/CT is available (Figure 2-27). The exams are completed simultaneously, rather than separately, using fusion software after the exams are completed using the two different modalities.

PET/CT with hybrid imaging demonstrates increased sensitivity, especially for lymph node staging. Additional training may be required for the hybrid technologist who is responsible for producing these special images to assure the use of the lowest radiation dose. Also, more education may be required to correctly demonstrate anatomic structures or molecular-physiologic relationships.

REVIEW QUESTIONS

1. Ultrasound depends on the echo of the high-frequency sound waves produced by the transducer. Tissue that produces a strong reflection is known as _____.
   A. hypoechoic
   B. anechoic
   C. isoechoic
   D. hyperechoic or echogenic

2. Ultrasound is limited by acoustic barriers, such as _____.
   A. liver and splenic tissue
   B. air and bone
   C. urine in the bladder
   D. gallstones or kidney stones

3. The modality that views tissue from multiple angles using a narrow x-ray beam is _____.
   A. CT
   B. SPECT
   C. PET
   D. MRI

4. The CT technique using continuous scanning while the table moves the patient through the gantry is _____.
   A. helical scanning
   B. conventional single-slice scanning
   C. high-resolution scanning
   D. CTA

5. Currently the term multidetector CT indicates _____.
   A. multitransducer crystals
   B. a 2-detector array
   C. 8- to 64-detector array
   D. 128- to 256-channel array

6. To create an image in MRI, the technology depends on _____.
   A. hydrogen atoms and their response to radiofrequency pulses
   B. x-radiation attenuation
   C. radiopharmaceuticals
   D. electrical stimulation of transducer crystals

7. Multiple-pulse sequences may be required to illustrate pathophysiologic changes. Examples of MRI pulse sequences are _____.
   A. T1- and T2-weighted images
   B. positron emission (gamma)
   C. single-photon emission
   D. 2 MHz to 15 MHz images

8. Nuclear medicine and SPECT imaging rely on scintillation cameras to detect _____.
   A. multiple-photon emission
   B. electron annihilation
   C. gamma rays
   D. photoelectric interaction

9. PET imaging is especially useful to evaluate _____.
   A. chest for pneumothorax
   B. reproductive organs for cysts
   C. preradiation and postradiation or chemotherapy
   D. cerebral ventricle displacement

10. Hybrid imaging equipment combines _____.
    A. two image modalities using software to fuse images
    B. two images comparatively viewed side by side
    C. two modalities simultaneously producing one set of images
    D. two technologists and radiologists viewing images

BIBLIOGRAPHY

Ultrasound

Hagen-Ansert SL: *Text of diagnostic ultrasonography,* St Louis, 2001, Mosby.

Mittelstaedt CA: *Abdominal ultrasound,* New York, 1987, Churchill Livingstone.

Rumack CM, Wilson SR, Charborneau JW: *Diagnostic ultrasound,* St Louis, 2005, Mosby.

Sarti DA: *Diagnostic ultrasound: text and cases,* St Louis, 1987, Mosby.

Computed Tomography

Greenberg M, Greenberg BM: *Essentials of body computed tomography,* Philadelphia, 1983, Saunders.

Lee JKT, Sagel SS, Stanley RJ: *Computed body tomography with MRI correlation,* New York, 1989, Raven Press.

Moss AA, Gamsu G, Genant HK: *Computed tomography of the body,* Philadelphia, 1992, Saunders.

Seeram E: *Computed tomography: physical principles, clinical applications and quality control,* Philadelphia, 2001, Saunders.

Magnetic Resonance Imaging

Edelman RR, Hesselink JR: *Clinical magnetic resonance imaging,* Philadelphia, 1990, Saunders.

Stark DD, Bradley WG: *Magnetic resonance imaging,* St Louis, 1993, Mosby.

Westbrook C, Kaut C: *MRI in practice,* Malden, Mass, 1998, Blackwell Science.

Nuclear Medicine, SPECT, and PET

Hood KH: *Single-photon computed tomography (SPECT),* http://cfii.lbl.gov/budinger/medIechdocs/SPECT.html.

Scarfone C: *SPECT image acquisition and processing,* Duke University Medical Center, 1995, www.bae.ncsu.edu/bae/courses/bae590f/ 1995/scarfone/gen.html.

SPECT of the brain, http://jura.stir.ac.uk/teaching/spect/tomographic.html.

TRIUMF (Canada's national laboratory for particle and nuclear physics): *Positron emission tomography (PET),* 1998, www.triumf.ca/welcome/petscan.html.

RESPIRATORY *System*

Chapter Outline

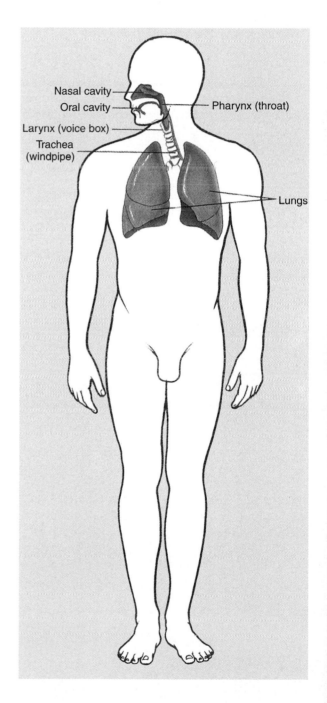

Key Terms

adenocarcinomas

adult respiratory distress
  syndrome (ARDS)

alveolar, or air-space, pneumonia

asthma

bronchial adenomas

bronchiectasis

bronchioalveolar carcinoma

bronchiolar (alveolar cell)
  carcinoma

bronchogenic carcinoma

bullae

chronic bronchitis

emphysema

extrinsic asthma

interstitial pneumonia

intrinsic asthma

pulmonary mycosis

small cell (oat cell) carcinomas

squamous carcinoma

surfactant

Prerequisite Knowledge

The student should have a basic knowledge of the anatomy and physiology of the respiratory system. In addition, proper learning and understanding of the material will be facilitated if the student has some clinical experience in chest radiography and image evaluation, including a concept of the changes in technique required to compensate for density differences produced by the underlying pathologic conditions.

Goals

To acquaint the student radiographer with the pathophysiology and radiographic manifestations of all of the common and some of the unusual disorders of the respiratory system.

Objectives

After reading this chapter, the reader will be able to:

1. Classify the more common diseases in terms of their attenuation of x-rays
2. Explain the changes in technical factors required to obtain optimal quality radiographs for patients with various underlying pathologic conditions
3. Define and describe all bold-faced terms in this chapter
4. Describe the physiology of the respiratory system
5. Identify anatomic structures on both diagrams and radiographs of the respiratory system
6. Differentiate the more common pathologic conditions affecting the respiratory system and their radiographic manifestations

RADIOGRAPHER *Notes*

Proper positioning and the correct exposure factors are especially important in radiography of the respiratory system because to make a precise diagnosis, radiologists must be able to detect subtle changes in pulmonary and vascular structures. Ideally, follow-up studies should be performed with the same exposure factors used when making the initial radiographs. By maintaining exposure factors, any density changes can be attributed to true pathologic findings rather than to mere technical differences.

All chest radiography should be performed with the patient in full inspiration (inhalation), except when expiration images are used for those few pathologic conditions requiring expiration images. In an ideal image, the upper 10 posterior ribs should be visualized above the diaphragm. Poor expansion of the lungs may cause a normal-sized heart to appear enlarged and makes it difficult to

evaluate the lung bases. To obtain a full-inspiration radiograph, the patient should be instructed to take a deep breath, exhale, and inhale again (thus accomplishing maximal inspiration), at which time the exposure should be made. This technique avoids the *Valsalva effect*, which is a forced expiration against the closed glottis that increases the intrapulmonary pressure. The Valsalva effect results in compression and a large decrease in the size of the heart and adjacent blood vessels, and thus it is difficult to evaluate heart size and pulmonary vascularity accurately.

The patient must be precisely positioned for chest radiography to ensure symmetry of the lung fields and a true appearance of the heart and pulmonary vasculature. Whenever possible, all chest radiographs should be taken with the patient in the erect position. The only exception is for the patient with a suspected pathologic condition that

RADIOGRAPHER *Notes—Cont'd*

requires a lateral decubitus position. Although recumbent radiographs may be necessary in immobile or seriously ill patients, they are less than satisfactory because in this position the abdominal contents tend to prevent the diaphragm from descending low enough to permit visualization of well-expanded lung bases or fluid levels. A 72-inch source-image receptor distance should be used when possible to minimize magnification of the heart and mediastinal structures. Correct positioning with absence of rotation in the frontal projection can be demonstrated by symmetry of the sternoclavicular joints. The shoulders must be rolled forward (anteriorly) to prevent the scapulas from overlying the lungs. In large-breasted women, it is often necessary to elevate and separate the breasts to allow good visualization of the lung bases. Nipple shadows of both men and women occasionally appear as soft tissue masses. If the nature of these soft tissue masses is unclear, it may be necessary to repeat the examination using small lead markers placed on the nipples. Collimation of the radiograph is required to reduce scattered radiation, although it is essential that both costophrenic angles be visualized. However, the radiographer obtains a diagnostic image, and it is necessary to label the image appropriately.

Radiographs exhibiting a long scale of contrast are necessary to visualize the entire spectrum of densities within the thoracic cavity (including those of the mediastinum, heart, lung markings, and pulmonary vasculature) and the surrounding bony thorax. Most authorities agree that a minimum of 120 kilovolts-peak (kVp) should be used with an appropriate ratio grid for all adult chest radiography. If it is necessary to decrease the overall density, this should be accomplished by reduction of the milliampere seconds (mAs) rather than of the kVp. Decreasing the kVp tends to enhance the bony thorax, which may obscure vascular details and cause underpenetration of the mediastinal structures. In general the density and contrast should be such that the thoracic vertebrae and intervertebral disk spaces are faintly visible through the shadow of the mediastinum without obscuring the lung markings and pulmonary vascularity. When producing radiographs for line placement, make sure to use the appropriate technical factors to demonstrate the line and possible chest pathology (pneumothorax or hemothorax) that may result from line placement.

Short exposure times (10 msec or less) must be used in chest radiography because longer times may not eliminate the involuntary motion of the heart. Automatic exposure devices are generally recommended, and they help to ensure that follow-up studies will have a similar film density. An exception is the expiration (exhalation) chest radiograph, which should be exposed with a manual technique because the preset density of an automatic exposure device may cause excessive overexposure of the lungs and thus obscure a small pneumothorax.

Compensatory filters are sometimes needed to overcome the broad range of different tissue densities within the chest. They are especially important to allow good visualization of the mediastinum without overexposing the lungs. The use of compensatory filters generally requires that the radiographic exposure be twice that used in the absence of additional filtration.

To demonstrate fluid levels, the patient should be in an erect position for a minimum of 5 minutes (preferably 10 to 15), and a horizontal x-ray beam must be used. Any angulation of the beam prevents a parallel entrance to the air-fluid interface and obscures the fluid level. In some clinical situations (e.g., when there is a small pneumothorax or pleural thickening as opposed to free pleural fluid), it is necessary to use a horizontal beam with the patient placed in the lateral decubitus position.

Certain pathologic conditions of the respiratory system require that the radiographer alter the routine technical factors. Some disorders produce increased density, which attenuates more of the x-ray beam, whereas others decrease the density of the lungs so there is less attenuation by the pulmonary tissue. It is important to remember that these changes may vary for a single disease because the chest structures attenuate more or less of the x-ray beam depending on the stage of the disease process. Unless the radiographer has access to previous films with recorded techniques, the initial exposures should be made using a standard technique chart. Adjustments and technical factors can then be made, if necessary, on subsequent films. See the box in Chapter 1 labeled Relative Attenuation of X-Rays in Advanced Stages of Diseases for a list of the changes in attenuation factors expected in advanced stages of various disease processes.

Physiology of the Respiratory System

The major role of the respiratory system is the oxygenation of blood and the removal of the body's waste products in the form of carbon dioxide. The upper respiratory system, which consists of the nasopharynx, oropharynx, and larynx, provides structure for the passage of air into the lower respiratory system. The lower respiratory system, which consists of the trachea, bronchi, and bronchioles, is composed of tubular structures responsible for conducting air from the upper respiratory structures. The smallest unit where gas exchange occurs consists of the terminal bronchiole, alveolar ducts, and alveolar sacs. With the use of the upper and lower respiratory structures, the air from outside the body enters the lungs. The single trachea branches out into two bronchi (one to each lung) at the carina (last segment of the trachea), which in turn branch out into progressively smaller bronchioles to produce a structure termed the bronchial tree because its appearance resembles an inverted tree. The tracheobronchial tree is lined with a mucous membrane (the respiratory epithelium) containing numerous hairlike projections called cilia. During inspiration, the air is moistened and warmed as it enters the lungs. The cilia act as miniature sweepers to prevent dust and foreign particles from reaching the lungs. When the ciliary blanket works correctly, the particles are moved away from the lungs to be coughed up or swallowed. Any damage to the respiratory epithelium and its cilia permits particles (entering with the inspired or inhaled air) to proliferate and produce a disease process.

The vital gas exchange within the lung (called external respiration) takes place within the alveoli, extremely thin-walled sacs surrounded by blood capillaries, which represent the true parenchyma of the lung. Oxygen in the inhaled air diffuses from the alveoli into the blood capillaries, where it attaches to hemoglobin molecules in red blood cells and circulates to the various tissues of the body (called internal respiration). Carbon dioxide, a waste product of cellular metabolism, diffuses in the opposite direction, passing from the blood capillaries into the alveoli and then exiting the body during expiration (or exhalation). Because individual alveoli are extremely small, chest radiographs can demonstrate only a cluster of alveoli and their tiny terminal bronchioles, which are the basic anatomic units of the lung. A cluster of alveoli is termed the acinus.

Respiration is controlled by a center in the medulla at the base of the brain. The level of carbon dioxide in the blood regulates the respiratory center. Even a slight increase in the amount of carbon dioxide in the blood increases the rate and depth of breathing, such as when an individual exercises. The accumulation of waste gases that must be removed from the body (and the body's need for additional oxygen) causes the respiratory center to stimulate the muscles of respiration—the diaphragm and the intercostal muscles between the ribs. Contraction of the muscles of respiration causes the volume of the chest cavity to increase. This decreases the pressure within the lungs and forces air to move into the lungs through the tracheobronchial tree. As the respiratory muscles relax, the volume of the chest cavity decreases, and air is forced out of the lungs. Special muscles of expiration (abdominal and internal intercostal muscles) may be needed for difficult breathing or in patients with decreased gas exchange as occurs in emphysema.

Unlike most other organs, the lung has two different blood supplies. The pulmonary circulation is a low-pressure, low-resistance system through which oxygen enters and carbon dioxide exits the circulatory system. The bronchial circulation, which is a part of the high-pressure systemic circulation, supplies oxygenated blood to nourish (or support) the lung tissue itself.

A double-walled membrane consisting of two layers of pleura encases the lungs. The visceral pleura is the inner layer that adheres to the lung, whereas the parietal pleura lines the inner chest wall (the thoracic cavity). Between the two layers of pleura is a potential space (pleural space), which normally contains only a small amount of fluid to lubricate the surfaces to prevent friction as the lungs expand and contract. The airtight space between the lungs and the chest wall has a pressure a bit less than that in the lungs. This difference in pressure acts like a vacuum to prevent the lungs from collapsing. An inflammatory or neoplastic process that involves the pleura may produce fluid within the potential space (a pleural effusion).

Congenital/Hereditary Diseases

Cystic Fibrosis

Cystic fibrosis (mucoviscidosis) is a hereditary disease characterized by the secretion of excessively viscous mucus by all the exocrine glands; it is caused by a defective gene in the middle of chromosome 7. Cystic fibrosis is the most common clinically important genetic disorder among Caucasian children. This disorder also affects the pancreas and digestive system. However, 90% of the morbidity and mortality related to cystic fibrosis occurs as a result of respiratory involvement.

In the lungs, thick mucus secreted by mucosa in the trachea and bronchi blocks the air passages. The thick mucus is the result of an imbalance of sodium and chloride production and reabsorption. These mucous plugs lead to focal areas of lung collapse. Recurrent pulmonary infections are common because bacteria that are normally carried away by mucosal secretions adhere to the sticky mucus produced in this condition. Due to the recurring nature of the disease, by age 10 many children will have widespread bronchiectasis with the formation of large cysts and abscesses. In the pancreas, blockage of the ducts by mucous plugs prevents pancreatic enzymes from entering the duodenum. This impairs the digestion of fat, resulting in failure of the child to gain weight and the production of large, bulky, foul-smelling stools. In about 10% of newborns with cystic fibrosis, the thick mucus causes obstruction of the small bowel (meconium ileus) (Figure 3-1). Bowel perforation with subsequent fatal peritonitis may occur.

Involvement of the sweat glands in cystic fibrosis causes the child to perspire excessively. This leads to a loss of large amounts of salt (sodium, potassium, and chloride), two to three times the normal amount. This makes the patients extremely susceptible to heat exhaustion in hot weather. The presence of excessive chloride on the skin is the basis for the "sweat test," a simple and reliable test for cystic fibrosis.

Radiographic Appearance

Radiographically, cystic fibrosis causes generalized irregular thickening of linear markings throughout the lungs that, when combined with the almost invariable hyperinflation, produces an appearance similar to that of severe chronic lung disease in adults (Figure 3-2). Computed tomography (CT) screening to detect structural lung damage and assess disease progression is becoming more accepted by the clinicians. There is a concern regarding the radiation dose if CT were used on a routine basis (yearly), especially since affected persons are living into their 30s.

Treatment

Patient well-being depends on the use of prophylactic antibiotics, chest physiotherapy (percussions), and improved airflow. Prophylactic antibiotics reduce the risk of lung infections that may cause permanent lung damage or bronchiectasis. Chest physiotherapy (hand tapping against the chest) prevents lungs from filling with viscous mucus by keeping the mucus moving. Improved airflow depends on the use of bronchodilators. A new drug to help control pulmonary infections, administered by inhalation used in clinical trials, is deoxyribonuclease (DNase), an enzyme that digests the DNA of bacterial and inflammatory cells in the lungs. The newest research trials focus on methods to control the production and reabsorption of sodium and chloride. In the future, gene therapy will be a viable alternative for patients with cystic fibrosis.

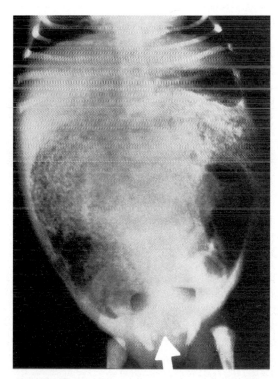

FIGURE 3-1 Meconium ileus in cystic fibrosis. Massive small bowel distention with profound soap-bubble effect of gas mixed with meconium.

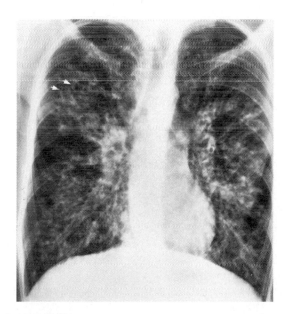

FIGURE 3-2 Cystic fibrosis. Multiple small cysts superimposed on diffuse, coarse, reticular pattern.

SUMMARY of FINDINGS for Congenital/Hereditary Disorders

disorder	location	radiographic appearance	treatment
Cystic fibrosis	Bronchi	Irregular thickening of linear markings throughout lung Hyperinflation CT demonstrates structural lung damage and disease progression	Prophylactic antibiotics Chest physiotherapy Bronchodilators
Hyaline membrane disease	Alveoli	Minute granular densities in parenchyma Air bronchogram	Artificial surfactant administered into the lungs via a saline solution Positive pressure ventilation

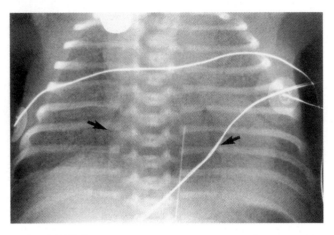

FIGURE 3-3 Hyaline membrane disease. Diffuse granular pattern of pulmonary parenchyma associated with air bronchograms (*arrows*).

Hyaline Membrane Disease

Hyaline membrane disease, also known as idiopathic respiratory distress syndrome (IRDS), is one of the most common causes of respiratory distress in the newborn. It primarily occurs in premature infants, especially those who have diabetic mothers or who have been delivered by cesarean section. Hypoxia and increasing respiratory distress may not be immediately evident at birth, but almost always appear within 6 hours of delivery.

The progressive underaeration of the lungs in hyaline membrane disease results from a lack of **surfactant** and immature lungs. Surfactant consists of a mixture of lipids, proteins, and carbohydrates that creates a high surface tension requiring less force to inflate and maintain the alveoli. Normally the alveolar cell walls produce lipoprotein, which maintains the surface tension within the alveoli. This permits the alveoli to remain inflated so that atelectasis does not occur. This disease process results from surfactant deficiency resulting from cell immaturity or birth trauma.

Radiographic Appearance

In addition to pronounced underaeration, the radiographic hallmark of hyaline membrane disease is a finely granular appearance of the pulmonary parenchyma (Figure 3-3). A peripherally extending air bronchogram develops because the small airways dilate and stand out clearly against the atelectasis in the surrounding lung.

Treatment

New treatment advances for this disease include the use of an artificial surfactant, which offers the best therapy to reduce morbidity and mortality from this disease process. The artificial surfactant is administered into the airways via a saline solution.

The treatment of hyaline membrane disease includes the use of positive-pressure ventilators that pump air (often with high concentrations of oxygen) into the lungs through an endotracheal tube. The positive-pressure ventilator ensures satisfactory levels of tissue oxygenation. The high ventilator pressure may cause leakage of air from overinflated alveoli or small terminal bronchioles, leading to interstitial emphysema, pneumothorax, and pneumopericardium, all of which further decrease the expansion of the lungs.

Inflammatory Disorders of the Upper Respiratory System

Croup

Croup is primarily a viral infection of young children that produces inflammatory obstructive swelling localized to the subglottic portion of the trachea. The edema causes inspiratory stridor or a barking cough, depending on the degree of laryngeal obstruction.

Radiographic Appearance

Frontal radiographs of the lower neck show a characteristic smooth, fusiform, tapered narrowing (hourglass shape) of the subglottic airway caused by the

SUMMARY
FINDINGS *for* Inflammatory Disorders of the Upper Respiratory System

disorder	location	radiographic appearance	treatment
Croup	Subglottic trachea Larynx	Smooth, tapered narrowing	Steam, mist tent, O_2
Epiglottitis	Supraglottic area or supraglottis	Rounded thickening epiglottic shadow	ER—intubation Antibiotic for infection

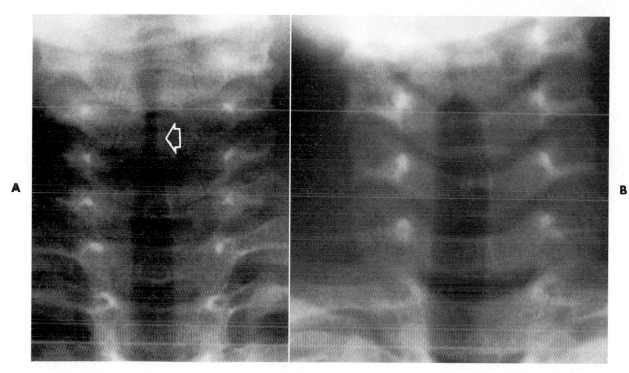

A

B

FIGURE **3-4** Croup. **A,** Arrow indicates smooth, tapered narrowing of subglottic portion of trachea (the Gothic arch sign). **B,** Normal trachea with broad shouldering in subglottic region.

edema (Figure 3-4, *A*), which is unlike the broad shouldering normally seen (Figure 3-4, *B*).

Treatment
A cool mist helps alleviate the breathing difficulty in patients with croup. At home, many patients use the steam from a hot shower for 15- to 20-minute intervals. When breathing continues to be difficult, medical attention should be sought. Corticosteroid treatment is used in severe cases to help reduce swelling.

Epiglottitis
Acute infections of the epiglottis, most commonly caused by *Haemophilus influenzae* in children, cause thickening of epiglottic tissue and the surrounding pharyngeal structures. The incidence of epiglottitis has decreased dramatically since the inception of

the *Haemophilus influenzae* group B (HiB) vaccine as a routine childhood immunization.

Radiographic Appearance
On lateral projections of the neck using soft tissue techniques, a rounded thickening of the epiglottic shadow gives it the configuration and approximate size of an adult's thumb (Figure 3-5), in contrast to the normal, narrow epiglottic shadow resembling an adult's little finger.

Treatment
Prompt recognition of acute epiglottitis is imperative because the condition may result in sudden complete airway obstruction. Because of its severity, epiglottitis requires hospitalization so the patient may be monitored. Intubation may become necessary to restore

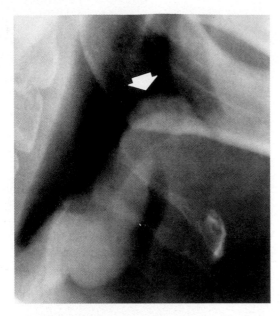

FIGURE 3-5 Epiglottitis. Lateral radiograph of neck demonstrates wide, rounded configuration of inflamed epiglottis *(arrow)*.

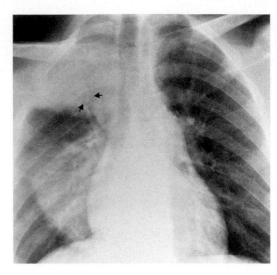

FIGURE 3-6 Alveolar pneumonia (pneumococcal). Homogeneous consolidation of right upper lobe and medial and posterior segments of right lower lobe. Note associated air bronchograms *(arrows)*.

normal respiration. Also, antibiotics may have to be administered to treat the infection, and corticosteroids to reduce the swelling.

Inflammatory Disorders of the Lower Respiratory System

Pneumonia

Acute pneumonia is an inflammation of the lung that can be caused by a variety of organisms, most commonly bacteria and viruses. Regardless of the cause, pneumonias tend to produce one of three basic radiographic patterns.

Alveolar Pneumonia

Alveolar, or **air-space, pneumonia,** exemplified by pneumococcal pneumonia, is produced by an organism that causes an inflammatory exudate that replaces air in the alveoli so that the affected part of the lung is no longer air containing but rather appears solid, or radiopaque (Figure 3-6). The inflammation spreads from one alveolus to the next by way of communicating channels, and it may involve pulmonary segments or an entire lobe (lobar pneumonia).

Radiographic Appearance

Consolidation of the lung parenchyma with little or no involvement of the airways produces the characteristic air-bronchogram sign (Figure 3-7). The sharp contrast between air within the bronchial

tree and the surrounding airless lung parenchyma permits the normally invisible bronchial air column to be seen radiographically. The appearance of an air bronchogram requires the presence of air within the bronchial tree, which suggests that the bronchus is not completely occluded at its origin. An air bronchogram excludes the diagnosis of a pleural or mediastinal lesion because there are no bronchi in these regions. Because air in the alveoli is replaced by an equal or almost equal quantity of inflammatory exudate and because the airways leading to the affected portions of the lung remain open, there is no evidence of volume loss in alveolar pneumonia.

Bronchopneumonia

Bronchopneumonia, typified by staphylococcal infection, is primarily an inflammation that originates in the bronchi or the bronchiolar mucosa and spreads to adjacent alveoli. Because alveolar spread of the infection in the peripheral air spaces is minimal, the inflammation tends to produce small patches of consolidation. Bronchial inflammation causing airway obstruction leads to atelectasis with loss of lung volume.

Radiographic Appearance

The small patches of consolidation may be seen radiographically as opacifications that are scattered throughout the lungs, but are separated by an abundance of air-containing lung tissue (Figure 3-8); air bronchograms are absent. If consolidation causes obstructed airways, atelectasis is evident.

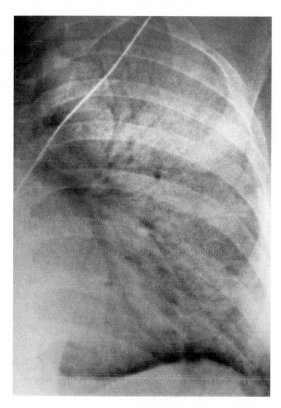

FIGURE 3-7 Air-bronchogram sign in pneumonia. Frontal chest radiograph demonstrates air within intrapulmonary bronchi in patient with diffuse alveolar pneumonia of left lung.

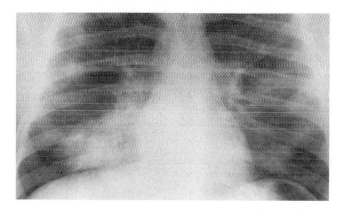

FIGURE 3-8 Bronchopneumonia (staphylococcal). Ill-defined consolidation at right base.

Interstitial Pneumonia

Interstitial pneumonia is most commonly produced by viral and mycoplasmal infections. In this type of pneumonia, the inflammatory process involves predominantly the walls and lining of the alveoli and the interstitial supporting structures of the lung, the alveoli septa.

Radiographic Appearance

The interstitial dispersal of the infection produces a linear or reticular pattern (Figure 3-9). When seen on

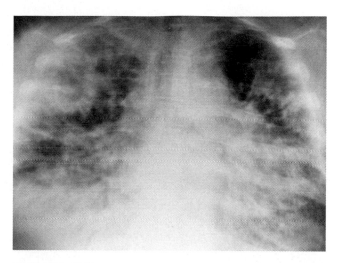

FIGURE 3-9 Interstitial pneumonia (viral). Diffuse peribronchial infiltrate with associated air-space consolidation obscures heart border (shaggy heart sign). Patchy alveolar infiltrate is present in right upper lung.

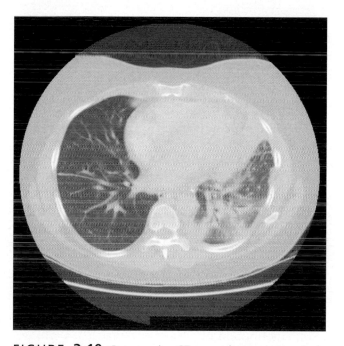

FIGURE 3-10 Pneumonia. CT scan demonstrates single lobe infiltrate by increased density of lung tissue on the left side.

end, the thickened interstitium may appear as multiple small nodular densities. Left untreated, interstitial pneumonia may cause "honeycomb lung," which is demonstrated by CT as cystlike spaces and dense fibrotic walls (Figure 3-10).

Treatment

Extensive inflammation of the lung can cause a mixed pattern of alveolar, bronchial, and interstitial pneumonias, and this pattern appears as opacifications representing pulmonary consolidation. Treatment for these

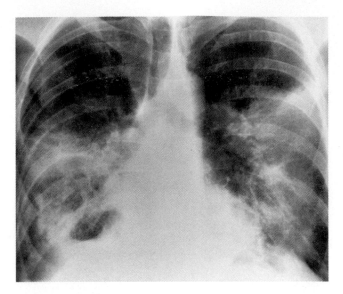

FIGURE 3-11 Aspiration pneumonia. Bilateral, nonsegmental air-space consolidation.

types of pneumonias usually includes regimented doses of an antibiotic to eradicate the cause. Rest, hydration, and deep-breathing techniques (supportive therapy) help in treating the infectious process.

Aspiration Pneumonia

The aspiration of esophageal or gastric contents into the lung can lead to the development of pneumonia. Aspiration of esophageal material can occur in patients with esophageal obstruction (e.g., tumor, stricture, and achalasia), diverticula (Zenker's), or neuromuscular swallowing disturbances. Aspiration of liquid gastric contents is most often related to general anesthetic, tracheostomy, coma, or trauma.

Radiographic Appearance

Both types of aspiration cause multiple alveolar densities, which may be distributed widely and diffusely throughout both lungs (Figure 3-11). Because the anatomic distribution of pulmonary changes is affected by gravity, the posterior segments of the upper and lower lobes are most commonly affected, especially in debilitated or bedridden patients.

Treatment

For effective treatment, early diagnosis of aspiration pneumonia and the prompt institution of corticosteroid and antibiotic therapy are essential to improve the otherwise grave prognosis.

Anthrax

Anthrax is caused by the sporelike microbe known as *Bacillus anthracis*. Since the mid-1970s, there have been no incidences until the biologic threat in the

fall of 2001. Anthrax is considered a highly volatile microbe because of its ease of transmission and high fatality rate. The organism can survive for decades in the soil in extreme conditions (heat and cold), without the need for a host.

There are three ways to contract anthrax: cutaneous, through an opening in the skin; inhalation (lungs), which is usually fatal (75%) if not treated in the early stages; and gastrointestinal. The cutaneous form is the most common type (75%) and is contracted by working with animals or animal byproducts (hides). Inhaled *B. anthracis* germinates in the lung tissue and lymph nodes, producing deadly toxins. These toxins cause cellular edema and disruption of normal cell function. Early signs are similar to influenza; however, progressive infection may cause labored breathing, shock, or even death. The gastrointestinal type, which causes intestinal inflammation, is usually caused by the consumption of contaminated meat.

Radiographic Appearance

Inhalation anthrax causes mediastinal widening and often pleural effusion without infiltrates on a chest image. Rarely, infiltrates may develop. Gastrointestinal involvement presents as mesenteric adenopathy on CT.

Treatment

Although high-dose antibiotics in the early stages attack the bacteria, the anthrax toxins are still produced and sometimes cause death. Vaccines are highly effective and available for limited use. They are not employed routinely in the United States because the last known reported incidence was 1976 (until the bioterror attacks in 2001).

Lung Abscess

A lung abscess is a necrotic area of pulmonary parenchyma containing purulent (puslike) material. A lung abscess may be a complication of bacterial pneumonia, bronchial obstruction, aspiration, a foreign body, or the hematogenous spread of organisms to the lungs either in a patient with diffuse bacteremia or as a result of septic emboli. Aspiration, which is the most common cause of lung abscesses, frequently occurs in the right lung because the right main bronchus is more vertical and larger in diameter than the left. The necrotic parenchyma becomes encapsulated by a fibrous wall, which encases the necrotic material. Unlike abscesses involving other organs, lung abscesses create an opening into the airway that can expand the extent of the infection.

Clinically a patient with a lung abscess has a fever and cough, and produces copious amounts of foul-smelling sputum. An important complication of

SUMMARY of FINDINGS for Inflammatory Disorders of the Lower Respiratory System

disorder	location	radiographic appearance	treatment
Pneumococcal pneumonia	Lobar/segment	Lobe/segment opacification	Antibiotic
Staphylococcal pneumonia	Bronchial airway/alveoli	Patchy opacification with air bronchogram	Antibiotic
Viral or mycoplasmic pneumonia	Alveolar/interstitial	Linear or reticular pattern	Antibiotic
Aspiration pneumonia	Alevolar (lobe/segment)	Patchy opacification	Corticosteroid and antibiotic
Anthrax	Throughout both lungs	Mediastinal widening with associated pleural effusions without infiltrates	High-dose antibiotics and vaccination
Lung abscess	Most common in right lung	Encapsulated opaque mass with air-fluid level	Appropriate antibiotic for specific organism, aid in expectoration of purulent material

lung abscess is the development of a brain abscess, which is produced by infected material carried by the blood from the lung to the left side of the heart and then on to the brain.

Radiographic Appearance

The earliest radiographic finding of lung abscess is a spherical density that characteristically has a dense center with a hazy, poorly defined periphery. If there is communication with the bronchial tree, the fluid contents of the cavity are partly replaced by air, producing a typical air-fluid level within the abscess (Figure 3-12). A cavitary lung abscess usually has a thickened wall with a shaggy, irregular inner margin. CT can assist in the diagnostic process to demonstrate an ill-defined outer wall and rule out empyema (Figure 3-13).

Treatment

The treatment for lung abscesses varies according to the cause. Specific therapy to control and eradicate the underlying organism is used along with supplemental treatment to alleviate possible complications. The patient also receives supportive therapy to help the lung mobilize the purulent material and to ensure pulmonary volume.

Tuberculosis

Tuberculosis is caused by *Mycobacterium tuberculosis*, a rod-shaped bacterium with a protective waxy coat that permits it to live outside the body for a long time. Tuberculosis spreads mainly by droplets in the air, which are produced in huge numbers by the coughing of an infected patient. Therefore it is essential that

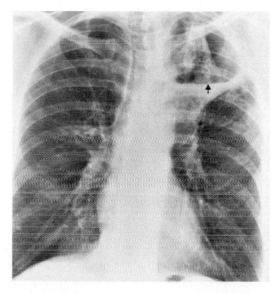

FIGURE 3-12 Lung abscess (bacterial pneumonia). Large, thick-walled left upper lobe abscess with air-fluid level *(arrow)* and associated infiltrate.

respiratory precautions be followed when radiographing patients with active disease. The organisms may be inhaled from sputum that has dried and turned into dust. They are rapidly killed by direct sunlight, but may survive a long time in the dark. Tuberculosis also may be acquired by drinking the milk of infected cows. However, routine pasteurization of milk has virtually eliminated this route of infection.

Unlike most bacteria, mycobacteria do not stain reliably by Gram's method. However, once stain is taken up, it is difficult to decolorize mycobacteria by either acid or alcohol, and thus the organisms are often called acid-fast bacilli.

Tuberculosis is primarily a disease of the lungs, although it can spread to involve the gastrointestinal, genitourinary, and skeletal systems. In the initial tuberculous infection (the primary lesion), a collection of inflammatory cells collects around a clump of tuberculosis bacilli to form a small mass (tubercle) that is visible to the naked eye. The outcome of this initial infection depends on the number of bacilli and the resistance of the infected tissue. If the resistance is good and the dose is small, the proliferation of fibrous tissue around the tumor limits the spread of infection and produces a mass of scar tissue. In the lung, tuberculous scars are commonly found in the posterior apical segments. They often contain calcium, which is deposited as healing occurs.

A larger dose of bacilli or lower patient resistance tends to permit the disease to progress slowly. Within the center of the tubercle, the bacilli kill inflammatory cells, so that the core becomes a necrotic, Swiss cheese–like mass (caseation). The caseous material may eventually become liquefied to form a cavity. Coalescence of several small cavities can result in the formation of a large cavity, which may contain an air-fluid level. Rupture of blood vessels crossing a cavity causes bleeding and the coughing up of blood (hemoptysis). An overwhelming infection with low resistance causes diffuse destruction throughout the lung, with the formation of huge cavities and often a fatal outcome.

The tuberculin skin test can detect previous tuberculous infection. The purified protein derivative (PPD) of the tuberculosis bacillus is injected into the skin and the injection site examined 2 to 3 days later. A visible and palpable swelling 10 mm in diameter or larger indicates that the individual has developed antibodies to a previous exposure to the bacilli. If there is no such reaction, the individual has either not been exposed to the tuberculosis bacilli or is anergic (i.e., immunologically nonreacting). The tuberculin test is not positive during an acute infection or for several weeks thereafter. One must consider the 3- to 6-week incubation period and the fact that the tuberculin skin test does not become positive until 2 to 10 weeks after infection.

Primary Tuberculosis

Primary pulmonary tuberculosis has traditionally been considered a disease of children and young adults. However, with the dramatic decrease in the prevalence of tuberculosis (especially in children and young adults), primary pulmonary disease can develop at any age. The current decline is the result of wider screening and prevention programs.

Radiographic Appearance

There are four basic radiographic patterns of primary pulmonary tuberculosis. (1) The infiltrate may be seen as a lobar or segmental air-space consolidation that is usually homogeneous, dense, and well defined (Figure 3-14). The apical lordotic projection best demonstrates the apices without superimposition of bony structures (Figure 3-15). (2) Associated enlargement of hilar or mediastinal lymph nodes is very common (Figure 3-16). (3) Indeed, the combination of a focal parenchymal lesion and enlarged hilar or mediastinal lymph nodes produces the classic primary complex (the Ghon lesion), an appearance strongly suggestive of primary tuberculosis. (4) Pleural effusion is common, especially in adults

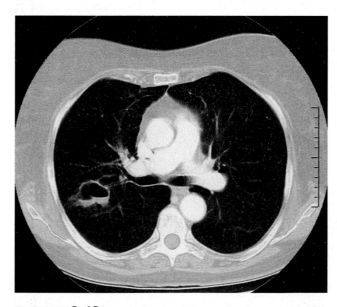

FIGURE 3-13 Lung abscess. CT scan demonstrates multiloculated capsule with air-fluid level.

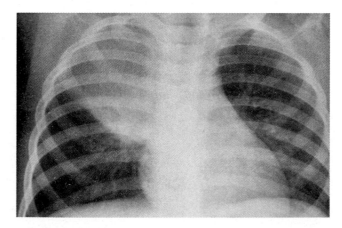

FIGURE 3-14 Primary tuberculosis. Consolidation of right upper lobe.

(Figure 3-17). Most primary tuberculous effusions are unilateral and clear rapidly with treatment.

Miliary tuberculosis refers to dissemination of the disease by way of the bloodstream. Radiographically, this produces innumerable fine discrete nodules (granulomas) distributed uniformly throughout both lungs (Figure 3-18).

Tuberculous pneumonia may resolve completely and leave a normal lung. However, if necrosis and caseation develop, some fibrous scarring occurs. Calcification may develop within both the parenchymal and the nodal lesions, and this may be the only residue of primary tuberculous infection on subsequent films. If the disease responds poorly to therapy and continues to progress (especially in patients with

immunodeficiency or diabetes and in those receiving steroid therapy), the pneumonia may break down into multiple necrotic cavities or a single large abscess filled with caseous material (Figure 3-19).

Secondary (Reactivation) Tuberculosis

Reactivation of organisms from previously dormant tubercles is termed a secondary lesion or reinfection tuberculosis. At times, the tuberculosis bacillus may remain inactive for many years before a secondary lesion develops, often because of a decrease in the body's immune defense. The diffuse, poorly defined lesion develops areas of caseous necrosis. Necrosis

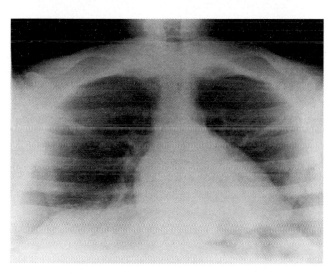

FIGURE **3-15** Apical lordotic projection. Lung apices can be seen without bony superimposition.

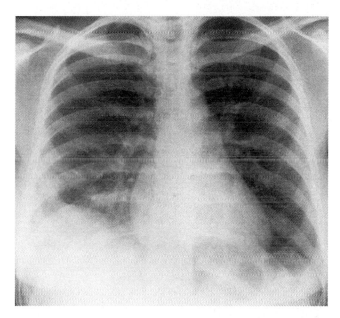

FIGURE **3-17** Primary tuberculosis. Unilateral right tuberculous pleural effusion without parenchymal or lymph node involvement.

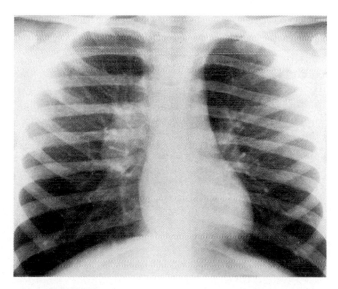

FIGURE **3-16** Primary tuberculosis. Enlargement of right hilar lymph nodes without discrete parenchymal infiltrate.

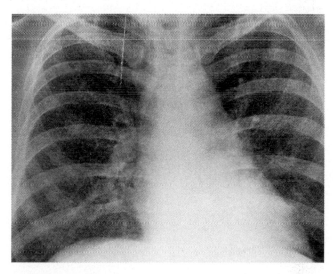

FIGURE **3-18** Miliary tuberculosis. Fine discrete nodules uniformly throughout both lungs.

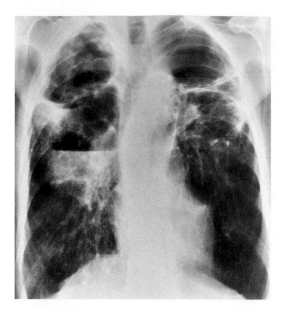

FIGURE 3-19 Tuberculosis. Multiple large cavities with air-fluid levels in both upper lobes. Notice chronic fibrotic changes and upward retraction of hila.

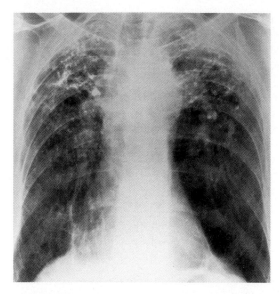

FIGURE 3-20 Secondary tuberculosis. Bilateral fibrocalcific changes at apices. Notice upward retraction of hila.

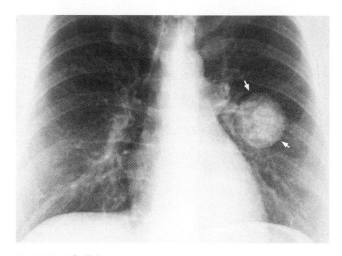

FIGURE 3-21 Calcified tuberculoma. Large soft tissue mass in left lung *(arrows)* that contains dense central calcification.

and liquefaction commonly lead to the development of tuberculous cavities, which typically have thick walls with ill-defined inner margins. Secondary pulmonary tuberculosis heals slowly with extensive fibrosis. Contraction of the fibrous scars causes loss of volume of the involved segment or lobe and a decrease in the size of the hemithorax. The trachea and other mediastinal structures are retracted to the involved side; in upper lobe disease the hilum is elevated.

Radiographic Appearance

Secondary tuberculosis most commonly affects the upper lobes, especially the apical and posterior segments (Figure 3-20). It is initially seen as a nonspecific, hazy, poorly marginated alveolar infiltrate that often radiates outward from the hilum.

Because of the difficulty of radiographically determining the activity of secondary tuberculosis, comparison with previous films is essential. An unchanged appearance of fibrosis and calcification on serial films usually indicates evidence of "healing" of the tuberculous process. Nevertheless, even densely calcified lesions can contain central areas of necrosis in which viable organisms can still be found even after long periods of apparent inactivity. Of course, new cavitation or an increasing amount of pulmonary infiltrate indicates active disease.

Tuberculoma

A tuberculoma is a sharply circumscribed parenchymal nodule, often containing viable tuberculosis bacilli that can develop in either primary or secondary

disease. Although the residual localized caseation may remain unchanged for a long period or permanently, a tuberculoma is potentially dangerous because it may break down at any time and lead to dissemination of the disease.

Radiographic Appearance

Radiographically, tuberculomas appear as single or multiple pulmonary nodules, usually 1 to 3 cm in diameter. They can occur in any part of the lung, but are most common in the periphery and in the upper lobes. A central nidus of calcification (which may be detectable only on tomograms) is strongly suggestive of the lesion representing a tuberculoma (Figure 3-21). However, the lack of calcification is of no diagnostic value.

SUMMARY of FINDINGS for Tuberculosis

disorder	location	radiographic appearance	treatment
Primary tuberculosis	Lobar or segmental	Consolidation is homogenous, dense, and well defined	For all active cases of tuberculosis, treatment is a two-drug regimen for 2 months or longer (isoniazid, rifampin, and pyrazinamide)
	Hilar and mediastinal lymph nodes	Hilar enlargement without parenchymal involvement	
	Parenchymal, hilar, and mediastinal nodes	Demonstrates Ghon lesion	
	Pleural cavity	Pleural effusion	For persons exposed to active tuberculosis, prophylactic treatment is suggested.
Miliary tuberculosis	Throughout lungs, and possible spread to other organs	Innumerable fine discrete nodules uniformly throughout lungs	
Tuberculous pneumonia	Parenchymal and nodal	Necrotic cavities or large abscess	
Secondary tuberculosis	Upper lobes and posterior segments	Extensive fibrotic changes with possible calcification	
Tuberculoma	Any part of lung, commonly in periphery and upper lobes	Single or multiple nodules, 1-3 cm	

Treatment

Currently, two groups of patients receive therapy. One consists of those who have active tuberculosis; the other are those who have been exposed to active tuberculosis and are at risk. For persons with active tuberculosis, treatment begins with a two-drug regimen to help prevent drug resistance through mutation. The most common drugs used today are isoniazid, rifampin, and pyrazinamide. The effectiveness of the treatment is evaluated regularly to be sure the patient's strain of *M. tuberculosis* has not become resistant to the drugs of choice. The treatment may take as long as 6 to 12 months. For the second group, prophylactic treatments are determined by the strain of tuberculosis to which the person has been exposed.

Pulmonary Mycosis

The term **pulmonary mycosis** means fungal infection of the lung. The two most common systemic fungal infections found in North America are histoplasmosis (endemic in the Mississippi and Ohio River valleys) and coccidioidomycosis (seen in the southwestern United States).

Histoplasmosis

Histoplasmosis, caused by the fungus *Histoplasma capsulatum,* is a common disease that often produces a radiographic appearance simulating that of tuberculosis. The primary form of histoplasmosis is usually relatively benign and often passes unnoticed.

Histoplasmosis can incite progressive fibrosis in the mediastinum. This can cause obstruction of the superior vena cava, pulmonary arteries, and pulmonary veins, as well as severe narrowing of the esophagus.

Diffuse calcification in the liver, spleen, and lymph nodes is virtually diagnostic of histoplasmosis, especially in areas in which the disease is endemic (e.g., the Mississippi and Ohio River valleys). These calcifications tend to be small, multiple, dense, and discrete, although occasionally they appear as moderately large, solidly calcified granulomas.

Coccidioidomycosis

Coccidioidomycosis is caused by a fungus, *Coccidioides immitis,* which is found in the desert soil of the southwestern United States. Coccidioidomycosis can develop from an acute infection to chronic or disseminated forms. The infection is transmitted through fungal spores in the air. Immunosuppressed patients are more susceptible, and the disease may progress rapidly in those with a compromised immune system.

Acute coccidioidomycosis has few or no symptoms in most cases. The symptoms emulate influenza. As in histoplasmosis, those who are infected often remain undiagnosed and the immune system builds antibodies to fight the infection. In chronic disease, the infection results in lung abscesses, which may rupture and infect the mediastinum and pleural cavity. The disease processes of chronic and disseminated coccidioidomycosis are similar to and may be indistinguishable from those of chronic histoplasmosis.

SUMMARY of FINDINGS for Pulmonary Mycosis

disorder	location	radiographic appearance	treatment
Primary histoplasmosis	Lower lung Hilar lymph nodes	Pulmonary infiltration Granulomatous nodule Hilar lymph node enlargement and/or calcification	<1% require treatment; amphotericin B Fluconazole for patients with acquired immunodeficiency syndrome (AIDS)
Chronic histoplasmosis	Upper lobe	Zones of parenchymal consolidation Cavitation Calcified granulomas	<1% require treatment; amphotericin B Fluconazole for AIDS patients
Acute coccidioidomycosis	Peripheral parenchyma	Pneumonia appearance Coccidioidoma (granuloma)	None needed unless grave; amphotericin B
Chronic coccidioidomycosis	Peripheral parenchyma	Lung abscesses	None needed unless grave; amphotericin B

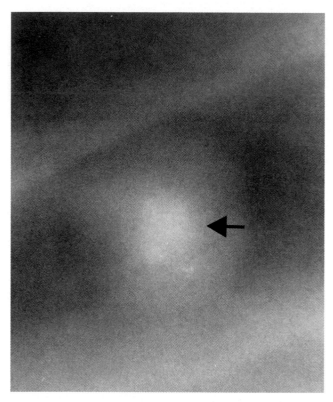

FIGURE 3-22 Histoplasmoma. Central calcification *(arrow)* in solitary pulmonary nodule.

Radiographic Appearance

Chest radiographs may demonstrate single or multiple areas of pulmonary infiltration; these most often appear in the lower lung and are frequently associated with hilar lymph node enlargement in primary histoplasmosis. Although this pattern simulates the primary complex of tuberculosis, pleural effusion rarely occurs with histoplasmosis. In children, striking hilar adenopathy,

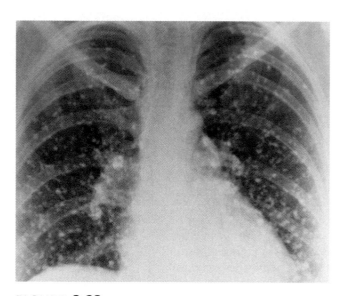

FIGURE 3-23 Histoplasmosis. Diffuse calcifications in lungs produce snowball pattern.

which may cause bronchial compression, may develop without radiographic evidence of parenchymal disease. Hilar lymph node calcification commonly occurs in adults and produces a "popcorn" radiographic appearance. Pulmonary histoplasmosis frequently manifests as a solitary, sharply circumscribed, granulomatous nodule (histoplasmoma), which is usually less than 3 cm in diameter and found most often in a lower lobe. Central, rounded calcification within the mass (the target lesion) is virtually pathognomonic (characteristic) of this disease (Figure 3-22). Multiple soft tissue nodules scattered throughout both lungs may simulate miliary tuberculosis. These shadows may clear completely or may fibrose and persist, often appearing on subsequent chest radiographs as widespread punctate calcifications (Figure 3-23).

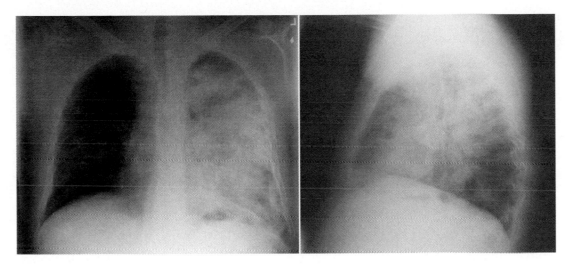

FIGURE 3-24 Coccidioidomycosis. Posteroanterior and lateral views demonstrate consolidation caused by fungus in the left lung.

Coccidioidomycosis typically produces small pulmonary consolidations in the periphery of the parenchyma resembling extensive pneumonia (Figure 3-24).

Chronic histoplasmosis and advanced chronic coccidioidomycosis closely simulate the radiographic appearance of reinfection tuberculosis because they both commonly exhibit cavitation and are found in an upper lobe.

Treatment

Fewer than 1% of patients with primary or chronic histoplasmosis or with coccidioidomycosis require any drug treatment. Restricted activity and bed rest are encouraged. When drug treatment is required, the drug of choice is amphotericin B.

Respiratory Syncytial Virus

Respiratory syncytial virus (RSV) affects approximately 3 to 4 million infants annually (2005) and of those affected, approximately 100,000 required hospitalization. Of all bronchiolitis cases, 80% occur as a result of an RSV infection. RSV attacks the lower respiratory tract and causes necrosis of the respiratory epithelium of the bronchi and bronchioles, which leads to bronchiolitis. The necrotic material and edema from the infection cause bronchial obstruction. Bronchiolitis produces bronchial spasm, and interstitial pneumonia occurs as a result of the obstruction. The patient has only cold or flulike symptoms and is not managed with the appropriate infection control procedures. Therefore the virus has caused a high rate of nosocomial infection. Fomites carry the virus through droplets from the nose or

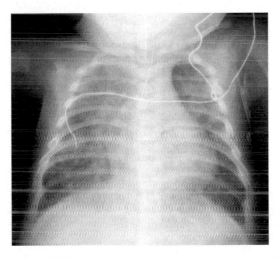

FIGURE 3-25 Respiratory syncytial virus. Bilateral fluffy pulmonary infiltrates, associated with hyperinflation, the features being consistent with respiratory syncytial virus pneumonia.

throat, and the virus has the ability to persist for many hours on surfaces. Healthcare workers must use appropriate protective personal devices and dispose of them properly to protect themselves and others.

Radiographic Appearance

Hyperinflation with diffuse increased interstitial markings is the most common finding on chest images. The necrosis of the respiratory epithelium, if severe, appears radiographically as an interstitial pneumonia (Figure 3-25). In the most severe cases, focal areas of atelectasis are apparent.

SUMMARY of FINDINGS for Viruses

disorder	location	radiographic appearance	treatment
Respiratory syncytial virus (RSV)	Bronchial epithelium	Hyperinflation with diffuse increased interstitial markings Interstitial pneumonia Severe cases will demonstrate focal areas of atelectasis	No treatment needed in most cases Antibiotic and antiviral drugs (ribavirin)
Severe acute respiratory syndrome (SARS)	Throughout both lungs	Early focal infiltrates progressing to generalized patchy interstitial infiltrates	Bacterial and antiviral agents, other treatment regimens similar to those for atypical pneumonia

Treatment

Many children do not need drug therapy and recover simply through their immune response. Those children who require hospitalization receive antibiotics for infectious complications, and they may also be given the antiviral drug ribavirin aerosol. Children may require oxygen therapy and, in the most severe cases, mechanical ventilation. Most infected adults recover without treatment.

Severe Acute Respiratory Syndrome

Severe acute respiratory syndrome (SARS) caused global concern in 2003 as a result of the 8000 cases diagnosed according to the World Health Organization (WHO). The first cases appeared in China. SARS, a SARS-*coronavirus* of unknown etiology, may survive in the environment many days. Person-to-person or droplet contact causes upper and lower respiratory infections that begin with a nonproductive cough and progress to hypoxemia. Severe SARS requires intubation and mechanical ventilation, and is associated with a fatality rate of about 3%. Other symptoms are similar to those in community-acquired atypical pneumonia.

Radiographic Appearance

On chest images, the lungs appear normal in the early stages. As the disease progresses into the lower respiratory region, there is the development of early focal infiltrates that may progress to generalized, patchy interstitial infiltrates. Eventually, areas of consolidation may be seen.

Treatment

Most persons with less than 10% of the lung infected on the seventh day survive the disease. Follow-up images play a vital role in determining whether treatment is appropriate or requires a more aggressive approach. Currently, antibacterial and antiviral agents are used to combat the disease. There is no known curative treatment, and SARS is treated the same as other atypical pneumonia.

Diffuse Lung Disease

Chronic Obstructive Pulmonary Disease

Chronic obstructive pulmonary disease (COPD) includes several conditions in which chronic obstruction of the airways leads to an ineffective exchange of respiratory gases and makes breathing difficult. In many cases, two disease processes coexist to cause the obstructive process. **Chronic bronchitis** is characterized by excessive tracheobronchial mucus production leading to the obstruction of small airways. **Emphysema** refers to the distention of distal air spaces as a result of the destruction of alveolar walls and the obstruction of small airways. **Asthma** occurs when the bronchioles go into spasm, causing decreased airflow and sometimes obstruction of the airway. Chronic dilatation of the bronchi or bronchioles indicates **bronchiectasis**. Factors that predispose to COPD include cigarette smoking, infection, air pollution, and occupational exposure to harmful substances, such as asbestos.

Chronic Bronchitis

Chronic inflammation of the bronchi leads to severe coughing with the production of sputum. Bronchitis may be a complication of respiratory infection or the result of long-term exposure to air pollution or cigarette smoking. Of all chronic bronchitis cases, 90% are associated with cigarette smoking. The severity of the disease and how quickly the symptoms can be relieved are directly related to the number of cigarettes smoked.

The walls of the bronchi and bronchioles thicken and produce viscous mucus. Over an extended period, the mucous glands become hyperplastic.

Radiographic Appearance

About half the patients with chronic bronchial disease demonstrate no changes on chest radiographs. The most common radiographic abnormality in chronic bronchitis is a generalized increase in bronchovascular markings ("dirty chest"), especially in the lower lungs (Figure 3-26). Thickening of bronchial walls and peribronchial inflammation can cause parallel or slightly tapered tubular line shadows ("tram lines") or may appear as thickening of bronchial shadows when viewed end on.

Eventually, excessive production of mucus and swelling of the bronchial mucosa may lead to narrowing of the airways and overinflation of the lungs (emphysema). Chest radiographs demonstrate hyperinflated lungs and a depressed diaphragm.

Treatment

In general, the treatment for chronic bronchitis is designed to improve symptoms, decrease any reversible processes, and prevent progression of the disease. Prophylactic antibiotic therapy reduces infections. Bronchial dilators reduce spasm and open airways. Expectorants assist in keeping the lungs clear. Although currently no cure exits, appropriate therapy can be expected to reduce severe flare-ups and minimize progression of the disease.

Emphysema

Emphysema is a crippling and debilitating condition in which obstructive and destructive changes in small airways (the acini or terminal bronchioles) lead to a dramatic increase in the volume of air in the lungs. In many patients, the development of emphysema is closely associated with heavy cigarette smoking. Other predisposing factors are chronic bronchitis, air pollution, and long-term exposure to irritants of the respiratory tract.

Irritating smoke, fumes, and pollutants injure the fine hairs (cilia) of the respiratory mucosa, which can no longer sweep away foreign particles. This causes mucosal inflammation and the secretion of excess mucus that plugs up the air passages and leads to an increase in airway resistance. Collateral air drift permits the ventilation of lung parenchyma served by the obstructed airways. Continuous bronchial narrowing and loss of elasticity, exacerbated by cigarette smoking, make it very difficult for the patient to exhale the stale air. The resulting air trapping and overinflation of the lung lead to alveolar distention and eventually to the rupture of alveolar septa. As the walls between alveoli are destroyed, these tiny air sacs become transformed into large air-filled spaces called **bullae**. With the loss of alveolar septa, the surface for gas exchange decreases, limiting the transfer of oxygen into the bloodstream. As the lungs become less efficient, the heart tries to compensate. This places excessive strain on the heart, which eventually enlarges. The large air sacs (bullae) may rupture, leading to air entering into the pleural space (spontaneous pneumothorax) and causing collapse of the lung (atelectasis).

Radiographic Appearance

The major radiographic signs of emphysema are related to pulmonary overinflation, alterations in the pulmonary vasculature, and bullae formation.

The hallmark of pulmonary overinflation is flattening of the domes of the diaphragm (Figure 3-27). Another important sign seen on lateral chest radiographs is an increase in the size and lucency of the retrosternal air space, the distance between the posterior side of the sternum and the anterior wall of the ascending aorta. The anteroposterior (AP) diameter of the chest increases and the chest becomes more barrel shaped as the disease progresses. Air trapping may be detected fluoroscopically as a decrease in the normal movement of the diaphragm during respiration.

The major vascular change in patients with emphysema is a reduction in the number and size of the peripheral arteries. As the pressure in the pulmonary arteries increases, the main and central pulmonary arteries become more prominent, which further accentuates the appearance of rapid tapering of peripheral vessels.

Bullae appear as air-containing cystic spaces whose walls are usually of hairline thickness. They range in size from 1 to 2 cm in diameter up to an entire hemithorax (Figure 3-28). These large, radiolucent,

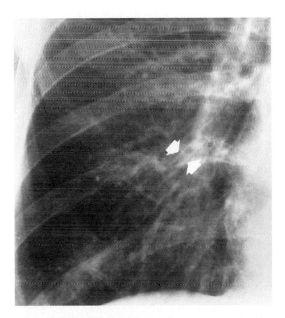

FIGURE 3-26 Chronic bronchitis. Coned view of right lower lung demonstrates an increase in coarseness in interstitial markings. Arrows point to characteristic parallel line shadows ("tram lines") outside the boundary of the pulmonary hilum.

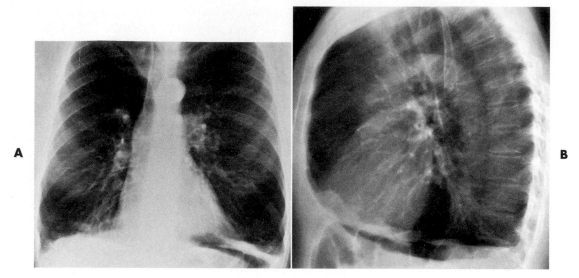

FIGURE 3-27 Emphysema. Frontal **(A)** and lateral **(B)** projections of the chest demonstrate severe overinflation of lungs along with flattening and even a superiorly concave configuration of the hemidiaphragms. Also, the size and lucency of the retrosternal air space are increased, the AP diameter of the chest is increased, and the number and caliber of peripheral pulmonary arteries are reduced.

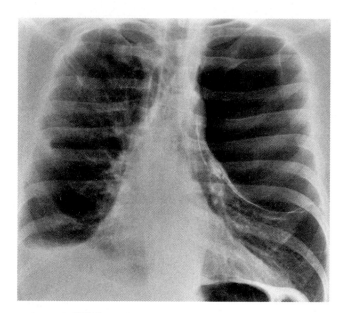

FIGURE 3-28 Giant emphysematous bulla. Air-containing mass fills most of the left hemithorax.

air-filled sacs are found predominantly at the apices or at the bases and may become so large that they cause respiratory insufficiency by compressing the remaining relatively normal lung.

A less common radiographic appearance of emphysema is the increased markings pattern. Instead of being narrowed, the vascular markings in this condition are more prominent than normal and tend to be irregular and indistinct, producing a "dirty chest" appearance.

Emphysema occasionally occurs in young patients who have hereditary disorders of connective tissue (osteogenesis imperfecta). Striking lower lobe predominance develops in young patients who have a deficiency of the enzyme α-antitrypsin, which leads to destruction of elastic and connective tissue in the lungs.

When patients have advanced stages of pulmonary emphysema and have large amounts of air trapped in their lungs (more radiolucent), the radiographer should reduce exposure factors for chest radiography. CT demonstrates large blebs and destruction of the lung parenchyma, and it can detect any spontaneous pneumothorax (Figure 3-29).

Treatment
Currently there is no cure for emphysema. Treatment assists only in relieving symptoms and in preventing progressive destruction by the disease.

Asthma
Asthma is a very common disease in which widespread narrowing of the airways develops because of an increased responsiveness of the tracheobronchial tree to various stimuli (allergens). Common allergens include house dust, pollen, molds, animal dander, certain fabrics, and various foods **(extrinsic asthma)**. Exercise, heat or cold exposure, and emotional upset can also cause an asthma attack **(intrinsic asthma)**. The hypersensitivity reaction to one or more of these allergens leads to swelling of the mucous membranes of the bronchi, excess secretion of mucus, and spasm

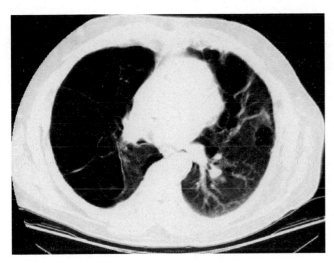

FIGURE 3-29 Emphysematous blebs. CT scan shows the destruction of lung parenchyma.

of the smooth muscle in the bronchial walls, all of which lead to severe narrowing of the airways. This makes breathing (especially expiration) difficult and results in the characteristic wheezing sound that is produced by air passing through the narrowed bronchial tubes. Untreated or uncontrolled asthma permanently scars the bronchial structure, causing progressive disease.

Radiographic Appearance

Early in the course of the disease, chest radiographs obtained between acute episodes demonstrate no abnormalities. During an acute asthmatic attack, bronchial narrowing and difficulty in expiration lead to an increased volume of the hyperlucent lungs with flattening of the hemidiaphragms and an increase in the retrosternal air space. In asthma, unlike in emphysema, the pulmonary vascular markings remain normal. In patients with chronic asthma, especially those with a history of repeated episodes of superinfection, thickening of bronchial walls can produce prominence of interstitial markings and the "dirty chest" appearance (Figure 3-30). The results of the chest radiograph taken in the emergency room determine if the asthma has progressed to pneumonia.

Treatment

Those patients with allergy-induced asthma can use preventive (cromolyn sodium or necromil sodium inhaler) and rescue (β-2 stimulants) bronchodilators. Allergy shots may build up natural antibodies. Asthmatics with exercise-induced problems may take oral medication to decrease bronchiomuscular spasm, in addition to preventive and rescue bronchodilators. Keeping airways open helps prevent infections, which asthmatics are prone to contract. New inhaled

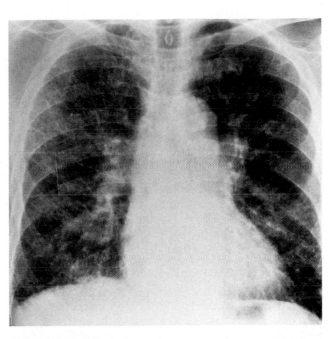

FIGURE 3-30 Asthma. Recurrent pulmonary infections have led to the development of diffuse pulmonary fibrosis and prominence of interstitial markings in lungs.

steroid drugs help control the inflammatory process and decrease the potential for developing pulmonary infection.

Bronchiectasis

Bronchiectasis refers to permanent abnormal dilation of one or more large bronchi as a result of destruction of the elastic and muscular components of the bronchial wall. Bronchitis, a destructive process, is a common complication of bronchiectasis and is nearly always the result of a bacterial infection. The infection may be either a severe necrotizing pneumonia or a result of a local or systemic abnormality that impairs the body's defense mechanisms and promotes bacterial growth. Since the advent of antibiotic therapy and vaccines, the incidence of bronchiectasis has substantially decreased.

The patient with bronchiectasis typically has a chronic productive cough, often associated with recurrent episodes of acute pneumonia and hemoptysis. The disease usually involves the basal segments of the lower lobes, and it is bilateral in about half of the cases. Pulmonary function tests assist in the diagnostic process by determining any evidence of decreased gas exchange.

Radiographic Appearance

Plain chest radiographs may show coarseness and loss of definition of interstitial markings caused by peribronchial fibrosis and retained secretions (Figure 3-31). In more advanced disease, oval or

SUMMARY of FINDINGS for Diffuse Lung Disease

disorder	location	radiographic appearance	treatment

Chronic bronchitis	Bronchi/bronchioles
	Mucus gland
	  hyperplasia
		No image change in 50%
		Increased bronchovascular markings
		Hyperinflation and depressed
		  diaphragm
			Prophylactic antibiotics
			Bronchial dilators
			Expectorants
			No cure

Emphysema	Destroyed alveolar septa	Pulmonary hyperinflation Bulla formation Flattened diaphragm Radiolucent retrosternal space	Treat symptoms No cure
Asthma	Bronchi	No evidence unless during acute attack Bronchial narrowing/hyperlucent lungs Exclude other processes	Preventive and rescue bronchial dilators

Bronchiectasis	Basal segments of
	  lower lobes
		Coarseness and decreased interstitial
		  markings
			Vaccines or antibiotic
			  drugs

Advanced bronchiectasis	Basal segments of
	  lower lobes
		Oval/circular cystic spaces	Bronchodilator to increase
			  pulmonary function

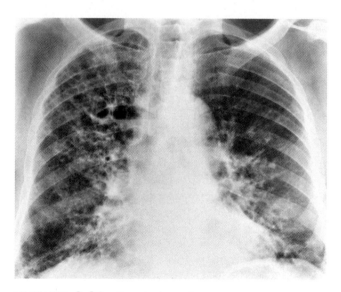

FIGURE 3-31 Chronic bronchiectasis. Severe coarsening of interstitial markings involves the bases and right upper lobe. Oval and circular cystic spaces, which produce a honeycomb-like pattern, are best seen in right upper lobe.

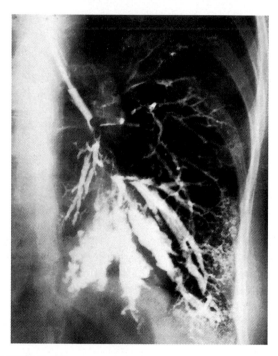

FIGURE 3-32 Chronic bronchiectasis. Bronchogram shows severe dilatation of the basal bronchi of the left lower lobe.

circular cystic spaces can develop. These cystic dilatations can be up to 2 cm in diameter and often contain air-fluid levels. In very severe cases, coarse interstitial fibrosis surrounding local areas of dilatation can produce a honeycomb pattern.

Although plain radiographs may strongly indicate bronchiectasis, bronchography is necessary to fill the dilated cystic spaces with contrast material and to establish the diagnosis unequivocally (Figure 3-32).

Treatment

Vaccines prevent many of the bacterial and viral infections that led to bronchiectasis in the past. Treatment of bronchiectasis consists of therapy to decrease the symptoms and an antibiotic based on the specific bacterial cause.

Pneumoconiosis

Prolonged occupational exposure to certain irritating particulates can cause severe pulmonary disease and a spectrum of radiographic findings. Inhaled foreign substances retained permanently in the acini cause irreversible damage. These inhaled particles cause a chronic interstitial inflammation that leads to pulmonary fibrosis and a diffuse nonspecific radiographic pattern of linear streaks and nodules throughout the lungs. The inflammation initially causes injury to the mucosal lining; long-term exposure may injure the pulmonary parenchyma and even lead to the development of a malignant neoplasm. The severity of the pneumoconiosis depends on the size of the particles, the length of exposure, and the concentration of particulates in the atmosphere (type of exposure). The more severe the exposure, the more fibrotic the lung becomes and the greater the resultant shortness of breath. The most common of the pneumoconioses are silicosis, asbestosis, and anthracosis (coal worker's disease). Other causes include exposure to such dusts as tin, iron oxide, barium, and beryllium. As many as 40 minerals cause lung lesions when inhaled, although most do not produce morphologic or functional abnormalities.

Silicosis

Silicosis is the most common and best-known work-related lung disease. The inhalation of high concentrations of silicon dioxide (crystalline silica) primarily affects workers engaged in mining, foundry work, and sandblasting. Quartz dust, the most frequent cause of inhalation silicosis, is the second most common element in the earth's crust. The lung reacts to the silica by producing a fibroblast-stimulating factor that results in extensive fibrosis. Acute silicosis can develop within 10 months of exposure in workers exposed to sandblasting in confined spaces. Most radiographic changes are the result of 15 to 20 years of long-term, less intense exposure. As the disease progresses, death occurs as a result of lung or heart failure.

Radiographic Appearance

The classic radiographic pattern in silicosis consists of multiple nodular shadows scattered throughout the lungs. These nodules, usually fairly well circumscribed and of uniform density, may become calcified (Figure 3-33). As the pulmonary nodules increase in size, they tend to coalesce and form conglomerates of irregular masses in excess of 1 cm in diameter (progressive massive fibrosis) (Figure 3-34). These masses are usually bilateral and relatively symmetric, and they almost always occur in the upper lobes or segments of the lungs. Occasionally a single large homogeneous mass in the perihilar area of one lung may closely simulate bronchogenic carcinoma. Hilar lymph node enlargement is common. The deposition of calcium salts in the periphery of enlarged lymph nodes produces the characteristic eggshell appearance (Figure 3-35), which is virtually pathognomonic of silicosis.

Asbestosis

Asbestosis may develop in improperly protected workers engaged in manufacturing asbestos products, in handling building materials, or in working with insulation composed of asbestos. In the 1980s, many public buildings, such as schools, with fireproof

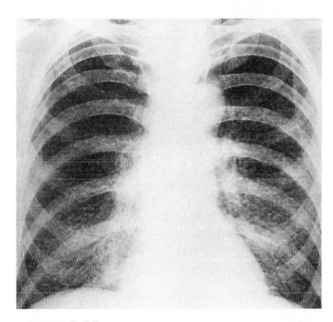

FIGURE **3-33** Silicosis. Calcification in miliary nodules is scattered throughout both lungs.

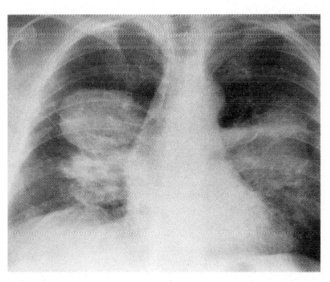

FIGURE **3-34** Progressive massive fibrosis in silicosis. Large, irregular nodules can be seen in both perihilar regions.

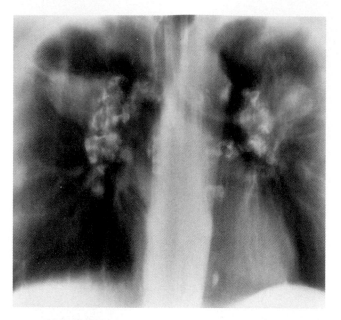

FIGURE 3-35 Silicosis. Chest tomogram demonstrates the characteristic eggshell lymph node calcification associated with bilateral perihilar masses.

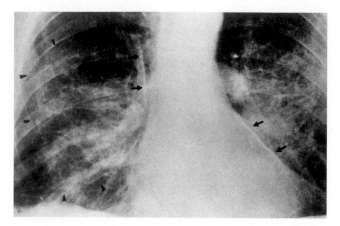

FIGURE 3-36 Asbestosis. Frontal film shows en face pleural calcifications on right (*arrowheads*), linear calcifications in profile in mediastinal reflection of pleura on right and in pericardium on left (*horizontal arrows*), and linear calcification in left diaphragmatic pleura (*vertical arrowhead*).

plasterboard and ceiling panels containing asbestos were reconstructed, removing the asbestos to prevent excessive public exposure to this particulate. Asbestos particles occur as long, thin fibers that cause little dust, but produce major fibrosis in the lung. The disease presents as alveolitis, with asbestos deposits at the bifurcation of the alveolar ducts. These deposits activate the fibrogenic and growth factors and result in extensive fibrosis. The major complication of asbestosis is mesothelioma, a highly malignant pleural tumor.

Radiographic Appearance

The radiographic hallmark of asbestosis is involvement of the pleura. Initially, pleural thickening appears as linear plaques of opacification, which are most often along the lower chest wall and diaphragm. Calcification of the pleural plaques is virtually pathognomonic of asbestosis, especially when the calcified plaques appear in the form of thin, curvilinear densities conforming to the upper surfaces of the diaphragm bilaterally (Figure 3-36). This pleural calcification generally does not develop until at least 20 years after the first exposure to asbestos (Figure 3-37). High-resolution CT best demonstrates the developing pleural plaques.

In the lungs, round or irregular opacities produce a combined linear and nodular pattern that may obscure the heart border, producing the so-called shaggy heart. Pleural mesothelioma appears as an irregular scalloped or nodular density within the

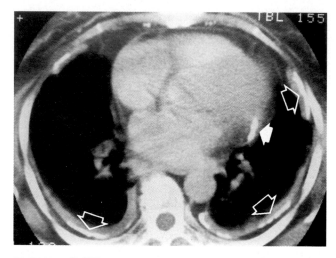

FIGURE 3-37 Asbestosis. CT scan shows calcified pleural plaques along lateral and posterior chest wall (*open arrows*) and adjacent to heart (*solid arrow*).

pleural space. It is frequently associated with a large pleural effusion that may obscure the underlying tumor. CT demonstrates the precise tumor involvement of the lung tissue. In addition to mesothelioma, bronchogenic carcinoma is also unusually common in patients with asbestosis, especially those who are cigarette smokers.

Anthracosis (Coal Worker's Pneumoniosis)

Coal miners, especially those working with anthracite (hard coal), have increased susceptibility to developing pneumoconiosis by inhaling high concentrations of coal dust. Anthracite collects in the walls of the respiratory bronchioles, causing weakened

SUMMARY of FINDINGS for Pneumoconiosis

disorder	location	radiographic appearance	treatment
Silicosis	Most often upper lobes Lung parenchyma	Multiple, well-defined, scattered nodules of uniform density	For all cases of pneumoconiosis: Prevent further exposure Breath clean air Treat complications
Asbestosis	Pleural lining	Pleural thickening with calcified plaques	
Anthracosis	Throughout lungs	Multiple less well-defined nodules of granular density	

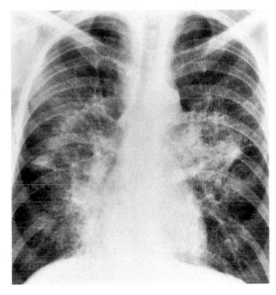

FIGURE 3-38 Coal worker's pneumoconiosis. Diffuse reticular pattern throughout both lungs is associated with ill-defined masses of fibrous tissue in the perihilar region that extend to the right base.

musculature and dilatation. The deposition of anthracite particles changes the lung tissue to a dark color, leading to the term black lung.

Radiographic Appearance

Initially, multiple small, irregular opacities produce a reticular pattern similar to that of silicosis (Figure 3-38). However, the nodules tend to be somewhat less well defined than those of silicosis, and they tend to have a granular density unlike the homogeneous density of silicosis nodules. With advanced disease, the pattern of progressive massive fibrosis can develop. In progressive massive fibrosis, one or more masses of fibrous tissue with smooth, well-defined lateral borders gradually migrate toward the hilum, leaving a zone of hyperinflated emphysematous lung between the fibrous mass and the chest wall. A single large homogeneous mass in the perihilar area of one lung may simulate bronchogenic carcinoma; an occupational history is necessary to make the proper diagnosis of pneumoconiosis.

Treatment

Today, there is no effective treatment for pneumoconiosis. Once the particles have embedded in the pulmonary tissue, the lungs deteriorate and lose the ability to remove them. The best available treatment is simply to avoid further exposure. Breathing clean air may assist in halting progression of the disease and reducing the severity of the symptoms. Treatment is limited to addressing complications of the disease. Patients who progress from asbestosis to mesothelioma may require lung resection to remove the cancerous tissue, radiation therapy to shrink the tumor, or chemotherapy.

Neoplasms

Solitary Pulmonary Nodule

The asymptomatic solitary pulmonary nodule seen as an incidental finding on a screening chest radiograph poses a diagnostic dilemma because it could represent a benign granuloma or neoplastic process, a primary bronchogenic carcinoma, or a solitary metastasis. In persons under the age of 30, a small, round, sharply defined solitary pulmonary nodule is associated with a minimal risk of cancer (less than 1%). However, this risk rises to about 15% in individuals between the ages of 30 and 45, and to approximately 50% in those older than age 50.

Radiographic Appearance

The presence of central dense or popcorn calcification is diagnostic of a benign process, and a low kVp technique may be required to demonstrate the calcification to best advantage (Figure 3-39). Another characteristic of a benign tumor is the absence of growth of the lesion on serial chest films over 2 years (therefore comparison films must be eagerly sought).

A CT scan can demonstrate the size, density, position, and borders of the lesion, which helps determine the diagnosis. Although malignant tumors generally have ill-defined, irregular, or fuzzy borders

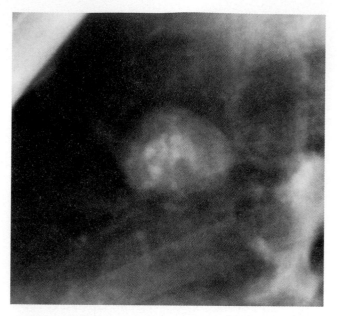

FIGURE 3-39 Benign solitary pulmonary nodule (tuberculoma). Notice central calcification characteristic of this benign lesion.

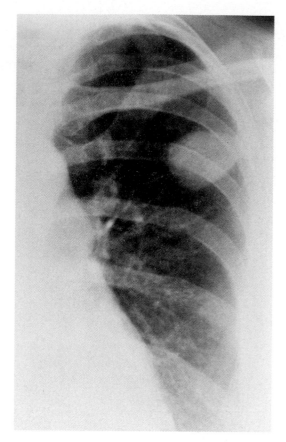

FIGURE 3-41 Benign solitary pulmonary nodule (tuberculoma). Notice sharp, well-defined borders of this left upper lobe mass.

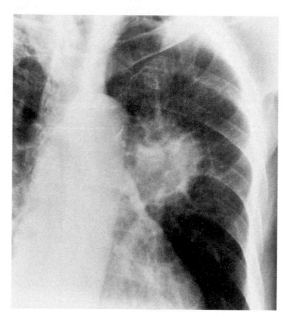

FIGURE 3-40 Malignant solitary pulmonary nodule (bronchogenic carcinoma). Notice fuzzy, ill-defined margins.

(Figure 3-40) in contrast to the sharp margins of benign lesions (Figure 3-41), there are many exceptions to this rule. CT may best differentiate the smooth, sharp margins of a benign tumor (Figure 3-42) from the spiculated, ill-defined contour of a malignant nodule (Figure 3-43). The growth rate (or doubling time) of a solitary pulmonary nodule has been used to determine the likelihood of its being malignant. A pulmonary nodule that doubles in volume in less than 1 month or more than

18 months is usually benign. However, the overlapping of growth rates of benign and malignant lesions, particularly among rapidly growing nodules, makes the use of doubling time unreliable as an absolute indicator of malignancy. In the patient older than 35 to 40 years of age, a solitary pulmonary nodule should be resected unless it can be unequivocally demonstrated to be benign. If the diagnosis is equivocal, CT is required. This modality may demonstrate additional nodules not visible on plain chest radiography (suggesting metastases), or it may detect hilar or mediastinal metastases (indicating a malignant process). Positron emission tomography (PET) may be employed to show increased metabolic activity of the lesion suggestive of malignancy (Figure 3-44). At times, percutaneous fine-needle aspiration biopsy (FNAB) may be required to provide a definitive diagnosis (Figure 3-45).

Bronchial Adenoma

Bronchial adenomas are neoplasms of low-grade malignancy that constitute about 1% of all bronchial neoplasms. They are equally common in men and women. Bronchial adenomas appear in a younger age

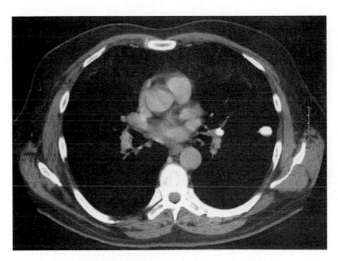

FIGURE 3-42 Benign solitary pulmonary nodule (granuloma). CT scan demonstrates a discrete homogeneous lobulated mass in the left lung periphery.

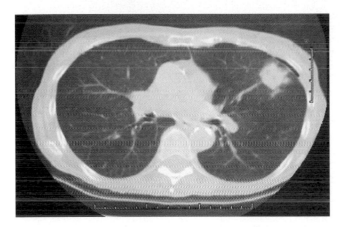

FIGURE 3-43 Malignant solitary pulmonary nodule (adenocarcinoma). CT scan demonstrates spiculated mass with ill-defined contour.

group than bronchogenic carcinoma. Hemoptysis and recurring pneumonia are the most common symptoms. They arise in the same glandular structures in the bronchi in which malignant neoplasms develop.

Radiographic Appearance

About 80% of bronchial adenomas occur centrally in major or segmental bronchi and cause obstruction. The most common radiographic findings are peripheral atelectasis and pneumonitis due to bronchial obstruction. This characteristically produces a homogeneous increase in density corresponding exactly to a lobe or one or more segments, usually with a substantial loss of volume. If large enough, a central bronchial adenoma causing peripheral atelectasis and pneumonia may be identifiable as a discrete, lobulated, soft tissue mass. A tumor too small to obstruct the lumen may

not be detectable on the chest radiograph. Tomography may demonstrate the rounded tumor mass within an air-filled bronchus (Figure 3-46). Peripheral bronchial adenomas do not cause bronchial obstruction and appear as nonspecific solitary pulmonary nodules (Figure 3-47).

Bronchogenic Carcinoma

Primary carcinoma of the lung arises from the mucosa of the bronchial tree. The most common primary malignant lung neoplasm is bronchogenic carcinoma. Although its precise cause remains unknown, bronchogenic carcinoma has been closely linked to smoking and to the inhalation of cancer-causing agents (carcinogens), such as air pollution, exhaust gases, and industrial fumes. A major form of bronchogenic carcinoma is the solitary pulmonary nodule within the lung parenchyma.

The most common type of lung cancer is **squamous carcinoma**, which typically arises in the major central bronchi and causes gradual narrowing of the bronchial lumen. **Adenocarcinomas** usually arise in the periphery of the lung rather than in the larger central bronchi. The least common type of lung tumor is **bronchiolar (alveolar cell) carcinoma**. Non–small cell lung cancers (i.e., the three types of lung cancer just listed) make up 80% of all lung cancers. **Small cell (oat cell) carcinomas** characteristically cause bulky enlargement of hilar lymph nodes, often bilaterally, and are responsible for the remaining 20% of primary pulmonary malignancies.

Although bronchogenic carcinoma may be diagnosed by detection of cancer cells in the sputum, a precise diagnosis usually requires biopsy of the tumor during bronchoscopy (i.e., direct visualization of the tracheobronchial tree using a tube inserted through the nose) or a needle biopsy in the radiology department under CT or fluoroscopic guidance.

Radiographic Appearance

Bronchogenic carcinoma produces a broad spectrum of radiographic abnormalities that depend on the site of the tumor and its relationship to the bronchial tree. The tumor may appear as a discrete mass, or it may be undetectable and identified only by virtue of secondary changes resulting from an obstruction caused by the tumor within or compressing the bronchus.

Airway obstruction by bronchogenic carcinoma may cause atelectasis of a segment of lung and often leads to pneumonia that develops in the lung distal to the obstructed bronchus. An important radiographic sign differentiating this postobstructive pneumonia from simple inflammatory disease is the absence of an air bronchogram in the former. The air bronchogram

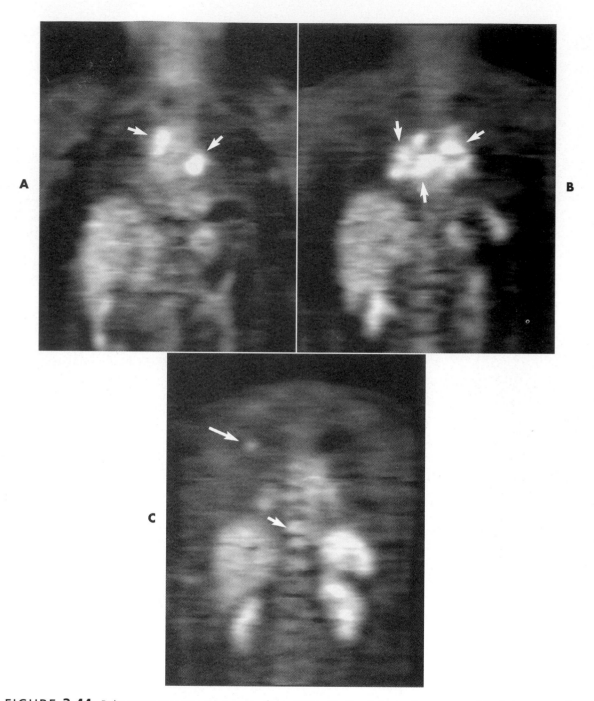

FIGURE 3-44 Pulmonary metastases. Images from PET with fluorodeoxyglucose reveal foci demonstrating metastases. **A,** Intense radionuclide-labeled foci in each perihilar region. **B,** The posterior mediastinal focus was identified in conjunction with additional bilateral perihilar radionuclide-labeled foci. **C,** The thoracic vertebral radionuclide-labeled foci were identified in conjunction with a posterior right upper lobe focus that demonstrated a positive finding, noted by arrows on each image. PET confirmed the presence of metastasis; the patient was referred to the medical oncologist for consideration of chemotherapy.

can be detected only if there is an open airway leading to the area of consolidation.

Unilateral enlargement of the hilum, best appreciated on serial chest radiographs, may be the earliest sign of bronchogenic carcinoma. The enlarged hilum represents either a primary carcinoma arising in the major hilar bronchus or metastases to enlarged pulmonary lymph nodes from a small primary lesion elsewhere in the lung (Figure 3-48). CT is far superior to plain radiographs in detecting hilar and mediastinal lymphadenopathy and bronchial narrowing resulting from bronchogenic carcinoma.

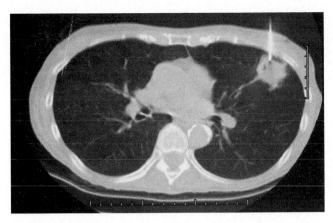

FIGURE **3-45** CT-guided FNAB of peripheral lung nodule in left lower lobe. CT scan demonstrates the needle position. Cells were sent for cytologic testing, and the results indicated infiltrating, poorly differentiated adenocarcinoma.

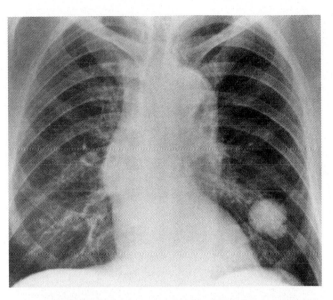

FIGURE **3-47** Peripheral bronchial adenoma. Nonspecific solitary pulmonary nodule at the left base.

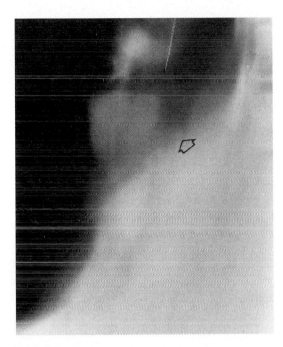

FIGURE **3-46** Central bronchial adenoma. Tomogram shows ill-defined mass causing high-grade obstruction of right lower lobe bronchus *(arrow)*.

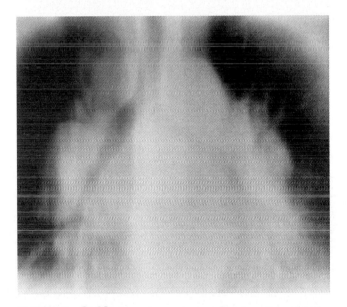

FIGURE **3-48** Bronchogenic carcinoma. Tomography demonstrates bilateral bulky hilar adenopathy typical of oat cell carcinoma.

Treatment of Pulmonary Neoplastic Diseases

For **bronchial adenomas**, the most common treatment involves surgical resection of the lobe.

The prognosis for **bronchogenic carcinoma** is poor, except when the tumor is in the form of a solitary pulmonary nodule that can be surgically removed. Direct lymphatic spread of a tumor can cause enlargement of hilar or mediastinal lymph nodes (Figure 3-50). Distant metastases most frequently involve the bones, where they cause osteolytic destruction. Metastases to the liver, brain, and adrenal glands commonly develop.

Cavitation commonly occurs in bronchogenic carcinoma. It most often involves upper lung lesions and represents central necrosis of the neoplasm. The cavities usually resemble acute lung abscesses and have thick walls with irregular, often nodular, inner surfaces (Figure 3-49).

Bronchiolar (alveolar cell) carcinoma has a spectrum of appearances, which can vary from a well-circumscribed, peripheral solitary nodule to a poorly defined mass simulating pneumonia or multiple nodules scattered throughout both lungs.

Squamous carcinoma, adenocarcinoma, and **bronchioalveolar carcinoma** grow more slowly than small cell carcinomas. Surgical resection has a cure rate of about 10%. Radiation therapy (which has a low cure rate) and chemotherapy are generally used for palliative treatment.

Pulmonary Metastases

Up to one third of patients with cancer develop pulmonary metastases; in about half of these patients, the only demonstrable metastases are confined to the lungs. Pulmonary metastases may develop from hematogenous or lymphatic spread, most commonly from musculoskeletal sarcomas, myeloma, and carcinomas of the breast, urogenital tract, thyroid, and colon. Carcinomas of the breast, esophagus, or stomach may directly extend to involve the lungs because of anatomic proximity. Primary lung lesions may metastasize by spread through the bronchial tree.

Radiographic Appearance

Hematogenous metastases typically appear radiographically as multiple, relatively well-circumscribed, round or oval nodules throughout the lungs (Figure 3-51). The pattern may vary from fine miliary nodules (Figure 3-52) produced by highly vascular tumors (e.g., kidney or thyroid gland carcinomas, sarcoma of bone, and trophoblastic disease) to huge, well-defined masses (cannonball lesions) caused by metastatic sarcomas. Carcinoma of the thyroid gland typically causes a snowstorm of metastatic deposits yet radiographically remains unchanged for a prolonged period because of a very low grade of malignancy.

Solitary metastases, which occur in about 25% of cases, may be indistinguishable from primary bronchogenic carcinomas or benign granulomas (Figure 3-53). In such cases, CT may permit the detection of additional pulmonary masses that cannot be seen on standard chest radiographs but aid in determining the choice of treatment. The emerging technology of PET scanning, which images cellular activity, has been used in the search for

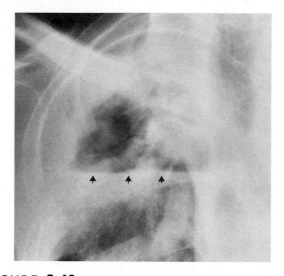

FIGURE 3-49 Bronchogenic carcinoma. Large cavitary right upper lobe mass with air-fluid level *(arrows)* and associated rib destruction.

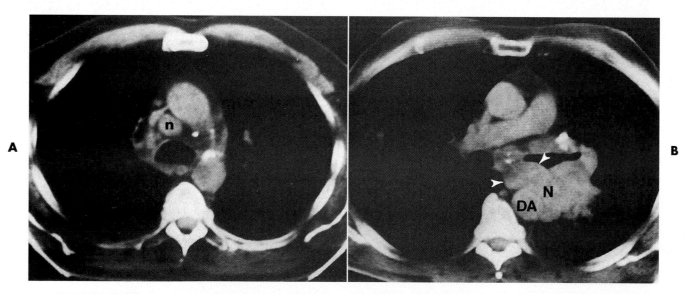

FIGURE 3-50 Spread of bronchogenic carcinoma to mediastinum. **A,** CT scan shows enlarged lymph node *(n)* in pretracheal region, a finding consistent with the diagnosis of unresectable mediastinal spread. **B,** In another patient, CT scan shows obliteration of fat plane around descending aorta *(DA)* by adjacent neoplasm *(N)*. In addition, tumor extends deep into the mediastinum *(arrowheads)* behind the left mainstem bronchus and in front of the descending aorta.

SUMMARY of FINDINGS for Pulmonary Neoplasms

disorder	location	radiographic appearance	treatment
Solitary pulmonary nodule	Throughout lungs	Solitary nodule Dense or popcorn calcification—benign Continued growth—malignancy	Depends on diagnosis (benign or malignant)
Bronchial adenoma	Glandular structure of major/segmental bronchi	Peripheral atelectasis (obstruction) Obstructive pneumonia	Surgical resection
Bronchogenic carcinoma	Lung parenchyma	Solitary lesion, ill-defined Atelectasis with obstruction Hilar enlargement Cavitation in upper lung	Surgical resection (cure) Radiation therapy (cure and palliative) Chemotherapy (palliative)
Pulmonary metastases	Throughout lungs	Multiple nodules, sharp margins Miliary/snowstorm nodules Solitary nodule Coarsened interstitial markings	All treatments palliative Surgical resection Radiation therapy Chemotherapy

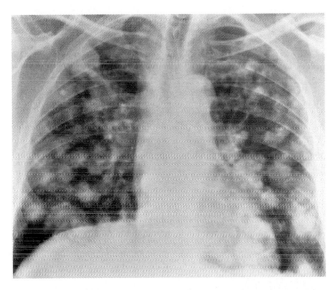

FIGURE 3-51 Hematogenous metastases. Multiple, well-circumscribed nodules scattered diffusely throughout both lungs.

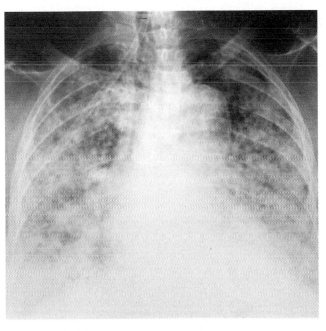

FIGURE 3-52 Metastatic thyroid carcinoma. Multiple fine miliary nodules throughout both lungs.

metastases when CT is inconclusive, as well as in determining whether a solitary pulmonary nodule is benign (when PET detects low cellular activity) or malignant (when PET detects high cellular activity) (Figure 3-54). Lymphangitic metastatic spread throughout the lungs is most commonly a complication of carcinoma of the breast, stomach, thyroid, pancreas, larynx, cervix, or prostate. The radiographic appearance consists of coarsened interstitial markings that have an irregular contour and are poorly defined (Figure 3-55). These coarsened markings are most prominent in the lower lobes and may simulate interstitial pulmonary edema.

Treatment

The treatment of pulmonary metastases includes surgical resection, radiation therapy, and chemotherapy; however, these serve only a palliative purpose.

Vascular Diseases

Pulmonary Embolism

Pulmonary embolism, a potentially fatal condition, is by far the most common pathologic process involving the lungs of hospitalized patients. In about

80% of patients with this disorder, the condition does not cause symptoms and thus remains unrecognized because the emboli are too small or too few to occlude blood flow to a substantial portion of the lung. Even when symptomatic, pulmonary embolism may be difficult to diagnose. More than 95% of pulmonary emboli arise from thrombi that develop in the deep venous system of the lower extremities because of venous stasis. The remainder come from thrombi that occur in the right side of the heart or in brachial or cervical veins and are trapped by the capillaries in the pulmonary artery circulation. Thrombi originating in the left side of the heart can embolize to the peripheral systemic arterial circulation, where they are trapped in the arterioles or capillaries before they can return in the venous blood to the heart and the pulmonary circulation. Most embolic occlusions occur in the lower lobes because of the preferential blood flow to these regions.

The physiologic consequences of embolic occlusion of the pulmonary arteries depend on the size of the embolic mass and the general state of the pulmonary circulation. In young persons with good cardiovascular function and adequate collateral circulation, the occlusion of a large central vessel may cause minimal, if any, functional impairment. In contrast, in patients with cardiovascular disease or severe debilitating illnesses, pulmonary vascular occlusion often leads to infarction.

Radiographic Appearance

For most patients with thromboembolism without infarction, the findings on the chest radiograph are normal. Nevertheless, some subtle yet distinctive abnormalities on plain radiographs can be strongly suggestive of this diagnosis. A large-vessel pulmonary embolism causes a focal reduction in blood volume without a substantial change in air or tissue volume. This leads to focal pulmonary oligemia and relative lucency of the involved portion of lung. Another sign of pulmonary embolism is enlargement of the ipsilateral main pulmonary artery caused by distention of the vessel by the bulk of the thrombus. Serial radiographs may demonstrate progressive enlargement of the affected vessel.

Pulmonary embolism with infarction appears radiographically as an area of lung consolidation. A highly characteristic, though somewhat uncommon, appearance of pulmonary infarction is the so-called Hampton's hump (Figure 3-56). This pleura-based, wedge-shaped density has a rounded apex and is most commonly seen at the base of the lung, often in the costophrenic sulcus. In many instances an infarction merely produces a nonspecific parenchymal density that simulates acute pneumonia. A pleural effusion often develops (Figure 3-57).

Because the findings on the chest radiograph are usually either normal or nonspecific, the radionuclide lung scan (or ventilation-perfusion ratio [V/Q] scan) is generally considered the most effective screening procedure for significant pulmonary embolism. On a radionuclide

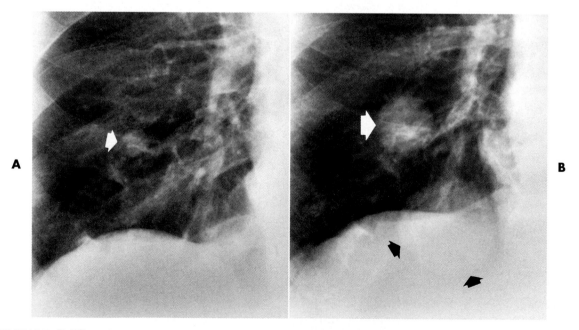

FIGURE 3-53 Pulmonary metastases. **A,** Solitary metastasis *(arrow).* **B,** Repeat examination 5 months later shows rapid growth of previous solitary nodule *(white arrow).* Second huge nodule *(black arrows)* was not appreciated on previous examination because it projected below the right hemidiaphragm.

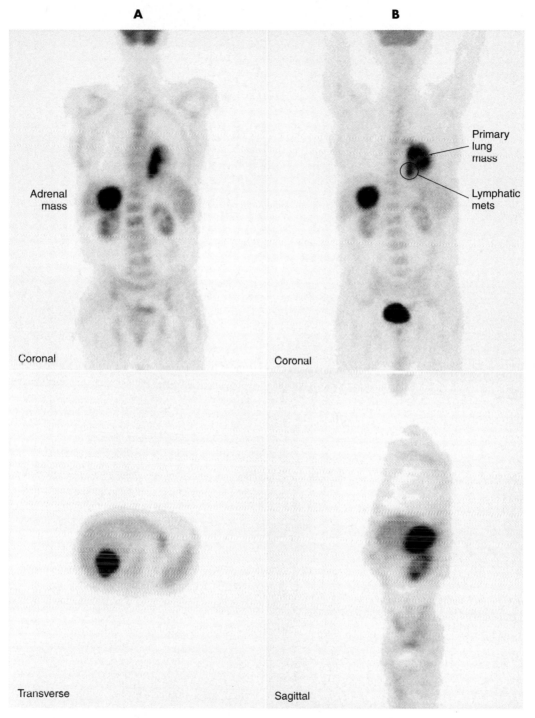

A

B

Adrenal
mass

Coronal

Transverse

Primary
lung
mass

Lymphatic
mets

Coronal

Sagittal

FIGURE 3-54 Non–small cell carcinoma. PET lung scan performed for initial staging. Following the injection of fluorodeoxyglucose, metabolically active metastases are suggested in the left hilum with lymphatic involvement **(B)** and in the right adrenal gland with hepatic involvement **(A)**.

perfusion scan that measures blood flow to the lungs, the area of lung distal to an embolus appears as a defect (Figure 3-58). Unfortunately, false-positive scan results may be recorded in portions of the lung that are poorly perfused because of impaired ventilation, even if no obstructing vascular lesion is present. Therefore ventilation lung scans are also performed to increase the diagnostic accuracy. The results of the ventilation scan are usually relatively normal in patients with pulmonary embolism, whereas they generally demonstrate defects corresponding to areas of decreased perfusion in patients with chronic pulmonary disease.

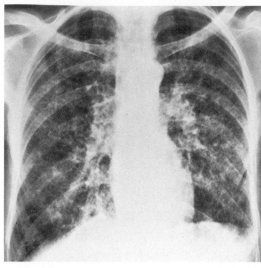

FIGURE 3-55 Lymphangitic metastases. Coarsened bronchovascular markings of irregular contour and poor definition are seen on the chest radiograph in this patient with metastatic carcinoma of stomach.

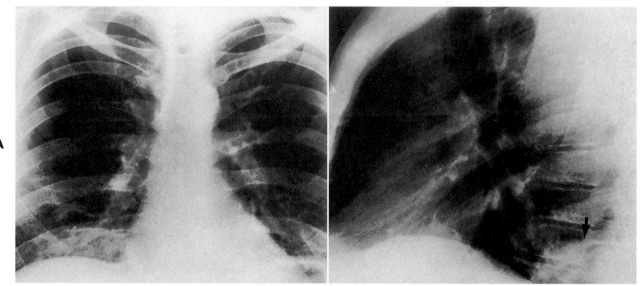

FIGURE 3-56 Pulmonary embolism. Frontal **(A)** and lateral **(B)** projections of the chest demonstrate fairly well-circumscribed shadow of homogeneous density occupying the posterior segment of the right lower lobe. On lateral projection, the pleural-based density has the shape of a truncated cone and is convex toward the hilum (Hampton's hump; *arrow*).

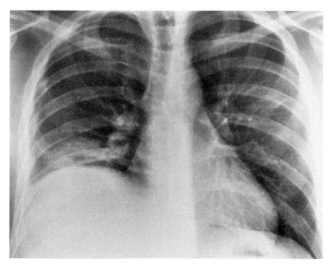

FIGURE 3-57 Pulmonary embolism. Plain chest radiograph demonstrates atelectasis at the right base; this is associated with elevation of the right hemidiaphragm and represents a large subpulmonic effusion.

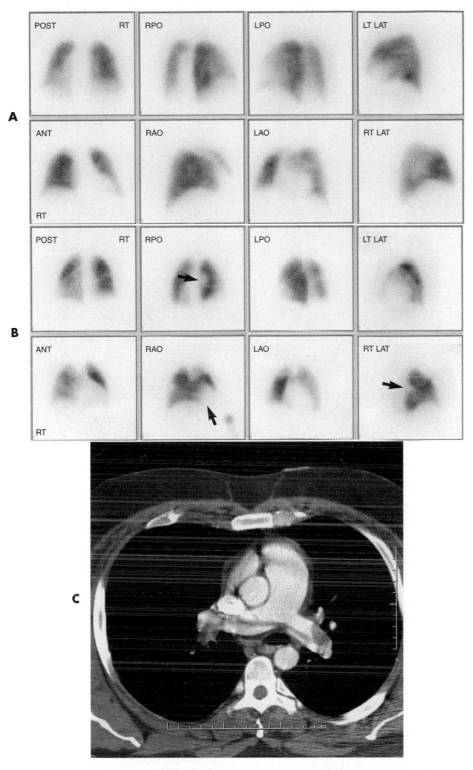

FIGURE 3-58 Pulmonary embolism. **A,** Normal radionuclide perfusion lung scan with uniform uptake in both lungs. **B,** A different patient with multiple wedge-shaped areas without isotope uptake *(arrows)*. **C,** CT scan (correlating with lung scan in **B**) demonstrates pulmonary emboli in both right and left pulmonary arteries. Note that the emboli are connected—a "saddle" embolus.

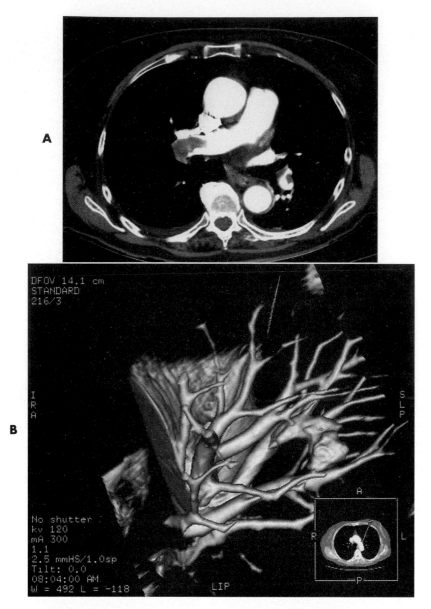

FIGURE 3-59 Pulmonary embolism. A filling defect of the right pulmonary artery demonstrated on a high-resolution spiral CT scan **(A)**. Using 3D-volume rendering, CT can visualize a smaller pulmonary embolus **(B)**.

High-resolution CT has now replaced lung scanning in many institutions as the preferred imaging modality for detecting and excluding pulmonary emboli. Following the injection of a contrast agent, cross-sectional images of the lung are obtained from the base of the heart to the top of the aortic arch. CT demonstrates pulmonary embolus either as a filling defect within the pulmonary artery (Figure 3-59) or as an abrupt cutoff indicating complete obstruction of a pulmonary vessel (Figure 3-60).

Pulmonary arteriography is the definitive technique for evaluating the patient with suspected pulmonary embolism (Figure 3-61). However, this invasive procedure carries a small but definite risk of morbidity and mortality. The unequivocal arteriographic diagnosis of pulmonary embolism requires the demonstration of an abrupt occlusion (cutoff) of a pulmonary artery or a persistent intraluminal filling defect within it. More recently, magnetic resonance imaging has been used to show a pulmonary embolus either as a moderate- to high-intensity signal within the black flow void of the normal pulmonary artery or as a generalized increased signal intensity caused by slow blood flow in an obstructed pulmonary vessel.

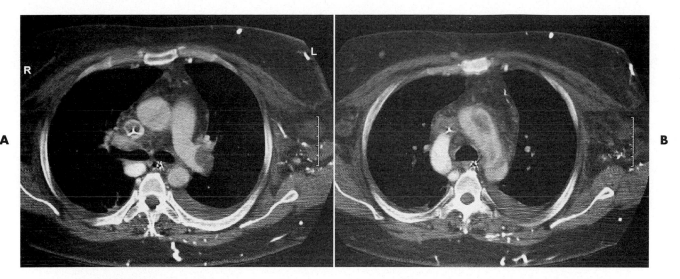

FIGURE 3-60 Pulmonary embolism. **A,** CT scan illustrates a filling defect in the left main pulmonary artery on a 41-year-old woman. **B,** The patient also has a thrombus located in the ascending aorta and aortic arch.

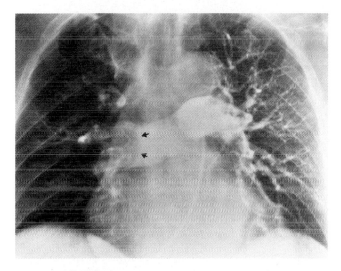

FIGURE 3-61 Pulmonary arteriogram shows virtually complete obstruction *(arrows)* of the right pulmonary artery.

Treatment

The first line of treatment is anticoagulant therapy, which limits the extent of infarction of the affected lung tissue and decreases the likelihood of more emboli to the lung. The patient may be required to take the anticoagulants for an extended period. If the patient does not respond to anticoagulant therapy, thrombolytics can assist in dissolving the emboli. In patients with large clot burdens, thrombolytic therapy may be the first line of treatment. The most invasive treatment is the placement of a filter in the vena cava, which is indicated if the anticoagulant or thrombolytic therapy is contraindicated or ineffective.

Septic Embolism

Septic embolism refers to a shower of bacteria that enter the pulmonary circulation and remain trapped within the lung. Septic emboli arise primarily from either the heart (bacterial endocarditis) or the peripheral veins (septic thrombophlebitis). Many patients have a clinical history of intravenous drug abuse.

Radiographic Appearance

Septic emboli, almost always multiple, appear radiographically as ill-defined, round or wedge-shaped opacities in the periphery of the lung. They often present a migratory pattern, first appearing in one area and then in another as the older lesions resolve. Cavitation frequently develops (Figure 3-62).

Treatment

Patients with septic embolism require regimented doses of antibiotics to destroy the underlying bacterial infection.

Pulmonary Arteriovenous Fistula

Pulmonary arteriovenous fistula is an abnormal vascular communication from a pulmonary artery to a pulmonary vein. Pulmonary arteriovenous fistulas are multiple in about one third of patients; up to two thirds of patients with these pulmonary malformations have similar arteriovenous communications elsewhere (hereditary hemorrhagic telangiectasia). Very large or multiple fistulas can cause so much shunting of blood from the pulmonary arteries to the pulmonary veins that the blood cannot be adequately oxygenated and cyanosis results.

SUMMARY of FINDINGS for Pulmonary Vascular Diseases

disorder	location	radiographic appearance	treatment
Pulmonary embolism	Most often lower lobes	Serial films demonstrating progressive enlargement of the affected vessel	Anticoagulants Thrombolytics Vena cava filter placement
Septic embolism	Lung periphery	Peripheral opacities	Regimented antibiotics until bacterial infection eradicated
Pulmonary arteriovenous fistula	Most often lower lobes	Defined soft tissue mass	Surgical removal Embolization

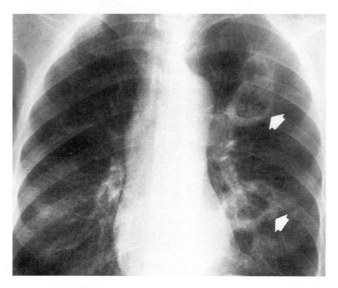

FIGURE 3-62 Septic pulmonary emboli. Large cavitary lesions *(arrows)* in the left lung of an intravenous drug abuser with septic thrombophlebitis.

Radiographic Appearance

A pulmonary arteriovenous fistula typically appears as a round or oval, lobulated soft tissue mass that is most commonly situated in the lower lobes. A pathognomonic finding is a feeding artery and a draining vein (Figure 3-63, *A*). This may be difficult to demonstrate on plain radiographs and often requires tomography or angiography (Figure 3-63, *B*).

Treatment

Before surgical removal, a pulmonary angiogram can confirm the diagnosis and detect smaller, unsuspected vascular malformations that cannot be identified on routine radiographs. Another treatment for arteriovenous fistula is the placement of a detachable balloon (embolization) to block the flow of blood through the fistulous connection.

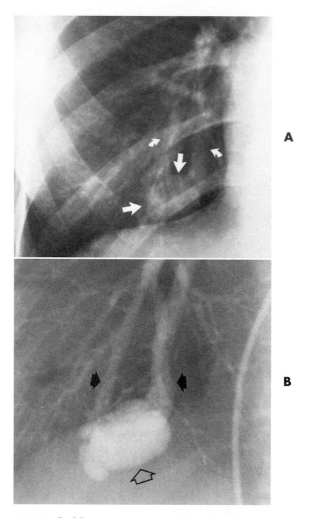

FIGURE 3-63 Pulmonary arteriovenous fistula. **A,** Radiographic film of right lung shows round soft tissue mass *(straight arrows)* at the base. Feeding and draining vessels *(curved arrows)* extend to the lesion. **B,** Arteriogram clearly shows feeding artery and draining veins *(solid arrows)* associated with arteriovenous malformation *(open arrow)*.

Miscellaneous Lung Disorders

Atelectasis

Atelectasis refers to a condition in which there is diminished air within the lung associated with reduced lung volume. Most commonly this results from bronchial obstruction, which may be attributable to a neoplasm, foreign body (e.g., peanut, coin, or tooth), or mucous plug. Mucoid obstruction may be attributable to an excessive secretion in patients with chronic bronchitis, or it may be a complication of abdominal surgery. As a result of surgery, mucus collects in the bronchi because of the irritative effect of anesthesia. Normal coughing, which would mobilize the secretions, is decreased because of the pain of the abdominal wound. Compression of the lung by pneumothorax, pleural fluid, a tumor, a lung abscess, or a large emphysematous bulla may result in atelectasis. Regardless of the precise cause, air cannot enter that part of the lung supplied by the obstructed bronchus. As the air trapped in the lung is absorbed into the bloodstream, the lung collapses.

An important iatrogenic cause of atelectasis is the improper placement of an endotracheal tube below the level of the tracheal bifurcation. Because of geometric factors, the endotracheal tube tends to enter the right mainstem bronchus, effectively blocking the left bronchial tree and causing collapse of part or all of the left lung (Figure 3-64).

Radiographic Appearance

The most common radiographic sign of atelectasis is a local increase in density caused by the airless lung, which may vary from thin plate-like streaks (Figure 3-65) to lobar collapse (Figure 3-66). An important direct sign of atelectasis is displacement of interlobar fissures, which shift and become bowed, conforming to the contour of the collapsed segment. Indirect signs of atelectasis reflect an attempt by the remaining lung to compensate for the loss of the collapsed portion. These signs include elevation of the ipsilateral hemidiaphragm; displacement of the heart, mediastinum, and hilum toward the atelectatic segment; and compensatory overinflation of the remainder of the ipsilateral lung.

Treatment

The goal of the treatment of atelectasis is the removal of pulmonary secretions and reexpansion of the affected lung tissue. To accomplish this, positioning or incentive spirometry (measurement of air capacity in the lungs) is employed. Positioning uses gravity to assist in expanding the affected lung tissue, and incentive spirometry directly increases lung volume by positive pressure.

Adult Respiratory Distress Syndrome

The term **adult respiratory distress syndrome (ARDS)** describes a clinical picture of severe, unexpected, and life-threatening acute respiratory distress that develops in patients who have a variety of medical and surgical disorders but no major underlying lung disease. As it occurs most commonly in patients with nonthoracic trauma who develop hypotension and shock, it is often called "shock lung." Other conditions that may lead to ARDS include severe pulmonary infection, aspiration or inhalation of toxins and irritants, and drug overdose. Regardless of

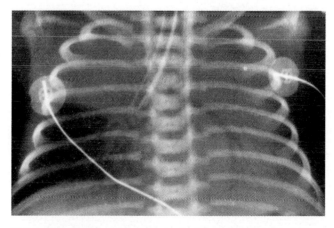

FIGURE 3-64 Malpositioned endotracheal tube. Excessively low position of endotracheal tube in the bronchus intermedius causes collapse of right upper lobe and entire left lung.

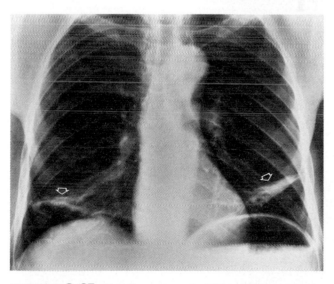

FIGURE 3-65 Platelike atelectasis. Horizontal linear streaks of opacity (arrows) can be seen in lower portions of both lungs.

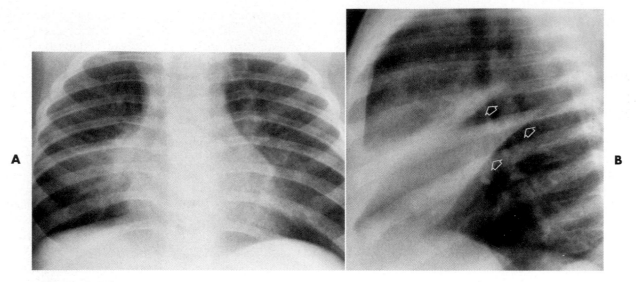

FIGURE 3-66 Right middle lobe and lingular collapse. **A,** Frontal chest radiograph demonstrates obliteration of right and left borders of the heart. **B,** Lateral projection demonstrates collapse of right middle lobe and lingula *(arrows).*

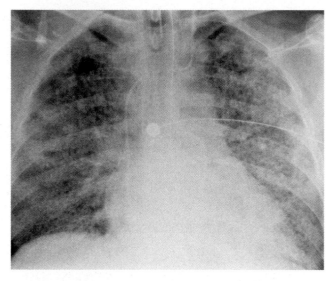

FIGURE 3-67 ARDS. Ill-defined areas of alveolar consolidation scattered throughout the lungs.

the cause, the structure of the lung completely breaks down, leading to massive leakage of cells and fluid into the interstitial and alveolar spaces. The structural breakdown results in severe hypoxemia caused by a pronounced respiratory impairment in the ability to oxygenate blood.

Radiographic Appearance

Patchy, ill-defined areas of alveolar consolidation are scattered throughout both lungs (Figure 3-67). Unlike pulmonary edema caused by heart failure, in ARDS the size of the heart usually remains normal, and there is no evidence of redistribution of blood flow to the upper zones.

Treatment

The hypoxemia in ARDS may be fatal, even with intensive medical therapy. Drug treatment may consist of diuretics to decrease the fluid load and possible fluid buildup in the lung tissue. Oxygen therapy and ventilation may assist the patient in breathing, which helps prevent further capillary and alveolar destruction. Continuous positive-pressure ventilation may cause air to enter the interstitium of the lung and lead to pneumothorax and pneumomediastinum. Diffuse interstitial and patchy air-space fibrosis may produce a coarse reticular pattern. If the patient recovers completely, the radiographic abnormalities may clear completely, and there may be only a mild decrease in pulmonary function.

Intrabronchial Foreign Bodies

The aspiration of solid foreign bodies into the tracheobronchial tree occurs almost exclusively in young children. Although some foreign bodies are radiopaque and easily detected on plain chest radiographs, most aspirated foreign bodies are not opaque and can be diagnosed only by observation of secondary signs in the lungs caused by partial or complete bronchial obstruction. Obstruction almost always involves the lower lobes, the right more often than the left.

Radiographic Appearance

The complete obstruction of a major bronchus leads to resorption of trapped air, alveolar collapse, and atelectasis of the involved segment or lobe. Extensive volume loss causes a shift of the heart and mediastinal structures toward the affected side along with

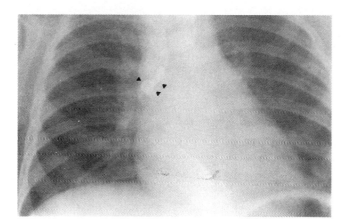

FIGURE 3-68 Intrabronchial foreign body. A nail *(arrows)* lies in the right mainstem bronchus.

elevation of the ipsilateral hemidiaphragm and narrowing of the intercostal spaces.

Partial bronchial obstruction may produce air trapping as a result of a check-valve phenomenon. Air freely passes the partial obstruction during inspiration, but remains trapped distally as the bronchus contracts normally during expiration (Figure 3-68). Hyperaeration of the affected lobes causes a shift of the heart and mediastinum toward the normal, contralateral side. This finding is accentuated during forced expiration because the hyperaerated segment does not contract. This classic appearance of partial bronchial obstruction is dramatically demonstrated with fluoroscopy as the mediastinum shifts away from the affected side during deep expiration and returns toward the midline on full inspiration.

A malpositioned endotracheal tube can act as an intrabronchial foreign body. The tube tends to extend down the right mainstem bronchus, causing hyperlucency of the right lung and obstructive atelectasis of the left lung.

Treatment

The treatment of intrabronchial foreign bodies includes expectoration, intervention, and surgery. The simplest is expectoration, which requires the patient to cough hard enough to dislodge the foreign body and spit it out. More invasive interventional techniques employ a bronchoscope to retrieve the object blocking the airway. The most invasive procedure is direct surgical removal of the foreign body.

Mediastinal Emphysema (Pneumomediastinum)

Air within the mediastinal space may appear spontaneously, or it may result from chest trauma, from perforation of the esophagus or tracheobronchial

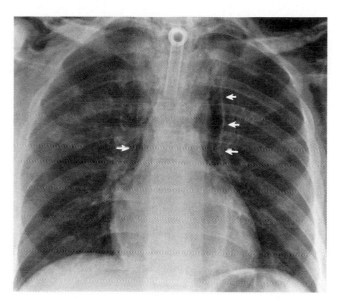

FIGURE 3-69 Mediastinal emphysema. Mediastinal pleura is displaced laterally and appears as a long linear opacity *(arrows)* parallel to the heart border but separated from it by gas.

tree, or from the spread of air along fascial planes in the neck, peritoneal cavity, or retroperitoneal space. Spontaneous pneumomediastinum usually results from a sudden rise in intraalveolar pressure (because of, for example, severe coughing, vomiting, or straining) that causes alveolar rupture and the dissection of air along blood vessels in the interstitial space to the hilum and mediastinum. Air may also extend peripherally and rupture into the pleural space, causing an associated pneumothorax.

Radiographic Appearance

On frontal chest radiographs, air causes lateral displacement of the mediastinal pleura, which appears as a long linear opacity that runs parallel to the heart border, but is separated from it by the air (i.e., the bronchovascular sheath) (Figure 3-69). On lateral projections, air is typically seen to have collected behind the sternum, extending in streaks downward and anterior to the heart. Chest radiographs may also demonstrate air outlining the pulmonary arterial trunk and aorta, and dissecting into the soft tissue of the neck.

In infants, mediastinal air causes elevation of the thymus. Loculated air confined to one side produces an appearance similar to that of a windblown sail. Bilateral mediastinal air elevates both thymic lobes to produce an angel-wings configuration (Figure 3-70).

Subcutaneous Emphysema

Subcutaneous emphysema is caused by penetrating or blunt injuries that disrupt the lung and parietal pleura and force air into the tissues of the chest wall.

SUMMARY of FINDINGS for Miscellaneous Lung Disorders

disorder	location	radiographic appearance	treatment
Atelactasis	Obstruction of segment/ lobe or lung collapse	Local increased density; platelike streaks	Positioning of patient Incentive spirometry
Acute respiratory distress syndrome	Lung structure breakdown	Patchy, ill-defined areas of consolidation	Diuretics to decrease fluid build up Oxygen therapy and ventilation
Intrabronchial foreign body	Lower lobes, most often right	Appears as atelectasis with possible shift	Removal of foreign body Expectoration, intervention, surgery
Mediastinal emphysema	Air in bronchovascular sheath	Radiolucency running parallel to heart border	If minimal, no treatment Surgical resection to prevent more air escape
Subcutaneous emphysema	Air in surrounding muscle bundles	Air streaks in muscle bundles	If minimal, no treatment Surgical resection to prevent more air escape

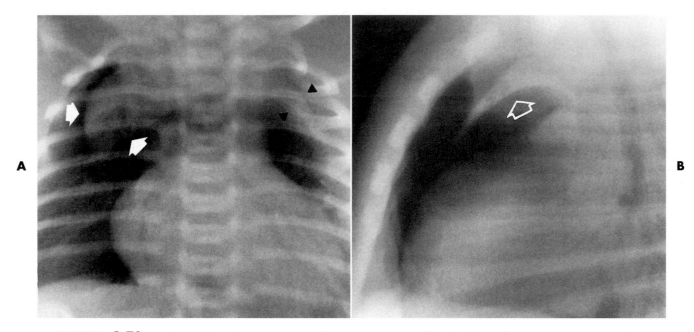

FIGURE 3-70 Mediastinal emphysema in an infant. **A,** Elevation of both lobes of thymus by mediastinal air *(arrows)* produces angel-wings sign. **B,** Lateral projection shows mediastinal air lifting thymus off pericardium and great vessels *(arrows and arrowheads).*

When palpating the skin, one might hear or feel crepitation (a crackling sound or sensation).

Radiographic Appearance

The radiographic appearance is bizarre, with streaks of lucency outlining muscle bundles (Figure 3-71).

Treatment of Mediastinal and Subcutaneous Emphysema

If the emphysema appears minimal and does not progress, no treatment may be needed. If the air in the mediastinum or subcutaneous tissue does not absorb, or if it increases in amount, surgical resection to block off the source of air may be required.

Disorders of the Pleura

Pneumothorax

Pneumothorax, the presence of air in the pleural cavity, results in a partial or complete collapse of the lung (Figure 3-72). It most commonly results from rupture of a subpleural bulla, either as a complication of emphysema or as a spontaneous event in an otherwise healthy young adult. Other causes of pneumothorax include trauma (e.g., stabbing, gunshot, or fractured rib) and iatrogenic causes (e.g., after lung biopsy or the introduction of a chest tube for thoracentesis), or it may be a complication of neonatal hyaline membrane disease and require prolonged assisted ventilation. Regardless of the cause, the increased air in the pleural cavity compresses the lung and causes it to collapse. This may cause the patient to experience sudden, severe chest pain and dyspnea (difficulty in breathing).

Radiographic Appearance

A pneumothorax appears radiographically as a hyperlucent area in which all pulmonary markings are absent. The radiographic hallmark of pneumothorax is the demonstration of the visceral pleural line, which is outlined centrally by air within the lung and peripherally by air within the pleural space. A large pneumothorax can cause collapse of an entire lung. Chest radiographs for pneumothorax should be taken with the patient in the upright position, as it may be very difficult to identify this condition in the supine patient. In addition to routine full-inspiration films, a posteroanterior (PA) radiograph, or an AP radiograph, should be obtained with the lung in full expiration to allow identification of small pneumothoraxes (Figure 3-73). This maneuver causes the lung to decrease in volume and become relatively denser, whereas the volume of air in the pleural space remains constant and is easier to detect. Very small

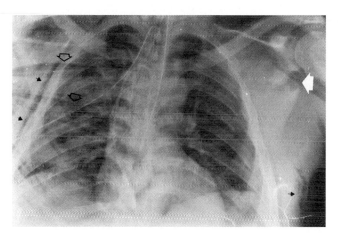

FIGURE 3-71 Subcutaneous emphysema. Frontal chest radiograph of severely injured patient shows streaks and bubbles of subcutaneous air *(black arrows)* in soft tissues along lateral borders of thorax, and broad lucencies outlining muscle bundles *(open arrows)* overlying the anterior chest wall. Note fracture of left scapula *(white arrows)* and multiple rib fractures.

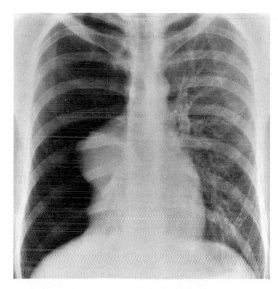

FIGURE 3-72 Spontaneous pneumothorax. Complete collapse of right lung.

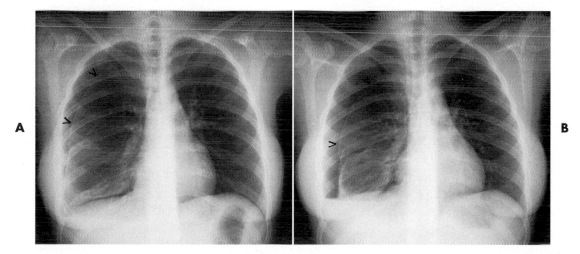

FIGURE 3-73 Pneumothorax. **A,** On routine frontal chest film, a faint rim of pleura *(arrows)* at the right apex is separated from the thoracic wall by an area containing air but no pulmonary vasculature. **B,** On expiratory film, right pneumothorax *(arrows)* is clearly seen.

pneumothoraxes may be evident on lateral decubitus films. In this position, air rising to the highest point in the hemithorax is more clearly visible over the lateral chest wall than on erect views, in which a small amount of air in the apical region may be obscured by overlying bony densities. Whenever an expiration radiograph is being obtained, the use of an automatic exposure control is *not* recommended because the preset density may produce a radiographic film density capable of concealing a small pneumothorax. Using a manual technique, the exposure factor (in milliampere seconds) for an expiration radiograph should be about one third higher than that used for inspiration films.

Treatment

Small pneumothoraxes usually reabsorb spontaneously. Larger pneumothoraxes may require prompt chest tube drainage with suction to remove the air and prevent recurrence. Tension pneumothorax is a medical emergency in which air continues to enter the pleural space, but cannot exit. The accumulation of air within the pleural space causes complete collapse of the ipsilateral lung and depression of the hemidiaphragm (Figure 3-74). The heart and mediastinal structures shift toward the opposite side, severely compromising cardiac output because the elevated intrathoracic pressure decreases venous return to the heart. If a tension pneumothorax is not treated promptly, the resulting circulatory collapse may be fatal.

Pleural Effusion

The accumulation of fluid in the pleural space is a nonspecific finding that may be caused by a wide variety of pathologic processes. The most common causes include congestive heart failure, pulmonary embolism, infection (especially tuberculosis), pleurisy, neoplastic disease, and connective tissue disorders. Pleural effusion can also be the result of abdominal disease, such as recent surgery, ascites, subphrenic abscess, and pancreatitis.

Radiographic Appearance

The earliest radiographic finding in pleural effusion is blunting of the normally sharp angle between the diaphragm and the rib cage (the costophrenic angle) along with an upward concave border of the fluid level (or meniscus) (Figure 3-75). Because the costophrenic angles are deeper posteriorly than laterally, small pleural effusions are best seen on the routine lateral projection posteriorly. As much as 400 ml of pleural fluid may accumulate and still not produce blunting of the lateral costophrenic angles on erect frontal views of the chest. Larger amounts of pleural fluid produce a homogeneous radiolucency (or whiteness) that may obscure the diaphragm and adjacent borders of the heart. Massive effusions may compress the adjacent lung and even displace the heart and mediastinum to the opposite side (Figure 3-76).

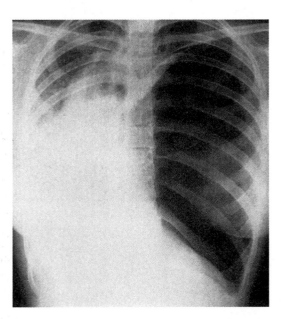

FIGURE 3-74 Tension pneumothorax. Left hemithorax is completely radiolucent and lacks vascular markings. There is a dramatic shift of the mediastinum to the right. Left hemidiaphragm is greatly depressed, and there is spreading of the left ribs.

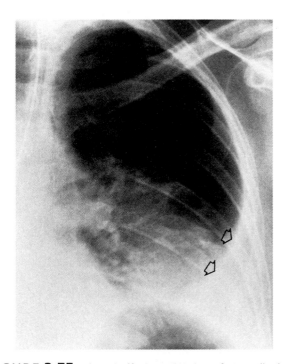

FIGURE 3-75 Pleural effusion. Blunting of normally sharp angle between diaphragm and rib cage *(arrows)* along with characteristic concave-upward fluid level (meniscus).

SUMMARY *of* FINDINGS *for* Pleural Disorders

disorder	location	radiographic appearance	treatment
Pneumothorax	Air in pleural cavity	Peripheral radiolucency without pulmonary markings	Small—none (reabsorbed) Large—chest tube with suction
Pleural effusion	Fluid in pleural cavity	Fluid level—best seen on lateral decubitus	Thoracentesis to remove fluid
Empyema	Infected fluid in pleural cavity	Lesion—loculated fluid; possible air–fluid level	Needle aspiration with possible drain placement

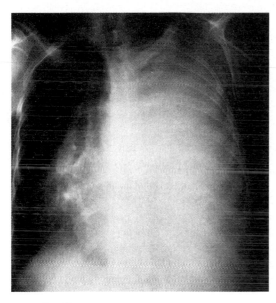

FIGURE 3-76 Pleural effusion causing shift of mediastinum. Left hemithorax is virtually opaque, and there is a shift of mediastinal structures to the right.

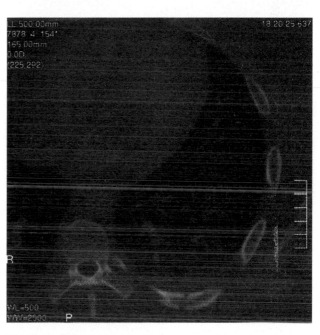

FIGURE 3-77 Pleural effusion caused by a left posterior rib fracture demonstrated on a CT

Small pleural effusions may be difficult to distinguish from pleural thickening and fibrosis, which results from previous pleural inflammation and appears radiographically as a soft tissue density along the lateral chest wall (Figure 3-77). The diagnosis of a small pleural effusion is best made using a horizontal x-ray beam with the patient in a lateral decubitus position with the affected side down. By placing the patient in a slight lateral Trendelenburg position, as little as 5 ml of pleural fluid can be seen as a layer of linear opacification along the dependent chest wall. At times, however, a collection of pleural fluid may be loculated (i.e., fixed in place by fibrous adhesions) and therefore will not form this layer in decubitus views.

Pleural effusions may produce less common appearances on chest radiographs. A pleural fluid collection that has become fixed by inflammatory fibrosis may mimic a solid mass. At times, pleural fluid may collect below the inferior surface of the lung (subpulmonic effusion) and give the radiographic appearance of an elevated hemidiaphragm (Figure 3-78). In patients with congestive heart failure, an effusion may develop in an interlobar fissure to produce a round or oval density resembling a solitary pulmonary nodule. As the patient's heart condition improves, repeat examinations demonstrate decreased size or complete resolution of these phantom tumors (see Figure 7-20).

Treatment

Thoracentesis is the procedure for removing fluid from the pleural cavity. Other treatments depend on the cause of the pleural effusion.

Empyema

Empyema refers to the presence of infected liquid or frank pus in the pleural space. Usually the result of the spread of an adjacent infection (e.g., bacterial

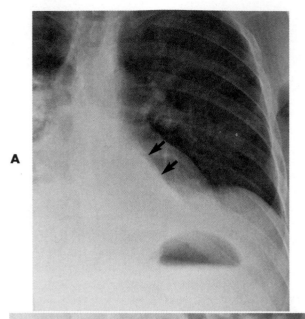

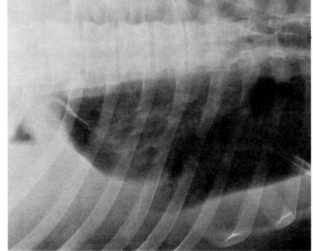

FIGURE 3-78 Pleural effusion. **A,** Frontal projection of chest demonstrates large distance between gastric air bubble and top of false left hemidiaphragm in this patient with large subpulmonic effusion. Note retrocardiac paraspinal density *(arrows)* that simulates left lower lobe infiltrate or atelectasis. **B,** Left lateral decubitus projection shows that retrocardiac density represents large amount of free pleural fluid.

pneumonia, subdiaphragmatic abscess, lung abscess, and esophageal perforation), empyemas may also occur after thoracic surgery, trauma, or instrumentation of the pleural space. Since the development of antibiotics, empyemas are rare.

Radiographic Appearance
Radiographically, an empyema is initially indistinguishable from pleural effusion. As the empyema develops, it becomes loculated and appears as a discrete mass that may vary in size from a large lesion

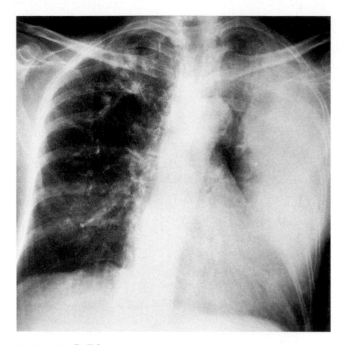

FIGURE 3-79 Empyema. Large soft tissue mass fills much of left hemithorax.

filling much of the hemithorax (Figure 3-79) to a small mass along the chest wall or in an interlobar fissure. Air within a free or loculated empyema causes an air-fluid level and indicates communication with a bronchus or the skin surface.

Treatment
Needle aspiration of an empyema may be performed under fluoroscopic guidance; when the loculated mass is situated adjacent to the chest wall, ultrasound may be used to guide the aspiration needle. A sinus tract or fistula may require drainage tube placement.

Mediastinal Masses

Because various types of mediastinal masses tend to occur predominantly in specific locations, the mediastinum is often divided into anterior, middle, and posterior compartments. The anterior compartment extends from the sternum back to the trachea and the anterior border of the heart. The middle mediastinum contains the heart and great vessels, the central tracheobronchial tree and lymph nodes, and the phrenic nerves. The posterior compartment consists of the space behind the pericardium.

Major lesions of the anterior mediastinum include thymomas (Figure 3-80), teratomas, thyroid masses, lipomas, and lymphoma. The middle mediastinum involves lymph node disorders (e.g., lymphoma, metastatic carcinoma, and granulomatous processes),

SUMMARY of FINDINGS for Mediastinal Masses

disorder	location	radiographic appearance	treatment
Thymoma Teratoma Thyroid mass Lipoma Lymphoma	Anterior mediastinum	Cystic masses—compress, producing multiloculated appearance Solid masses—compress and displace adjacent structures	Excision of lesion because of difficult differential diagnosis
Lymph node disorders Bronchogenic cysts Vascular anomalies	Middle mediastinum	Cystic masses—compress, producing multiloculated appearance Solid masses—compress and displace adjacent structures	Excision of lesion because of difficult differential diagnosis
Neurogenic tumors Neurogenic cysts Aneurysms Extramedullary hematopoiesis	Posterior mediastinum	Cystic masses—compress, producing multiloculated appearance Solid masses—compress and displace adjacent structures	Excision of lesion because of difficult differential diagnosis

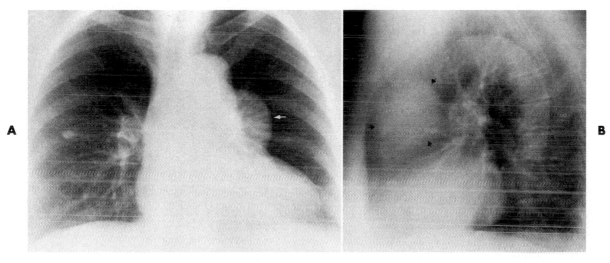

A

B

FIGURE 3-80 Anterior mediastinal mass. Frontal **(A)** and lateral **(B)** projections of chest demonstrate large mass (thymoma) in anterior mediastinum *(arrows)*.

bronchogenic cysts (Figure 3-81), vascular anomalies, and various masses situated in the anterior costophrenic angle (e.g., pericardial cysts and foramen of Morgagni hernia). The posterior mediastinum is the site of neurogenic tumors, neurogenic cysts (Figure 3-82), aneurysms of the descending aorta, and extramedullary hematopoiesis.

About one third of patients with mediastinal masses are asymptomatic, and the lesion is detected on a routine chest radiograph. Chest pain, cough, dyspnea, and symptoms caused by compression or invasion of structures in the mediastinum (e.g., dysphagia, hoarseness as a result of recurrent laryngeal nerve involvement, and superior vena cava obstruction) are highly suggestive of malignancy.

The configuration of a mediastinal mass depends to a large extent on its consistency. Cystic masses, often compressed between blood vessels and the tracheobronchial tree, produce a multiloculated appearance. In contrast, solid masses tend to compress and displace adjacent structures.

In addition to plain chest radiographs, conventional tomography and contrast studies of the esophagus may be of value in defining the anatomic location and borders of the mass. CT of the chest after the intravenous injection of contrast material may help in distinguishing between vascular and nonvascular lesions, and in determining whether a lesion is cystic and thus most probably benign (Figures 3-83 and 3-84).

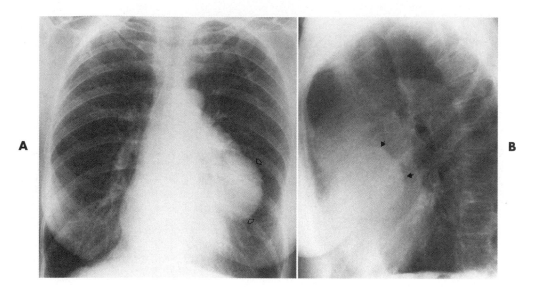

FIGURE 3-81 Middle mediastinal mass. Frontal **(A)** and lateral **(B)** projections of chest demonstrate a smooth-walled, spherical mediastinal mass *(arrows)* projecting into left lung and left hilum (found to be a bronchogenic cyst).

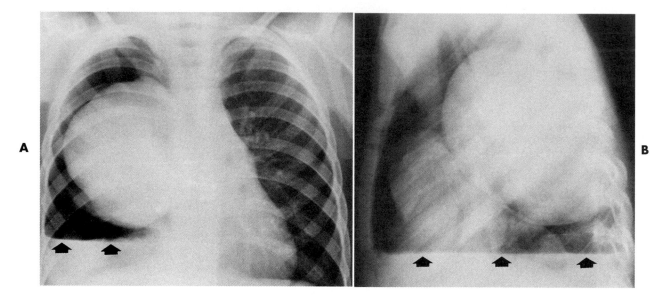

FIGURE 3-82 Posterior mediastinal mass. Frontal **(A)** and lateral **(B)** projections of chest demonstrate a large, oval, homogeneous mass in posterior mediastinum (neurenteric cyst). Note right hydropneumothorax *(arrows)* with long air-fluid level that developed as a complication of diagnostic needle biopsy.

Treatment

For all masses found in the mediastinal region, surgical excision of the neoplasm is suggested because of the difficulty in differentiating the cause and the possible complications associated with these lesions.

Disorders of the Diaphragm

The diaphragm is the major muscle of respiration separating the thoracic and abdominal cavities. Radiographically the height of the diaphragm varies considerably with the phase of respiration. On full inspiration, the diaphragm usually projects at about the level of the tenth posterior intercostal space. On expiration, it may appear two or three intercostal spaces higher. The average range of diaphragmatic motion with respiration is 3 to 6 cm, but in patients with emphysema this may be substantially reduced. The level of the diaphragm falls as the patient moves from a supine to an upright position. In an erect patient, the dome of the diaphragm tends to be about half an interspace higher on the right than on the left. However, in about 10% of normal individuals,

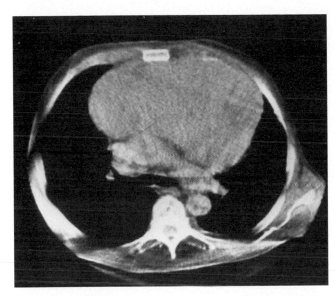

FIGURE **3-83** CT of anterior mediastinal mass. Enormous soft tissue mass (thymoma) causes posterior displacement of other mediastinal structures. No difference in density can be seen between the mass and the heart behind it.

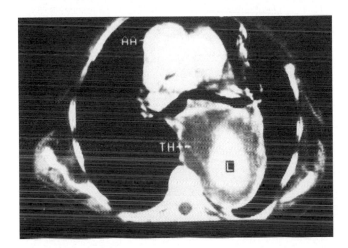

FIGURE **3-84** CT of posterior mediastinal mass. Contrast-enhanced scan at level just below carina shows large aneurysm of descending aorta. Large mural thrombus *(TH)* surrounds greatly dilated lumen of descending aorta *(L)*. Note also prominently dilated ascending aorta *(AA)*.

the hemidiaphragms are at the same height, or the left is higher than the right.

Diaphragmatic Paralysis

Elevation of one or both leaves of the diaphragm can be caused by paralysis resulting from any process that interferes with the normal function of the phrenic nerve. The paralysis may be attributable to accidental surgical transection of the phrenic nerve, involvement of the nerve by primary bronchogenic carcinoma or metastatic malignancy in the mediastinum, or a

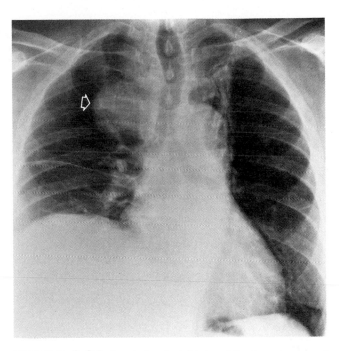

FIGURE **3-85** Paralysis of right hemidiaphragm caused by involvement of phrenic nerve by primary carcinoma of lung *(arrow)*.

variety of intrinsic neurologic diseases (Figure 3-85). Reduced lung volume results from this paralysis.

Radiographic Appearance

The radiographic hallmark of diaphragmatic paralysis is paradoxical movement of the diaphragm, which is best demonstrated at fluoroscopy by having the patient sniff. This rapid but shallow inspiration causes a quick downward thrust of a normal leaf of the diaphragm, whereas a paralyzed hemidiaphragm tends to rise with inspiration because of the increased intraabdominal pressure. During expiration, the normal hemidiaphragm rises and the paralyzed one descends. The demonstration of a pronounced degree of paradoxical motion is a valuable aid in differentiating paralysis of the diaphragm from limited diaphragmatic motion resulting from intrathoracic or intraabdominal disease.

Treatment

In most cases, diaphragmatic paralysis requires no treatment. If gravity does not provide enough lung volume, insertion of a diaphragmatic pacer may be necessary.

Eventration of the Diaphragm

Eventration of the diaphragm is a rare congenital abnormality in which one hemidiaphragm (very rarely both) is poorly developed and too weak to

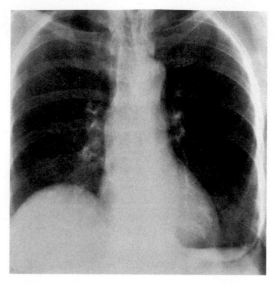

FIGURE 3-86 Eventration of right hemidiaphragm.

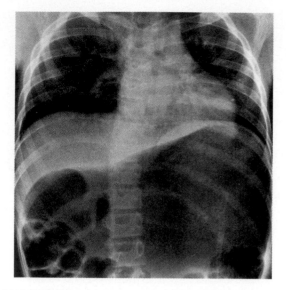

FIGURE 3-87 Diffuse elevation of both leaves of the diaphragm caused by severe, acute gastric dilatation.

SUMMARY of FINDINGS for Diaphragmatic Disorders

disorder	location	radiographic appearance	treatment
Diaphragmatic paralysis	Diaphragm motion	Sniff test to distinguish normal from abnormal	No treatment in most cases Diaphragmatic pacer
Diaphragmatic eventration	Diaphragm poorly developed and elevated	Diaphragm elevation	No treatment in most cases Plication possible
Other causes of diaphragmatic elevation	Elevation due to extrinsic cause	Diaphragm elevation	Treatment varies on the basis of cause

permit the upward movement of abdominal contents into the thoracic cage. The condition is usually asymptomatic and occurs more frequently on the left.

Radiographic Appearance

Eventration produces the radiographic appearance of a localized bulging or generalized elevation of the diaphragm (Figure 3-86). An eventration must be distinguished from a diaphragmatic hernia, through which abdominal contents are displaced into the chest. Oral administration of barium should permit the differentiation between the normal contours of the bowel below a diaphragmatic eventration and the crowding of these structures and narrowing of their afferent and efferent limbs when trapped in a hernia sac.

Treatment

Eventration rarely needs treatment. Infants in distress may require surgical plication to shorten the diaphragm by removing a fold.

Other Causes of Elevation of the Diaphragm

Diffuse elevation of one or both leaves of the diaphragm can be caused by ascites, obesity, pregnancy, or any other process in which the intraabdominal volume is increased (Figure 3-87). Intraabdominal inflammatory diseases, such as subphrenic abscess, can lead to elevation of a hemidiaphragm with severe limitations of diaphragmatic motion. Cystic or tumor masses arising in the upper quadrants can cause localized or generalized bulging of the diaphragm. Acute intrathoracic processes (e.g., chest-wall injury, atelectasis, and pulmonary embolism) can produce diaphragmatic elevation caused by splinting of the diaphragm.

Radiographic Appearance

An apparent elevation of a hemidiaphragm may be caused by a subpulmonic pleural effusion, which can be correctly diagnosed on a chest radiograph performed with a horizontal x-ray beam and the patient in a lateral decubitus position.

REVIEW QUESTIONS

1. _____ is a disease of newborns character- ized by progressive underaeration of the lungs and a granular appearance.

2. _____ is a hereditary disease in which thick mucus is secreted by all the exocrine glands.

3. A necrotic area of pulmonary parenchyma con- taining purulent or puslike material is called a(n) _____.

4. What radiographic procedure is often required to confirm the diagnosis of bronchiectasis when the results of routine chest radiographs are inconclusive?

5. Flattening of the domes of the diaphragm, in- creased AP diameter of the chest, and increased lucency of the retrosternal air space are sugges- tive of a diagnosis of _____.

6. The three most common pneumoconioses are _____, _____, and _____.

7. An abnormal vascular communication between a pulmonary artery and a pulmonary vein is termed a(n) _____.

8. What medical emergency has occurred when air continues to enter the pleural space and cannot escape, leading to complete collapse of a lung and shift of the heart and mediastinal structures?

9. Pus in the pleural space is called _____.

10. A lung inflammation caused by bacteria or vi- ruses is called a(n) _____.

11. Name two common types of pulmonary mycoses.

12. For the radiographer's safety, it is important to remember that tuberculosis is spread mainly by _____, which produces infectious _____.

13. What medical term is used to describe the entry of air into the pleural space?

14. An increased volume of air in the lungs is seen in _____.

15. Inhalation of irritating dusts leading to chronic inflammation and pulmonary fibrosis is called _____.

16. A malignant pleural neoplasm that results from asbestosis is _____.

17. The trapping of bacteria in the pulmonary circu- lation that occurs in patients with a history of in- travenous drug abuse is called _____.

18. Reduced air volume within a lung leading to col- lapse is termed _____.

19. Why do intrabronchial foreign bodies occur more frequently in the lower right lung?

20. Blunt or penetrating trauma to the chest can pro- duce _____, which appears as streaks of air that outline muscles of the thorax and some- times the neck.

21. At what costal interspace does the diaphragm lie when the lungs are fully inflated?
    A. eighth   C. tenth
    B. ninth   D. eleventh

22. Air collecting behind the sternum and dissect- ing up into the soft tissue of the neck is called _____.

23. An accumulation of fluid in the pleural space, sometimes caused by heart failure or pulmonary embolus, is called _____.
    A. empyema   C. effusion
    B. edema   D. abscess

BIBLIOGRAPHY

Centers for Disease Control: U.S. Department of Health and Human Services, www.cdc.gov.

Felson B: *Chest roentgenology,* Philadelphia, 1971, Saunders.

Heitzman ER: *The lung: radiologic-pathologic correlations,* St Louis, 1984, Mosby.

Krilov LR: *Respiratory syncytial virus infection,* eMedicine Specialties, 2004, www.emedicine.com.

National Institute of Allergy and Infectious Diseases: National Institute of Health, U.S. Department of Health and Human Services, www.niaid.nih.gov.

Paré JAP, Fraser RG: *Synopsis of diseases of the chest,* Philadelphia, 1983, Saunders.

Reed JC: *Chest radiology: patterns and differential diagnoses,* St Louis, 1981, Mosby.

World Health Organization (WHO): www.who.int.

SKELETAL*System*

Chapter Outline

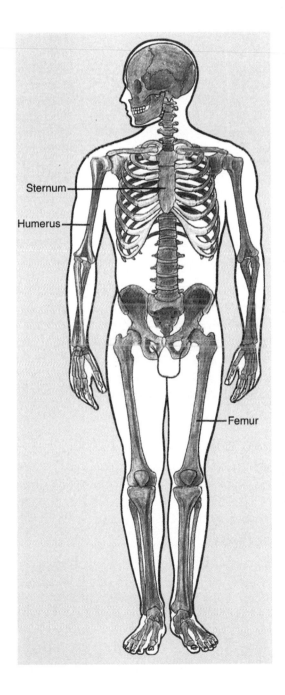

Key Terms

aneurysmal bone cyst
angulation
ankylosing spondylitis
appositional growth
avulsion fractures
bone islands
bowing fracture
boxer's fracture
butterfly fragment
cancellous (spongy) bone
cervical rib
chondrosarcoma
clay shoveler's fracture
closed fractures
Colles' fracture
comminuted fracture
compact bone
complete fracture
compound fracture
compression fracture
depressed fracture
diaphysis
dislocation
displacement
endosteum
epiphyseal cartilage

epiphyses
external fixation
external, or closed, reduction
Galeazzi fracture
giant cell tumor (osteoclastoma)
greenstick fracture
hangman's fracture
incomplete fracture
internal fixation
intramembranous ossification
Jefferson fracture
Jones fracture
marrow
medullary cavity
meningocele
metaphysis
Monteggia fracture
multiple myeloma
myelomeningocele
navicular
oblique fracture
open fracture
open reduction
ossification
osteoblasts
osteoclasts

osteogenic sarcoma
osteomas
pathologic fracture
periosteum
Pott's disease
psoriatic arthritis
resorption
seat belt fracture
segmental fracture
simple bone cyst (unicameral)
spina bifida occulta
spiral fracture
spondylolisthesis
spondylolysis
stable
stress, or fatigue, fracture
subluxation
torus (buckle) fracture
trabeculae
transitional vertebra
transverse fracture
tuberculous arthritis
undisplaced fracture
unstable

Prerequisite Knowledge

The student should have a basic knowledge of the anatomy and physiology of the skeletal system. In addition, proper learning and understanding of the material will be facilitated if the student has some clinical experience in skeletal radiography and image evaluation, including a concept of the changes in technique required to compensate for density differences produced by the underlying pathologic conditions.

Goals

To acquaint the student radiographer with the pathophysiology and radiographic manifestations of all the common and some of the unusual disorders of the skeletal system.

Objectives

After reading this chapter, the reader will be able to:
1. Classify the more common diseases in terms of their attenuation of x-rays
2. Explain the changes in technical factors required for obtaining optimal-quality radiographs in patients with various underlying pathologic conditions

3. Define all key terms in this chapter
4. Describe the physiology of the skeletal system
5. Identify anatomic structures on both diagrams and radiographs of the skeletal system
6. Differentiate the various pathologic conditions affecting the skeletal system and their radiographic manifestations

Physiology of the Skeletal System

The skeletal system is composed primarily of two highly specialized connective tissues: bone and cartilage. Bone consists of an organic matrix in which inorganic salts (primarily calcium and phosphate) are deposited. A fibrous membrane termed the **periosteum** covers the outer surfaces of bone, except at joint surfaces where articular cartilage covers the bone and acts as a protective cushion. The periosteum contains a network of blood vessels from which nutrient arteries penetrate into the underlying bone. The main shaftlike portion is termed the **diaphysis,** and the ends of the bone are called **epiphyses**. The hollow, tubelike structure within the diaphysis, known as

RADIOGRAPHER *Notes*

Three factors are critical in radiography of the skeletal system: (1) proper patient positioning; (2) correct alignment of the radiographic tube, the body part being imaged, and the image receptor; and (3) exposure factors chosen to produce optimal contrast and visibility of detail. In patients with suspected fractures, two projections as close as possible to 90 degrees to each other must always be obtained to demonstrate fracture relationships. A variety of projections (e.g., oblique, tangential, or coned-down) may be required to identify obscure fractures.

At times, the poor condition of a patient may require ingenuity on the part of the radiographer to obtain diagnostic radiographs when routine positioning methods cannot be accomplished. Patients with bone tumors, arthritis, or recent trauma are frequently in severe pain and extremely frightened of further injury or of suffering more discomfort. The radiographer must reassure the patient that positioning will be carefully accomplished with as little pain or discomfort as possible. Remember that a radiographer can easily cause further injury to the patient if the proper moving techniques are not used.

At times, the radiographer may need to perform cross-table or tube angulation projections to obtain the required images without moving the patient. In such cases, the radiographic tube must be perpendicular to the image receptor and the body part to prevent image distortion. Variations in this relationship can obscure pathologic bone conditions or lead to errors in interpretation of the alignment of fracture fragments.

Bone radiographs require a short scale of contrast to provide maximal visibility of detail. The periosteum, cortex, and internal bone structure (trabeculae) must be well demonstrated to detect the often subtle changes of fractures, demineralization, and bone destruction. For example, periosteal new bone formation may indicate underlying tumor, infection, or prior trauma, whereas minute juxtaarticular erosions are often seen in arthritis. The scale of contrast must also allow visualization of the soft tissues and muscles because soft tissue swelling, calcifications, opaque foreign bodies, muscle wasting, and the presence of gas are all important radiographic findings.

It is recommended that lower to mid kilovolt-peak (kVp) ranges be used in all skeletal radiography. To achieve the necessary scale of contrast, extremity radiographs should be exposed using an exposure in the 50 to 69 kVp range, whereas a range of 70 to 80 kVp is recommended for studies of the spine, pelvis, thoracic cavity, and shoulder. Appropriate ratio grids, or Bucky devices, should be used for all body parts 10 cm or greater.

Special techniques, such as magnification or tomography, may be necessary to detect subtle fractures or other pathologic bone conditions. For example, the navicular bone of the wrist typically requires the use of the magnification technique. For 2x linear or 4x area magnification, the object must be an equal distance from the radiographic tube and the image receptor. For 3x linear or 9x area magnification, the body part must be twice as far from the image receptor as from the x-ray tube. Close collimation is extremely important to prevent undercutting the image. A radiographic tube with a fractional focal spot of 0.3 mm or less is mandatory for a magnification factor of 2x or more to compensate for the excessive penumbra (geometric blur) that results from the object image receptor distance. Larger focal spot sizes cause excessive geometric blurred images that appear to have motion and lack recorded detail as a result of excessive geometric blur (penumbra).

Tomography may be required to make a definitive diagnosis if the plain radiographs are equivocal or to delineate precisely the extent of bone involvement. For example, tomography is frequently needed in the evaluation of fractures of the tibial plateau and spine. Computed tomography (CT) is the modality of choice for spinal injuries because it best demonstrates the vertebrae and fracture fragments that could impinge on the spinal cord or peripheral nerves. Magnetic resonance imaging (MRI) better demonstrates nontraumatic disk herniation or tumor impingement. In trauma cases, if CT is inconclusive, MR imaging may better delineate soft tissue injury.

In most cases, it is essential to prevent motion of the body part being radiographed. To accomplish this, make the patient as comfortable as possible, use immobilization devices when necessary, and use the shortest possible exposure times. However, a few portions of the skeletal system are better visualized using a motion technique. For three such areas (the sternum and the lateral thoracic spine, and to obtain a transthoracic lateral projection of the upper humerus), a shallow breathing technique is used while the patient remains immobilized. A minimum exposure time of about 5 seconds and a very low milliamperage should be used. The patient is instructed to breathe rhythmically during

Continued

RADIOGRAPHER *Notes—Cont'd*

the entire exposure to blur out overlying ribs and lung markings. An additional technique, the Ottonello (or "wagging jaw") method, is used to obtain an anteroposterior (AP) projection of the cervical spine. Movement of the jaw is used to blur out the image of the mandible, which otherwise would superimpose the upper portion of the cervical spine.

Certain pathologic conditions of the skeletal system require that the radiographer alter routine technical settings. Some disorders produce increased bone density (e.g., sclerosis and increased bone growth), which increases attenuation; others decrease the density of the bony structures (e.g., lytic bone destruction and loss of calcium from bone), and so they will attenuate x-rays less (see the box in Chapter 1 labeled Relative Attenuation of X-Rays in Advanced Stages of Diseases). It is important to remember that the necessary technical changes may vary depending on the stage of the underlying condition. However, do not change the technical factors to obscure or change the interpretation of the pathophysiologic changes.

the **medullary cavity,** or **marrow,** is lined by an inner membrane termed the **endosteum.**

There are two major types of bone. The outer layer consists of **compact bone,** which to the naked eye appears dense and structureless. Under the microscope, the matrix of compact bone consists of complex structural units called "haversian systems." **Cancellous (spongy) bone** is composed of a weblike arrangement of marrow-filled spaces separated by thin processes of bone, called **trabeculae,** which are visible to the naked eye. The relative amount of each type of bone depends on the degree of strength required and thus varies from bone to bone and in different portions of the same bone. For example, the shafts of long bones, such as the femur and tibia, have a thick outer layer of compact bone, whereas the layer of compact bone is relatively thin in irregular bones, such as vertebral bodies and facial bones, and in short bones, such as the carpal and tarsal bones.

Most bones form from models composed of hyaline cartilage (enchondral ossification). In a typical long bone, a primary ossification center appears in the center of the cartilage precursor in about the eighth week of intrauterine life, and bone formation extends so that the entire shaft is usually ossified before birth. Just before or after birth, secondary ossification centers appear in the epiphyses, the ends of developing long bones. Until the linear growth of bone is complete, the epiphysis remains separated from the diaphysis by a cartilaginous plate called the **epiphyseal cartilage.** The epiphyseal cartilage persists until the growth of the bone is complete. At that time, the epiphyseal plate ossifies, and the epiphysis and diaphysis fuse (at various ages depending on the specific bones). Where the diaphysis meets the epiphyseal growth plate is a slight flaring, known as the **metaphysis.**

The increase in length of a developing long bone occurs by growth of the epiphyseal cartilage followed by ossification. Bones grow in diameter by the combined action of two special types of cells called **osteoblasts** and **osteoclasts.** Osteoclasts enlarge the diameter of the medullary cavity by removing bone from the diaphysis walls. At the same time, osteoblasts from the periosteum produce new bone around the outer circumference. Osteoblasts and osteoclasts thus continuously resorb old bone and produce new bone. This constant process of remodeling occurs until the bone assumes its adult size and shape.

The radiographic determination of bone age is useful for evaluating physiologic age and growth potential, and for predicting adult stature. The most well known and widely accepted method of determining skeletal bone age (skeletal maturation) is that of Greulich and Pyle in their radiographic atlas compiled from thousands of examinations of American children at different ages. This atlas contains standard radiographs for age and sex that permit an assessment of bone age based on the presence or absence of ossification centers and their configuration, and the fusion of epiphyses in various portions of the hand and wrist.

Throughout life, bone formation **(ossification)** and bone destruction **(resorption)** continue to occur. They are in balance during the early and middle years of adulthood. After about 40 years of age, however, bone loss at the inner or endosteal surface exceeds bone gain at the outer margins. Thus in long bones, the thickness of compact bone in the diaphyses decreases, and the diameter of the medullary cavity increases. The bone eventually resembles a hollow shell and is less able to resist compressive and bending forces. This process may lead to collapse and loss of height of vertebral bodies, and fractures of long bones after relatively mild injury.

Bones can also develop within a connective tissue membrane **(intramembranous ossification).** The clavicles and flat bones of the skull have no cartilaginous stage and begin to take shape when groups of primitive cells differentiate into osteoblasts, which secrete matrix material and collagenous fibrils. Deposition of complex calcium salts in the organic bone matrix produces rodlike trabeculae that join in a network of interconnecting spicules to form spongy or cancellous bone. Eventually, plates of compact or dense bone cover the core layer of spongy bone. Flat bones grow in size by the addition of osseous tissue to their outer surfaces (**appositional growth**). They cannot grow by expansion, as enchondral bone does.

Bones perform five basic functions:

1. They serve as the supporting framework of the body.
2. Bones protect the vital organs (e.g., the skull protects the brain, and the rib cage protects the heart and lungs).
3. Bones serve as levers on which muscles can contract and shorten and thus produce movement at a joint.
4. Red bone marrow within certain bones (spinal column, upper humerus, and upper femur in the adult) is the major site of production of blood cells.
5. Bone serves as the major storehouse for calcium salts. The maintenance of a normal level of calcium, which is essential for survival, depends on a balance in the rates of calcium movement between the blood and bones.

Congenital/Hereditary Diseases of Bone

Vertebral Anomalies

A **transitional vertebra** is one that has characteristics of vertebrae on both sides of a major division of the spine.

Radiographic Appearance

Transitional vertebrae most frequently occur at the lumbosacral junction and contain expanded transverse processes, which may form actual unilateral or bilateral joints with the sacrum (Figure 4-1). When unilateral, this process often leads to degenerative change involving the opposite hip and the intervertebral disk space above it. At the thoracolumbar junction, the first lumbar vertebra may have rudimentary ribs articulating with the transverse processes. The seventh cervical vertebra may also have a rudimentary rib (Figure 4-2).

Treatment

Most vertebral anomalies remain unnoticed and are incidental findings on radiographs. A **cervical rib** may compress the brachial nerve plexus (causing pain or numbness in the upper extremity) or the subclavian artery (decreasing blood flow to the arm) and therefore require surgical removal.

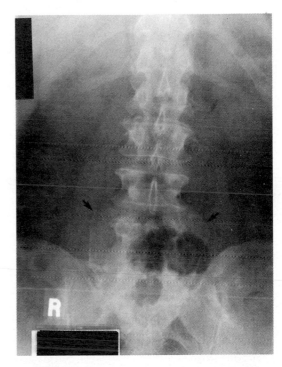

FIGURE 4-1 Transitional vertebrae. Expanded transverse process at the lumbosacral junction.

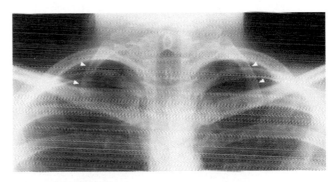

FIGURE 4-2 Bilateral cervical ribs *(arrowheads).*

Spina Bifida

Spina bifida refers to a posterior defect of the spinal canal resulting from failure of the posterior elements to fuse properly. A mild, insignificant form is **spina bifida occulta,** in which there is a splitting of the bony neural canal at the L5 or S1 level (Figure 4-3). Large defects are associated with spinal cord abnormalities and may lead to a variety of muscular abnormalities and lack of bladder or bowel control. In many cases a slight dimpling of the skin or a tuft of hair over the vertebral defect indicates the site of the lesion.

Large defects in the lumbar or cervical spine may be accompanied by herniation of the meninges **(meningocele),** or of the meninges and a portion of the spinal cord or nerve roots **(myelomeningocele).**

A patient with a meningocele may be asymptomatic. Other malformations associated with a meningocele include clubfeet, gait disturbances, and bladder incontinence. The myelomeningocele has associated neurologic deficits at and below the site of protrusion. Almost all patients with myelomeningocele have the Chiari II malformation, with caudal displacement of posterior fossa structures into the cervical canal. Hydrocephalus is a frequent complication.

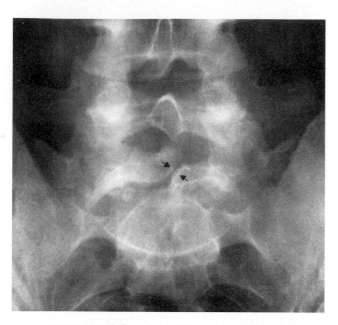

FIGURE 4-3 Spina bifida occulta *(arrows).*

Radiographic Appearance

These lesions are associated with large bony defects, absence of the laminae, and increased interpedicular distance (Figure 4-4). The herniated spinal contents are seen as a soft tissue mass posterior to the spine. Myelography, CT, or MRI can demonstrate the presence of spinal cord or nerve roots within the herniated sac. Prenatal real-time ultrasound can now demonstrate this serious malformation in utero. The sagittal spine fetal images determine the location and severity of the deformity.

Treatment

Prenatal intervention includes the daily supplement of folic acid, which has reduced the number of incidences of spina bifida. The ability to diagnose the fetus allows for fetal intervention, experimental surgery that helps to minimize nerve deficits. Spina bifida occulta and meningoceles usually require no treatment. Sometimes a meningocele requires surgical repair, depending on the size and location of the protrusion. A myelomeningocele generally requires surgical repair. When this repair is being completed, a shunt is placed to prevent hydrocephalus.

Osteopetrosis

Osteopetrosis (marble bones) is a rare hereditary bone dysplasia in which failure of the resorptive mechanism of calcified cartilage interferes with the normal replacement by mature bone. This prevents the bone

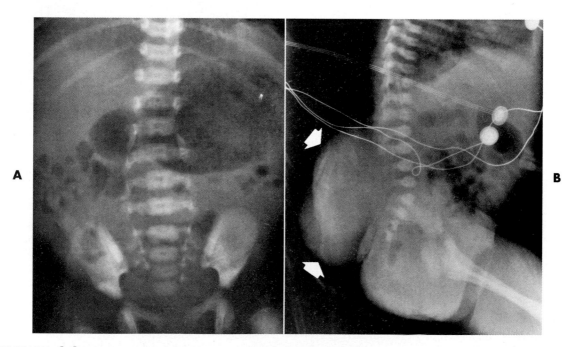

FIGURE 4-4 Meningomyelocele. **A,** Frontal projection of abdomen shows greatly increased interpedicular distance of lumbar vertebrae. **B,** In another patient, lateral projection demonstrates large soft tissue mass *(arrows)* situated posterior to spine. Notice absence of posterior elements in lower lumbar and sacral regions.

marrow from forming, so that the bones become very brittle and stress fractures occur often. The patient may also become anemic as a result of the lack of blood-producing bone marrow. Osteopetrosis varies in severity and age of clinical presentation from a fulminant, often fatal condition involving the entire skeleton at birth or in utero, to an essentially asymptomatic form that is an incidental radiographic finding.

Radiographic Appearance

Osteopetrosis results in a symmetric, generalized increase in bone density (Figure 4-5). To produce a diagnostic image, the radiographer must increase the exposure factors (milliampere seconds [mAs] and kilovolts peak [kVp]) to compensate for the increase in bone formation. The image may appear blurred because of the structural changes; in some cases, a good image may be difficult to produce.

Treatment

Currently, no effective treatment exists for osteopetrosis. Medications designed to increase bone resorption and increase blood cell production may help control the disease. For the most severe cases bone marrow transplant is the only way to improve the prognosis

of this pathologic disorder. For less severe cases, bone marrow transplants increase the production of blood cells to manage the anemia. Transplantation of osteoclastic precursors may help control the balance of bone formation and resorption.

Osteogenesis Imperfecta

Osteogenesis imperfecta (brittle bones) is an inherited generalized disorder of connective tissue characterized by multiple fractures and an unusual blue color of the normally white sclera of the eye. Due to imperfectly formed or inadequate bone collagen, adult patients are generally wheel chair bound because the skeletal structure does not support their body weight (Figure 4-6).

Radiographic Appearance

Patients with this condition suffer repeated fractures caused by the severe osteoporosis and the thin, defective cortices (Figure 4-7, *A*). The fractures often heal with exuberant callus formation (often so extensive as to simulate a malignant tumor), sometimes causing bizarre deformities. Because of the severe cortical bone loss in advanced stages of disease, producing a good image may require lowering the kilovoltage to compensate for the loss of bone quality. Ossification

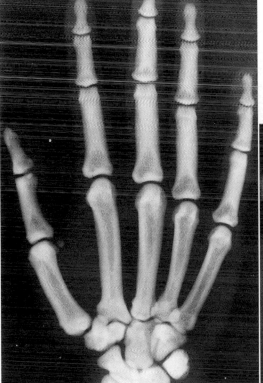
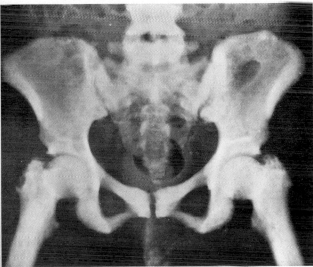

FIGURE 4-5 Osteopetrosis. **A,** Striking sclerosis of bones of hand and wrist. **B,** Generalized increased density of lower spine, pelvis, and hips.

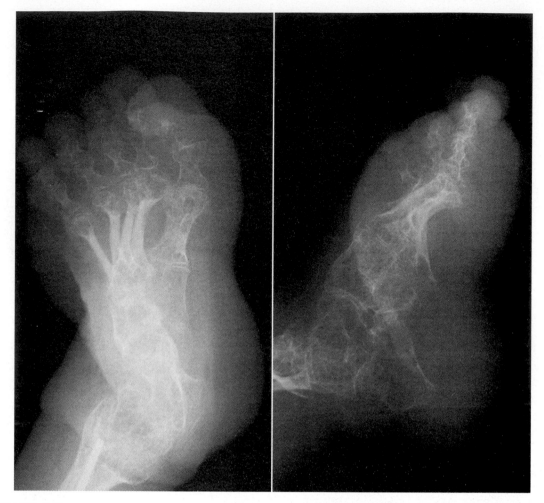

FIGURE 4-6 Osteogenesis imperfecta of adult foot. Demineralization and the lack of bony cortices are demonstrated on anteroposterior and lateral projections.

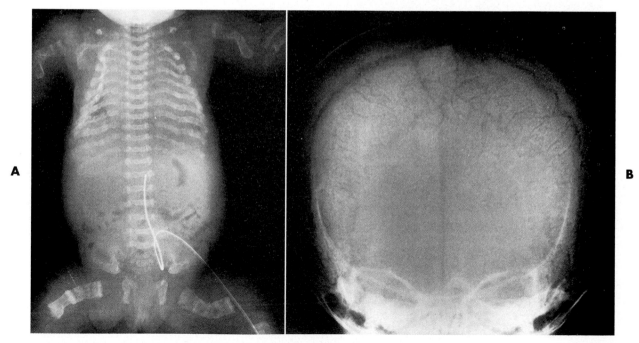

FIGURE 4-7 Osteogenesis imperfecta. **A,** Generalized flattening of vertebral bodies associated with fractures of multiple ribs and long bones in an infant. **B,** Multiple wormian bones.

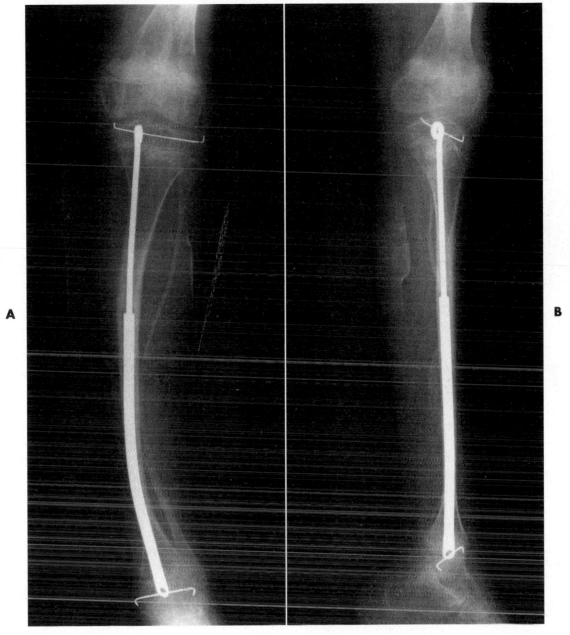

FIGURE 4-8 Osteogenesis imperfecta. Anteroposterior **(A)** and lateral **(B)** projections of the lower leg show extension rod placement to strengthen bone and decrease fracture possibility.

of the skull progresses slowly, leaving wide sutures and multiple juxtasutural accessory bones within a suture (wormian bones) that produce a mosaic appearance (Figure 4-7, *B*). "Child abuse" may be confused with osteogenesis imperfecta due to the presentation of multiple fractures in different stages of the healing process.

Treatment

The aim of treatment is to reduce fractures by using proper safety measures. Because of defective cortices in severe cases, the long bones become less supportive. Therefore in some instances, extendable

rods are surgically placed to provide more support, help prevent new fractures from occurring, and prevent bowing (Figure 4-8). Currently, drugs are prescribed to regulate the osteoclastic formation, thus keeping the bone density more normal. As research continues, stem cell transplants may become a viable cure.

Achondroplasia

Achondroplasia is the most common form of dwarfism; it results from diminished proliferation of cartilage in the growth plate (decreased enchondral bone formation). This autosomal dominant condition does not affect membranous bone formation. Therefore the individual has short limbs, which contrast with the nearly normal length of the trunk. Other characteristic physical features include a large head with frontal bulging, saddle nose, a prognathous (jutting) jaw, and prominent buttocks that give the false impression of lumbar lordosis.

Radiographic Appearance

Typical radiographic findings include progressive narrowing of the interpedicular distances from above

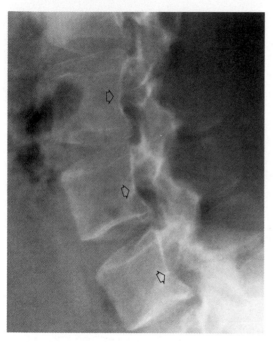

FIGURE 4-9 Achondroplasia. Posterior scalloping of multiple vertebral bodies *(arrowheads)*.

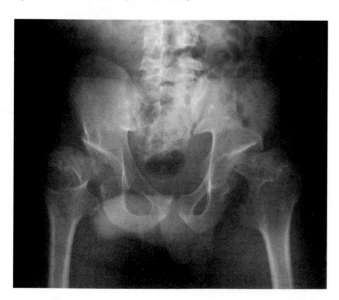

FIGURE 4-10 Achondroplasia. View of the pelvis demonstrates femoral head deformity caused by decreased endochondral bone formation.

downward, the opposite of normal, and scalloping of the posterior margins of the lumbar vertebral bodies (Figure 4-9). The decreased enchondral bone formation may make the long bones appear short and thick with a widened metaphysis (Erlenmeyer flask deformity) (Figure 4-10). CT is beneficial in demonstrating the degree of spinal narrowing caused by spondylosis and the changes in the vertebral column.

Treatment

Achondroplasia has no cure, and treatments address complications or deformities associated with the disease process. Those afflicted live normal independent and productive lives. With today's technology, the long bones can be surgically lengthened. Growth hormone treatment is still considered experimental; however, preliminary reports indicate positive results in increasing bone growth.

Congenital Hip Dysplasia (Dislocation)

Congenital hip dysplasia, also known as developmental hip dysplasia, results from incomplete acetabulum formation caused by physiologic and mechanical factors. Physiologically the fetus is exposed to increased hormone levels during delivery. Mechanically, as the fetus grows and occupies more space, the amount of amniotic fluid decreases, placing gentle pressure on the infant. Hip dysplasia is more common in females. Upon pediatric assessment of the hip, when the leg is flexed and abducted, the hip may "pop" out of joint and a "click" is felt or heard. The tendons and ligaments responsible for proper femoral head alignment are affected.

Radiographic Appearance

Anteroposterior (AP) pelvis and bilateral Cleaves (frog-leg) views are required to make a diagnosis (Figure 4-11). In many cases the AP image appears almost

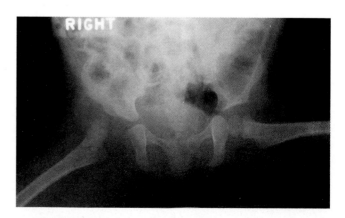

FIGURE 4-11 Hip dysplasia of the right hip in a 2-year-old child. Cleaves (frog-leg) view of the pelvis demonstrates superior and posterior displacement.

SUMMARY of FINDINGS for Congenital/Hereditary Bone Diseases

disorder	location	radiographic appearance	treatment
Vertebral anomalies	Lumbar Cervical	Unilateral or bilateral, L5 expanded transverse process Rudimentary C7 rib	Cervical—may require surgical removal for compression of brachial plexus or subclavian artery Prevention—folic acid supplements during pregnancy Fetal intervention—minimizing nerve damage
Spina bifida	Cervical, thoracic, or lumbar/sacral spine	Splitting of bony neural canal CT/MRI—soft tissue posterior mass with or without spinal cord and nerve roots US—fetal demonstration of location and severity of pathophysiology	Nonfusion requires no treatment Myelomeningocele is removed surgically
Osteopetrosis	Entire skeleton	Generalized increased bone density	No efficacious treatment Medications to increase bone resorption Possible transplant—bone marrow or osteoclastic precursors
Osteogenesis imperfecta	Long bones	Pathologic fracture, very thin cortical density	Fracture alignment External fixation—casting or braces Internal fixation—extension rods for long-bone support to reduce deformities Medications to reduce osteoclastic formation Stem cell transplants are on the horizon
Achondroplasia	Vertebrae (short stature), long bones	Progressive interpedicular distance from superior to inferior, and scalloping of posterior vertebral bodies Widened metaphysis (Erlenmeyer flask deformity) CT—demonstrates spinal narrowing due to spondylosis and vertebral column changes	Nonspecific Growth hormone therapy (experimental)
Hip dysplasia	Incomplete acetabulum formation	AP and Cleaves view of pelvis to demonstrate superior and posterior dislocation US—sonolucent femoral head in relationship to acetabulum (angle determination)	Immobilization by a harness or casting

US, Ultrasound.

normal with only a slightly larger joint space. On the bilateral Cleaves view, the hip is usually dislocated superiorly and posteriorly. Because the children will have a multitude of follow-up images to recheck development, it is very important to shield the gonadal anatomy.

Sonography now provides an alternative imaging method. The sonolucent femoral head can be viewed in relationship to the acetabulum to demonstrate the femoral angles. Previously, clinicians relied on two different x-ray projections.

Treatment

Treatment depends upon the type of femoral head movement: subluxation or dislocation. Children not diagnosed and treated before walking may appear to "waddle like a duck." Immobilization of the femoral head is the most common treatment. To accomplish this, a harness or pelvic cast is used. This allows the acetabulum to continue to form correctly before the infant begins to walk.

Inflammatory and Infectious Disorders

Rheumatoid Arthritis

Rheumatoid arthritis is a chronic systemic disease of unknown cause that appears primarily as a nonsuppurative (noninfectious) inflammatory arthritis of the small joints of the hands and feet. Women are affected about three times more frequently than men, and the average age of onset in adults is 40 years. Rheumatoid arthritis usually has an insidious origin and may either run a protracted and progressive course, leading to a crippling deformity of affected joints, or undergo spontaneous remissions of variable length. There is usually symmetric involvement of multiple joints, and the disease often progresses proximally toward the trunk until practically every joint in the body is involved.

Rheumatoid arthritis begins as an inflammation of the synovial membrane (synovitis) that lines the joints. The excessive exudate, a result of the inflammation, causes proliferation of the synovium. The resulting mass of thickened granulation tissue (pannus, meaning "covers like a sheet") causes erosion of the articular cartilage and underlying bony cortex, fibrous scarring, and even the development of ankylosis (bony fusion across a joint). The erosion occurs because the inflammatory cells produce lytic enzymes. A combination of the fusion of joint surfaces and an inflammatory laxity of ligaments leads to the development of crippling deformities in the end stage of the disease (Figure 4-12).

Radiographic Appearance

The earliest radiographic evidence of rheumatoid arthritis is fusiform periarticular soft tissue swelling caused by joint effusion and hyperplastic synovial inflammation. Disuse and local hyperemia (increased blood flow) lead to periarticular osteoporosis that initially is confined to the portion of bone adjacent to the joint but may extend to involve the entire bone (Figure 4-13). Extension of the pannus from the synovial reflections onto the bone causes characteristic small foci of destruction at the edges of the joint, where articular cartilage is absent. These typical marginal erosions have poorly defined edges without a sclerotic rim and sometimes may be seen only on oblique or magnification views. Destruction of articular cartilage causes narrowing of the joint space. The laying down of bony trabeculae across a narrow joint space may completely obliterate the joint cavity

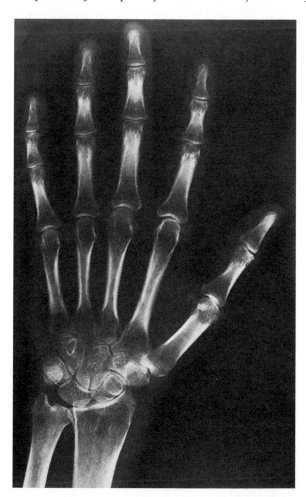

FIGURE 4-13 Rheumatoid arthritis. Striking periarticular osteoporosis.

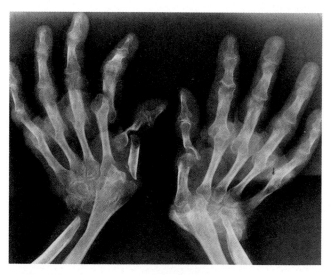

FIGURE 4-12 Mutilating rheumatoid arthritis. Severe, bilaterally symmetric destructive changes of hands and wrists with striking subluxations.

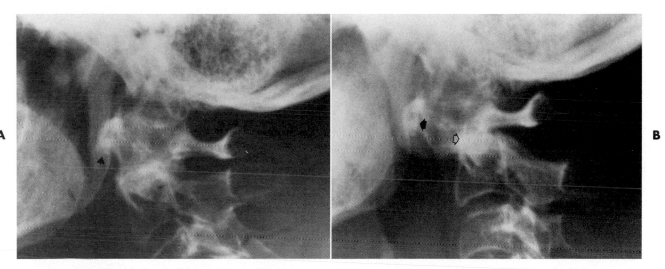

A

B

FIGURE 4-14 Subluxation of atlantoaxial joint in rheumatoid arthritis. **A,** Routine lateral film of cervical spine shows normal relationship between anterior border of odontoid process and superior portion of anterior arch of atlas *(arrowhead)*. **B,** With flexion, there is wide separation between the anterior arch of atlas *(solid arrow)* and the odontoid *(open arrow)*.

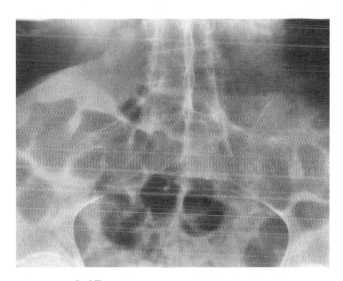

FIGURE 4-15 Ankylosing spondylitis. Bilateral, symmetric obliteration of sacroiliac joints and "bamboo spine."

and produce solid bony ankylosis, which most frequently involves the bones of the wrist.

Ligamentous involvement produces a variety of contractures and subluxations causing the common ulnar deviation of the hands. In the cervical spine, rheumatoid arthritis characteristically produces atlantoaxial subluxation (Figure 4-14), an increased distance between the anterior border of the odontoid and the superior border of the anterior arch of the atlas (normally less than 2.5 mm), which results from weakening of the transverse ligaments from synovial inflammation. The synovial inflammation appears as a soft tissue mass that causes a narrowing of the atlantoaxial articulation on CT images. CT

also demonstrates associated erosion of the odontoid (in about two thirds of patients).

Rheumatoid nodules are soft tissue masses that usually appear over the extensor surfaces on the ulnar aspect of the wrist or the olecranon, but occasionally are seen over other body prominences, tendons, or pressure points. These characteristic nodules, which develop in about 20% of patients with rheumatoid arthritis and do not occur in other diseases, aid in making the diagnosis.

Rheumatoid Variants: Ankylosing Spondylitis, Reiter's Syndrome, and Psoriatic Arthritis
Radiographic Appearance of Ankylosing Spondylitis

Ankylosing spondylitis almost always begins in the sacroiliac joints, causing bilateral and usually symmetric involvement. Blurring of the articular margins and patchy sclerosis generally progress to narrowing of the joint space and may lead to complete fibrous and bony ankylosis (Figure 4-15). The disease typically progresses from the lumbar spine upward.

Ossification in the paravertebral tissues and longitudinal spinal ligaments (poker spine) combines with extensive lateral bony bridges (syndesmophytes) between vertebral bodies to produce the characteristic "bamboo spine" of advanced disease (Figure 4-16, and see Figure 4-15). Limitation of activity leads to generalized skeletal osteoporosis and a tendency to fracture in response to the stress of minor trauma (Figure 4-17). CT demonstrates the fusion as a result of the intraarticular and ligamentous ossification, and any spinal stenosis caused by the displacement of the fractures.

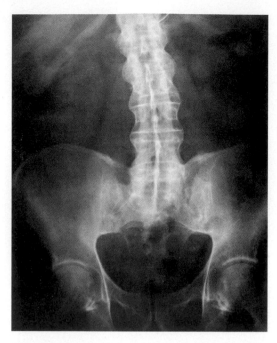

FIGURE 4-16 Lumbar spine. Severe vertebral fusion illustrates "bamboo spine."

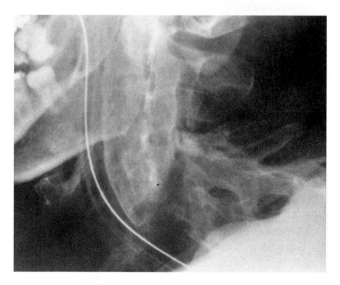

FIGURE 4-17 Ankylosing spondylitis. Oblique fracture of midcervical spine with anterior dislocation of superior segment is seen in patient who fell while dancing and struck his head. Fracture extends through lateral mass and lamina.

Radiographic Appearance of Reiter's Syndrome

Reiter's syndrome (reactive arthritis) is characterized by arthritis, urethritis, and conjunctivitis. It primarily affects young adult men and appears to occur after certain types of venereal or gastrointestinal infections. Reiter's syndrome most frequently involves the sacroiliac joints, heel, and toes (Figure 4-18). Unlike in ankylosing spondylitis, the sacroiliac involvement here is

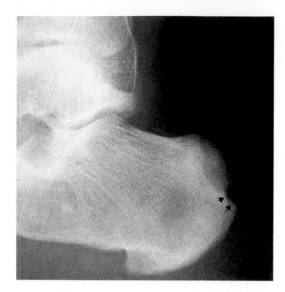

FIGURE 4-18 Reiter's syndrome. Striking bony erosion *(arrows)* at insertion of Achilles tendon on posterosuperior margin of calcaneus.

usually bilateral but asymmetric, and Reiter's syndrome tends to cause only minimal changes in the spine.

Although the radiographic changes in peripheral joints often mimic rheumatoid arthritis, Reiter's syndrome tends to be asymmetric and primarily involves the feet rather than the hands (Figure 4-19).

Radiographic Appearance of Psoriatic Arthritis

Psoriatic arthritis refers to a rheumatoid-like destructive process involving peripheral joints that develops in patients with typical skin changes of psoriasis (Figure 4-20). Unlike rheumatoid arthritis, psoriatic arthritis predominantly involves the distal rather than the proximal interphalangeal joints of the hands and feet, produces asymmetric rather than symmetric destruction, and causes little or no periarticular osteoporosis.

Characteristic findings include bony ankylosis of the interphalangeal joints of the hands and feet and resorption of the terminal tufts of the distal phalanges (Figure 4-21). Common characteristics of Reiter's syndrome and psoriatic arthritis include erosions and hypertrophic changes occurring in the origin and insertion of the tendons and ligaments.

Osteoarthritis (Degenerative Joint Disease)

Osteoarthritis is an extremely common generalized disorder characterized pathologically by loss of joint cartilage and reactive new bone formation. Part of the wear and tear of the aging process, degenerative joint disease tends to predominantly affect the weight-bearing

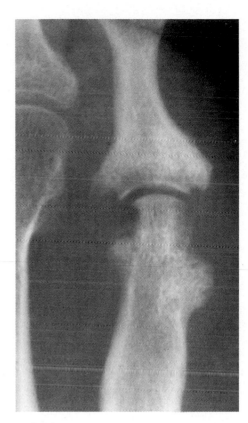

FIGURE 4-19 Reiter's syndrome. Erosive changes about the metatarsophalangeal joint of the fifth digit. Erosions involve juxtaarticular region, leaving articular cortex intact.

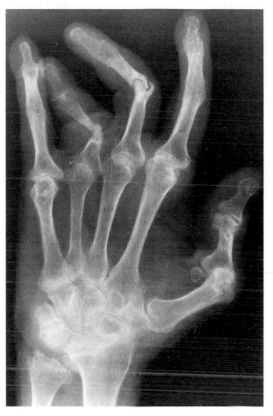

FIGURE 4-20 Psoriatic arthritis. Bizarre pattern of asymmetric bone destruction, subluxation, and ankylosis. Notice the particularly severe pencil-in-cup deformity of third proximal interphalangeal joint, and the bony ankylosis involving wrist and phalanges of second and fifth digits.

joints (spine, hip, knee, ankle) and the interphalangeal joints of the fingers. A secondary form of degenerative joint disease may develop in a joint that has been repeatedly traumatized or subjected to abnormal stresses because of orthopedic deformities, or it may be a result of a septic or inflammatory arthritis that destroys cartilage.

Radiographic Appearance

The earliest radiographic findings in degenerative joint disease are narrowing of the joint space, caused by thinning of the articular cartilage, and development of small bony spurs (osteophytes) along the margins of the articular edges of the bones. In contrast to the smooth, even narrowing of the joint space in rheumatoid arthritis, the joint space narrowing in degenerative joint disease is irregular and more pronounced in that part of the joint where weight-bearing stress is greatest and where degeneration of the articular cartilage is most noticeable. The articular ends of the bones become increasingly dense (periarticular sclerosis). Erosion of the articular cortex may produce typical irregular, cyst-like lesions with sclerotic margins in the subchondral bone near the joint. Calcific or ossified loose bodies may develop, especially at the

knee. With advanced disease, relaxation of the joint capsule and other ligamentous structures may lead to subluxation. Local osteoporosis does not occur unless pain causes prolonged disuse of the joint.

In the fingers, degenerative joint disease involves primarily the distal interphalangeal joints (Figure 4-22). Marginal spurs produce well-defined bony protuberances that appear clinically as the palpable and visible knobby thickening of Heberden's nodes. In the hip, the most prominent finding is asymmetric narrowing of the joint space that involves predominantly the superior and lateral aspects of the joint, where the greatest stress of weight bearing exists (Figure 4-23). Joint space narrowing is also asymmetric in the knee, where it predominantly involves the medial femorotibial compartment (Figure 4-24).

Infectious Arthritis

Pyogenic (pus-forming) organisms may gain entry into a joint by the hematogenous route, by direct extension from an adjacent focus of osteomyelitis, or from trauma to the joint (e.g., after surgery or needling). The onset of bacterial arthritis usually

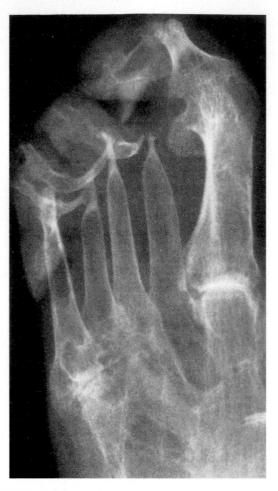

FIGURE 4-21 Psoriatic arthritis. Severe mutilating arthritis of foot and ankle. There is extreme pencil-like destruction of metatarsals and phalanges, with ankylosis of almost all tarsal joints.

presents abruptly with a high fever, shaking chills, and one or a few severely tender and swollen joints. The most common type today is a migratory arthritis from Lyme disease.

Radiographic Appearance

Soft tissue swelling is the first radiographic sign of acute bacterial arthritis. In children, fluid distention of the joint capsule may cause widening of the joint space and actual subluxation, especially about the hip and shoulder. Periarticular edema displaces or obliterates adjacent tissue fat planes (Figure 4-25, *A*). Rapid destruction of articular cartilage causes joint space narrowing early in the course of the disease. The earliest bone changes, which tend to appear 8 to 10 days after the onset of symptoms, are small focal erosions in the articular cortex. Because of the delay in bone changes, detection of the characteristic soft tissue abnormalities is essential for early diagnosis.

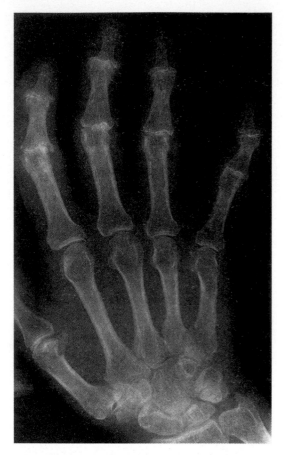

FIGURE 4-22 Osteoarthritis of fingers. Note narrowing of interphalangeal joints with spurring and erosions.

Severe, untreated infections cause extensive destruction and a loss of the entire cortical outline (Figure 4-25). With healing, sclerotic bone reaction results in an irregular articular surface. If the articular cartilage has been completely destroyed, bony ankylosis usually follows.

Radiographic Appearance of Tuberculous Arthritis

Tuberculous arthritis is a chronic, indolent (organic) infection that has an insidious (gradual) onset and a slowly progressive course (Figure 4-26). It usually involves only one joint, and it affects primarily the spine, hips, and knees. Most patients have a focus of tuberculosis elsewhere in the body, most commonly in the lungs.

A distinctive early radiographic feature of tuberculous arthritis is the extensive juxtaarticular (near a joint) osteoporosis that precedes bone destruction; this is in contrast to bacterial arthritis, in which osteoporosis is a relatively late finding. Joint effusion leads to a nonspecific periarticular soft tissue swelling. Cartilage and bone destruction occur relatively

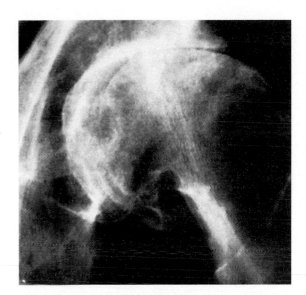

FIGURE 4-23 Osteoarthritis of the hip.

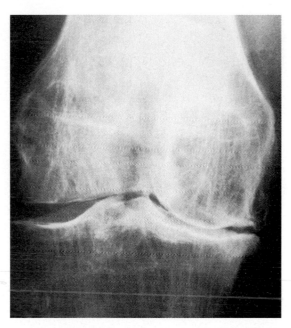

FIGURE 4-24 Osteoarthritis of the knee.

late in the course of tuberculous arthritis and tend to initially involve the periphery of the joint, sparing the maximal weight-bearing surfaces that are destroyed in pyogenic arthritis. Therefore, joint space narrowing occurs late in tuberculous arthritis in contrast to the early narrowing with bacterial infections. As in pyogenic arthritis, the earliest evidence of bone destruction is usually erosion at the margins of the articular ends of bone. With progressive disease, there is ragged destruction of the articular cartilage and subchondral cortex and disorganization of the joint, often with preservation of necrotic fragments of bone (sequestra) that may involve opposing surfaces ("kissing sequestra").

Treatment of Arthritis

Arthritis therapy should protect affected joints, maintain mobility, and strengthen muscles. For this to occur, lifestyle changes, use of support devices, drugs, and surgery may be necessary. For those with rheumatoid arthritis and osteoarthritis, which make up 90% of all cases diagnosed, rest and exercise are recommended to minimize inflammation and preserve the range of motion. The first-line medications are nonsteroidal antiinflammatory drugs (NSAIDs), which decrease the inflammatory response but do not affect the disease process. Prostaglandin inhibitors, such as aspirin and ibuprofen (salicylates), fall into this category of drugs that reduce the triggering of inflammation. A more aggressive group of drugs, disease-modifying antirheumatic drugs, are used in advanced stages to reduce symptoms. The antimetabolite methotrexate, a cytoxic drug, tempers cell division in the synovial joint. Invasive surgery includes replacing joints with new artificial joints

(Figure 4-27) to increase joint mobility. For infectious arthritis, antibiotics usually eradicate the infection and cure the arthritis. Aspiration may be needed if fluid accumulates in the bursa.

Bursitis

Bursitis refers to an inflammation of the bursae, small fluid-filled sacs located near the joints that reduce the friction caused by movement. Repeated physical activity commonly causes bursitis, but trauma, rheumatoid arthritis, gout, or infections also can cause this inflammation. Bursitis or tenosynovitis is usually not visualized on plain radiographs, but disorders of the bursa and synovium can be seen on ultrasound images (Figure 4-28). Plain films may exclude other disorders that cause similar symptoms.

Radiographic Appearance

The major radiographic manifestation of bursitis is the deposition of calcification in adjacent tendons, which is a common cause of pain, limitation of motion (frozen joints), and disability about a joint. Calcific tendinitis most commonly involves the shoulder, and calcification may be demonstrated radiographically in about half the patients with persistent pain and disability in the shoulder region (Figure 4-29). However, calcification may also be detected in asymptomatic persons, and severe clinical symptoms may occur without evidence of calcification. Calcific tendinitis appears as amorphous calcium deposits that most frequently occur about the shoulder in the supraspinatus tendon, where they are seen directly above the

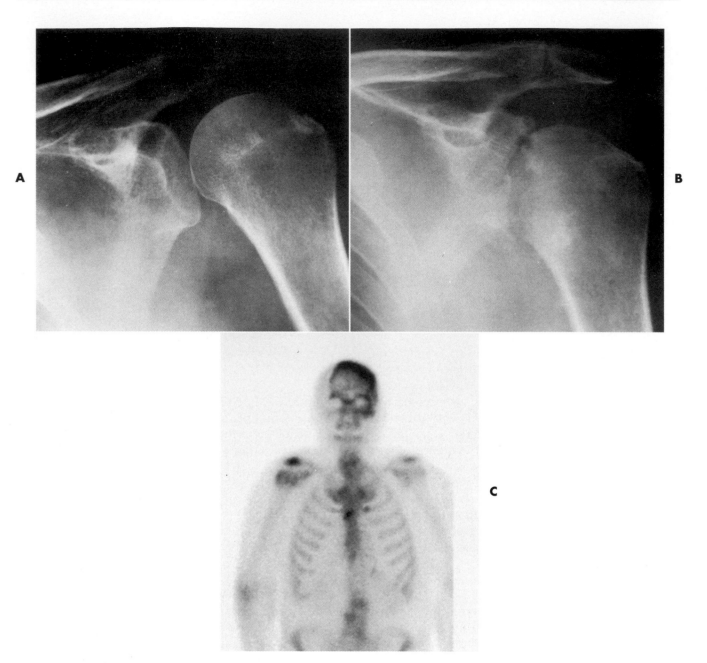

FIGURE 4-25 Acute staphylococcal arthritis. **A,** Several days after instrumentation of shoulder for joint pain, there is separation of humeral head from glenoid fossa caused by fluid in joint space. **B,** Six weeks later, pronounced cartilage and bone destruction are evident, with sclerosis on both sides of the glenohumeral joint. **C,** Septic arthritis. On a radionuclide bone scan, a focal area of increased activity in the right shoulder correlates with the clinical history of septic arthritis.

greater tuberosity of the humerus. The deposits vary greatly in size and shape, from thin curvilinear densities to large calcific masses.

In the acute early stages of bursitis, sonography demonstrates the bursa filled with synovial fluid having ill-defined margins. In true tendonitis, during the acute phase the thickened tendon has ill-defined margins. Both bursitis and tendonitis may demonstrate increased vascularity on Doppler ultrasound.

Treatment
First-line treatments for bursitis include application of heat, rest, and immobilization. NSAIDs are taken to reduce inflammation and relieve pain, as necessary. If the inflammation results from an infection, a regimen of antibiotics is appropriate. In recurring or severe bursitis, corticosteroid injections into the affected bursa may reduce the inflammation.

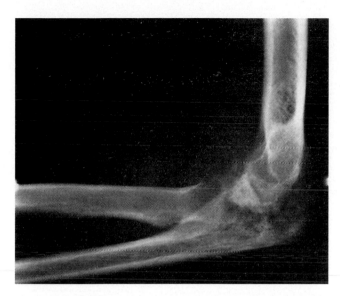

FIGURE 4-26 Tuberculous arthritis of the elbow with complete destruction of the joint space. A large chronic granulomatous mass can be seen in the antecubital region.

Rotator Cuff Tears

The rotator cuff of the shoulder is a musculotendinous structure composed of the teres minor, infraspinatus, supraspinatus, and subscapularis muscles. Rupture of the rotator cuff produces a communication between the shoulder joint and the subacromial bursa that can be demonstrated by arthrography (the injection of contrast material directly into the shoulder joint) (Figure 4-30). Currently, MRI is considered the modality of choice for demonstrating a rotator cuff disorder. The normal rotator cuff appears as a black structure, but tears cause it to have high signal intensity (Figure 4-31). However, ultrasound may be the preferred initial modality to demonstrate the tear of the tendon (Figure 4-32) because of its wider availability and lower cost.

Tears of the Menisci of the Knee

Meniscal tears are a common cause of knee pain. Although occasionally the result of acute trauma, meniscal tears more frequently reflect a degenerative process caused by the chronic trauma inherent in human knee function. In the past, meniscal tears were best demonstrated by arthrography, which is invasive; now, MRI is clearly the imaging modality of choice, as it is noninvasive and has an accuracy of 90% to 98%.

MRI demonstrates a tear as a sharply marginated line of high signal intensity (Figure 4-33) that crosses the normally dark, triangular meniscus. In addition, this modality can show the often-associated tears of the anterior and posterior cruciate ligaments and changes in the underlying bone. Ultrasound may

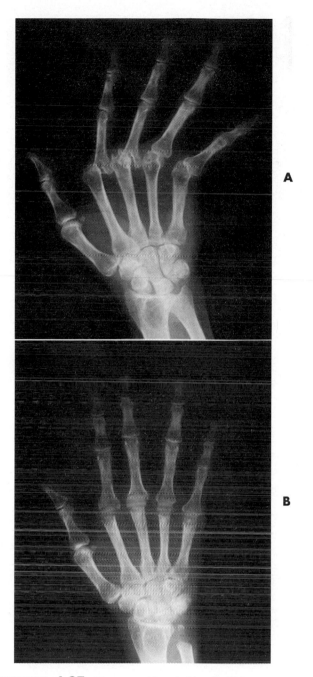

FIGURE 4-27 Rheumatoid arthritis. **A,** This posteroanterior image of the hand demonstrates dislocation and joint destruction of the second through fifth metacarpophalangeal joints. **B,** Postoperative image, with digits fully extended, illustrates joint implants.

demonstrate tenosynovitis of related tendons, which appears as a thickened synovial sheath (Figure 4-34).

Treatment for Intraarticular Components

Antiinflammatory medications and immobilization of the joint are the first line of treatment if the damage will repair itself. When the component is not completely destroyed, this treatment may result in cure (30% to 90%

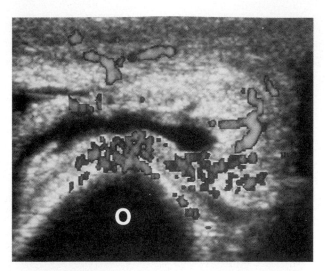

FIGURE **4-28** Bursitis. Transverse scan of the posterior aspect of the elbow shows the thick-walled, fluid-containing olecranon bursa. Power-mode color Doppler imaging shows the bursa's activity.

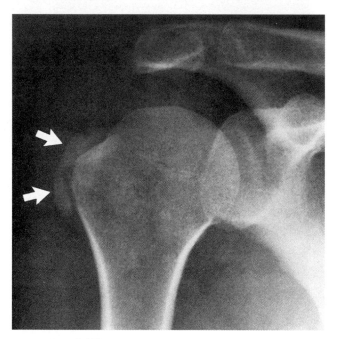

FIGURE **4-29** Calcific tendinitis. Frontal projection of shoulder demonstrates amorphous calcium deposits *(arrows)* in supraspinatus tendon.

of patients respond to nonsurgical treatment). When irreparable joint damage has occurred, the orthopedist performs arthroscopic surgery to remove a complete or nonhealing tear, or to attempt suture repair.

Bacterial Osteomyelitis

Bacterial osteomyelitis is an inflammation of the bone (osteitis) and bone marrow (myelitis) caused by a broad spectrum of infectious (most often gram-positive) organisms that reach bone by hematogenous

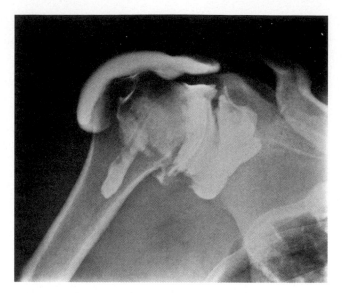

FIGURE **4-30** Shoulder arthrography of rotator cuff tear. Opacification of subacromial and subdeltoid bursae indicates abnormal communication between them and the glenohumeral joint cavity, thus confirming the diagnosis.

spread, by extension from an adjacent site of infection, or by direct introduction of organisms (after trauma or surgery). Acute hematogenous osteomyelitis tends to involve bones with rich red marrow. In infants and children, the metaphyses of long bones, especially the femur and tibia, are most often affected; staphylococci and streptococci are the most common organisms. Patients with acute osteomyelitis experience fever and localized warmth, swelling, and tenderness. In adults, acute hematogenous osteomyelitis primarily occurs in the vertebrae, causing localized back pain and muscle spasm, and it rarely involves the long bones. Although the incidence and severity of osteomyelitis have decreased since the advent of antibiotics, this disease has recently become more prevalent as a complication of intravenous drug abuse (in which case, gram-negative organisms are found). In diabetic patients and those with other types of vascular insufficiency, a soft tissue infection may spread from a skin abscess or a decubitus ulcer, usually in the foot, to cause cellulitis and eventually osteomyelitis in adjacent bones.

Osteomyelitis begins as an abscess of the bone. Pus produced by the acute inflammation spreads down the medullary cavity and outward to the surface. Once the infectious process has reached the outer margin of the bone, it raises the periosteum from the bone and may spread along the surface for a considerable distance.

Because the earliest changes of osteomyelitis are usually not evident on plain radiographs until about 10 days after the onset of symptoms, radionuclide

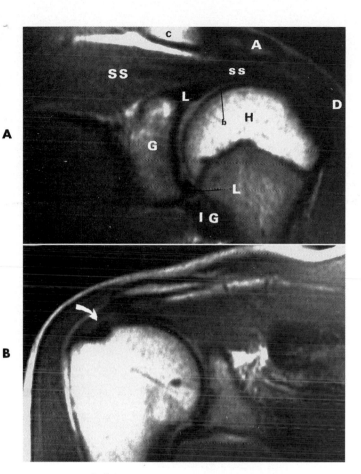

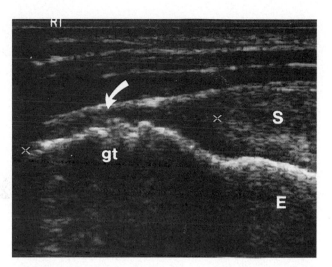

FIGURE **4-32** Horizontal full-thickness tear. The longitudinal ultrasound image through the supraspinatus tendons, *S*, shows 2-cm retraction of the torn tendon (the distance between the calipers [x]). Bursa and peribursal fat *(curved arrow)* rest directly on the irregular bone surface of the greater tuberosity *(gt)*. *E,* Humeral epiphysis.

FIGURE **4-31** MR image of rotator cuff tear. **A,** Normal shoulder. Notice the low signal intensity of the supraspinatus tendon *(ss)*. *A,* Acromion; *C,* clavicle; *D,* deltoid muscle; *G,* glenoid fossa; *H,* humeral head; *IG,* inferior glenohumeral ligament; *L,* glenoid labrum. **B,** Degenerative tear. A high signal intensity *(arrow)* can be seen within the rotator cuff.

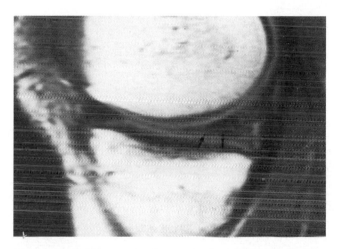

FIGURE **4-33** Meniscal tear. Sagittal MR scan of knee shows horizontal line of high signal intensity *(arrows)* crossing dark posterior horn of medial meniscus.

(gallium) bone scanning is the most valuable imaging modality for the early diagnosis of osteomyelitis. Increased nuclide uptake, reflecting the inflammatory process and increased blood flow, is evident within hours of the onset of symptoms (Figure 4-35).

Radiographic Appearance

On plain radiographs, the earliest evidence of osteomyelitis in a long bone is a localized, deep soft tissue swelling adjacent to the metaphysis. The inflammation causes displacement or obliteration of the normal fat planes adjacent to and between the deep muscle bundles, unlike in skin infections, where the initial swelling is superficial. The initial bony change appears as subtle areas of metaphyseal lucency reflecting resorption of necrotic bone. Soon, bone destruction becomes more prominent, producing a ragged, moth-eaten appearance (Figures 4-36 and 4-37). The more virulent the organism, the larger is the area of

destruction. Subperiosteal spread of inflammation elevates the periosteum and stimulates the deposition of layers of new bone parallel to the shaft. This results in a layered periosteal reaction that is characteristic of benign diseases, especially infection. Eventually, a large amount of new bone surrounds the cortex in a thick, irregular bony sleeve (involucrum). Disruption of cortical blood supply leads to bone necrosis. Segments of avascular dead bone (sequestra) remain as dense as normal bone and are clearly differentiated from the demineralized bone, infected granulation tissue, and pus around them (Figure 4-38). Power

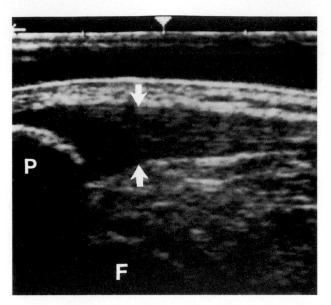

FIGURE 4-34 Acute patellar tendinitis. Longitudinal ultrasound scan shows thickening and decreased echogenicity of the upper two thirds of the tendon *(arrows)*. *F,* Femoral condyle; *P,* patella.

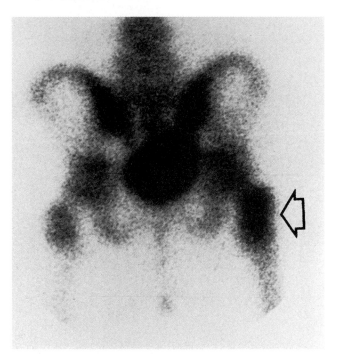

FIGURE 4-35 Osteomyelitis. Radionuclide bone scan (posterior projection) demonstrates increased uptake of radionuclide in trochanteric portion of right femur *(arrow)*. Plain film of pelvis and hips obtained at the same time showed no detectable abnormality.

Doppler ultrasound demonstrates increased vascularity in the inflammation elevating the periosteum.

After the acute infection has subsided, a pattern of chronic osteomyelitis develops. The bone appears thickened and sclerotic with an irregular outer

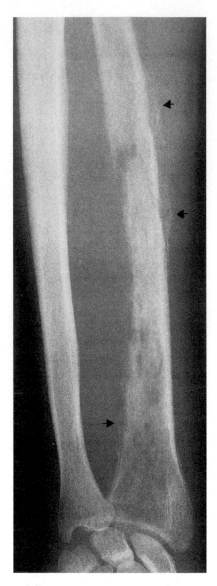

FIGURE 4-36 Osteomyelitis. Patchy pattern of bone destruction involves much of the shaft of the radius. Notice early periosteal new bone formation *(arrows)*.

margin. The cortex may become so dense that the medullary cavity is difficult to demonstrate. Reactivation of infection may appear as the recurrence of deep soft tissue swelling or periosteal calcification, or the development of lytic abscess cavities within the bone. However, plain radiographs are often inadequate to determine whether an active infection is present. Radionuclide scanning is much more sensitive and accurate for establishing recurrence.

The earliest sign of vertebral osteomyelitis is subtle erosion of the subchondral bony plate with loss of the sharp cortical outline. This may progress to total destruction of the vertebral body associated with a paravertebral soft tissue abscess (Figure 4-39). Unlike neoplastic processes, osteomyelitis usually affects the

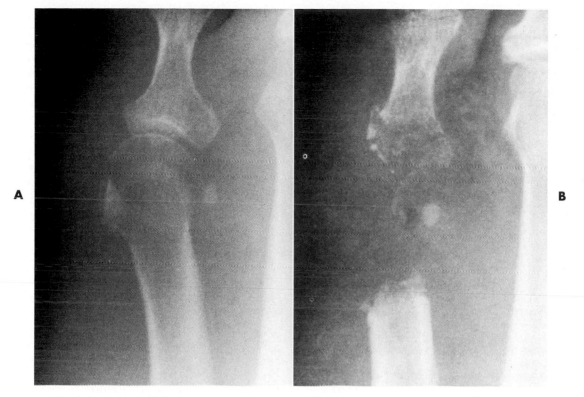

FIGURE 4-37 Staphylococcal osteomyelitis. **A,** Initial film of first metatarsophalangeal joint shows soft tissue swelling and periarticular demineralization caused by increased blood flow to region. **B,** Several weeks later, severe bony destruction about metatarsophalangeal joint can be seen.

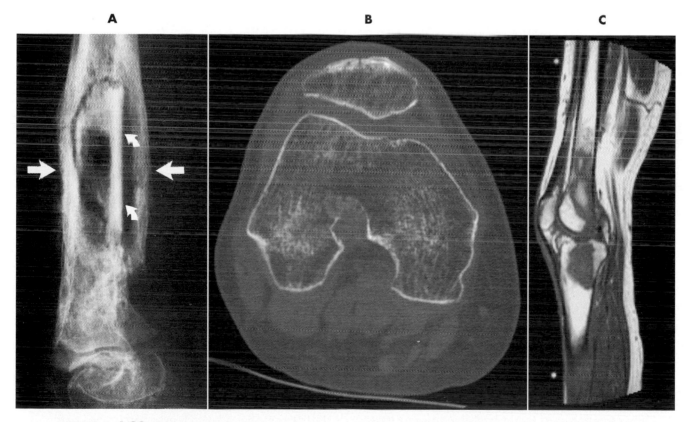

FIGURE 4-38 Chronic osteomyelitis. **A,** Involucrum *(straight arrows)* surrounds sequestra *(curved arrows).* **B,** After knee surgery, multiple foci can be seen to be lacking trabeculation in both femoral condyles in this 33-year-old woman. **C,** Sagittal MRI on the patient in **B** shows decreased signal intensity from the femoral condyle extending into the femoral shaft.

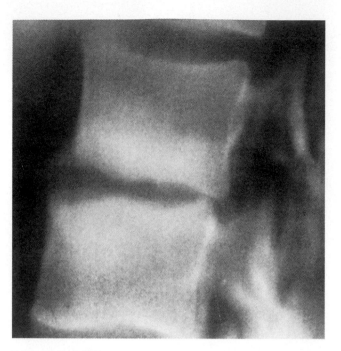

FIGURE 4-39 Bacterial vertebral osteomyelitis. Narrowing of intervertebral disk space with irregularity of end plates and reactive sclerosis.

intervertebral disk space and often involves adjacent vertebrae. Depending on the site of disease, anterior extension of osteomyelitis may cause retropharyngeal abscess, mediastinitis, empyema, pericarditis, subdiaphragmatic abscess, psoas muscle abscess, or peritonitis; posterior extension of inflammatory tissue can compress the spinal cord or produce meningitis if the infection penetrates the dura to enter the subarachnoid space.

CT can be of value in the diagnosis of osteomyelitis, especially that involving the spine. This modality can precisely define the size of the surrounding soft tissue mass, its relation to nearby vital structures (aorta, spinal cord), and the presence of abscess cavities requiring surgical drainage (see Figure 4-38, *B*). In acute osteomyelitis of long bones, the bone destruction and periosteal reaction produce a thin laminated periosteal reaction.

MRI can assist in determining whether an abscess has formed and in excluding cellulitis. Bone marrow changes caused by inflammatory exudate result in decreased signal intensity on T1-weighted images and increased signal intensity on T2-weighted images (see Figure 4-38, *C*).

Treatment
Antibiotics to eradicate gram-negative or gram-positive organisms should be taken for 4 to 8 weeks to prevent recurrence. Surgery may be required for débridement of necrotic tissue or for placement of a drain into an abscess. Bone grafts, usually of bone marrow, are placed to fill bony defects or to help bones heal. After surgery, the patient must continue to take antibiotics for approximately 3 weeks.

Tuberculous Osteomyelitis
Tuberculous osteomyelitis (which is rare today) most commonly involves the thoracic and lumbar spine. **Pott's disease** (tuberculosis of the spine) occurs in the midthoracic spine and thoracolumbar region. Irregular, poorly marginated bone destruction within the vertebral body is often associated with a characteristic paravertebral abscess, an accumulation of purulent material that produces a fusiform soft tissue mass about the vertebra. The spread of tuberculous osteomyelitis causes narrowing of the adjacent intervertebral disk and the extension of infection and bone destruction across the disk to involve the adjacent vertebral body. Unlike bacterial infection, tuberculous osteomyelitis is rarely associated with periosteal reaction or bone sclerosis.

Radiographic Appearance
The infection tends to begin in the anterior part of the vertebral body adjacent to the intervertebral disk (Figure 4-40, *A*). Caseous necrosis of the vertebral marrow produces a slow resorption of bony trabeculae, with bone destruction appearing 2 to 5 months after onset of infection. In the untreated patient, progressive vertebral collapse and anterior wedging lead to a characteristic sharp kyphotic angulation (gibbous deformity) (Figure 4-40, *B*). A radionuclide bone scan may demonstrate early activity, but cannot distinguish tumors or fractures. The gallium bone scan can help to define the total tissue involvement and determine response to therapy in tuberculous osteomyelitis. CT also may delineate the extent of soft tissue involvement and illustrate osseous destruction. Soft tissue calcifications identified on CT aid in distinguishing tuberculous osteomyelitis from other conditions. MRI scans demonstrate changes in the bone marrow, but are no more specific than the radionuclide bone scans.

Tuberculosis can, rarely, involve a low-grade chronic infection of the long bones that appears radiographically as a generally destructive lytic process with minimal or no periosteal reaction. The spectrum of radiographic appearances is wide, varying from localized, well-circumscribed, expansile lesions to diffuse, uniform, honeycomb-like areas of destruction that are often associated with pathologic fractures. Chronic draining sinuses may develop, especially in children.

SUMMARY of FINDINGS for Inflammatory and Infectious Disorders

disorder	location	radiographic appearance	treatment
Rheumatoid arthritis (ankylosing spondylitis, Reiter's syndrome, psoriatic arthritis)	Small joints symmetrically	All rheumatoid variants • Periarticular soft tissue swelling • Symmetric joint destruction and deformity RA—CT synovial inflammation (soft tissue mass) causes narrowing of atlantoaxial articulation Ankylosing spondylitis CT—fusion due to intraarticular and ligament ossification and spinal stenosis	NSAIDs Surgery is last resort Possible joint implants or replacements
Osteoarthritis	Weight-bearing joints	Irregular narrowing of joint space with small bony spurs (steophytes)	NSAIDs (timed release and coated)
Infectious arthritis	Any joint	Early joint narrowing with focal erosions	Antibiotics
Bursitis	Shoulder most common	Radiograph—calcific tendinitis in 50% US—thickened synovium or dense synovial fluid	Immobilization, heat, rest NSAIDs Antibiotics if infection related Corticosteroid injection for recurring incidences
Rotator cuff tear	Shoulder	US—tear in bursa and inflamed synovium	Nonsurgical: physical therapy, immobilization, and NSAIDs
Meniscal tear of the knee	Knee	MRI—tears have a high signal intensity (normal—black)	Surgery: rotator cuff repair or meniscus removal
Bacterial osteomyelitis	Child—long bones high in red marrow Adult—vertebra or bone associated with decubitus ulcer	Radiograph—soft tissue swelling with periosteal elevation Doppler US soft tissue vascularity elevating periosteum NM—bone scan most accurate at localizing process and recurrence CT—defines tissue involvement and thin laminated periosteal reaction MRI—demonstrates changes in bone marrow signal intensity	Antibiotics first-line treatment Surgery for débridement
Tuberculous osteomyelitis	Vertebra (Pott's disease)— thoracic and lumbar most common	Lytic lesion without periosteal elevation Collapsed vertebra with kyphosis	Nonoperative: antibiotics, antituberculous drug therapy, and bracing Surgical: spinal fusion and Harrington rod placement for stability

RA, Reumatoid arthritis; *US,* ultrasound; *NM,* nuclear medicine.

Treatment

Nonoperative treatments for tuberculous osteomyelitis include a regimen of antibiotics, antituberculous drug therapy, and possible bracing. Antibiotics help prevent abscess development, antituberculous drug therapy eradicates the tuberculosis bacilli, and bracing provides support. With this treatment combination, most patients do not require surgery. If the pain, neurologic deficits, and deformities progress, surgical intervention may be necessary. Spinal fusion or Harrington rod placement for stability may be performed.

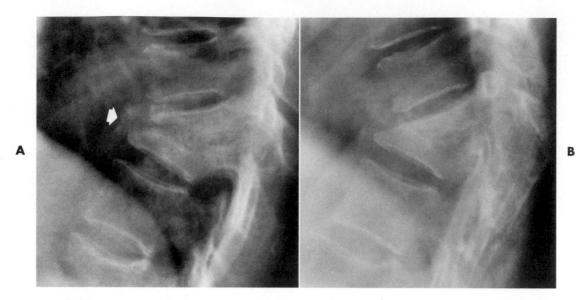

FIGURE 4-40 Tuberculous osteomyelitis. **A,** Initial film demonstrates vertebral collapse and anterior wedging of adjacent midthoracic vertebrae *(arrow)*. Residual intervertebral disk space can barely be seen. **B,** Several months later there is virtual fusion of collapsed vertebral bodies, producing characteristic sharp kyphotic angulation (gibbous deformity).

Metabolic Bone Disease

Osteoporosis

Osteoporosis is a generalized or localized deficiency of bone matrix in which the mass of bone per unit volume is decreased in amount but normal in composition. Bone is a living, constantly changing tissue, and normally a balance exists between the amount of old bone being removed (an osteoclastic process) and the amount of new bone replacement (an osteoblastic process). Osteoporosis is usually caused by accelerated resorption of bone, although decreased bone formation may lead to osteoporosis in some situations—for example, in Cushing's syndrome, after prolonged steroid administration, and after prolonged disuse or immobilization as in a casted extremity (Figure 4-41).

Loss of mineral salts causes osteoporotic bone to become more lucent than normal. This may be difficult to detect, because about 50% to 70% of the bone density must be lost before it can be demonstrated as a lucent area on routine radiographs. For patients with osteoporosis, it is essential to use the lowest practical kVp. This technique provides the extremely short scale of contrast necessary to visualize the demineralized osteoporotic bones. Today, quantitative CT (QCT), single-photon absorptiometry, and dual-energy x-ray absorptiometry (DEXA bone densitometry-qualitative) provide data that measure bone mineral content. A quantitative CT scan accurately demonstrates levels of bone mass

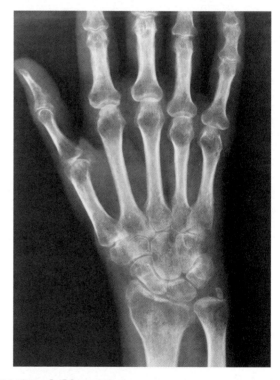

FIGURE 4-41 Disuse osteoporosis. Severe periarticular demineralization after prolonged immobilization of the hand.

and determines the rate of bone decay, which represents bone quantity. 3D-QCT is considered more sensitive and accurate than the other methods. QCT measurements are dependent on the trabecular bone, which demonstrates the earliest signs of osteoporosis. CT scans, because of their high radiation dose, are not

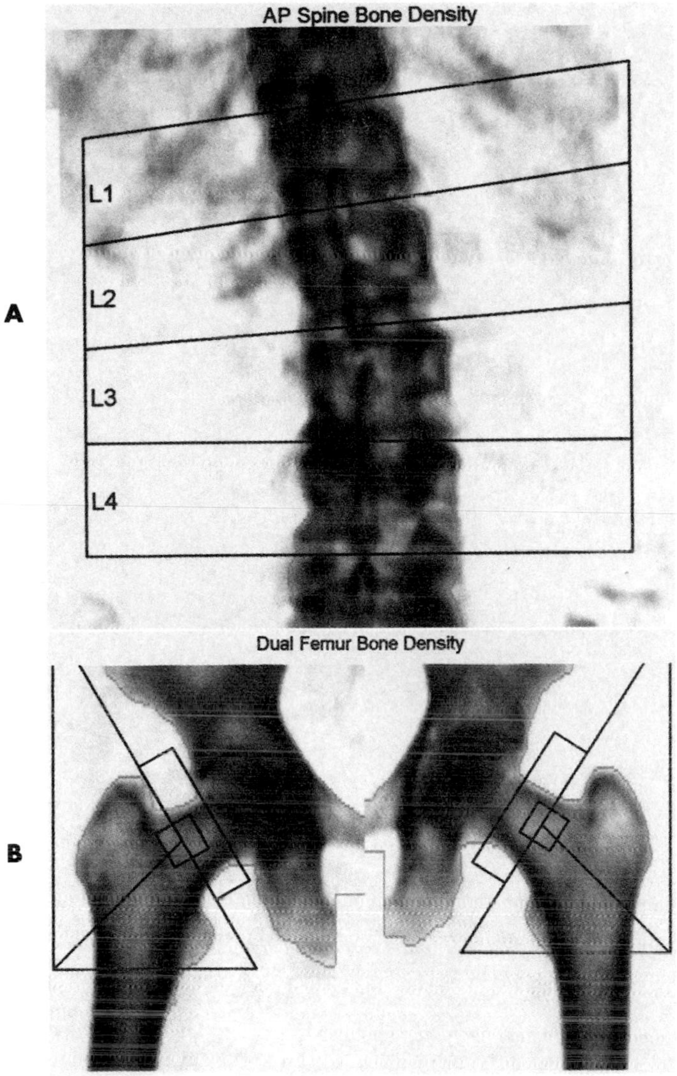

AP Spine Bone Density

A

L1

L2

L3

L4

Dual Femur Bone Density

B

FIGURE **4-42** Osteoporosis. Results of DEXA bone mineral density (BMD) of the spine. **A,** A T-score average of 3.3 demonstrates osteoporosis. **B,** The dual femur of this 65-year-old woman has a T-score average of 2.3, indicating osteopenia.

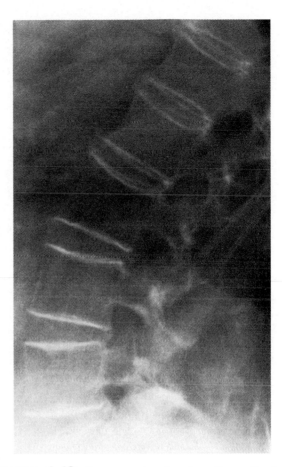

FIGURE **4-43** Osteoporosis of aging. Generalized demineralization of spine in postmenopausal woman. Cortex appears as a thin line that is relatively dense and prominent (picture-frame pattern).

done as frequently as bone densitometry. DEXA bone densitometry is used to image the hip and spine, assisting in determining bone quality. The patient's history is entered into the computer system and two images, usually an AP lumbar spine and an AP hip, are taken (Figure 4-42). The image data are compared with those of other individuals of the same race, age, and weight to determine a bone-quality value. This value indicates whether the patient has normal bone (T-score greater than −1.0 standard deviation [SD]), osteopenia (T-score between −1.0 and −2.5 SD), or osteoporosis (T-score less than −2.5 SD).

The major causes of generalized osteoporosis include aging and postmenopausal hormonal changes.

With increasing age, bones lose density and become more brittle, fracturing more easily and healing more slowly. Two factors contribute to this: elderly persons may become less active and they may have poor diets, often deficient in protein. In postmenopausal women, there is a deficiency in the gonadal hormonal levels that stimulate bone formation. This decreased bone formation plus an increase in bone resorption by a factor of three to five times results in a loss in density.

Radiographic Appearance

Regardless of the cause, the radiographic appearance is somewhat similar in all conditions producing osteoporosis. The most striking change is cortical thinning, with irregularity and resorption of the endosteal (inner) surfaces (Figure 4-43). These findings are most evident in the spine and pelvis. As the bone density of a vertebral body decreases, the cortex appears as a relatively dense and prominent thin line producing the typical picture frame pattern. Because

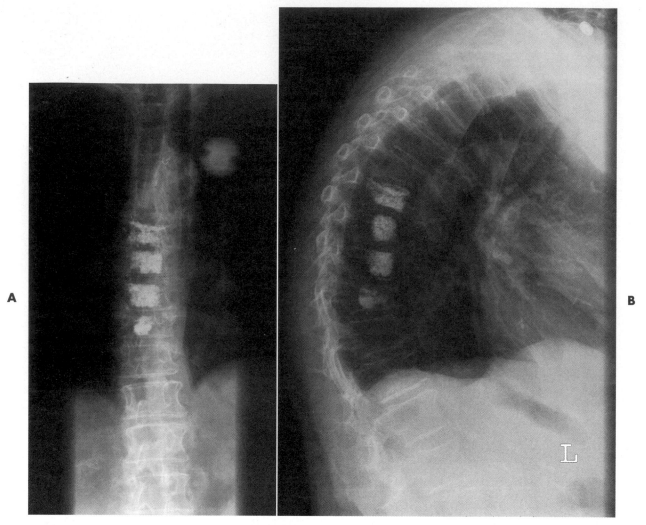

FIGURE 4-44 Thoracic vertebroplasty demonstrated on an 81-year-old female with osteoporosis to prevent vertebral collapse.

of the severe loss of bone density, anterior wedging or compression fractures of one or more vertebral bodies may result, most commonly in the middle and lower thoracic and upper lumbar areas. The intervertebral disk may expand into the weakened vertebral bodies and produce characteristic concave contours of the superior and inferior disk surfaces. In the skull, the calvaria may show a spotty loss of density, and there is commonly deossification (bone loss) of the floor of the sella turcica and dorsum sellae.

Treatment

To help prevent osteoporosis, weight-bearing exercises help build bone density and muscle mass. For postmenopausal osteoporosis, hormonal replacement therapy and dietary supplements of calcium and vitamin D may reduce development of the disease process. In severe cases, vertebroplasty (kyphoplasty) is done to prevent vertebral collapse (Figure 4-44).

Osteomalacia

Osteomalacia refers to insufficient mineralization of the adult skeleton. The lack of a balance between osteoid formation and mineralization influencing bone quality results in either excessive osteoid formation or, more frequently, insufficient mineralization. Proper calcification of osteoid requires that adequate amounts of calcium and phosphorus be available at the mineralization sites. In osteomalacia, failure of calcium and phosphorus deposition in bone matrix may be attributable to an inadequate intake of, or to a failure of absorption of, calcium, phosphorus, or vitamin D. Vitamin D is necessary for intestinal absorption of calcium and phosphorus and may have a direct effect on bone. At times, the level of vitamin D is sufficient but is not used because of resistance to the action of the vitamin at end organs, such as the kidneys. Other nonnutritional causes of osteomalacia

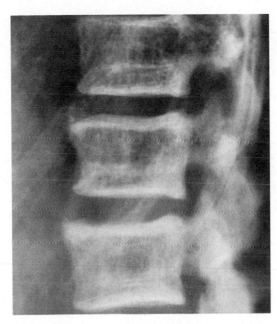

FIGURE 4-45 Osteomalacia. Striking prominence of cortices of vertebral bodies with increased trabeculation of spongy bone.

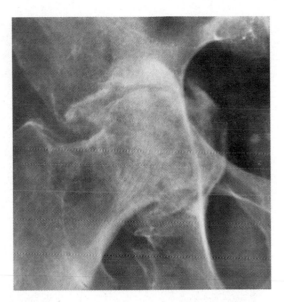

FIGURE 4-46 Protrusio acetabuli, as seen in osteomalacia and also in Paget's disease.

include chronic kidney failure and certain renal diseases in which calcium is lost to the urine and then bone breaks down as the body attempts to maintain a normal calcium level in the blood.

Radiographic Appearance

Regardless of the cause, osteomalacia appears radiographically as a loss of bone density because of the presence of nonmineralized osteoid. Although the cortex is thinned, it may stand out more prominently than normal because of the uniform deossification of medullary bone (Figure 4-45). In contrast to the situation in osteoporosis, the cortical borders in osteomalacia often appear indistinct. Fine-detail radiographs of the hands in patients with osteomalacia often demonstrate intracortical lines caused by local resorption or lack of mineralization, a finding not seen in osteoporosis.

Bones that are softened by osteomalacia may bend or give way as a result of weight bearing. Bowing deformities primarily involve the pelvis, vertebral column, thorax, and proximal extremities. In the pelvis, there may be a characteristic inward bending of the sidewalls with deepening of the acetabular cavities (protrusio acetabuli) (Figure 4-46).

Rickets

Rickets is a systemic disease of infancy and childhood that is the equivalent of osteomalacia in the mature skeleton. In this condition, calcification of growing skeletal elements is defective because of a deficiency of vitamin D in the diet or a lack of exposure to ultraviolet radiation (sunshine), which converts sterols in the skin into vitamin D. Rickets, most common in premature infants, usually develops between the ages of 6 months and 1 year.

Radiographic Appearance

The early radiographic changes in rickets are best seen in the fastest-growing portions of bone, such as the sternal ends of the ribs, the proximal ends of the tibia and humerus, and the distal ends of the radius and ulna. An overgrowth of noncalcified osteoid tissue appears radiographically as a characteristic increase in distance between the ossified portion of the epiphysis and the end of the shaft. In response to the pull of muscular and ligamentous attachments, the metaphyseal ends of the bone become cupped and frayed, and the normally sharp metaphyseal lines disappear (Figure 4-47). Lack of calcification leads to a delayed appearance of the epiphyseal ossification centers. Because of poor mineralization, bowing of weight-bearing bones (especially the tibia) develops once the infant begins to stand or walk. Extensive osteoid tissue in the sternal ends of the ribs produces a characteristic beading (rachitic rosary).

Softening of the vertebral bodies leads to the development of kyphosis. In females, narrowing of the pelvic inlet may make normal delivery impossible in later life.

Treatment for Osteomalacia and Rickets

Treatment consists of doses of vitamin D with calcium supplements. Other treatments are required if the calcium loss has a nonnutritional cause.

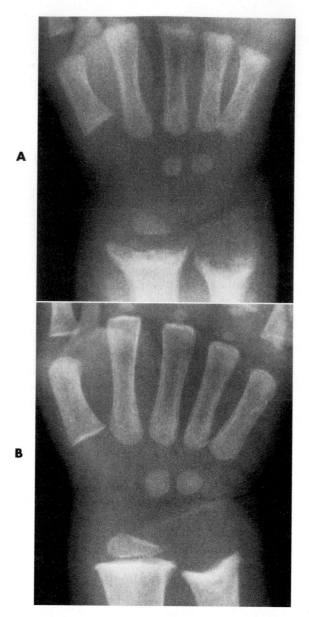

FIGURE 4-47 Rickets. **A,** Initial film of this wrist shows characteristic cupping and fraying of metaphyseal ends of the radius and ulna, with disappearance of normally sharp metaphyseal lines. **B,** After therapy with vitamin D, there is remineralization of metaphyseal ends of the radius and ulna, increased sharpness of metaphyseal lines, and a return of epiphyseal centers to normal density and sharpness of outline.

Gout

Gout is a disorder in the metabolism of purine (a component of nucleic acids) in which an increase in the blood level of uric acid leads to the deposition of uric acid crystals in the joints, cartilage, and kidney. Several inherited enzyme defects can cause overproduction of uric acid (primary gout). In secondary gout, hyperuricemia can be caused by an overproduction of uric acid, which in turn may be caused by increased turnover of

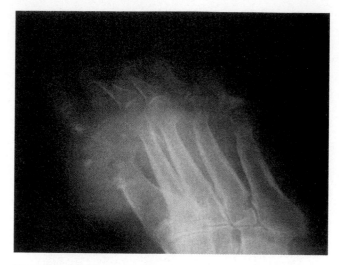

FIGURE 4-48 Gout. Effusion with tophi deposits at the first, fourth, and fifth metatarsophalangeal joints.

nucleic acids (e.g., as in metastatic carcinoma, myeloma, and hemolytic anemia), drugs (e.g., chemotherapy and thiazides used to treat hypertension), or a decrease in the excretion of uric acid resulting from kidney failure.

Radiographic Appearance

Acute gout primarily manifests as an exquisitely painful arthritis that initially attacks a single joint, primarily the first metatarsophalangeal joint (Figure 4-48). Radiographic changes develop late in the disease and only after repeated attacks. Therefore negative radiographs do not exclude gout and thus do not aid in early diagnostic evaluation.

Deposition of nonopaque urate crystals in the joint synovial membrane and on the surface of articular cartilage incites an inflammatory reaction that produces the earliest radiographic signs of joint effusion and periarticular swelling (Figure 4-49). Clumps of urate crystals (tophi) form along the margins of the articular cortex and erode the underlying bone, producing small, sharply marginated, punched-out defects at the joint margins of the small bones of the hand and foot. These erosions often have the appearance of cystlike lesions with thin sclerotic margins and characteristic overhanging edges ("rat bite" erosions) (Figure 4-50). In advanced disease, severe destructive lesions are associated with joint space narrowing and even fibrous ankylosis. Because patients are relatively free of symptoms between acute exacerbations of the disease, the bone density remains relatively normal, and diffuse osteoporosis is not part of the radiographic appearance.

Continued deposition of urate crystals in the periarticular tissues causes the development of the characteristic large, lumpy soft tissue swellings representing gouty tophi. In addition to the first metatarsophalangeal joints, other common sites of tophi include the ear,

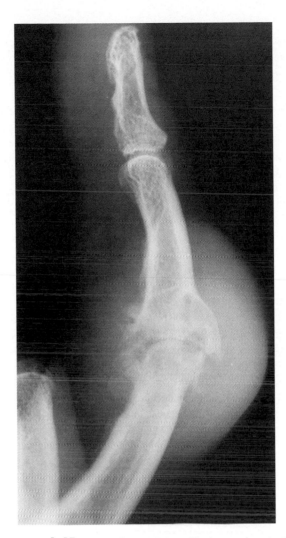

FIGURE 4-49 Gout. Severe joint effusion and periarticular swelling of proximal interphalangeal joint of finger. Note associated erosion of articular cartilage.

the olecranon bursa, and the insertion of the Achilles tendon. Tophi consisting of only sodium urate appear as a soft tissue density. Deposition of calcium in these urate collections causes the tophaceous periarticular masses to become radiopaque (Figure 4-51).

Although some renal dysfunction occurs in almost all patients with gouty arthritis, no radiographic abnormalities in the urinary tract can be demonstrated unless uric acid stones form. Nonradiopaque pure uric acid stones can be demonstrated only on excretory urograms, where they appear as filling defects in the pelvicalyceal system or ureter. Stones containing the calcium salts of uric acid can be detected on plain abdominal radiographs, where they appear radiopaque.

MRI produces various patterns, although regions of persistent low signal intensity are characteristic.

Treatment
Patients receiving doses of antihyperuricemic drugs rarely experience tophi. Untreated gout may lead to decreased renal excretion because of renal damage resulting from crystal deposits in the interstitial tissue. Eventually, this causes obstruction of the renal tubules and renal failure.

Paget's Disease
Paget's disease (osteitis deformans) is one of the most common chronic metabolic diseases of the skeleton. Destruction of bone, followed by a reparative process, results in weakened, deformed, and thickened bony structures that tend to fracture easily. The disease, seen most commonly during middle life, affects men twice as often as women and has been reported to occur in about 3% of all persons older than 40 years of age. Although the destructive phase often predominates

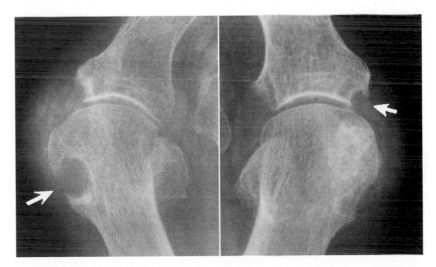

FIGURE 4-50 Two examples of typical "rat bite" erosions about first metatarsophalangeal joint *(arrows)*. The cystlike lesions have thin sclerotic margins and characteristic overhanging edges.

initially, there is more frequently a combination of destruction and repair in the pelvis and weight-bearing bones of the lower extremities. The reparative process may begin early and may be the prominent feature, often involving multiple bones. Paget's disease affects particularly the pelvis, femurs, skull, tibias,

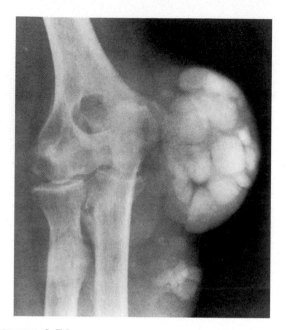

FIGURE 4-51 Gout. Massive deposition of calcium in long-standing tophaceous lesion about elbow.

vertebrae, clavicles, and ribs. The radionuclide bone scan is the most efficient method to visualize multi-centric lesions (Figure 4-52, *A*).

Radiographic Appearance

In the skull, Paget's disease begins as an area of sharply demarcated radiolucency (osteoporosis circumscripta) that represents the destructive phase of the disease (see Figure 4-52, *B*). During the reparative process, the development of irregular islands of sclerosis and cortical thickening results in a mottled, cotton-wool appearance (see Figure 4-52, *C*). In the spine, Paget's disease characteristically causes enlargement of the vertebral body. Increased trabeculation, which is most prominent at the periphery of the bone, produces a rim of thickened cortex and a picture-frame appearance. Uniform dense sclerosis of one or more vertebral bodies (ivory vertebrae) may occur.

The pelvis is the most common and often the initial site of Paget's disease. A distinctive early sign is coarsening of the trabeculae along the iliac margins, which produces thickening of the pelvic brim (Figure 4-53).

In the long bones, the destructive phase almost invariably begins at one end of the bone and extends along the shaft for a variable distance before ending in a typical, sharply demarcated, V-shaped configuration (blade of grass appearance). In the reparative stage, the bone is enlarged with an irregularly

SUMMARY of FINDINGS for Metabolic Bone Disease

disorder	location	radiographic appearance	treatment
Osteoporosis	Loss of bone mass in entire skeleton (accelerated bone resorption)	Cortical thinning appears as a relatively dense and prominent thin line DEXA BMD T-scores: • Normal, ≥−1.0 SD • Osteopenia, −1.0 to −2.25 SD • Osteoporosis, ≤−2.5 SD	Weight-bearing exercise Postmenopausal—hormonal replacement therapy Vitamin D and calcium supplements
Osteomalacia	Insufficient mineralization of adult skeleton (deossification of medullary bone)	Loss of bone density Cortex becomes thin and often indistinct	Vitamin D supplements with calcium
Rickets	Insufficient mineralization of immature skeleton	Cupped and frayed metaphysis in long bones	Vitamin D with calcium supplements
Gout	First metatarsophalangeal joint May attack any joint	Joint inflammation (effusion) Urate crystals (tophi) in joint space	Antihyperuricemic drugs
Paget's disease	Destruction and reparative process in pelvis, weight-bearing bones, and skull	Radiolucencies in destructive phase Cotton-wool appearance in reparative phase CT–lytic stage—washed out lesions with bone deformity and sclerosis with irregularity in the reparative stage	No known cure Bisphosphonates and calcitonin to slow bone resorption Antiinflammatory drugs

BMD, Bone mineral density; *DEXA,* dual-energy x-ray absorptiometry; *SD,* standard deviation.

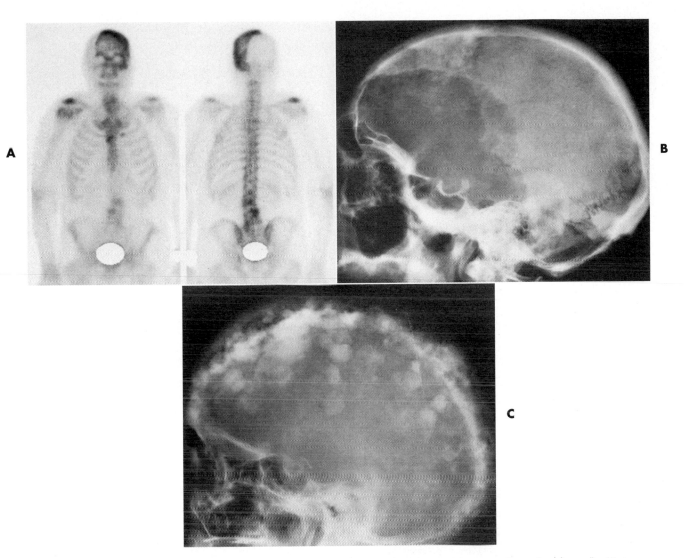

FIGURE 4-52 Paget's disease of the skull. **A,** Nuclear medicine bone scan demonstrating a "cold spot" within a "hot spot" in the skull. The cold spot represents the initial destructive phase, whereas the hot spot is a result of the reparative process. **B,** Radiograph obtained during the destructive phase of the disease demonstrates an area of sharply demarcated radiolucency (osteoporosis circumscripta) that involves primarily the frontal portion of the calvaria. **C,** During the reparative phase in another patient, irregular areas of sclerosis produce the characteristic cotton-wool appearance of the skull.

widened cortex and coarse, thickened trabeculae (Figure 4-54). Although dense, the bones are soft and weakened, and deformities are common. On CT, the lytic stage produces a washed-out appearance with cortical bone deformity. During the reparative process, the sclerosis appears as increased irregular cortical thickening and enlargement.

Paget's disease may lead to severe clinical complications. The downward thrust of the heavy head on the softened bone of the spine may compress the brainstem and cause numerous cranial nerve deficits. Expansion and distortion of softened vertebral bodies, sometimes with pathologic fractures, may compress the spinal cord and produce nerve root deficits.

Multiple microscopic arteriovenous malformations in pagetoid bone may result in high-output cardiac failure. The most serious complication of Paget's disease, the development of osteosarcoma, fortunately occurs in less than 1% of patients with this condition. MRI and CT provide the most accurate imaging if osteosarcoma is suspected.

Treatment

No known cure exists for Paget's disease; however, the process may be slowed by the administration of bisphosphonates, which bind to the bone to minimize the resorption, and calcitonin, which inhibits the activity of the osteoclasts (resorption cells). Sometimes

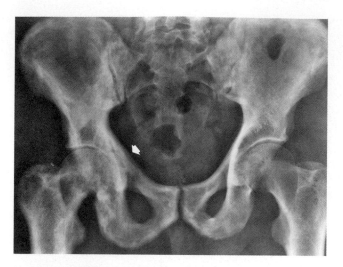

FIGURE 4-53 Paget's disease of the pelvis. Diffuse sclerosis with cortical thickening involves the right femur and both iliac bones. Note characteristic thickening and coarsening of the iliopectineal line *(arrow)* on the involved right side.

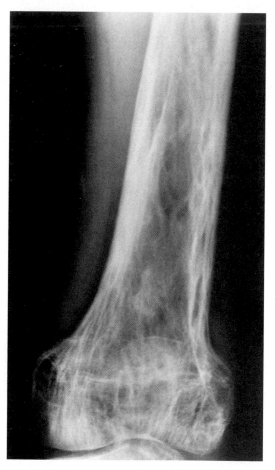

FIGURE 4-54 Paget's disease of knee. Note characteristic cortical thickening, destruction of fine trabeculae, and accentuation of secondary trabeculae.

antiinflammatory drugs reduce the inflammation caused by cell breakdown.

Fibrous Dysplasia

Fibrous dysplasia, a disorder that usually begins during childhood, is characterized by the proliferation of fibrous tissue within the medullary cavity. This proliferation causes loss of trabecular markings and widening of the bone. The disease may be confined to a single bone (monostotic) or the bones of one extremity, which is the most common form when it occurs in adults. The other form, in which the disease is widely distributed throughout the skeleton (polyostotic—among patients with this form, 25% have involvement of half the skeleton with more than 25% involvement of the skull), is present in children and occurs most often in females. Fibrous dysplasia involves primarily the long bones (especially the femur and tibia), ribs, and facial bones.

Radiographic Appearance

Fibrous replacement of the medullary cavity typically produces a well-defined radiolucent area, which may vary from completely radiolucent to a homogeneous ground-glass density, depending on the amount of fibrous or osseous tissue deposited in the medullary cavity (Figure 4-55). Irregular bands of sclerosis may cross the cystlike lesion, giving it a multilocular appearance (Figure 4-56). The bone is often locally expanded (suggesting a balloon), and the cortex may be eroded from within, predisposing to pathologic fractures. In severe and long-standing disease, affected bones may become bowed or deformed. CT images have a similar appearance to diagnostic x-rays, a cross-sectional perspective demonstrating sclerotic formation with radiolucent lesions. CT better demonstrates the location of the lesion, the cause (tissue type—lucent or sclerotic), and the degree of expansion. For the most definitive diagnosis, CT complements radiographic findings.

Fibrous dysplasia is the most common cause of an expansile focal rib lesion, which usually has a ground-glass or soap-bubble appearance.

Treatment

Treatment consists of curettage, repair of fractures, and prevention of deformities.

Ischemic Necrosis of Bone

Ischemic necrosis of bone results from loss of the blood supply, which in turn can result from such varied conditions as thrombosis, vasculitis, disease of surrounding bone, or single or repeated episodes

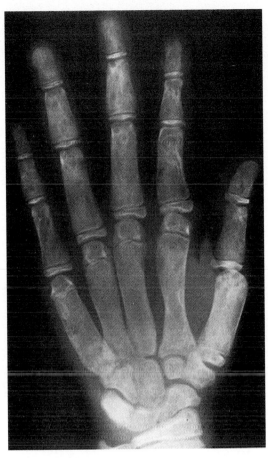

FIGURE 4-55 Fibrous dysplasia. Note smudgy, ground-glass appearance of medullary cavities with failure of normal modeling.

of trauma. Among the many conditions associated with ischemic necrosis are acute trauma (fracture or dislocation), steroid therapy or Cushing's disease, hemolytic anemia (especially sickle cell disease), chronic alcoholism and chronic pancreatitis, Gaucher's disease, radiation therapy, and caisson disease (a complication of underwater diving, the so-called bends).

Radiographic Appearance

The femoral head is the most common site of ischemic necrosis. Initially, the ischemic bone may appear denser than adjacent viable bone. The first sign of structural failure is the development of a radiolucent subcortical band (the crescent sign) representing a fracture line (Figure 4-57, A). As the disorder progresses, fragmentation, compression, and resorption of dead bone, along with proliferation of granulation tissue, revascularization, and production of new bone, produce a pattern of lytic and sclerotic areas with flattening of the femoral head and periosteal new bone, formation (Figure 4-57, B). Mechanical distortion about the hip leads to uneven weight bearing and accelerated secondary osteoarthritis.

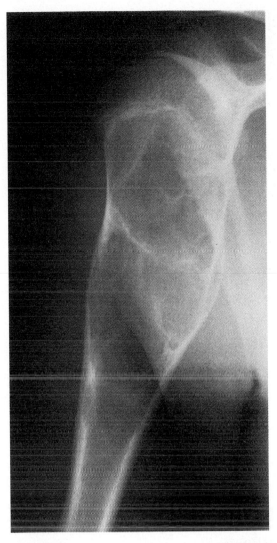

FIGURE 4-56 Fibrous dysplasia. An expansile lesion of the humerus contains irregular bands of sclerosis, giving it a multilocular appearance

It is often necessary to obtain two radiographs in patients with ischemic necrosis. The first is taken with normal density, whereas the second is made with an increased kilovolt peak to allow for adequate penetration of the more opaque sclerotic ischemic bone.

Radionuclide bone scanning is more sensitive than plain radiography for detecting changes of ischemic necrosis. In the initial stages of infarction, nuclide activity is absent in the area of involvement. As the disease progresses, this area of decreased activity may become rimmed by a zone of increased activity as a result of the reparative process.

MRI may be even more sensitive than radionuclide bone scanning for detecting ischemic necrosis. Infarction at the end of a bone causes changes in the fatty marrow, sharply reducing the normally intense

SUMMARY of FINDINGS for Fibrous Dysplasia and Ischemic Necrosis

disorder	location	radiographic appearance	treatment
Fibrous dysplasia	Monostotic—single bone or entire extremity Polyostotic—widely distributed	Well-defined radiolucent area, homogeneous ground-glass density or soap-bubble appearance CT—demonstrates the degree of sclerotic regions and radiolucent areas	Curettage Repair of fractures Prevention of deformities
Ischemic necrosis	Femoral head most common	Crescent sign, lytic/sclerotic areas with flattening of femoral head NM—bone scan—cold spot in lytic phase; cold spot rimmed by increased activity in reparative phase MRI—In T1-weighted images the infracted marrow appears gray or black	Immobilization Antibiotics Analgesics

T1-weighted signal from the marrow so that the infarcted area becomes gray or black (Figure 4-58).

In addition to ischemic changes in the subchondral areas of bone, infarction may involve the shaft of a long bone. In many cases, this type of bone infarction is asymptomatic and is detected only on radiographs obtained for another purpose. A mature infarct in the shaft of a bone appears as a densely calcified area in the medullary cavity (Figure 4-59). It may be sharply limited by a dense sclerotic zone or associated with dense streaks extending from the central region. Bone infarction must be differentiated from a calcified enchondroma, which contains amorphous, spotty calcific densities; is not surrounded by a sclerotic rim; and may expand the bone.

Treatment

Immobilization is accomplished with braces (pelvic for femoral head necrosis) to prevent further erosion and necrosis. Antibiotics may be useful if the necrosis results from infection. Analgesics are appropriate if inflammation is caused by vasculitis or trauma.

Benign Bone Tumors

Benign bone neoplasms generally displace soft tissue, whereas malignant bone tumors produce true soft tissue swelling. When there is bone expansion, an intact cortex with a sclerotic margin usually indicates a benign lesion. Benign bone neoplasms occur much less often than do bone metastases.

Radiographic Appearance of Osteochondromas

Osteochondroma (exostosis) is a benign projection of bone with a cartilaginous cap that arises in childhood or the teen years, especially about the knee. The exostosis occurs in the epiphyseal plate (the ring of Ranvier) and grows laterally from the epiphysis. A true osteochondroma must exhibit the cortex and medullary portion (spongiosa) as continuous bone growth. The cartilaginous cap of the lesion may convert to a malignancy if the cartilage cap becomes thicker and contains disorganized calcifications (chondrosarcoma or osteosarcoma). Ultrasound is a safe, quick, and inexpensive method to evaluate the thickness of the cartilaginous cap. A hereditary form of osteochondroma (autosomal dominant) produces multiple lesions and has an increased risk of malignancy.

A radiograph is the preferred method to demonstrate that the cortex of an osteochondroma blends with that of normal bone. The long axis of the tumor characteristically runs parallel to the parent bone and points away from the nearest joint (Figure 4-60). The best modality to demonstrate the thickness of the cartilaginous cap and thus rule out malignant conversion is MRI with long TR pulses (increased signal). On T2-weighted spin-echo images, the cartilaginous cap produces a high signal intensity.

Radiographic Appearance of Enchondromas

Enchondromas begin as slow-growing benign cartilaginous tumors arising in the medullary canal (ectopic cartilaginous growth). This tumor destroys normal bone by erupting as a mixture of calcified and uncalcified hyaline cartilage. They are most frequently found in children and young adults, and they involve primarily the small bones of the hands and feet. Enchondromas are often multiple.

As the well-demarcated tumor grows, it expands bone locally, causing thinning and endosteal scalloping of the cortex. This often leads to a pathologic fracture with only minimal trauma (Figure 4-61).

FIGURE 4-57 Ischemic necrosis of femoral head. **A,** An arclike radiolucent cortical band (the crescent sign) *(arrow)* in the femoral head represents the fracture line. **B,** Eventually there is combination of lytic and sclerotic areas with severe flattening of the femoral head.

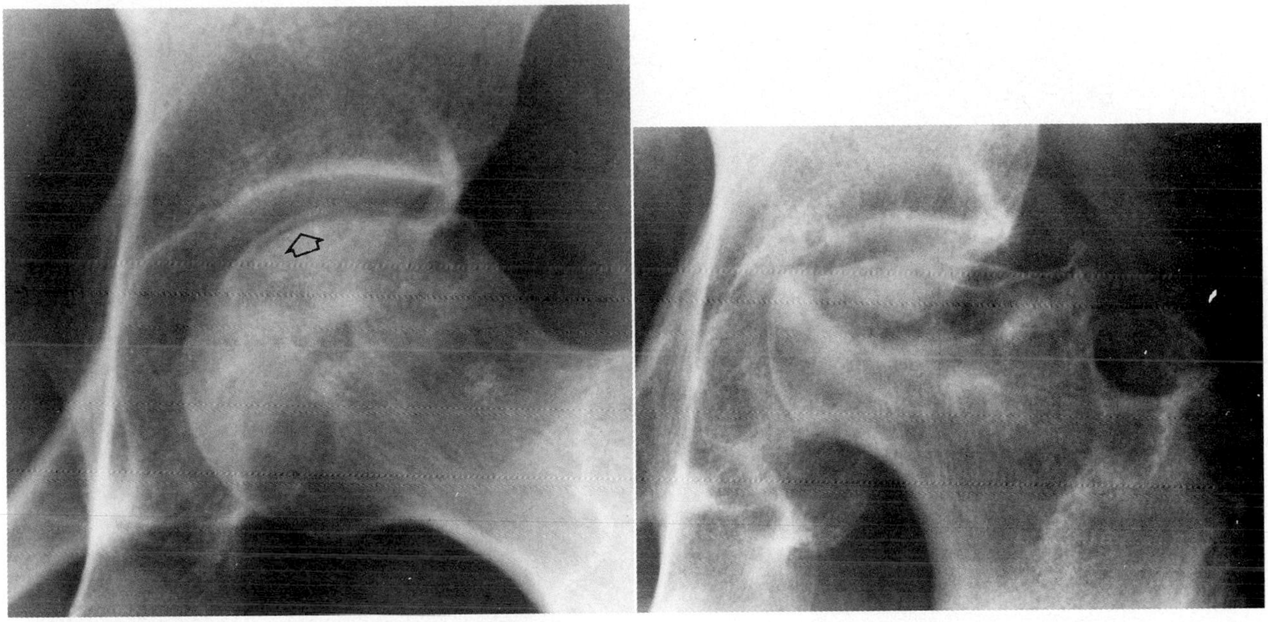

A characteristic finding of enchondroma is stippled, speckled, and ringlike or arclike calcifications within the lucent matrix because of the tumor composition. This radiographic appearance is also seen on CT images.

T2-weighted MR images demonstrate a lesion having lobulated borders from the endosteal scalloping and containing focal areas of high signal intensity. On T1-weighted images, enchondromas have low to intermediate signal intensity.

Nuclear medicine bone scans are usually negative in cases of enchondromas, ruling out the possibility of malignancy.

Radiographic Appearance of Giant Cell Tumors

Giant cell tumor (osteoclastoma) typically arises at the end of the distal femur or proximal tibia of a young adult after epiphyseal closure (20- to 40-year olds). It begins as an eccentric lucent lesion in the metaphysis, and it characteristically extends to the immediate subarticular cortex of the bone, but does not involve the joint (Figure 4-62). MRI is used to determine intraarticular extension, soft tissue involvement, and bone marrow changes. When the results are combined with x-ray images, the accuracy is especially high. A few giant cell tumors may be premalignant or actually malignant.

As the tumor expands toward the shaft, it produces the characteristic radiographic appearance of multiple large bubbles separated by thin strips of bone.

Radiographic Appearance of Osteomas

Osteomas most often arise in the outer table of the skull, the paranasal sinuses (especially frontal and ethmoid), and the mandible. Diagnosis of these tumors may be incidental on radiographs taken because of the pain produced by bone expansion.

Osteomas appear radiographically as well-circumscribed, extremely dense, round lesions that are rarely larger than 2 cm in diameter (Figure 4-63).

Radiographic Appearance of Osteoid Osteomas

Osteoid osteoma usually develops in teenagers or young adults and produces the classic clinical symptom of local pain that is worse at night and is dramatically relieved by aspirin. Most osteoid osteomas occur in the femur and tibia, originate from osteoblastic cells, and are less than 1.5 cm in diameter. A radionuclide bone scan can help differentiate osteoid osteoma from osteomyelitis; osteoid osteoma has a double density, whereas osteomyelitis demonstrates only an outline because of the avascularity of the inner structure. Preoperatively, nuclear medicine studies localize the tumor for complete excision.

The tumor is typically seen as a small, round or oval, lucent center (the nidus), less than 1 cm in

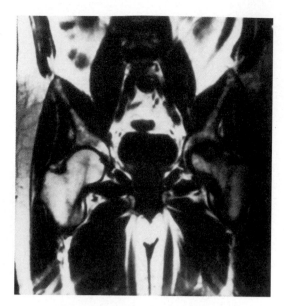

FIGURE 4-58 Ischemic necrosis. On this T1-weighted image, the ischemic left femoral head has lost its normal bright signal intensity and appears dark.

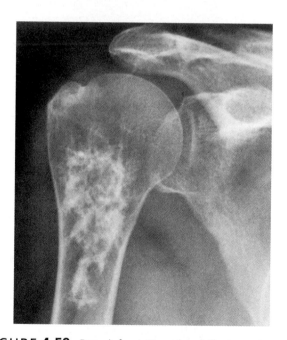

FIGURE 4-59 Bone infarct. Densely calcified area in medullary cavity of humerus with dense streaks extending from central region.

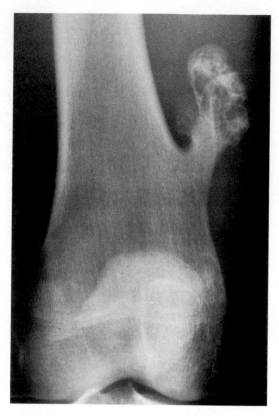

FIGURE 4-60 Osteochondroma. The long axis of the tumor is parallel to that of the femur and points away from the knee joint.

diameter, that is surrounded by a large, dense sclerotic zone of cortical thickening (Figure 4-64). The nidus may not be visualized depending on the bone structure involved (cortical versus cancellous). Because this dense reaction may obscure the nidus on conventional radiographs, overpenetrated films or tomography (conventional or computed) may be necessary to demonstrate it. CT is commonly used if there is need to demonstrate the central radiolucent nidus for percutaneous ablation. The nidus enhances following contrast enhancement. T1-weighted MR images demonstrate the nidus as isoechoic to muscle (same intensity as muscle). CT is considered the definitive diagnostic modality.

Radiographic Appearance of Simple Bone Cysts

A **simple bone cyst (unicameral)** is a true fluid-filled cyst with a wall of fibrous tissue, which most often occurs in the proximal humerus or femur at the metaphysis. Although not a true neoplasm, a simple bone cyst may resemble one radiographically and clinically. Solitary bone cysts are asymptomatic and often discovered either incidentally or after pathologic fracture.

The simple bone cyst appears as an expansile lucent lesion that is sharply demarcated from adjacent normal bone and may have a thin rim of sclerosis around it. It has an oval configuration, with its long axis parallel to that of the host bone and may cause cortical bone thinning (Figure 4-65). CT appearance is very similar to radiographs, so is usually unnecessary. Simple bone cysts produce low signal intensity on T1-weighted MR images (high signal intensity on

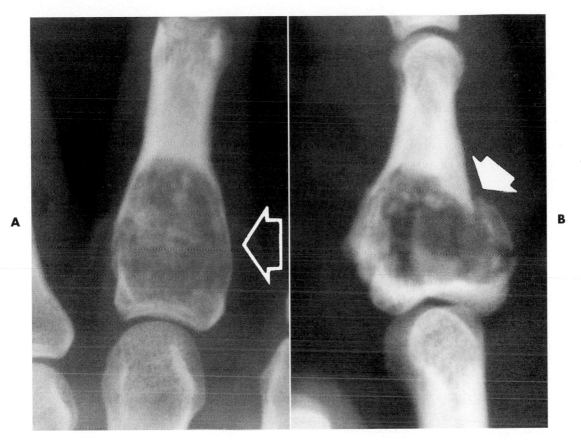

FIGURE 4-61 Enchondroma. **A,** Well-demarcated tumor *(arrow)* expands bone and thins cortex. **B,** Pathologic fracture *(arrow)*.

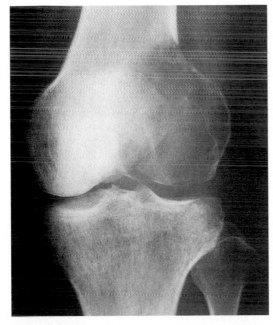

FIGURE 4-62 Giant cell tumor. Typical eccentric lucent lesion in distal femoral metaphysis extends to the immediate subarticular cortex. Surrounding cortex, although thinned, remains intact.

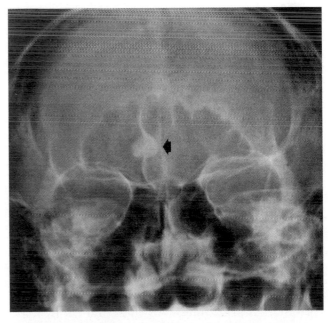

FIGURE 4-63 Osteoma *(arrow)* in a frontal sinus.

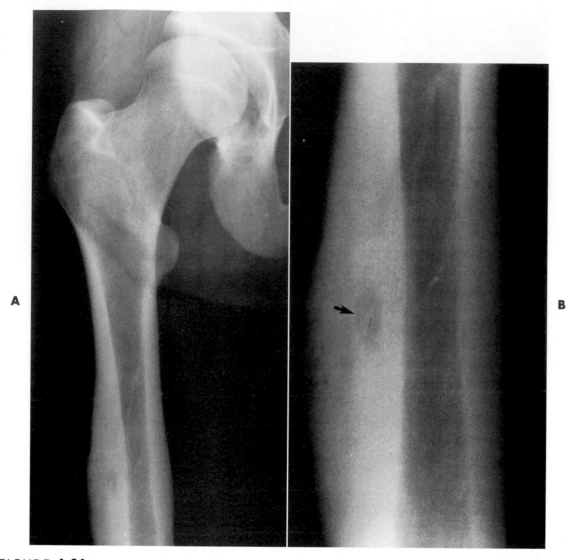

FIGURE 4-64 Osteoid osteoma. Full **(A)** and coned **(B)** projections of the midshaft of the femur demonstrate a dense sclerotic zone of cortical thickening laterally, which contains a small oval lucent nidus *(arrow)*.

T2-weighted images). MRI will determine if septations exist that may not be visible on the radiograph to aid in determining proper treatment.

Radiographic Appearance of Aneurysmal Bone Cysts

An **aneurysmal bone cyst,** rather than being a true neoplasm or cyst, consists of numerous blood-filled arteriovenous communications thought to be caused by trauma.

In long bones, an aneurysmal bone cyst is an expansile, eccentric, cystlike lesion that causes pronounced ballooning of the thinned cortex (Figure 4-66). In some cases, the cystlike lesion may present with internal separations. At times, the cortex may be so thin that it is invisible on plain radiographs,

and thus this benign lesion may be mistaken for a malignant bone tumor. A CT scan may assist in defining the well-lobulated lesion, but MRI better shows the internal loculations and fluid levels that produce a low signal on T2-weighted images. On T1-weighted images, the cyst has a low to intermediate signal intensity, but contains high signal intensity if there has been acute hemorrhage.

Bone islands are solitary, sharply demarcated areas of dense compact bone that occur most commonly in the pelvis and upper femur. They appear in every bone except the skull (Figure 4-67). Although almost half of the bone islands enlarge over a period of years and many show activity on radionuclide scans, bone islands are asymptomatic and completely benign and must be distinguished from osteoblastic metastases.

SUMMARY of FINDINGS for Benign Bone Tumors (Neoplasia)

disorder	location	radiographic appearance	treatment
Osteochondroma	Epiphyseal plate growing laterally in long bones	Tumor runs parallel to long bone and points away from nearest joint US—determines cartilage cap thickness MRI—cartilage cap produces a high signal intensity on T2-weighted spin-echo images	Surgical removal only when mechanical impingement occurs
Enchondroma	Arises in the medullary canal of hands and feet	Cortical thinning and endosteal scalloping Calcifications within lesion appear stippled, speckled, ringlike, or arclike MRI—T2-weighted image shows lobulated endosteal scalloping with focal high-intensity signals	Curettage of lesion
Giant cell tumor (osteoclastoma)	Metaphysis extends into subarticular cortex; does not involve the joint	Multiple large bubbles separated by strips of bone MRI—demonstrates tumor extension with soft tissue involvement and bone marrow changes	Curettage and local resection
Osteoma	Outer table of the skull	Well-circumscribed extremely dense round lesions less than 2 cm in diameter	No treatment required
Osteoid osteoma	Femur and tibia, osteoblastic cells	Round or oval lesion with lucent center (nidus), sometimes surrounded by dense sclerotic zone; less than 1 cm CT—contrast enhancement to demonstrate nidus	Surgical removal includes nidus to be successful Percutaneous ablation
Simple bone cyst	Most common in proximal humerus and femur at the metaphysis	Expansile lucent lesion with a thin rim of sclerosis MRI—low signal intensity on T1-weighted images and demonstrates septations within the cyst	Many require no treatment Curettage with implantation of bone chips
Aneurysmal bone cyst	Metaphysis or long bones	Pronounced ballooning with thinned cortex (internal separations) MRI—T2-weighted image demonstrates loculated lesions producing low signal intensity; T1-weighted image produces high signal intensity if cyst is hemorrhagic in nature	Curettage
Bone island	Every bone except the skull	Sharply defined, dense compact lesion	No treatment required

US, Ultrasound.

Treatment of Benign Bone Tumors

An osteochondroma requires treatment only when mechanical friction (joint mobility) impinges on nerves, blood vessels, or muscles. For an enchondroma, curettage of the lesion is the common treatment. The treatment for giant cell tumor includes curettage of the bone and local resection. About 50% of giant cell tumors recur. Surgical excision of the nidus of an osteoid osteoma is essential for cure; it is not necessary to remove the reactive calcification, although it may form the major part of the lesion. CT-guided percutaneous radiofrequency ablation (destruction) may provide the best treatment. Simple bone cyst treatment depends on the size and location of the cyst. If the cyst continues to develop, surgical curettage and implantation of bone chips is performed. Aneurysmal bone cysts require curettage to prevent further destruction from occurring. Bone islands require no treatment.

Malignant Bone Tumors

Malignant bone neoplasms generally cause soft tissue swelling and cortical bone erosion that has a poorly defined or absent margin. The neoplasm extends into the soft tissue through spiculations (fingerlike projections). Plain radiographs may identify a single lesion. A radionuclide bone scan or positron emission tomography (PET) scan can detect silent lesions when minimal cellular destruction has occurred. Discovering additional lesions determines

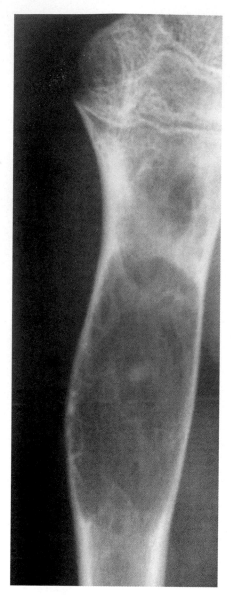

FIGURE 4-65 Simple bone cyst. This cyst in the proximal humerus has an oval configuration, with its long axis parallel to that of host bone.

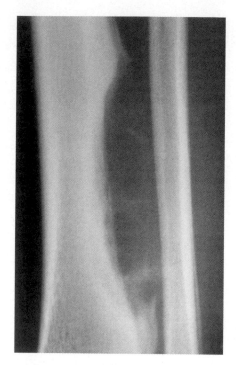

FIGURE 4-66 Aneurysmal bone cyst. This expansile, eccentric, cystic lesion of the tibia has multiple fine internal septa. Because severely thinned cortex is difficult to detect, the tumor resembles a malignant process.

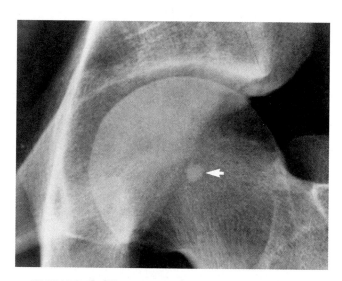

FIGURE 4-67 Bone island *(arrow)* in femoral head.

the treatment and prognosis. CT and MRI can precisely define the location of a malignant bone tumor and its extension into the medullary cavity and spread to surrounding structures (Figures 4-68 and 4-69).

Radiographic Appearance of Osteogenic Sarcoma

Osteogenic sarcoma generally occurs in the end of a long bone in the metaphysis (especially about the knee). This tumor consists of osteoblasts, which produce osteoid and spicules of calcified bone. Most osteogenic sarcomas arise in persons between 10 and 25 years old, although a smaller peak incidence is seen in

older persons who have a preexisting bone disorder, particularly Paget's disease. The usual initial complaints are local pain and swelling, sometimes followed by fever, weight loss, and secondary anemia. Pulmonary metastases develop early, and a plain chest radiograph should be obtained to exclude this unfavorable prognostic sign. If no metastases to the lung are detected by this modality, CT or a PET scan should be performed.

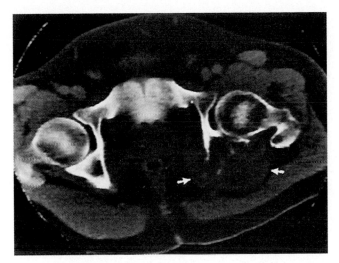

FIGURE 4-68 Osteogenic sarcoma. CT scan through the level of the femoral head shows destruction of the left ischium, which was seen on plain radiographs. In addition, CT scan demonstrates large soft tissue mass *(arrows)* in area covered by gluteus maximus muscle and separated from rectum. Mass was not clinically palpable.

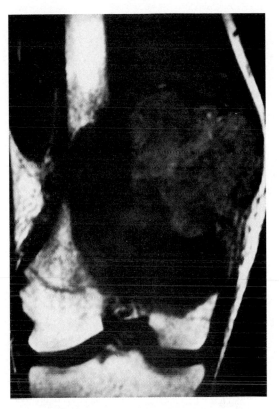

FIGURE 4-69 MRI of osteogenic sarcoma. Coronal image shows the intramedullary and soft tissue extent of the mass.

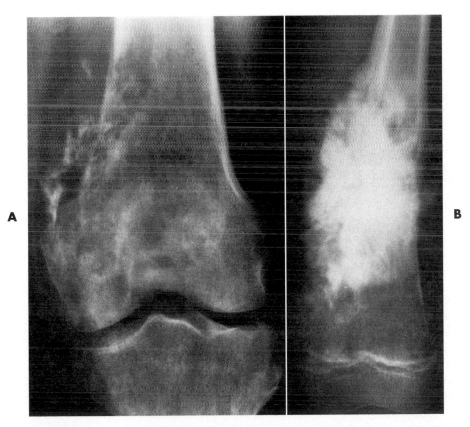

FIGURE 4-70 Osteogenic sarcoma. **A,** Predominantly destructive lesion with irregular periosteal reaction. **B,** Classic sunburst pattern with bony spicules extending outward in radiating fashion.

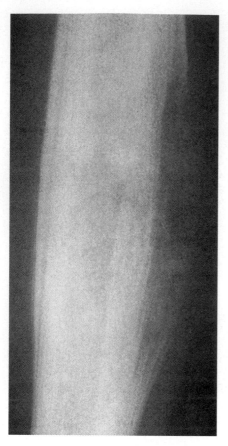

FIGURE 4-71 Codman's triangle. Thin periosteal elevation and subsequent new bone formation at periphery of this neoplastic lesion.

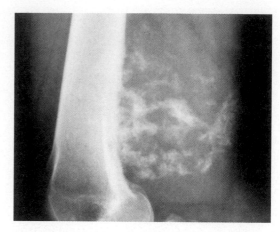

FIGURE 4-72 Chondrosarcoma. Prominent dense calcification in large neoplastic mass.

The typical radiographic appearance of osteogenic sarcoma is a mixed destructive and sclerotic lesion associated with a soft tissue mass, irregular periosteal reaction, and reactive new bone formation (Figure 4-70, *A*). In the classic sunburst pattern, horizontal bony spicules extend in radiating fashion into the soft tissue mass (Figure 4-70, *B*). A characteristic finding is elevation of the periosteum at the periphery of a lesion, with subsequent new bone formation (Codman's triangle) (Figure 4-71). CT images are beneficial in demonstrating this finding in flat bones, where periosteal change is more difficult to visualize. MRI of the entire length of the bone is important to rule out skip lesions, and this modality is more accurate to visualize the tissue extension and medullary involvement. To determine the longitudinal involvement, specifically in the medullary cavity, T1-weighted images using a spin-echo sequence are best. The STIR (short-tau inversion recovery) sequence produces high-intensity signals. Both signal sequences are required because the T1-weighted images are slightly more specific, whereas the STIR sequence produces images that are slightly more sensitive.

Radiographic Appearance of Chondrosarcoma

Chondrosarcoma is a malignant tumor of cartilaginous origin that may originate anew or within a preexisting cartilaginous lesion (e.g., osteochondroma and enchondroma). Tumor grading of this particular neoplasm depends on the maturity and differentiation of the cells. Chondrosarcomas commonly occur in long bones, but often originate in a rib, scapula, or vertebra. The tumor is about half as common as osteogenic sarcoma; it develops at a later age (peak incidence in 35- to 60-year-olds), grows more slowly, and metastasizes later.

In addition to the bone destruction seen with all malignant tumors, chondrosarcoma often contains punctate or amorphous calcification within its cartilaginous matrix (Figure 4-72). On CT, as on radiographs, chondrosarcomas demonstrate endosteal scalloping and cortical destruction. To evaluate for possible pulmonary metastases, CT is the modality of choice. On T2-weighted MR images, the lobulated lesions have high signal intensity, whereas the septations appear as low signal intensity.

Radiographic Appearance of Ewing's Sarcoma

Ewing's sarcoma is a primary malignant tumor arising in the bone marrow of long bones. A tumor of children and young adults, Ewing's sarcoma has a peak incidence in the midteens and is rare in persons over 30 years of age. The major clinical complaint is local pain, often of several months' duration, that persistently increases in severity and may be associated with a tender soft tissue mass. Patients with this tumor characteristically have malaise and appear sick, often with fever and leukocytosis, suggestive of osteomyelitis.

The classic radiographic appearance of Ewing's sarcoma is an ill-defined permeative area of bone destruction that involves a large central portion of the shaft of

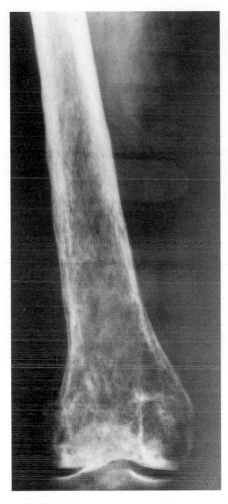

FIGURE 4-73 Ewing's sarcoma. Diffuse permeative destruction with mild periosteal response involving distal half of femur.

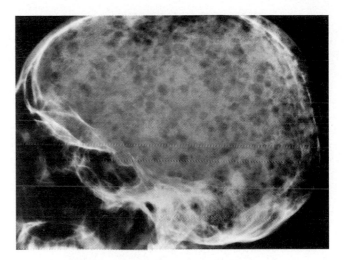

FIGURE 4-74 Multiple myeloma. Diffuse punched-out osteolytic lesions scattered throughout skull.

a long bone (underlying medullary destruction) and is associated with a fusiform layered periosteal reaction (onionskin appearance) parallel to the shaft (Figure 4-73). Tumor cells invade the cortical bone and spread into the soft tissue. For staging and follow-up, MRI is the modality of choice. MRI best demonstrates the soft tissue involvement on T1-weighted images, where the tumor has a low signal intensity when compared with normal bone marrow. On T2-wighted imaging, the tumor has a higher signal intensity than muscle, so fat-saturation sequences are best (STIR sequences provide an alternative when fat saturation is unavailable).

Radiographic Appearance of Multiple Myeloma

Multiple myeloma is a disseminated (widespread) malignancy of plasma cells that may be associated with bone destruction, bone marrow failure, hypercalcemia, renal failure, and recurrent infections. The disease affects primarily persons between 40 and 70 years of age. This frequently occurring primary bone tumor attacks the intramedullary canal of the diaphysis. Typical laboratory findings include an abnormal spike of monoclonal immunoglobulin and the presence of Bence Jones protein in the urine.

The classic radiographic appearance of multiple myeloma is multiple punched out osteolytic lesions scattered throughout the skeletal system and best seen on lateral views of the skull (Figures 4-74 and 4-75). Because the bone destruction is attributable to the proliferation of plasma cells distributed throughout the bone marrow, the flat bones containing red marrow (vertebrae, skull, ribs, pelvis) are primarily affected. The appearance may be indistinguishable from that of a metastatic carcinoma, although the lytic defects in multiple myeloma tend to be more discrete and uniform in size. Extensive plasma cell proliferation in the bone marrow with no tendency to form discrete tumor masses may produce generalized skeletal deossifications simulating postmenopausal osteoporosis. In the spine, decreased bone density and destructive changes in multiple myeloma are usually limited to the vertebral bodies, sparing the pedicles (which lack red marrow and are frequently destroyed by metastatic disease). The severe loss of bone substance in the spine often results in multiple vertebral compression fractures (Figure 4-76).

Because multiple myeloma causes little or no stimulation of new bone formation, radionuclide bone scans may be normal even with extensive skeletal infiltration. On T1-weighted MR images, low-intensity tumor tissue replaces the normal high-intensity fatty marrow.

Treatment of Malignant Bone Tumors

The treatment of osteogenic sarcoma includes surgical removal with or without chemotherapy and/or radiation therapy. Although osteogenic sarcoma is usually

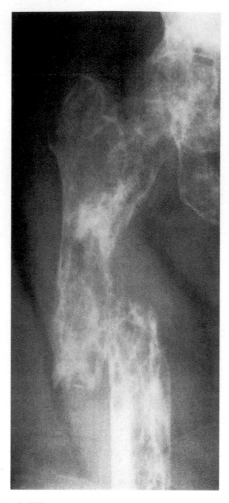

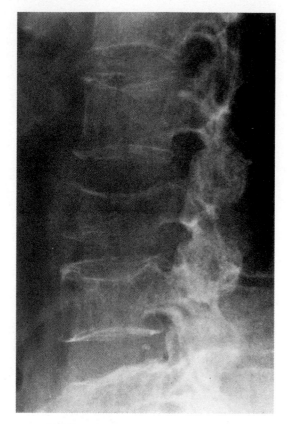

FIGURE 4-76 Multiple myeloma. Diffuse myelomatous infiltration has caused generalized demineralization of vertebral bodies and compression fracture of L2.

FIGURE 4-75 Diffuse destructive bone lesion that has led to pathologic fracture of femur.

fatal, about 30% of patients receiving chemotherapy are cured. For chondrosarcoma lesions, the treatment usually includes surgical excision. Because of poor response, chemotherapy and radiation therapy are not suggested. The more differentiated the involved cells, the higher the survival rate. Chondrosarcoma tumors are not sensitive to chemotherapy. Ewing's sarcoma and multiple myeloma are treated with radiation therapy and chemotherapy. Chemotherapy for Ewing's sarcoma increases the survival rate to about 30%. Multiple myeloma (Figure 4-77) patients have a grim prognosis, most dying within 3 to 4 years.

Bone Metastases

Metastases are the most common malignant bone tumors, spreading by means of the bloodstream or lymphatic vessels or by direct extension. The most common primary tumors are carcinomas of the breast, lung, prostate, kidney, and thyroid. Favorite sites of metastatic spread are bones containing red marrow,

such as the spine, pelvis, ribs, skull, and the upper ends of the humerus and femur. Metastases distal to the knees and elbows are infrequent but do occur, especially with bronchogenic (lung) tumors.

The detection of skeletal metastases is critical in the management of patients with known or suspected neoplastic disease, both at the time of initial staging and during the period of continuing follow-up care. The presence of metastases may exclude some patients from the radical "curative" therapy that is offered to those without disseminated disease, thus sparing them from fruitless, high-morbidity procedures for a nonremediable condition.

The best screening examination for the detection of asymptomatic skeletal metastases is the radionuclide bone scan (Figure 4-78) or the PET scan (Figure 4-79), which is unquestionably more sensitive than the radiographic skeletal survey. Because almost half the mineral content of a bone must be lost before the loss is detectable on plain radiographs, the skeletal survey should be abandoned as a general screening examination for the detection of asymptomatic skeletal metastases. False-negative findings on bone scans occur only with aggressively osteolytic lesions, especially

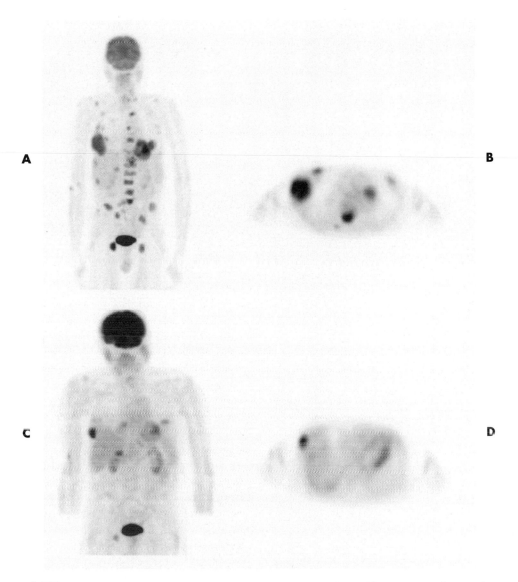

FIGURE 4-77 Multiple myeloma. The PET oncologic survey is positive, with a pattern of extensive metaboli-cally active tumor metastases demonstrated throughout the axial skeleton and in both lower lung fields on coronal **(A)** and transverse **(B)** images. After 4 months, when the patient is in his last cycle of chemotherapy, the survey images (**C** and **D**) still demonstrate persistent, viable, metabolically active neoplasm. However, a dramatic improve-ment in the overall pattern is seen when compared with the earlier scan.

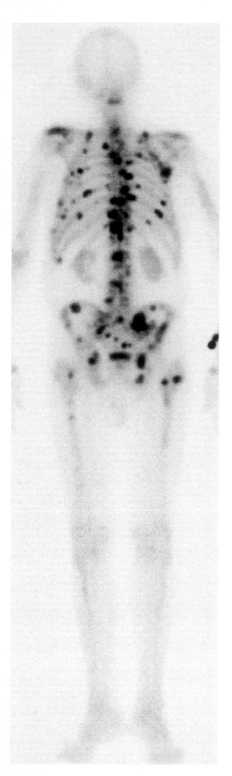

FIGURE 4-78 Screening radionuclide bone scan. Multiple focal areas of radionuclide uptake in axial skeleton, representing metastases from prostate carcinoma.

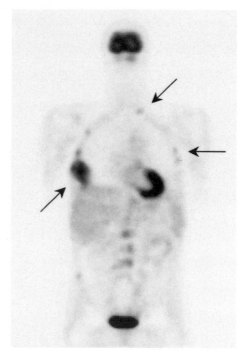

FIGURE 4-79 PET scan showing metastases. Arrows point to metabolic activity in the skeletal system (ribs) on the fluorodeoxyglucose-PET scan.

in patients with multiple myeloma. The role of plain radiographs in screening for metastases is to further evaluate focal abnormalities detected on radionuclide scanning because a variety of lesions (e.g., infections, benign tumors, fibrous dysplasia, and bone islands) can also show positive findings on bone scans. Because the presence of multiple focal abnormalities is typical of metastatic disease, it is necessary to radiographically examine only a single lesion or area to confirm the diagnosis. In addition, because of the occasional false-negative results on a bone scan, it is imperative that all symptomatic sites in patients with neoplastic disease be examined by plain radiographs unless the radionuclide bone scan unequivocally demonstrates diffuse metastatic disease.

Radiographic Appearance

Metastatic disease may produce a broad spectrum of radiographic appearances: osteolytic, sclerotic, or mixed. Osteolytic metastases cause destruction without accompanying bone proliferation. They develop from tumor embolic deposits in the medullary canal and eventually extend to destroy cortical bone. The margins of the lucent lesions are irregular and poorly defined, rarely sharp and smooth. The most common primary lesions causing osteolytic metastases are carcinomas of the breast, kidney, and thyroid. Metastases from carcinomas of the kidney and thyroid typically produce a single large metastatic focus that may appear as an

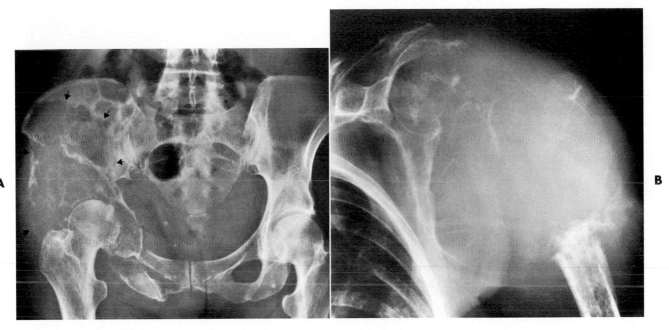

FIGURE 4-80 Blowout metastases. **A,** Lytic expansile destruction of left ilium *(arrows)* in metastatic thyroid carcinoma. **B,** Osteolytic metastasis to humerus from carcinoma of kidney.

SUMMARY of FINDINGS for Malignant Bone Tumors (Neoplasia)

disorder	location	radiographic appearance	treatment
Osteogenic sarcoma	Metaphysis of long bone Most common in knee	Mixed destructive/sclerotic lesion with soft tissue mass "Sunburst" pattern Codman's triangle CT—best to visualize periosteal changes in flat bones MRI—T1-weighted spin echo and STIR sequences demonstrate longitudinal medullary bone involvement	Surgical excision, with/without chemotherapy or radiation therapy
Chondrosarcoma	Metaphysis of long bone or flat bones	Punctate or amorphous calcification in cartilaginous matrix CT—endosteal scalloping and cortical destruction MRI—T1-weighted image produces high signal intensity with low signal intensity of septations	Surgical excision
Ewing's sarcoma	Bone marrow of long bones	Medullary destruction with "onionskin" periosteal reaction MRI—T1-weighted image has a low intensity signal when compared to bone marrow; T2-weighted image produces a higher signal intensity than muscle	Radiation therapy Chemotherapy
Multiple myeloma	Intramedullary canal of the diaphysis	Multiple punched-out lesions MRI—tumor tissue has a low signal intensity (replacing high signal intensity of fatty marrow)	Radiation therapy Chemotherapy
Bone metastases	Entire skeleton	Irregular, poorly defined lucent lesions or poorly defined increased densities depending on site of origin	Radiopharmaceuticals to reduce bone pain Radiation therapy Chemotherapy

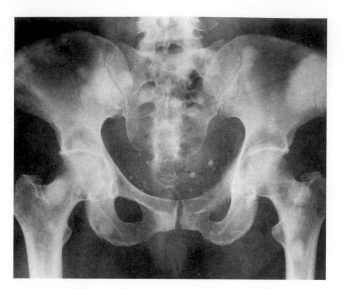

FIGURE **4-81** Osteoblastic metastases. Multiple areas of increased density involving pelvis and proximal femurs representing metastases from carcinoma of urinary bladder.

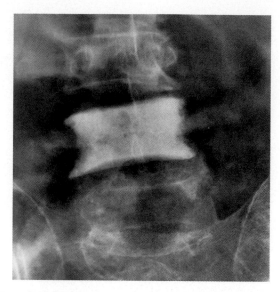

FIGURE **4-82** Ivory vertebra. Diffuse sclerosis of L4 vertebral body from metastatic carcinoma of prostate.

expansile trabeculated lesion (a "blowout") (Figure 4-80). Metastases from breast carcinoma are most often multiple when first detected.

In the spine, osteolytic metastases tend to involve not only the vertebral bodies but also the pedicles and posterior arches. Destruction of one or more pedicles may be the earliest sign of metastatic disease and may help in differentiating this process from multiple myeloma, in which the pedicles are much less often involved. Because cartilage is resistant to invasion by metastases, preservation of the intervertebral disk space may help to distinguish metastases from an inflammatory process. Pathologic collapse of vertebral bodies frequently occurs in advanced disease.

Osteoblastic metastases are generally considered evidence of slow growth in a neoplasm that has allowed time for a proliferation of reactive bone. In men, osteoblastic metastases are usually a result of carcinoma of the prostate gland; carcinoma of the breast is the most common primary site of osteoblastic metastases in women. These lesions initially appear as ill-defined areas of increased density that may progress to complete loss of normal bony architecture. They may vary from small, isolated round foci of sclerotic density to a diffuse sclerosis involving most or all of a bone (Figure 4-81). In the spine, this may produce the characteristic uniform density of an "ivory" vertebral body (Figure 4-82).

The combination of destruction and sclerosis in the mixed type of metastasis causes the affected bone to have a mottled appearance, with intermixed areas of lucency and increased density.

Bone destruction by metastases and associated extension of tumor in the adjacent soft tissues can be well demonstrated by CT and MRI (Figure 4-83). A PET scan can quickly determine if the patient has a solitary metastatic lesion or multiple lesions. New fusion technology (superimposition of two imaging modality scans, such as PET and MRI) can further define the number, size, and location of metastatic lesions, influencing the type of treatment best suited for the patient.

Treatment

Radiopharmaceuticals are increasing in use to reduce painful bone metastases. Radiation therapy and chemotherapy are the most common types of treatment, but they are generally only palliative because patients diagnosed with bone metastasis have a poor prognosis.

Fractures

Fractures are the most common skeletal abnormality seen in a general radiology practice. A fracture is defined as a disruption of bone caused by mechanical forces applied either directly to the bone or transmitted along the shaft of a bone. Although often obvious, some fractures are subtle and difficult to detect. A fracture typically appears as a radiolucent line crossing the bone and disrupting the cortical margins. However, the fracture line may be thin and easily overlooked, whereas overlap of fragments may produce a radiopaque line. Secondary signs of an underlying fracture include joint effusion, soft tissue swelling, and interruption of the normal pattern of bony trabeculae.

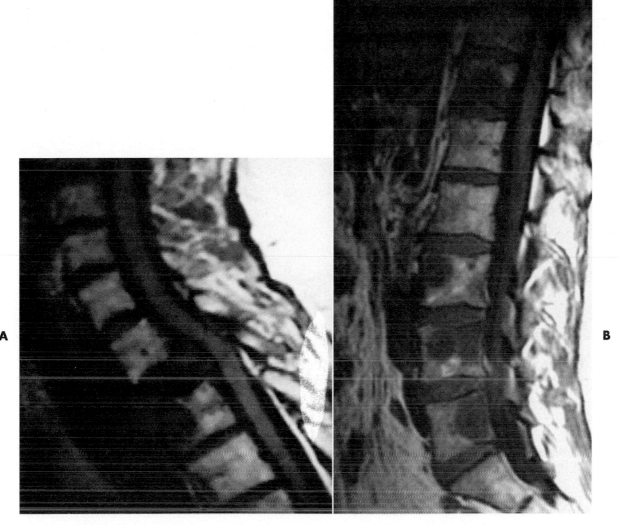

FIGURE 4-83 **A,** MR image of metastases. Sagittal scan shows gross metastatic destruction and replacement of the body of T2, which has collapsed. The metastasis has a lower signal intensity than that of vertebral marrow or the spinal cord. The spinal cord is focally indented and displaced posteriorly by the tumor. Also, a low-signal-intensity lytic metastasis involves the anterior portion of T3. **B,** Vertebral metastasis of breast carcinoma. Many lytic lesions are evident on this MR scan of the lumbar region.

Types of Fractures

Fractures are described and classified by their extent, direction, and position; the number of fracture lines; and the integrity of the overlying skin (Figure 4-84). A fracture that results in discontinuity between two or more fragments is a **complete fracture;** an **incomplete fracture** causes only partial discontinuity, with a portion of the cortex remaining intact. In **closed fractures,** the overlying skin is intact; if the overlying skin is disrupted, the fracture is **open,** or **compound.** Although it is a clinical distinction, the radiographic demonstration of bone clearly protruding through the skin and the presence of air and soft tissues about the fracture site on radiographs obtained immediately after the injury are highly suggestive of an open fracture.

The direction of a fracture is determined by its relationship to the long axis of long and short bones and to the longest axis of irregular bones (e.g., the talus or carpal navicular). A **transverse fracture** runs at a right angle to the long axis of a bone and most commonly results from a direct blow or is a fracture within pathologic bone. An **oblique fracture** runs a course of approximately 45 degrees to the long axis of the bone and is caused by angulation or by both angulation and compression forces. A **spiral fracture** encircles the shaft, is generally longer than an oblique fracture, and is caused by torsional forces. **Avulsion fractures** are generally small fragments torn from bony prominences; they are usually the result of indirectly applied tension forces within attached ligaments and tendons rather than direct blows.

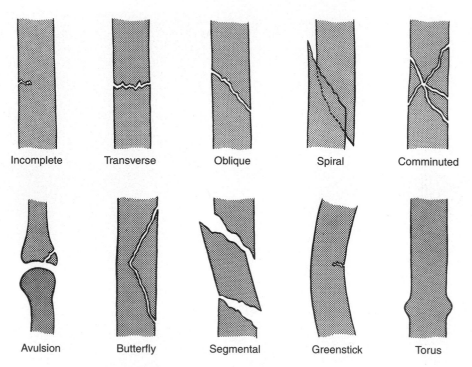

Incomplete   Transverse   Oblique   Spiral   Comminuted

Avulsion   Butterfly   Segmental   Greenstick   Torus

FIGURE 4-84 Classification of fractures.

A **comminuted fracture** is composed of more than two fragments. A **butterfly fragment** is an elongated triangular fragment of cortical bone generally detached from two other larger fragments of bone. A **segmental fracture** consists of a segment of the shaft isolated by proximal and distal lines of fracture.

A **compression fracture** results from a compression force that causes compaction of bone trabeculae and results in decreased length or width of a portion of a bone. Compression fractures most commonly occur in the vertebral body as a result of flexion of the spine; they may also be seen as impacted fractures of the humeral or femoral heads. A **depressed fracture** occurs in the skull or tibial plateau. In the skull, a small object with great force can produce a comminuted fracture, with portions of the fracture fragments driven inward. In the knee, the relatively hard lateral femoral condyle may impact on the relatively soft lateral tibial plateau with sufficient force to push the cortical surface of the tibia into the underlying cancellous bone.

A **stress, or fatigue, fracture** is the response of bone to repeated stresses, none of which is sufficient to cause a fracture. The earliest pathologic process in a stress fracture is osteoclastic resorption, followed by the development of periosteal callus in an attempt to repair and strengthen the bone. A **pathologic fracture** occurs in bone at an area of weakness caused by such processes as tumor, infection, or metabolic bone disease.

A **greenstick fracture** is an incomplete fracture with the opposite cortex intact. Greenstick fractures are found almost exclusively in infants and children because of the softness of their cancellous bone. A **torus (buckle) fracture** is one in which one cortex is intact with buckling or compaction of the opposite cortex. A **bowing fracture** is a plastic deformation caused by a stress that is too great to permit a complete recovery of normal shape, but is less than the stress required to produce a fracture.

An **undisplaced fracture** occurs when a plane of cleavage exists in the bone without angulation or separation. **Displacement** refers to separation of bone fragments; the direction of displacement describes the relationship of the distal fragment with respect to the proximal fragment and is usually measured in terms of the thickness of the shaft. **Angulation** indicates an angular deformity between the axes of the major fragments and also describes the position of the distal fragment with respect to the proximal one. **Dislocation** refers to the displacement of a bone that is no longer in contact with its normal articulation. If there is only partial loss of continuity of the joint surfaces, the displacement is called a **subluxation**.

Radiographic Appearance

Radiographs are essential in the diagnosis and management of fractures. Initially, a radiograph documents the clinically suspected fracture and determines whether the underlying bone is normal or whether the fracture is pathologic and has occurred in abnormal bone. After the orthopedic reduction of a fracture, repeat radiographs determine whether the fracture fragments are in anatomic position. Over the next several weeks or months, additional radiographs are obtained to assess fracture healing and to exclude possible complications.

In all cases of trauma, it is essential to have at least two projections of the injured part, preferably taken at 90 degrees to each other to determine fracture continuity or displacement in the anterior or posterior, medial or lateral, and superior or inferior direction. It is also important to demonstrate the joint above and below the fracture to search for a dislocation or a second fracture that may have resulted from transmission of the mechanical force. An example of this mechanism is the fracture or dislocation of the head of the fibula that frequently occurs with a fracture of the distal part of the tibia at the ankle.

Treatment

The overall goal of fracture treatment is to restore function and stability with an acceptable cosmetic result and a minimum of residual deformity. In **external, or closed, reduction** the fracture is treated by manipulation of the affected body part without surgical incision. **Open reduction** is a surgical procedure using direct or indirect manipulation of the fracture fragments and usually involving the application or insertion of some type of appliance or device to achieve and maintain the reduction (Figure 4-85). **External fixation** is accomplished by the use of splints or casts; **internal fixation** uses metal plates and screws, wires, rods, or nails, either alone or in combination, to maintain the reduction.

Most reduced fractures are immobilized or protected by an overlying cast. Fiberglass casting material causes less attenuation than plaster and thus produces less artifact. The radiopaque cast causes some obscuration of fine bony detail and, in severely osteoporotic bone, may make it difficult to visualize the fracture site. Therefore if there is a question of healing that requires the demonstration of early callus formation or if there is a possibility of osteomyelitis, it is essential that the cast be removed by the physician before obtaining radiographs so that there is sufficient visibility of bone detail to resolve these questions. The radiographer must increase exposure factors to compensate for the use of plaster or fiberglass casting and whether the cast is wet or dry. Depending on the resource, some authorities recommend an increase in mAs while others indicate an increase in kVp; it is recommended that one follow department protocol to produce the best images possible.

Fracture Healing

The radiographic evidence of fracture healing is a continuous external bridge of callus (calcium deposition) that extends across the line of fracture and unites the fracture fragments (Figure 4-86). The

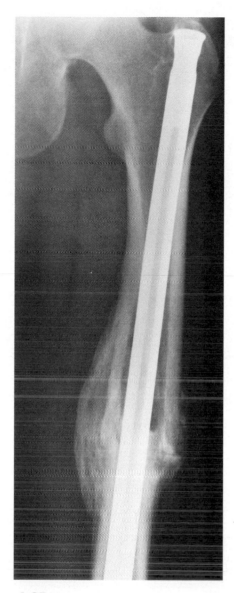

FIGURE 4-85 Open reduction with internal fixation. Intramedullary rod has been placed across a fracture of the femoral shaft. Note extensive callus formation about fracture site.

callus uniformly ossifies and approaches the density of normal bone. It is essential that at least two views be taken (preferably 90 degrees to each other) to ensure that there is callus about the fracture line in all directions. Proper exposure of the radiograph is required because underexposed films may produce the illusion of obliteration of the fracture line by bony trabeculae, whereas a properly exposed film would demonstrate the continued presence of the fracture line and a lack of healing. If the findings are equivocal, either computed or conventional tomography may be required to determine the degree of union. "Stress" films, a series of radiographs obtained with the injured part in the neutral position and during the

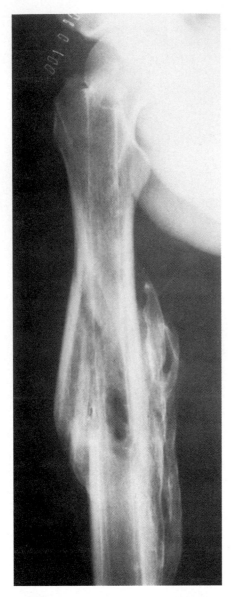

FIGURE 4-86 Normal union of a fracture. There is dense callus formation bridging the previous fracture of the mid-shaft of the femur. The original fracture line is completely obliterated.

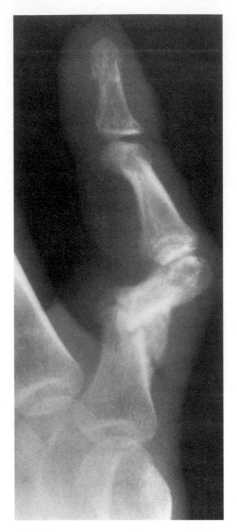

FIGURE 4-87 Malunion. Healing of proximal phalangeal fracture in poor position led to impairment of normal function.

application of stress by a physician or designated assistant on the distal fragment or part in the plane of suspected motion, may demonstrate a change in the alignment of the fragment, which indicates a lack of union.

Malunion is the healing of fracture fragments in a faulty position. This leads to impairment of normal function or a cosmetic appearance that may require surgical correction (Figure 4-87).

Delayed union is an ill-defined term arbitrarily applied to any fracture that takes longer to heal than the average fracture at that anatomic location. Delayed union may result from infection, from inadequate immobilization, from limited blood supply, or from loss of bone at the fracture site.

Nonunion refers to a condition in which the fracture healing process has completely stopped and the fragments remain ununited even with prolonged immobilization. Radiographically, nonunion characteristically appears as smooth, well-defined sclerosis about the fracture margins with occlusion of the medullary canal by sclerotic bone (Figure 4-88). A persistent defect, consisting of fibrous tissue and cartilage, appears between the fragments. Nonunion occurs predominantly in adults, is rare in children, and requires operative intervention to reinitiate the healing process.

Pathologic Fractures

Pathologic fractures are those occurring in bone that has been weakened by a preexisting condition. The most common underlying process is metastatic malignancy

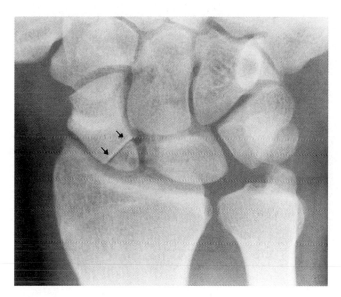

FIGURE 4-88 Nonunion of fracture of carpal navicular bone. Twenty years after initial injury, there is a smooth, well-defined line of sclerosis *(arrows)* about the fracture margin.

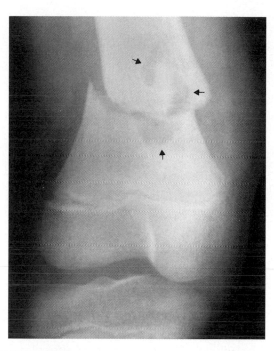

FIGURE 4-89 Pathologic fracture. A transverse fracture crosses the large benign tumor *(arrows)* of the distal femur.

or multiple myeloma. In children, developmental diseases, such as osteogenesis imperfecta or osteopetrosis, or nutritional deficiencies (rickets, scurvy) may result in pathologic fractures. Pathologic fractures also may occur when there is a benign cause of weakened bone, such as simple bone cyst, enchondroma, aneurysmal bone cyst, and fibrous dysplasia. Metabolic disorders causing a diffuse loss of bone substance (osteoporosis, osteomalacia, hyperparathyroidism) also make the skeleton more susceptible to injury.

Radiographic Appearance

Clinically, pathologic fractures arise from minor trauma that would not affect normal bone. Radiographically the fracture crosses an area of abnormal thinning, expansion, or bone destruction (Figure 4-89). The most common sites of pathologic fractures are the spine, femur, and humerus, areas in which metastatic disease is most common. In the spine, a pathologic fracture results in collapse of the vertebral body; indeed, a compressed vertebra in a patient older than 40 years should indicate underlying myeloma or metastatic disease.

CT or MRI scanning may detect a subtle change in the abnormal bone that is obscured by an abnormal lytic area or by sclerotic changes on plain radiographs.

Remember that patients with suspected pathologic fractures must be handled with extreme care lest the radiographer cause either further injury to the bone in question or an additional pathologic fracture in another area.

Treatment

Treatment of a pathologic fracture varies depending on the cause. Patients with malignant causes of fracture receive palliative therapy with possible surgery to place an orthotic fixation device, joint replacement, or amputation. For benign lytic lesions (cysts), surgical bone grafts or implantation of bone chips may be required to increase bone strength and structure.

Stress Fractures

Stress (fatigue) fractures are the result of repeated stresses to a bone that would not be injured by isolated forces of the same magnitude. The type of stress fracture and the site where it occurs vary with the activity. Regardless of location, the activities resulting in stress fractures are usually strenuous, often new or different, and repeated with frequency before producing pain. Stress fractures frequently occur in soldiers during basic training ("march" fracture). The most common sites are the shafts of the second and third metatarsals, the calcaneus, the proximal and distal shafts of the tibia and fibula, the shaft and neck of the femur, and the ischial and pubic rami.

Radiographic Appearance

Initially, plain radiographs of the symptomatic area are within normal limits (Figure 4-90). The stress fracture is first visualized 10 to 20 days after the onset of symptoms as either a thin line of transverse or occasionally

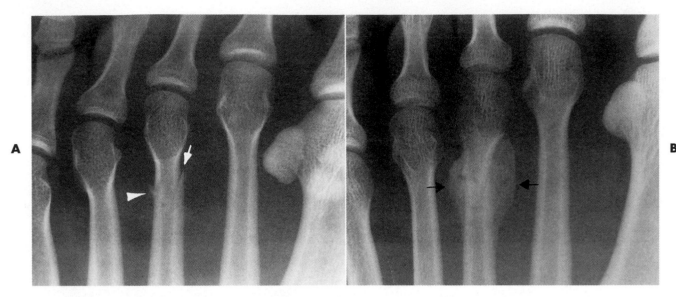

FIGURE 4-90 Stress fracture of third metatarsal. Initial radiograph was within normal limits. **A,** Radiograph obtained 14 days after onset of symptoms demonstrates thin oblique lucency *(arrow)* interrupting one cortex, and a small amount of fluffy periosteal callus formation *(arrowhead)* along the opposite cortex. There is no evidence of complete fracture line. **B,** Repeat radiograph 3 weeks later shows dense callus formation *(arrows)* about fracture site.

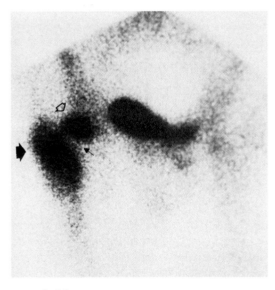

FIGURE 4-91 Radionuclide bone scan of stress fracture. Greatly increased radionuclide uptake in femoral neck *(open arrow)* and intertrochanteric region *(solid arrow)*, with lack of uptake at actual fracture site *(thin arrow)*. Plain radiograph and tomograms showed only minimal trabecular disruption and slight callus formation.

oblique radiolucency or as fluffy periosteal callus formation without evidence of a fracture line. When this radiographic appearance is detected at a site common to stress fractures, a history of athletic or other unusual activity should be elicited as the underlying cause.

Radionuclide bone scans using a triple-phase technique to maximize specificity can demonstrate a stress fracture before it can be detected on plain radiographs

(Figure 4-91). MRI, used only for cases with indeterminate radiographic findings, is highly sensitive for detecting stress fractures. In some cases, MRI has higher specificity than radionuclide bone scans. Early stress fractures produce low signal intensity on T1-weighted images; there is a progressive increase in signal intensity with increased T2-weighting. A fat-saturation (fat-suppressing) technique may demonstrate associated medullary edema or hemorrhage, which produces a high signal compared with the fat-suppressed background.

Treatment
Immobilization of the injured area prevents further injury and gives the stressed area time to heal.

Battered-Child Syndrome
The battered-child syndrome refers to multiple, repeated, physically induced injuries in young children caused by parents or guardians. The facility treating the suspected battered child, also known as suspected nonaccidental trauma (SNAT), has a legal responsibility to report suspicious cases to child protective services. While the child is being evaluated, diagnosed, and treated, the environment must be protective for the child.

Shaken-baby syndrome, Munchausen syndrome by proxy, and sudden infant death syndrome are all situations investigated to prove or disprove abusive injury. A skeletal series is performed in such instances and includes an AP view of each extremity and the pelvis. AP and lateral projections of the chest and skull are also required.

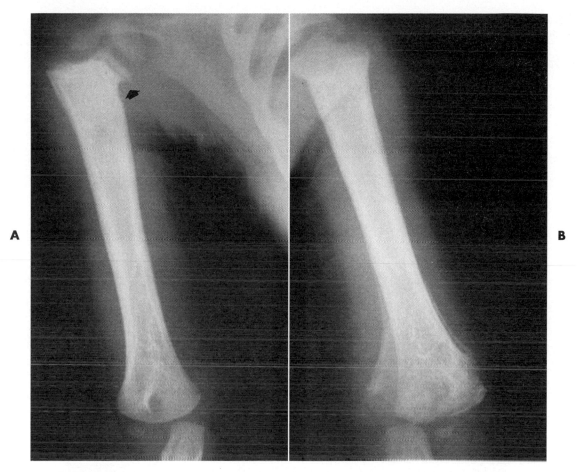

FIGURE 4-92   Battered-child syndrome. **A,** Frontal radiograph of right arm demonstrates corner fracture *(arrow)* of proximal humerus. **B,** Frontal radiograph of left arm shows healing displaced fracture of distal humerus.

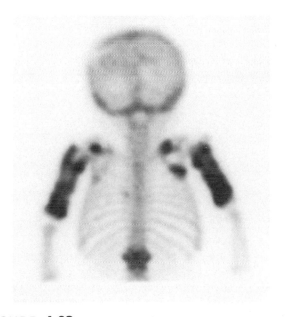

FIGURE 4-93 Bone scan of upper body with multiple hot spots indicating fracture sites in the humerus, clavicle, and scapula.

Radiographic Appearance

The radiographic findings in this syndrome include multiple fractures of varying age in various stages of healing, fractures of the corners of metaphyses with or without associated epiphyseal displacement, and exuberant subperiosteal new bone formation along the shafts of long bones (Figure 4-92). Skull fractures or widening of the cranial sutures are commonly associated. Another highly suggestive finding is one or more fractures at otherwise unusual sites (usually fractured only by direct blows), such as the ribs, scapula, sternum, spine, or lateral ends of the clavicles (Figure 4-93).

Treatment

Prompt and accurate diagnosis of battered-child syndrome is essential to minimize the extent of physical and psychological damage and sometimes to prevent a fatal injury.

Common Fractures and Dislocations

Colles' fracture is a transverse fracture through the distal radius with dorsal (posterior) angulation and often overriding of the distal fracture fragment

SUMMARY of FINDINGS for Fractures

fracture type	location	radiographic appearance	treatment
Trauma	All skeletal bones	Fragments, bone separation, and/or discontinuity	Reduction with immobilization—external/cast, internal/surgical fixation
Pathologic	Diseased bone	Vertebral collapse Bone destruction—radiolucency due to underlying cause	Treat cause Immobilization
Stress	Site of increased stress activity	Bone discontinuity Radiolucent, transverse, or oblique line Fluffy periosteal callus formation without fracture line MRI—low signal intensity on T1-weighted images; progressive increased signal intensity on T2-weighted images	Immobilization Reduce cause of stress
Battered-child syndrome	Skull, long bones, flat bones	Multiple fractures of varying age in various stages of healing	Minimize physical and psychological damage

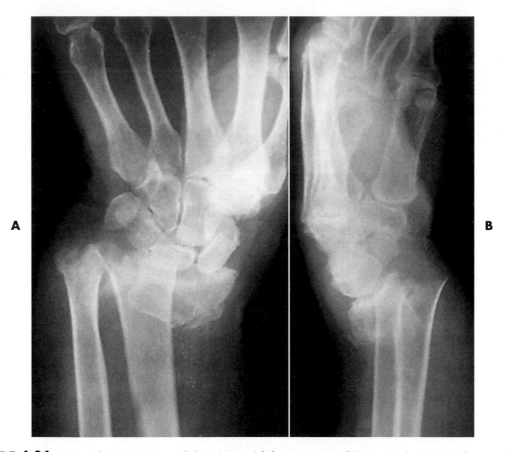

FIGURE 4-94 Colles' fracture. Frontal **(A)** and lateral **(B)** projections of the wrist show overriding and dorsal displacement of distal fragment. There is also a displaced fracture of the distal ulna.

(Figure 4-94). In more than half the cases, there is an associated avulsion fracture of the ulnar styloid process. Colles' fracture is usually caused by a fall on the outstretched hand and is the most common fracture of the wrist.

Navicular (scaphoid) fractures are the most common fractures involving the carpal bones. They are usually transverse and occur through the central part (the waist) of the bone. Although most navicular fractures can be identified on routine

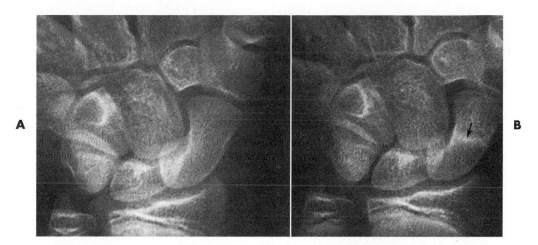

FIGURE **4-95** Navicular fracture. **A,** On a radiograph obtained immediately after injury, fracture cannot be detected. **B,** On the repeat radiograph obtained 3 weeks later, fracture is clearly identified by sclerotic band *(arrow)* of opaque internal callus.

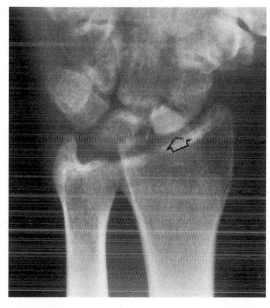

FIGURE **4-96** Avascular necrosis of navicular fracture. Increased bone density is seen in the avascular proximal fragment *(arrow)*.

frontal projections of the wrist, subtle fractures may require specific oblique and angulated projections or films made using magnification techniques. In some cases, a navicular fracture cannot be detected on the initial examination despite strong clinical suspicion (Figure 4-95, *A*). In this situation, the wrist should be placed in a cast or plaster splint and reexamined (out of plaster) in 7 to 10 days. At this time, resorption of bone at the margins of the fracture widens the fracture line and makes it more apparent radiographically (Figure 4-95, *B*).

Nonunion is a serious complication of navicular fractures (see Figure 4-88). Its incidence increases with motion or displacement of the fracture fragments resulting from either poor immobilization or neglect. Because the blood supply to the navicular bone comes primarily from the distal portion, the proximal fragment may become avascular and undergo ischemic necrosis. This is seen as an increase in bone density associated with collapse of bone or loss of volume in the affected fragment (Figure 4-96).

A **boxer's fracture** is a transverse fracture of the neck of the fifth metacarpal with volar (palmar) angulation of the distal fragment (Figure 4-97). This injury is typically the result of a blow struck with the fist.

In the detection of fractures about the elbow, a valuable clue is displacement of the normal elbow fat pads (the fat pad sign). On lateral projections of the elbow, the anterior fat pad normally appears as a radiolucency closely applied to the anterior surface of the distal end of the humerus. The posterior fat pad, normally hidden in the depths of the olecranon fossa, should not be visible on standard lateral projections of the elbow. Any process producing synovial or hemorrhagic effusion within the elbow joint displaces the fat pads. The normally hidden posterior fat pad, posteriorly displaced, becomes visible as a crescentic lucency behind the lower end of the humerus (Figure 4-98). The anterior fat pad becomes more rounded and further separated from the underlying bone. The posterior fat pad is by far the more sensitive indicator of an elbow joint effusion. Its presence on the lateral projection of the patient with elbow trauma strongly suggests an underlying fracture, especially of the radial head, and indicates

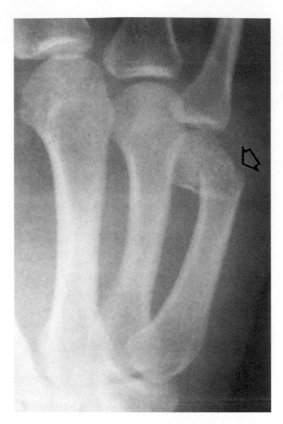

FIGURE 4-97 Boxer's fracture. There is a fracture at the neck of the fifth metacarpal *(arrow)* with volar angulation of distal fragment.

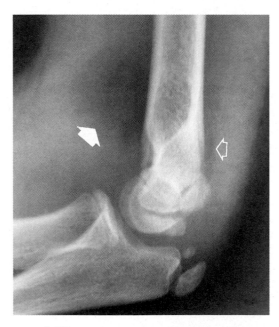

FIGURE 4-98 Fat pad sign in the elbow. Anterior fat pad *(solid arrow)* is clearly lifted from its fossa as a result of a large joint effusion in this child with a supracondylar fracture of the distal humerus. The normally hidden posterior fat pad is posteriorly displaced by effusion *(open arrow)*.

the need for oblique projections if no fracture is seen on standard projections. If no fracture is identified, a repeat radiograph obtained 2 weeks or more after appropriate immobilization often shows a fracture by demonstrating a fracture line or callus formation indicating healing.

Most fractures of the forearm involve both the radius and the ulna. If only one bone fractures, it is essential to examine both the elbow and the wrist to exclude the possibility of proximal or distal joint dislocation. A **Monteggia fracture** (Figure 4-99) is an isolated fracture of the shaft of the ulna associated with anterior dislocation of the radius at the elbow. A **Galeazzi fracture** is the combination of a fracture of the shaft of the radius and a dorsal (posterior) dislocation of the ulna at the wrist.

Pott's fracture involves both malleoli (i.e., of tibia and fibula) with dislocation of the ankle joint. A bimalleolar fracture is one involving both the medial and the lateral malleoli (Figure 4-100). Because of the mechanism of injury, the fracture on one side is transverse, whereas the fracture on the opposite side is oblique or spiral. Trimalleolar fractures involve the posterior lip of the tibia in addition to the medial and lateral malleoli and usually represent fracture dislocations.

One of the most frequent injuries to the foot is a transverse fracture at the base of the fifth metatarsal (a **Jones fracture**) (Figure 4-101). This fracture represents an avulsion injury that results from plantar flexion and inversion of the foot, as occurs when stepping off a curb or falling while walking on stairs. It is important to distinguish this fracture from the longitudinally oriented apophysis that is normally found in children at the lateral margin of the base of the fifth metatarsal.

The shoulder is by far the most commonly dislocated joint in the body (Figure 4-102). About 95% of shoulder dislocations are anterior, resulting from external rotation and abduction of the arm. As the anterior displacement occurs, the posterolateral surface of the humeral head impacts against the anterior or anteroinferior surface of the glenoid fossa and may result in a compression fracture of the humeral head, a fracture of the glenoid rim, or both. In most cases, the humeral head is displaced medially and anteriorly and comes to rest beneath the coracoid process.

Dislocations of the hip, with or without associated fracture of the acetabulum, are caused by severe injuries, such as automobile collisions, pedestrian accidents, or falls from a great height. Unlike in the shoulder, posterior dislocations of the hip are far more common than anterior dislocations and account for 85% to 90% of the cases (Figure 4-103).

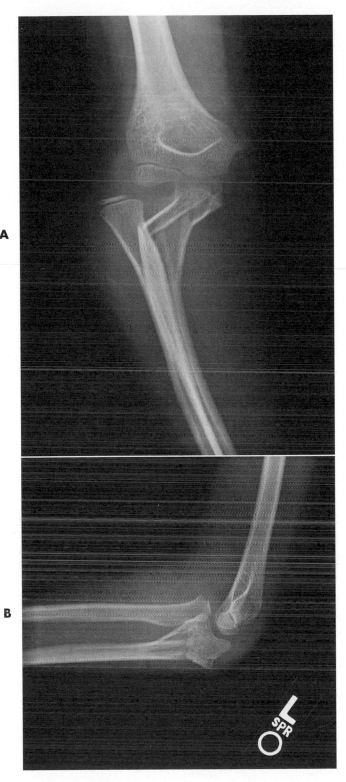

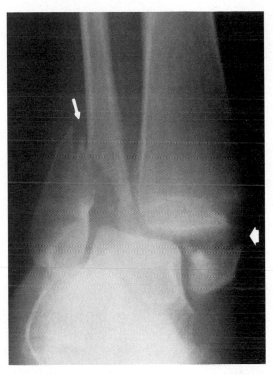

FIGURE 4-100 Bimalleolar fracture of ankle. A transverse fracture of the medial malleolus *(broad arrow)* is associated with a low oblique fracture of distal fibula *(thin arrow)*.

FIGURE 4-99 Monteggia fracture. Displaced fracture of the proximal ulna is associated with anterior dislocation of radial head.

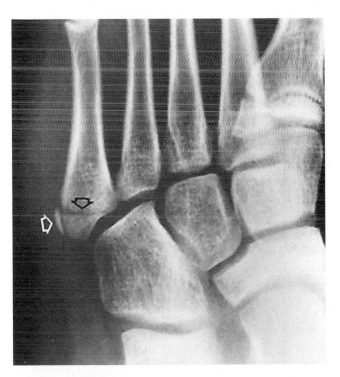

FIGURE 4-101 Jones fracture of base of fifth metatarsal. Note that the fracture line is transverse *(black arrow)* on the base of the fifth metatarsal, whereas the normal apophysis in this child has vertical orientation *(white arrow)*.

A

B

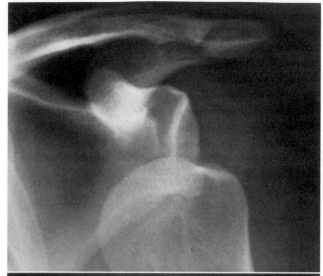

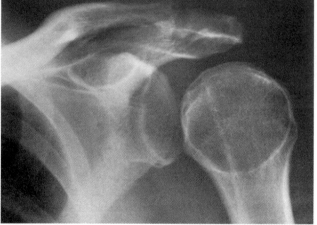

FIGURE 4-102 Dislocation of shoulder. Anterior **(A)** dislocation seen with inferior and medial displacement of the humeral head, and posterior **(B)** dislocation demonstrated by the increased distance between the anterior glenoid rim and the humeral head.

Fractures and Dislocations of the Spine

Fractures and dislocations of the spine may be the result of direct trauma, hyperextension-flexion injuries (whiplash), or normal stresses in abnormal bone (osteoporosis, metastatic destruction). In the patient with spinal injury, the major goal of the radiographic evaluation is to determine whether a fracture or dislocation is present and whether the injury is stable or unstable. The spine can be considered as consisting of two major columns. The anterior column consists of the vertebral bodies, intervertebral disks, and anterior and posterior longitudinal ligaments. The facets, apophyseal joints, pedicles, laminae, spinous processes, and all the intervening ligaments form the

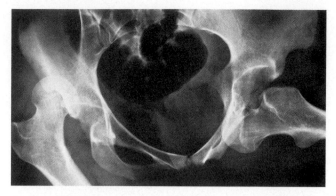

FIGURE 4-103 Dislocations of hip. Frontal radiograph of teen-aged girl injured in motor vehicle collision demonstrates right posterior dislocation and left anterior dislocation of hip. Right posterior dislocation is characterized by typical superolateral displacement of femoral head, fixed adduction, and internal rotation (lesser trochanter superimposed on femoral shaft). Left anterior dislocation is manifested by characteristic inferomedial displacement of femoral head, which has come to overlie obturator foramen; fixed abduction; and external rotation (lesser trochanter depicted in profile).

posterior column. If one of the two columns remains intact, the injury is considered **stable**. If both columns are disrupted, the injury is considered **unstable**.

If there is a strong suspicion of injury to the cervical spine, the initial radiograph should be a horizontal-beam lateral projection with the patient supine. This cross-table lateral radiograph must be checked by the physician before obtaining any other projections (Figure 4-104). It is essential to include all seven cervical vertebrae on the film lest the relatively common injuries of C6 and C7 be overlooked (Figure 4-105). This may require supine oblique projections or films made in the swimmer's position in which one arm of the patient is extended over the head while the other arm remains by the side so as to slightly oblique the upper torso and permit visualization of the cervicothoracic junction. A frontal projection of the spine and an open-mouth projection of the atlas and axis (C1 and C2) should be obtained next. In an acutely injured patient, oblique or flexion and extension projections should be performed only under the direct supervision of the attending physician. Computed or even conventional tomography may be used to confirm the presence or absence of a fracture (especially of the posterior elements) and to visualize otherwise obscured areas of the spine, such as the craniovertebral and cervicothoracic junctions. CT can precisely localize fracture fragments in relation to the spinal canal and detect otherwise obscure fractures of the posterior elements. Myelography may be performed in patients with a spinal cord injury in the absence of an obvious fracture or dislocation to identify

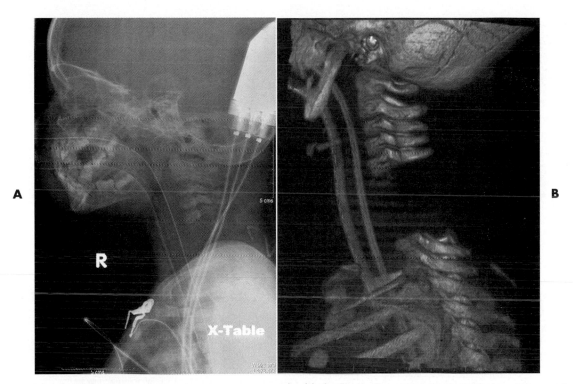

FIGURE 4-104 Cross-table C-spine on a 23-month-old demonstrating internal decapitation **(A)**. **B,** The volume-rendered CT, which better delineates the separation of C5-C6.

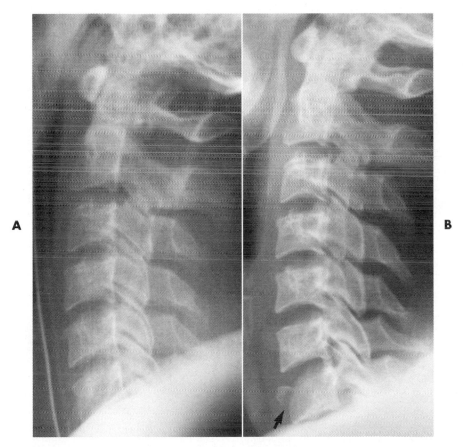

FIGURE 4-105 Fracture of C7 vertebral body. **A,** On initial lateral radiograph, only upper six cervical vertebrae can be seen. Patient's shoulders overlie seventh cervical vertebra. **B,** With shoulders pulled down to expose seventh cervical vertebra, anterosuperior fracture *(arrow)* is clearly identified.

a condition amenable to surgical removal or repair (e.g., a herniated disk fragment or an epidural hematoma of the spinal cord).

Several types of fractures are peculiar to the cervical spine. A **Jefferson fracture,** a comminuted fracture of the ring of the atlas, involves both the anterior and the posterior arches and causes displacement of the fragments. The characteristic appearance on frontal radiographs or tomograms is a bilateral offset or spreading of the lateral articular masses of C1 in relation to the opposing articular surfaces of C2 (Figure 4-106).

Fractures of the odontoid process are usually transverse and located at the base of the dens at its junction with the body (Figure 4-107). On an open-mouth view, a lucency between the upper central incisor teeth often overlaps the dens; this must be differentiated from a rare vertical fracture of the dens.

The **hangman's fracture** is the result of acute hyperextension of the head on the neck. This appears as a fracture of the arch of C2 anterior to the inferior facet and is usually associated with anterior subluxation

of C2 on C3 (Figure 4-108). Although originally described in patients who had been hanged, this injury is now far more commonly the result of motor vehicle collisions.

Clay shoveler's fracture is an avulsion fracture of a spinous process in the lower cervical or upper thoracic spine. The fracture is difficult to demonstrate on emergency cross-table lateral radiographs because the shoulders frequently obscure the lower cervical region. The diagnosis can be made on the frontal view by noting the double shadow of the spinous processes caused by the caudal displacement of the avulsed fragment (Figure 4-109). This

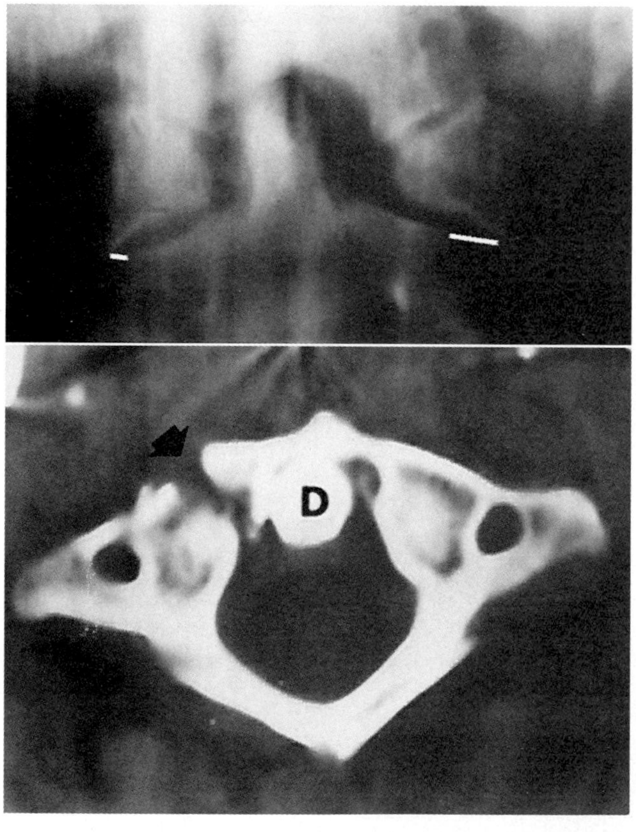

FIGURE 4-106 Jefferson fracture. **A,** On frontal projection, there is lateral displacement of lateral masses of C1 bilaterally *(white lines).* **B,** CT scan in another patient shows unilateral break in arch of C1 *(arrow). D,* Dens.

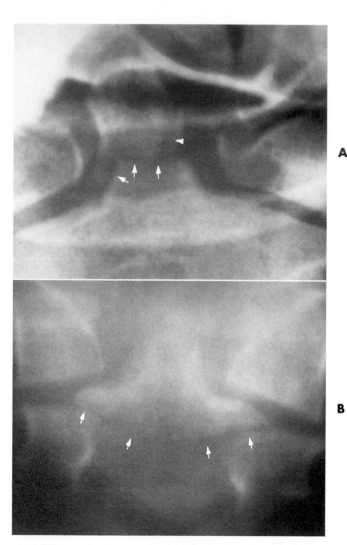

FIGURE 4-107 Fracture of odontoid process. **A,** Open-mouth frontal projection shows combined oblique and transverse fracture at base of dens *(arrows).* There is also separate cortical fragment on left *(arrowhead),* which most likely remains attached to alar ligament. **B,** In another patient, frontal tomogram shows low fracture *(arrows)* through body of C2.

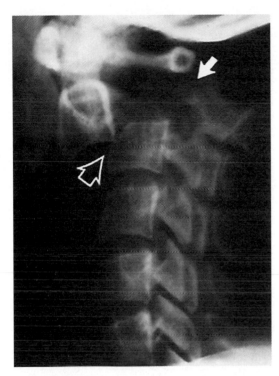

FIGURE 4-108 Hangman's fracture. Neural arch fracture *(solid arrow)* associated with complete C2-3 subluxation *(open arrow)*.

double-spinous-process sign must be differentiated from a bifid spinous process, which usually lies at a higher level and on a more horizontal plane.

Most fractures of the thoracolumbar spine are attributable to compressive forces that cause anterior wedging or depression of the superior end plate of a vertebral body (Figure 4-110). The **seat belt fracture** is a transverse fracture of a lumbar vertebra that is often associated with significant visceral injuries (Figure 4-111). In this condition, a horizontal fracture of the vertebral body extends to involve some or all of the posterior elements.

Herniation of Intervertebral Disks

The intervertebral disks act as shock absorbers between the vertebrae, cushioning the movements of the spine. They consist of a fibrous outer cartilage (annulus) surrounding a central nucleus pulposus, which is the essential part of the disk. The nucleus pulposus is a highly elastic, semifluid mass compressed like a spring between the vertebral surfaces. In youth, it contains a large amount of fluid to cushion the motion of the spine. With increasing age, the fluid and elasticity gradually diminish, leading to degenerative changes and back pain. Protrusion, or herniation,

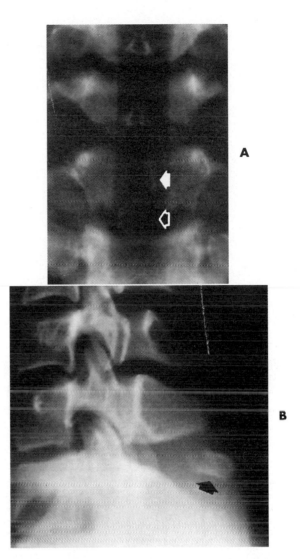

FIGURE 4-109 Clay shoveler's fracture. **A,** Frontal projection of cervical spine shows characteristic double-spinous-process sign resulting from caudal displacement of avulsed fragment *(open arrow)* with respect to normal position of major portion of spinous process *(solid arrow)*. **B,** Lateral projection clearly shows avulsed fragment *(arrow)*.

of a lumbar intervertebral disk is the major cause of severe acute, chronic, or recurring low back and leg pain. It most frequently involves the L4-5 and L5-S1 levels in the lumbar region, where it often causes sciatica, pain that radiates down the sciatic nerve to the back of the thigh and lower leg. Other major sites are the C5-6 and C6-7 levels in the neck and the T9-12 levels in the thoracic region.

Radiographic Appearance

Although plain radiographs show characteristic narrowing of the intervertebral disk spaces with hypertrophic spur formation, bony sclerosis, spurs impinging on the neural foramina, and the vacuum

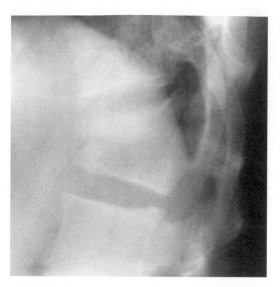

FIGURE 4-110 Vertebral body fracture. Characteristic anterior wedging of superior end plate of L1 vertebral body.

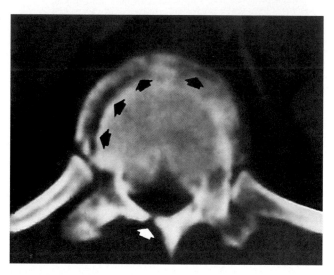

FIGURE 4-111 Seat belt fracture. CT scan shows fracture of lumbar vertebral body *(black arrows)* associated with laminar fracture at the same level *(white arrow).*

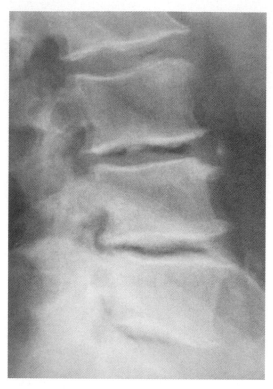

FIGURE 4-112 Degenerative disk disease. Hypertrophic spurring, intervertebral disk space narrowing, and reactive sclerosis. Note linear lucent collections (vacuum phenomenon) overlying several intervertebral disks.

phenomenon (lucent collections overlying the intervertebral disks), these findings are nonspecific and frequently occur in patients with minimal symptoms (Figure 4-112). The diagnosis of herniation of an intervertebral disk requires CT, MRI, or myelography to demonstrate impression of the disk on the spinal cord or individual nerve roots (Figures 4-113 to 4-118).

Treatment
Patients with symptoms suggestive of disk herniation are initially treated conservatively with bed rest, muscle relaxants, and analgesics before being subjected to radiographic studies. If conservative treatment is unsuccessful, surgery may be necessary to remove the cause of impingement and alleviate the pain and symptoms.

Spondylolysis and Spondylolisthesis

Spondylolysis refers to a cleft in the pars interarticularis that is situated between the superior and inferior articular processes of a vertebra. Occurring in about 5% of the population, these clefts are usually bilateral, most commonly involve the fifth lumbar vertebra, and predispose to the forward displacement of one vertebra on the other that may cause chronic back pain. *Spondylolysis* is the term for a defect in the pars interarticularis without displacement; if displacement occurs, the condition is called **spondylolisthesis**.

Radiographic Appearance
A plain lateral radiograph of the lower lumbar spine clearly shows any spondylolisthesis and may demonstrate the lucent cleft in the pars interarticularis even if no displacement has occurred (Figure 4-119). In grading spondylolisthesis of the lumbosacral

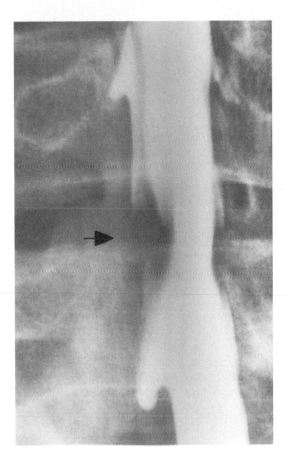

FIGURE 4-113 Lumbar disk herniation. Myelogram shows extradural lesion *(arrow)* at level of intervertebral disk space. Note amputation of nerve root by disk compression.

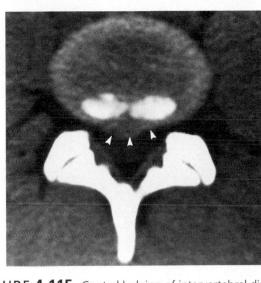

FIGURE 4-115 Central bulging of intervertebral disk. CT scan shows convex posterior border of the disk *(arrowheads)*. Note preservation of epidural fat.

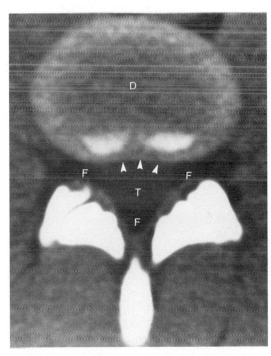

FIGURE 4-114 CT of normal lumbar disk *(D)*. The normal lumbar intervertebral disk has a concave posterior border *(arrowheads)*. Note normal epidural fat *(F)* surrounding the thecal sac *(T)*.

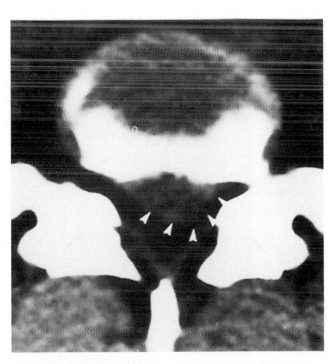

FIGURE 4-116 Disk herniation at L5-S1 level. CT shows herniation of disk *(arrowheads)* to the left with obliteration of epidural fat.

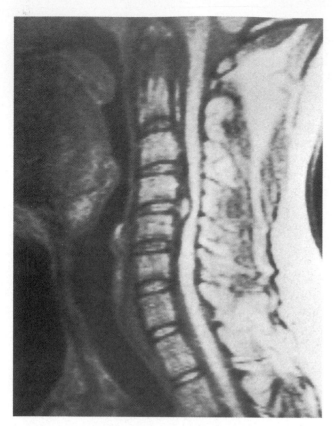

FIGURE **4-117** MR image of intervertebral disk herniation in cervical region. Note extradural impression on spinal cord.

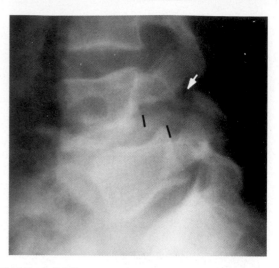

FIGURE **4-119** Spondylolisthesis. Lateral view of lower lumbar spine shows break in pars interarticularis *(arrow)*, with resultant anterior slippage of L4 with respect to L5. Vertical black lines indicate posterior margins of vertebral bodies.

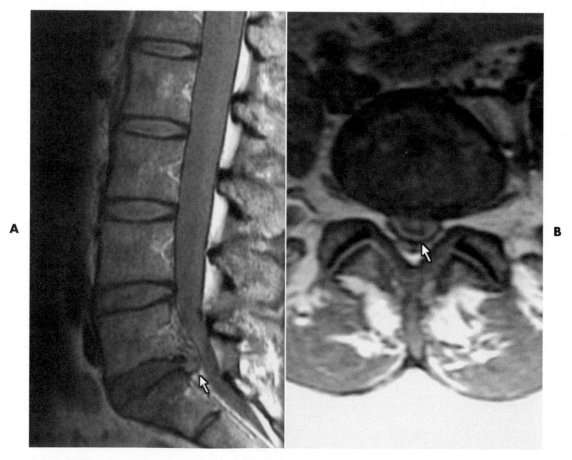

FIGURE **4-118** Lumbar disk herniation. MR image illustrating a torn annulus fibrosis and nucleus pulposus of L5-S1 *(arrows)* in sagittal **(A)** and transverse **(B)** planes.

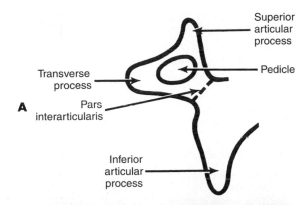

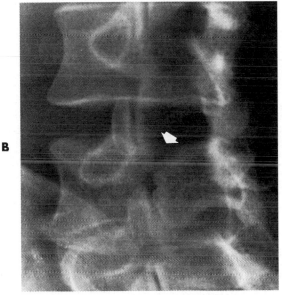

junction on the lateral projection, the superior surface of the sacrum is divided into four equal parts. A forward displacement of the fifth lumbar vertebra up to one fourth the thickness of the sacrum is called a first-degree spondylolisthesis; half the thickness, a second-degree spondylolisthesis; and so on.

The diagnosis of spondylolysis without displacement may require an oblique projection of the lumbar spine, in which the appearance of the posterior elements has been likened to that of a Scotty dog (Figure 4-120). The pedicle and transverse process form the eye and nose; the superior and inferior articular processes form the ear and leg; and the pars interarticularis forms the neck, which is "fractured" in a patient with spondylolysis.

Treatment

Passive treatment includes bracing, physical therapy, restricted activity, and nonnarcotic analgesics to control pain to a tolerable level. Conservative therapy works for the majority of patients. Surgical treatment is necessary only when passive treatment is unsuccessful for controlling pain. A complete laminectomy, usually with spinal fusion, is performed to free the peripheral nerves and stabilize spinal movement.

FIGURE 4-120 Spondylolysis. **A,** Diagram of Scotty dog sign. **B,** Oblique projection of lumbar spine demonstrates a defect in the pars interarticularis, which appears as a fracture through the neck of the Scotty dog *(arrow).*

SUMMARY of FINDINGS for Common Spinal Disorders

disorder	location	radiographic appearance	treatment
Disk herniation	Cervical and lumbar spine regions	CT and MRI—disk impingement on nerve or spinal cord	Conservative—bed rest, muscle relaxants, and analgesics Aggressive—surgical removal of disk
Spondylolysis Spondylolisthesis	Fifth lumbar vertebra, lumbosacral junction	Defect in pars interarticularis without displacement Forward displacement with pars interarticularis defect	Nonoperative—bracing, physical therapy, restricted activity, and nonnarcotic analgesics Surgical—complete laminectomy with spinal fusion

REVIEW QUESTIONS

1. The shaft of any long bone is termed the _____.
   - A. epiphysis
   - B. diaphysis
   - C. metaphysis
   - D. periosteum

2. The end of a long bone is referred to as the _____.
   - A. epiphysis
   - B. diaphysis
   - C. metaphysis
   - D. periosteum

3. The special types of cells responsible for the diameter growth of bones are _____.
   - A. osteoblasts
   - B. osteoclasts
   - C. chondroblasts
   - D. both A and B

4. The common area(s) of the body radiographed to determine bone age is/are _____.
   - A. skull
   - B. wrist
   - C. hand
   - D. both B and C

5. What pathologic condition is present if the posterior elements of one or more vertebrae fail to unite?
   - A. meningocele
   - B. spina bifida
   - C. myelomeningocele
   - D. spondylolisthesis

6. Aging and postmenopausal hormonal changes are the major causes of generalized _____.
   - A. osteogenesis imperfecta
   - B. osteoporosis
   - C. osteopetrosis
   - D. osteomalacia

7. An inherited generalized disorder of connective tissue characterized by multiple fractures and a bluish color of the sclera of the eye is _____.
   - A. osteogenesis
   - B. osteoporosis
   - C. osteopetrosis imperfecta
   - D. osteomalacia

8. Lack of vitamin D in the diet of infants and children can cause a systemic disease called _____.
   - A. achondroplasia
   - B. rickets
   - C. osteomalacia
   - D. osteopetrosis

9. A disorder of metabolism causing an increased blood level of uric acid is called _____.
   - A. achondroplasia
   - B. rickets
   - C. gout
   - D. uremia

10. A benign projection of bone with a cartilage-like cap occurring around the knee in children or adolescents is _____.
    - A. osteochondroma
    - B. enchondroma
    - C. achondroplasia
    - D. osteoma

11. An example of a malignant bone tumor is _____.
    - A. osteogenic
    - B. chondrosarcoma
    - C. Ewing's sarcoma
    - D. all of the above

12. The form of noninfectious arthritis characterized by osteoporosis, soft tissue swelling, and erosions of the metacarpophalangeal joints and ulnar styloid processes is _____.
    - A. Reiter's
    - B. rheumatoid
    - C. psoriatic
    - D. osteoarthritis

13. The extremely common form of arthritis that is characterized by loss of joint cartilage and reactive new bone growth and that is part of the normal wear of aging is _____.
    - A. Reiter's
    - B. rheumatoid
    - C. psoriatic
    - D. osteoarthritis

14. Inflammation of the small fluid-filled sacs that are located around joints and that reduce friction is termed _____.
    - A. tendinitis
    - B. arthritis
    - C. bursitis
    - D. both A and C

15. In what type of fracture is the skin broken?
    - A. butterfly
    - B. compound
    - C. comminuted
    - D. both A and C

16. What type of fracture consists of more than two fragments?
    - A. open
    - B. compound
    - C. comminuted
    - D. both A and B

17. What term applies to the new calcium deposits that unite fracture sites?
    - A. bone
    - B. callus
    - C. periosteum
    - D. both A and C

18. What type of fracture occurs in bone weakened by some preexisting condition, such as a metastatic lesion or multiple myeloma?
    - A. stress
    - B. Colles'
    - C. Pott's
    - D. pathologic

19. What is the name for the type of fracture that can occur from falling on the outstretched hand and that involves the distal portion of the radius?
    A. stress
    B. Colles'
    C. Pott's
    D. pathologic

20. What name is applied to a fracture involving both malleoli?
    A. stress
    B. Colles'
    C. Pott's
    D. pathologic

21. What is the name applied to the fracture resulting from acute hyperextension of the head on the neck that usually affects C2 and C3?
    A. Hangman's
    B. Jefferson
    C. Boxer's
    D. Monteggia

22. What area of the spine does a clay shoveler's fracture involve?
    A. lower thoracic and upper lumbar
    B. lumbar only
    C. lower cervical and upper thoracic
    D. cervical only

23. Diagnosis of an intervertebral disk herniation requires which radiographic procedure(s)?
    A. myelography
    B. CT
    C. MRI
    D. A or B or C

24. What medical term refers to a cleft in the pars interarticularis commonly involving the fifth lumbar vertebra?
    A. spondylolisthesis
    B. spondylolysis
    C. spondylitis
    D. A or B or C

25. What pathologic condition sometimes occurs after trauma, causing an interrupted blood supply to a bone?
    A. vasculitis
    B. ischemic necrosis
    C. Cushing's
    D. stress fracture

BIBLIOGRAPHY

Brower AC: *Arthritis in black and white,* Philadelphia, 1988, Saunders.

Burgener FA, Kormano M: *Differential diagnosis in computed tomography,* New York, 1996, Thieme.

Callen PW: *Ultrasonography in obstetrics and gynecology,* ed 4, Philadelphia, 2000, Saunders.

eMedicine>Specialties>Radiology>Musculoskeletal: www.emidicine.com.

Greenfield GB: *Radiology of bone diseases,* ed 4, Philadelphia, 1990, Lippincott.

Greenspan A: *Orthopedic radiology: a practical approach,* Philadelphia, 1992, Lippincott.

Griffiths HJ: *Basic bone radiology,* Norwalk, 1987, Appleton & Lange.

Helms CA: *Fundamentals of skeletal radiology,* Philadelphia, 1989, Saunders.

Pressel DM: Evaluation of physical abuse in children, *Am Fam Physician,* May 15, 2000; aafp.org/aft/20000515/37.57.html.

Resnick D, Niwayama G: *Diagnosis of bone and joint disorders,* Philadelphia, 1988, Saunders.

Rogers LF: *Radiology of skeletal trauma,* New York, 1992, Churchill Livingstone.

Rumack CM, Wilson SR, Charbonneau JW: *Diagnostic ultrasound,* ed 3, St Louis, 2005, Mosby.

GASTROINTESTINAL *System*

Chapter Outline

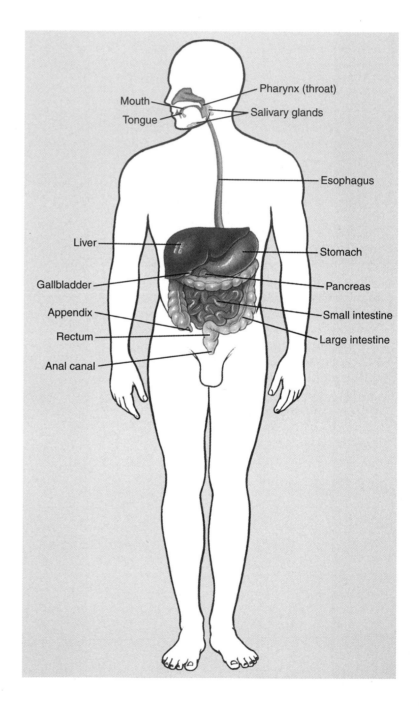

Pancreas
Acute Pancreatitis
Chronic Pancreatitis
Pancreatic Pseudocyst
Cancer of the Pancreas
Pneumoperitoneum
Spleen
Enlargement
Rupture

Key Terms

alcoholic gastritis
bacterial (phlegmonous) gastritis
chronic atrophic gastritis
chyme
colonic ileus
congenital tracheoesophageal (TE) fistulas
constipation
corrosive gastritis
deglutition
diarrhea
diarrheogenic islet cell tumors
emulsifier
epiphrenic diverticula
glycogen
infectious gastritis
infiltrating
insulinoma
irritable bowel syndrome
localized ileus
malabsorption disorder
Mallory-Weiss syndrome
mastication
pancreatitis
peristalsis
polypoid
traction
ulceration
ulcerogenic islet cell tumors (gastrinomas)
villi
Zenker's diverticula

Prerequisite Knowledge

The student should have a basic knowledge of the anatomy and physiology of the gastrointestinal system. In addition, proper learning and understanding of the material will be facilitated if the student has some clinical experience in gastrointestinal radiography and image evaluation, including a concept of the changes in technique required to compensate for density differences produced by a few of the underlying pathologic conditions.

Goals

To acquaint the student radiographer with the pathophysiology and radiographic manifestations of all of the common and some of the unusual disorders of the gastrointestinal system.

Objectives

After reading this chapter, the reader will be able to:
1. Classify the more common diseases in terms of their attenuation of x-rays
2. Explain the changes in technical factors required for obtaining optimal quality radiographs in patients with various underlying pathologic conditions
3. Define all key terms in this chapter
4. Describe the physiology of the gastrointestinal system
5. Identify anatomic structures on both diagrams and radiographs of the gastrointestinal system
6. Differentiate the various pathologic conditions affecting the gastrointestinal system and their radiographic manifestations

As in other body systems, certain pathologic conditions in the gastrointestinal system require alterations in the technical factors chosen for imaging. In patients with ascites, a common complication of advanced cirrhosis, an increased kilovolt peak (kVp) is required to penetrate the additional fluid content of the abdomen. On the other hand, a decreased kVp is needed in patients with suspected large or small bowel obstruction because of the excessive amount of gas in the abdominal cavity.

The radiographer is usually called on to assist the radiologist during fluoroscopic examinations of the gastrointestinal tract. Indeed, it is generally the radiographer's task to coerce the patient into drinking (and not vomiting) the rather unpleasant tasting contrast material and to urge the patient to turn around several times to provide adequate mucosal coating for the double-contrast upper gastrointestinal series. Similarly, the radiographer may have to convince the patient to retain barium and air during the often uncomfortable barium enema examinations. It is frequently time well spent for the radiographer to explain fully to the patient both the mechanics of the procedure and the extreme importance of patient cooperation.

Physiology of the Digestive System

The basic function of the digestive system is to alter the chemical and physical composition of food so that it can be absorbed and used by body cells. This process

RADIOGRAPHER *Notes*

Plain abdominal radiographs and contrast studies of the digestive tract remain the most common imaging examinations of the gastrointestinal system. Ultrasound and computed tomography (CT) are the major imaging modalities for the pancreas and biliary tract, and magnetic resonance imaging (MRI) is now being used in some institutions to screen for hepatic metastases.

Plain abdominal radiographs must show an appropriate scale of contrast to demonstrate the many different densities in the abdominal cavity. Depending on the screen-film combination, this requires the use of a middle to high kV range (70 to 80 kVp). Bony structures, such as the lumbar spine and its transverse processes, must be well demonstrated along with soft tissue shadows of the liver, kidney, and psoas muscle. For barium studies of the gastrointestinal tract, adequate penetration of the dense barium solution requires a high kV range (about 120 kVp). For double-contrast (air-barium) studies, a kVp range of 90 to 100 kVp is needed to allow penetration of the barium combined with excellent visualization of mucosal detail. Gallbladder studies require a shorter scale of contrast than other abdominal examinations and therefore are usually performed using a kVp in the low to middle range (about 70 kVp). Computed radiography and direct imaging systems tend to be more dependent on the kVp and require the use of slightly higher ranges (approximately 10 kVp higher) to produce the same images as obtained on screen-film systems. The radiographer must select the proper algorithm (combination of procedure and position) to obtain an image with the proper contrast and density.

depends on secretions of the endocrine and exocrine glands and on the controlled movement of ingested food through the tract so that absorption can occur.

Digestion begins in the mouth with chewing **(mastication),** the mechanical breakdown of food. The secretion of saliva moistens the food in preparation for swallowing. Swallowing **(deglutition)** is a complex process that requires coordination of many muscles in the head and neck and the precise opening and closing of esophageal sphincters. Digestion continues in the stomach with the churning movement of gastric contents that have become mixed with hydrochloric acid and the proteolytic enzyme pepsin. The resulting milky white **chyme** is propelled through the pyloric sphincter into the duodenum by rhythmic smooth muscle contractions called **peristalsis.**

The greatest amount of digestion occurs in the duodenum, the first part of the small bowel. In addition to intestinal secretions containing mucus and enzymes, secretions of the pancreas and liver enhance digestion in this region. The pancreas secretes enzymes for the digestion of proteins (trypsin and chymotrypsin), fat (lipase), and carbohydrates (amylase). It also secretes an alkaline solution to neutralize the acid carried into the small intestine from the stomach. Bile is secreted by the liver, is stored in the gallbladder, and enters the duodenum through the common bile duct. Bile is an **emulsifier,** a substance that acts like soap by dispersing the fat into very small droplets that permit it to mix with water.

When digestion is complete, the nutrients are absorbed through the intestinal mucosa into blood capillaries and lymph vessels of the wall of the small bowel. The inner surface area of the small bowel is increased by the formation of numerous fingerlike projections **(villi),** which provide the largest amount of surface area possible for digestion and absorption.

Material that has not been digested passes into the colon, where water and minerals are absorbed, and the remaining matter is excreted as feces. If the contents of the lower colon and rectum move at a rate that is slower than normal, extra water is absorbed from the fecal mass to produce a hardened stool and **constipation. Diarrhea** results from increased motility of the small bowel, which floods the colon with an excessive amount of water that cannot be completely absorbed.

The vermiform (worm-shaped) appendix arises from the inferomedial aspect of the cecum about 3 cm below the ileocecal valve. Although the appendix has no functional importance in digestion, it is often classified as an accessory digestive organ merely because of its location.

The liver is the largest gland in the body and is responsible for several vital functions. Liver cells detoxify (make harmless) a variety of poisonous substances that enter the blood from the intestines. Toxic chemicals that are changed to nontoxic compounds in the liver include ammonia (converted to urea and excreted by the kidneys), alcohol, and barbiturates. Liver cells secrete about 1 pint of bile each day. As mentioned, bile is an emulsifier; it is essential for the digestion and absorption of dietary fat and the fat-soluble vitamins A, D, E, and K. Bile is a greenish liquid consisting of water, bile salts, cholesterol, and bilirubin (a breakdown product of hemoglobin).

Liver cells play a vital role in the metabolism of proteins, fats, and carbohydrates. The liver is the major site of synthesis of the enzymes necessary for various cellular activities throughout the body. Liver cells also synthesize blood proteins, such as albumin, which maintains the correct amount of fluid within blood vessels and the essential proteins required for blood clotting (fibrinogen and prothrombin). Therefore liver damage may result in edema (excess water in the soft tissues) and a serious bleeding tendency. The liver plays an important role in maintaining the proper level of glucose in the blood by taking up excess glucose absorbed by the small intestine and storing it as **glycogen**. When the level of circulating glucose falls below normal, the liver breaks down glycogen and releases glucose into the bloodstream. Liver cells also store iron and vitamins A, B$_{12}$, and D.

The gallbladder is a pear-shaped sac that lies on the undersurface of the liver. Its function is to store bile that enters by way of the hepatic and cystic ducts and to concentrate the bile by absorbing water. In response to the presence of dietary fat in the small bowel, the gallbladder contracts and ejects the concentrated bile into the duodenum.

The pancreas controls the level of circulating blood glucose by secreting insulin and glucagon in the islets of Langerhans. An increased concentration of glucose in the blood stimulates the beta cells to increase secretion of insulin, which decreases the blood glucose level probably by accelerating the transport of glucose into cells. A blood glucose concentration less than normal triggers the alpha cells to secrete glucagon, which accelerates the breakdown of glycogen into glucose by the liver.

As discussed, pancreatic secretions are vital for digestion. Pancreatic enzymes that pass through the pancreatic duct into the duodenum are necessary for the breakdown of proteins, carbohydrates, and fats.

Esophagus

Tracheoesophageal Fistula

Congenital Type
Congenital tracheoesophageal (TE) fistulas result from the failure of a satisfactory esophageal lumen to develop completely separate from the trachea. Esophageal atresia and TE fistulas are often associated with other congenital malformations involving the skeleton, cardiovascular system, and gastrointestinal tract.

Radiographic Appearance
In the second most common type of esophageal anomaly, type I, both the upper and lower segments of the esophagus are blind pouches. This anomaly can be differentiated from the type III lesion (the most common type) only by plain abdominal radiographs,

which demonstrate the absence of air below the diaphragm in the type I lesion and air below the stomach in the type III lesion.

In the type II form of TE fistula, the upper esophageal segment communicates with the trachea, whereas the lower segment ends in a blind pouch. Because there is no connection between the trachea and the stomach, there is no radiographic evidence of gas within the abdomen. Oral administration of contrast material in this condition immediately outlines the tracheobronchial tree.

The type III TE fistula (seen in 85% to 90% of cases) consists of an upper segment that ends in a blind pouch at the level of the bifurcation of the trachea or slightly above it, and a lower segment attached to the trachea by a short fistulous tract. Radiographic demonstration of the looping of a small esophageal feeding tube indicates that the proximal esophagus ends in a blind pouch (Figure 5-1, *A*). Plain radiographs of the abdomen demonstrate the presence of air in the bowel that has freely entered the stomach through the fistulous connection between the trachea and the distal esophagus.

There are two forms of type IV TE fistula. In one, the upper and lower esophageal segments end in blind pouches, both of which are connected to the tracheobronchial tree. In this form, gas is seen in the stomach, and oral contrast material outlines both fistulas and the bronchial tree. In the other form of type IV fistula (called an H fistula), both the trachea and the esophagus are intact. These two structures are connected by a single fistulous tract that can be found at any level from the cricoid cartilage of the trachea to the tracheal bifurcation (see Figure 5-1, *B*). Unlike the other forms of TE fistula, the H fistula may not be identified in infancy and, if it is small and only occasionally causes emptying of material into the lungs, can permit survival into adulthood.

Treatment
Immediate surgical repair will prevent the infant from dying of starvation. If a fistula exists, delayed surgical repair may result in aspiration pneumonia.

Acquired Type
About 50% of acquired fistulas between the trachea and esophagus are caused by malignancy in the mediastinum. Almost all the rest result from infectious processes or trauma.

Fistulization between the esophagus and the respiratory tract is a major late complication of esophageal carcinoma and is often a terminal event (Figure 5-2). A fistula can also be a complication of erosion into the esophagus by carcinoma of the lung arising near or metastasizing to the middle mediastinum, or by mediastinal metastases from other primary sites. Regardless

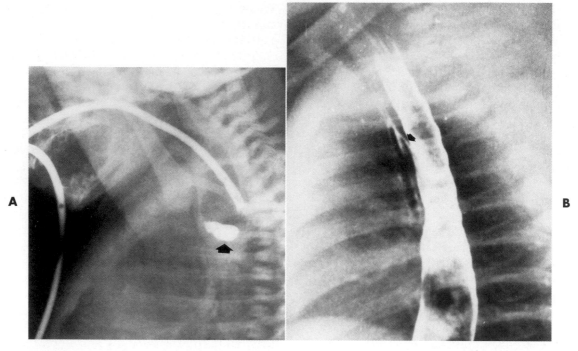

FIGURE 5-1 Congenital TE fistula. **A,** Type III fistula *(arrow),* in which contrast material (injected through a feeding tube) demonstrates occlusion of proximal esophageal pouch. **B,** Type IV, or H, fistula *(arrow).*

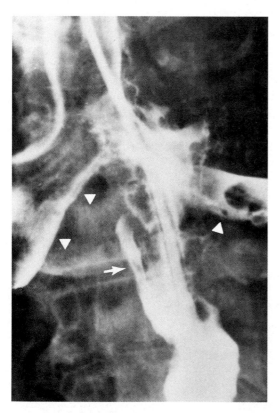

FIGURE 5-2 Esophagorespiratory fistula between esophagus *(arrow)* and bronchial tree *(arrowheads),* seen as complication of esophageal carcinoma.

of therapy, the overall prognosis of malignant TE fistulas is dismal, and more than 80% of patients with this complication die within 3 months from uncontrollable hemorrhage or from pulmonary infection caused by repeated episodes of aspiration pneumonia.

Fistulous communications between the esophagus and the tracheobronchial tree can be the result of esophageal instrumentation and perforation (Figure 5-3). This is most common after esophagoscopy, but may also occur after instrumental dilation of strictures by bougienage, pneumatic dilation of the esophagus for the treatment of achalasia, or even the insertion of a nasogastric tube. Blunt or penetrating trauma to the chest, especially after crush injury, can result in esophageal perforation and fistulization.

Radiographic Appearance
After traumatic perforation of the thoracic esophagus, chest radiographs may demonstrate air dissecting within the mediastinum and soft tissue, often with pleural effusion or hydropneumothorax. The introduction of an oral contrast agent may demonstrate the site of perforation and the extent of fistulization.

Treatment
For patients with unresectable metastases or esophageal malignancies, using an interventional technique to place a stent to maintain the lumen may be the best palliative treatment available. Surgery may be performed if the benefit outweighs the risk.

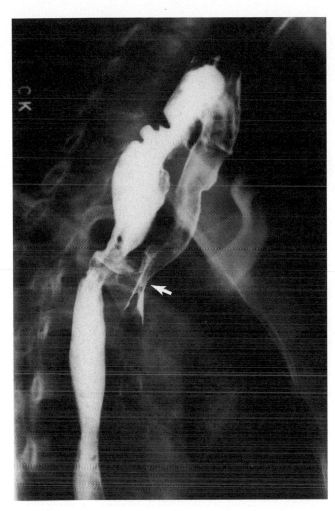

FIGURE 5-3 Acquired TE fistula. A 23-year-old female aspirated her dentures, causing an erosion through the esophagus. The esophagram demonstrates the fistula *(arrow)* between the esophagus and trachea.

Esophagitis

Reflux (Gastroesophageal Reflux Disease)

Although the reflux of gastric acid contents is the most common cause of acute esophagitis, infectious and granulomatous disorders, physical injury (caustic agents, radiation injury), and medication may produce a similar inflammatory response. Gastroesophageal reflux disease (GERD) describes any symptomatic condition or structural changes caused by reflux of the stomach contents into the esophagus. Alcohol, chocolate, caffeine, and fatty foods tend to decrease the pressure of the esophageal sphincter, allowing reflux to occur. Regardless of the cause, acute esophagitis produces burning chest pain that may simulate the pain of heart disease. Superficial ulcerations are most typical of reflux. The esophagus is often dilated, with a loss of effective peristalsis. Nonpropulsive peristaltic waves, ranging from mild

tertiary contractions to severe segmental spasms, are an early finding.

Reflux esophagitis develops when the lower esophageal sphincter fails to act as an effective barrier to the entry of gastric acid contents into the distal esophagus. Although there is a higher-than-normal likelihood of gastroesophageal reflux in patients with sliding hiatal hernias, reflux esophagitis can be endoscopically demonstrated in only about one fourth of these patients. On the other hand, esophagitis is often encountered in patients in whom no hiatal hernia can be demonstrated.

Several radiographic approaches have been suggested for the demonstration of gastroesophageal reflux. One procedure is to increase intraabdominal pressure by straight-leg raising or manual pressure on the abdomen, often with Valsalva's maneuver (forced expiration with the glottis closed). Turning the patient from prone to supine or vice versa may demonstrate reflux of barium from the stomach into the esophagus. It must be remembered, however, that the failure to demonstrate reflux radiographically does not exclude the possibility that a patient's esophagitis is related to reflux. As long as typical radiographic findings of reflux esophagitis are noted, there is little reason to persist in strenuous efforts to actually demonstrate retrograde flow of barium from the stomach into the esophagus.

Radiographic Appearance

The earliest radiographic findings in reflux esophagitis are detectable on double-contrast studies. They consist of superficial ulcerations or erosions that appear as streaks or dots of barium superimposed on the flat mucosa of the distal esophagus. In single-contrast studies of patients with esophagitis, the outer borders of the barium-filled esophagus are not sharply seen but rather have a hazy, serrated appearance with shallow, irregular protrusions indicating erosions of varying length and depth. Widening and coarsening of edematous longitudinal folds can simulate filling defects. In addition to diffuse erosion, reflux esophagitis can result in large, discrete, penetrating ulcers in the distal esophagus (Figure 5-4) or in a hiatal hernia sac (Figure 5-5). Fibrotic healing of diffuse reflux esophagitis or a localized penetrating ulcer may cause narrowing of the distal esophagus. Strictures resulting from reflux esophagitis tend to be smooth and tapering with no demonstrable mucosal pattern (Figure 5-6).

Barrett's Esophagus

Barrett's esophagus is a condition related to severe reflux esophagitis in which the normal squamous lining of the lower esophagus is destroyed and replaced by columnar epithelium similar to that of the stomach. Ulceration in Barrett's esophagus typically occurs at the squamocolumnar junction (Z-line).

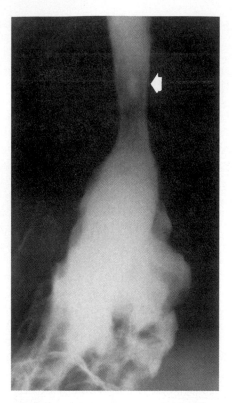

FIGURE **5-4** Large, penetrating ulcer *(arrow)* in reflux esophagitis.

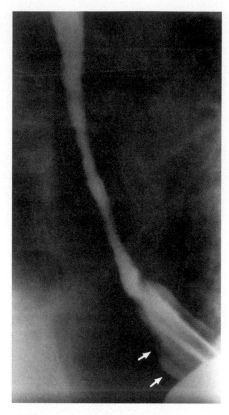

FIGURE **5-6** Long esophageal stricture caused by reflux esophagitis. Note the associated hiatal hernia *(arrows)*.

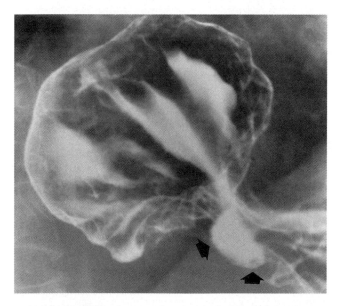

FIGURE **5-5** Ulcer *(arrows)* in large hiatal hernia sac.

In addition to exhibiting postinflammatory stricture, Barrett's esophagus has an unusually high propensity for developing malignancy in the columnar cell-lined portion. These tumors are almost always adenocarcinomas, which are otherwise very rare in the esophagus (comprising about 5% of esophageal cancers).

Radiographic Appearance

Although a hiatal hernia with gastroesophageal reflux is commonly demonstrated, Barrett's ulcer is usually separated from the hiatal hernia by a variable length of normal-appearing esophagus (Figure 5-7), in contrast to reflux esophagitis, in which the distal esophagus is abnormal down to the level of the hernia. As in reflux esophagitis, fibrotic healing of the ulceration in Barrett's esophagus often leads to a smooth, tapered stricture (Figure 5-8).

Because the distal esophagus consists of a gastric type of mucosa in Barrett's esophagus, it actively takes up the intravenously injected radionuclide pertechnetate. The demonstration of a continuous concentration of the isotope from the stomach into the distal esophagus to a level that corresponds approximately to that of the ulcer or stricture is indicative of Barrett's esophagus.

Candida *and Herpesvirus*

Candida (fungal) and herpesvirus are the organisms most often responsible for infectious esophagitis, which usually occurs in patients with widespread malignancy who are receiving radiation therapy, chemotherapy, corticosteroids, or other immunosuppressive agents. It also can develop in patients with acquired

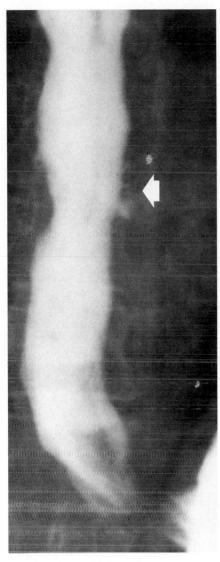

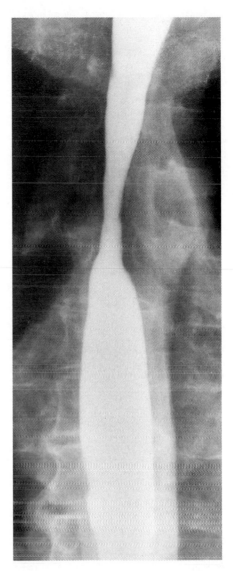

FIGURE 5-7 Barrett's esophagus. Ulcerations *(arrow)* have developed at a distance from esophagogastric junction.

FIGURE 5-8 Barrett's esophagus. Note smooth, tapered stricture in upper thoracic esophagus.

immunodeficiency syndrome (AIDS) and even in otherwise healthy adults who have received antibiotics (especially tetracycline) for upper respiratory infection.

Radiographic Appearance

The classic radiographic appearance is an irregular cobblestone pattern with a shaggy marginal contour of the esophagus caused by deep ulcerations and sloughing of the mucosa (Figure 5-9). *Candida* presents as plaques and nodules as a result of a superficial collection of fungi. Characteristics of herpetic esophagitis include small mucosal ulcers or plaques.

Treatment for Esophagitis

Modifications to lifestyle including weight loss, changes in diet to prevent decreased esophageal sphincter control, and medications to reduce acidity

are the first line of treatment. One technique called proton pump inhibitor therapy (using esomeprazole) can help control progression in reflux and Barrett's esophagitis. Other techniques used are photodynamic therapy and thermal ablation to destroy the Barrett's tissue. If these therapies do not work, surgical fundoplication (tucks in the stomach fundus and distal esophagus) is an option. Infectious esophagitis caused by *Candida* or herpesvirus may require a regimen of antifungal or antiviral drugs to eradicate the cause.

Ingestion of Corrosive Agents

The ingestion of alkaline or acidic corrosive agents produces acute inflammatory changes in the esophagus. Superficial penetration of the toxic agent results in only minimal ulceration. Deeper penetration of the

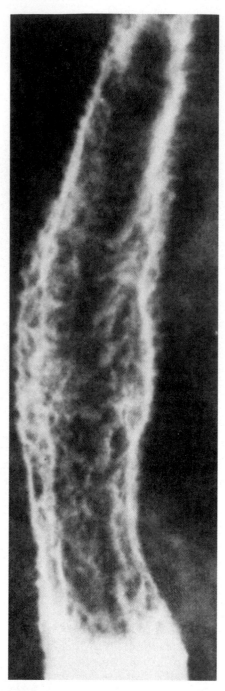

FIGURE 5-9 *Candida* esophagitis. Multiple ulcers and nodular plaques produce the grossly irregular contour of shaggy esophagus. This manifestation of far-advanced candidiasis has become infrequent because of earlier and better treatment of the disease.

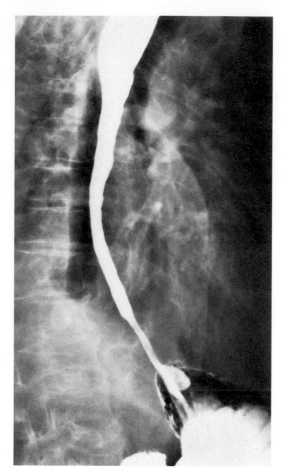

FIGURE 5-10 Corrosive stricture resulting from ingestion of lye.

submucosa and muscular layers causes sloughing of destroyed tissue and deep ulceration. Ingesting strong alkaline agents causes deeper lesions than ingesting strong acids, and only half of those who ingest an acid suffer severe injury. Drug-induced esophagitis may occur in patients who have delayed esophageal transit time, which permits prolonged mucosal contact with the ingested substance. The most common drug causing esophageal ulceration is potassium chloride in tablet form. Other medications that can cause esophagitis are weak caustic agents that are harmless when they pass rapidly through the esophagus.

Radiographic Appearance

Healing of the intense mucosal and intramural inflammation of acute esophagitis may lead to pronounced fibrosis and stricture formation. These benign strictures tend to be long lesions with tapered margins and relatively smooth mucosal surfaces (Figure 5-10), in contrast to the irregular narrowing, mucosal destruction, and overhanging margins that are generally associated with malignant processes.

Treatment

The type of agent ingested determines the therapy. Poison control is usually called for specific treatments if the situation is not drug induced. Vomiting is generally not induced because this would cause a repeated exposure to the esophagus. Dilution by administering milk or water is appropriate unless the corrosive agent is acidic (in this case, water should not be used as this would produce excessive heat).

Esophageal Cancer

Progressive difficulty in swallowing (dysphagia) in a person older than 40 years must be assumed to be caused by cancer until proven otherwise. Because the symptoms of esophageal carcinoma tend to appear late in the course of the disease, and because the lack of a limiting outer layer (serosa) commonly permits direct extension of the tumor by the time of the initial diagnosis, carcinoma of the esophagus has a dismal prognosis. Most carcinomas of the esophagus are of the squamous cell type and they occur most often at the esophagogastric junction. The incidence of carcinoma of the esophagus is far higher in men than in women. There is a strong correlation between excessive alcohol intake, smoking, and esophageal carcinoma.

Radiographic Appearance

The earliest radiographic evidence of infiltrating carcinoma of the esophagus appears on a double-contrast barium swallow film as a flat, plaquelike lesion, occasionally with central **ulceration,** that involves one wall of the esophagus (Figure 5-11). At this stage, there may be minimal reduction in the caliber of the lumen. Unless the patient is carefully examined in various positions, this earliest form of esophageal carcinoma can be missed. As the **infiltrating** cancer progresses, irregularity of the wall is seen, indicating mucosal destruction. Advanced lesions encircle the lumen completely, causing annular constrictions with overhanging margins and often some degree of obstruction. The lumen through the stenotic area is irregular, and mucosal folds are absent or severely ulcerated (Figure 5-12). Less commonly, carcinoma of the esophagus can appear as a localized **polypoid** mass, often with deep ulceration and a fungating appearance.

Luminal obstruction as a result of carcinoma causes proximal dilation of the esophagus and may result in aspiration pneumonia. Extension of the tumor to adjacent mediastinal structures may lead to fistula formation, especially between the esophagus and the respiratory tract (see Figure 5-16).

Wall thickening greater than 3 to 5 mm on a CT scan is suggestive of esophageal cancer. CT has become a major method of staging patients with esophageal

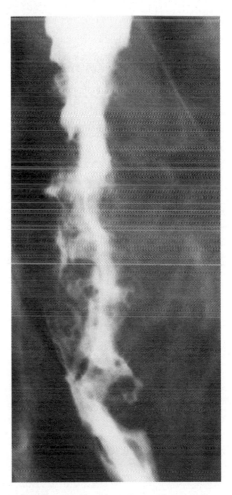

FIGURE 5-12 Carcinoma of esophagus. Irregular narrowing with ulceration involves an extensive segment of the thoracic portion of the esophagus.

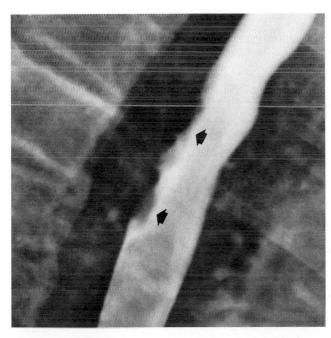

FIGURE 5-11 Early carcinoma of the esophagus. Flat, plaquelike lesion *(arrows)* involves the posterior wall of the esophagus.

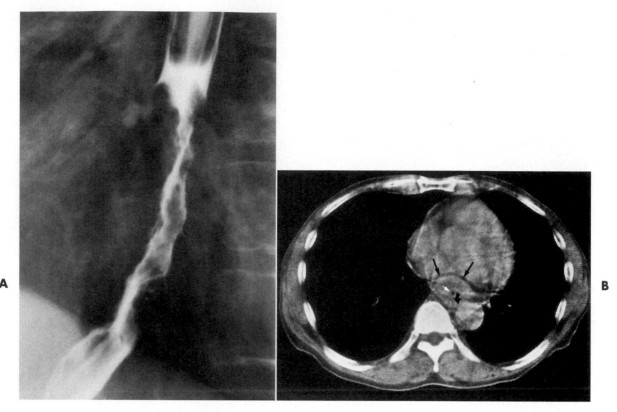

FIGURE 5-13 CT staging of esophageal carcinoma. **A,** Esophagram demonstrates infiltrating lesion causing irregular narrowing of the distal part of the esophagus. **B,** CT scan shows a mass of bulky carcinoma *(black arrows)* filling most of the lumen *(white arrow).* Obliteration of the fat plane adjacent to the aorta *(curved arrow)* indicates mediastinal invasion.

carcinoma (with 90% accuracy), providing information on tumor size, extension, and resectability that was previously available only at thoracotomy (Figure 5-13). Evidence of tumor spread includes the obliteration of fat planes between the esophagus and adjacent structures (left atrium, aorta), the formation of a fistula to the tracheobronchial tree, and recognition of metastatic disease (e.g., low-density masses in the liver, enlargement of draining lymph nodes). Using contrast enhancement improves the detail of tumor delineation.

Treatment

If the cancerous lesion has not extended into surrounding tissue, surgical resection may result in cure. When the cancerous lesion involves surrounding tissue, treatment becomes palliative surgery together with radiation therapy or chemotherapy. If the esophagus is severely narrowed, a technique known as bougienage can be employed; this is the introduction of a long instrument to dilate and help maintain an adequate lumen. Laser therapy aids in treating the dysphagia in patients with unresectable lesions. A newer technique, photodynamic therapy using

laser-activated chemicals, provides a method of destroying tumor tissue. The prognosis of the patient who is diagnosed in the late stages is extremely poor.

Esophageal Diverticula

Esophageal diverticula (outpouchings) are common lesions that either contain all layers of the wall (traction or true diverticula) or are composed of only mucosa and submucosa herniating through the muscular layer (pulsion or false diverticula). Small diverticula do not retain food or secretions and are asymptomatic. When the diverticulum fills with food or secretions, aspiration pneumonia may result.

Radiographic Appearance

Zenker's diverticula arise from the posterior wall of the upper (cervical) esophagus (Figure 5-14). Occasionally, they can become so large that they almost occlude the esophageal lumen. CT prominently demonstrates the cricopharyngeal muscle, which aids in locating the origin of Zenker's diverticula at the pharyngoesophageal junction. Diverticula of the thoracic portion of the esophagus are primarily found opposite the bifurcation of the trachea in the

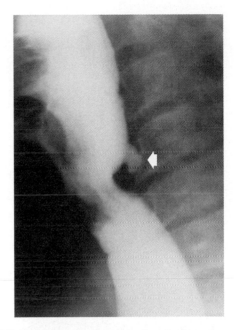

FIGURE 5-14 Small Zenker's diverticulum. Saccular out-pouching *(arrow)* arising posteriorly just proximal to an impression produced by the cricopharyngeal muscle.

region of the hilum of the lung (Figure 5-15). These **traction** diverticula reflect motor function disturbance and develop in response to the pull of fibrous adhesions after infection of the mediastinal lymph nodes. **Epiphrenic diverticula** arise in the distal 10 cm of the esophagus (Figure 5-16). They are associated with incoordination of esophageal peristalsis and sphincter relaxation, which increases the intraluminal pressure in this segment.

Treatment

Diverticula do not require treatment unless they interfere with swallowing. In Zenker's diverticulum, surgery consists of excision of the diverticulum and correction of any motility issues.

Esophageal Varices

Esophageal varices are dilated veins in the wall of the esophagus that are most commonly the result of increased pressure in the portal venous system (portal hypertension), which is in turn usually a result of cirrhosis of the liver. In patients with portal hypertension, much of the portal blood cannot flow along its normal pathway through the liver to the inferior vena cava and then on to the heart. Instead, it must go by a circuitous collateral route, and increased blood flow through these dilated veins causes the development of esophageal (and gastric) varices. Esophageal varices are infrequently demonstrated in the absence of portal hypertension. "Downhill"

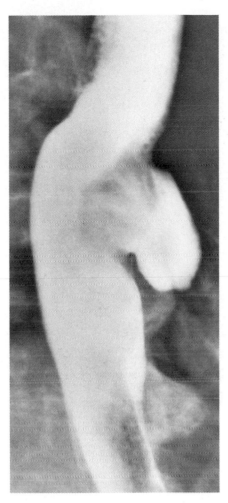

FIGURE 5-15 Traction diverticulum of the midthoracic portion of the esophagus.

varices are produced when venous blood from the head and neck cannot reach the heart because of an obstruction of the superior vena cava caused by tumors or inflammatory disease in the mediastinum. In this situation, blood flows "downhill" through the esophageal veins before eventually entering the portal vein, through which it flows to the inferior vena cava and the right atrium.

Radiographic Appearance

The characteristic radiographic appearance of esophageal varices is serpiginous (wavy border) thickening of folds, which appear as round or oval filling defects resembling the beads of a rosary (Figure 5-17). Precise technique is required to demonstrate esophageal varices. A double-contrast barium swallow best demonstrates the serpiginous and wormlike filling defect. Complete filling of the esophagus with barium may obscure varices, and powerful contractions of the esophagus may squeeze blood out of the varices

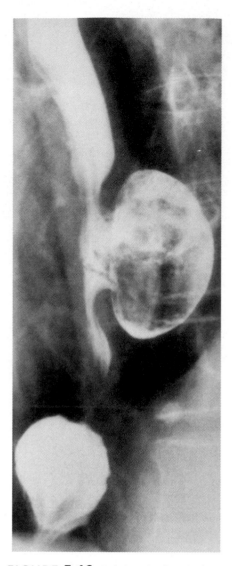

FIGURE 5-16 Epiphrenic diverticulum.

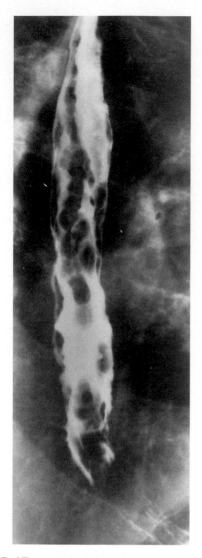

FIGURE 5-17 Esophageal varices. Note diffuse round and oval filling defects, which resemble rosary beads.

and make them impossible to detect. Upright and recumbent imaging may best demonstrate the varices dilated and empty, respectively.

Varices can be demonstrated with endoscopic ultrasound as compressible hypoechoic or cystic masses in the gastrointestinal tract from the outer to the submucosal layers.

The major complication of esophageal varices is bleeding. Their appearance in patients with cirrhotic liver disease implies significant portal venous hypertension and is an ominous sign because up to 90% of the deaths from liver disease in patients with cirrhosis occur within 2 years of the diagnosis of varices.

Treatment

Vasoconstrictor drugs to constrict the dilated vessels are commonly used to treat esophageal varices. Active bleeding can be controlled by a technique

called balloon tamponade, which creates pressure to stop the bleeding. If bleeding cannot be controlled, surgery is performed to tie off collateral vessels.

Hiatal Hernia

Hiatal hernia is the most common abnormality (occurring in 50% of the population) detected on upper gastrointestinal examination. Its broad radiographic spectrum ranges from large esophagogastric hernias, in which much of the stomach lies within the thoracic cavity and there is a predisposition to volvulus (twisting), to small hernias that emerge above the diaphragm only under certain circumstances (related to changes in intraabdominal or intrathoracic pressure) and easily slide back into the abdomen through the hiatus (sliding hiatal hernia). The symptoms associated with hiatal hernia

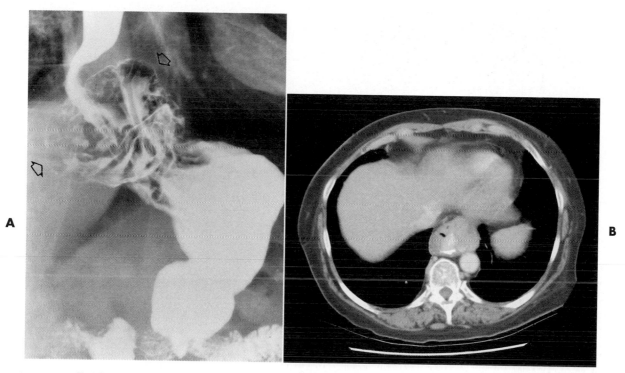

FIGURE 5-18 **A,** Large hiatal hernia *(arrows).* **B,** This 65-year-old woman had right lower quadrant pain. Hiatal hernia was an incidental finding on CT scan of the abdomen with oral contrast agent. The stomach was shown to be in the retrocardiac area.

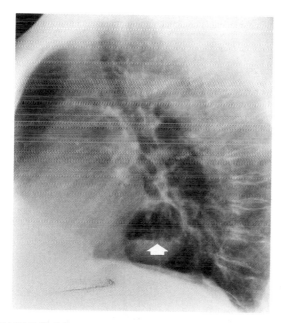

FIGURE 5-19 Air-fluid level *(arrow)* in a hiatal hernia seen on a lateral chest radiograph.

and its complications (esophagitis, esophageal ulcer, esophageal stenosis) are related to the presence of esophageal reflux rather than to the hiatal hernia itself. Most hiatal hernias do not produce symptoms and are clinically of no importance.

Radiographic Appearance

Although the diagnosis of hiatal hernia generally requires a barium study (Figure 5-18), at times a large hiatal hernia may appear on plain chest radiographs as a soft tissue mass in the posterior mediastinum, often containing a prominent air-fluid level (Figure 5-19). The esophagus and stomach are distinguished by their appearance; mucosal folds are linear and parallel in the esophagus, whereas in the stomach the folds appear numerous and thicker without a parallel orientation.

Treatment

In most cases, a hiatal hernia requires no treatment. If surgical intervention is necessary, the hiatus is tightened and the stomach secured below the diaphragm.

Achalasia

Achalasia is a functional obstruction of the distal section of the esophagus with proximal dilation caused by incomplete relaxation of the lower esophageal sphincter. It is related to a paucity or absence of ganglion cells in the myenteric neural plexuses of the distal esophageal wall.

Radiographic Appearance

On plain chest radiographs, the dilated, tortuous esophagus may produce a widened mediastinum (often with an air-fluid level) on the right side adjacent

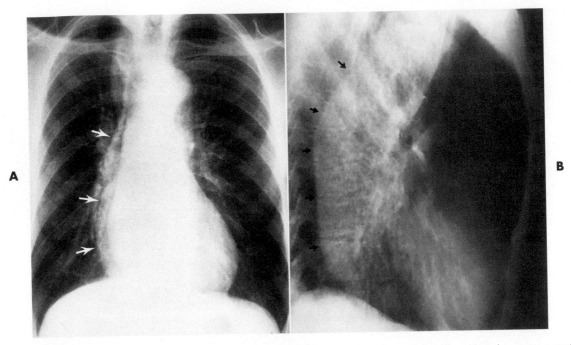

FIGURE 5-20 Achalasia. **A,** Frontal chest radiograph demonstrates the margin of a dilated tortuous aorta *(arrows)* parallel with the right border of the heart, producing a widened mediastinum. **B,** The lateral image demonstrates posterior widening of the mediastinum *(arrows)*.

to the cardiac shadow (Figure 5-20). The hallmark of achalasia, seen on barium studies, is a gradually tapered, smooth, conical, 1- to 3-cm narrowing of the distal esophageal segment (rat-tail or beak appearance) (Figure 5-21). On sequential radiographs, especially with the patient upright, only small spurts of barium pass through the narrowed distal segment to enter the stomach.

Treatment

Medications are given before meals to assist in relaxing the esophageal sphincter. If these do not control the symptoms, endoscopic balloon dilation with a bougienage may be helpful. A last resort is surgery (Heller's myotomy) to open the sphincter.

Foreign Bodies

A wide spectrum of foreign bodies can become impacted in the esophagus, usually in the cervical esophagus at or just above the level of the thoracic inlet (Figure 5-22). Symptomatically, the patient is unable to swallow without regurgitation. Most metallic objects, such as pins, coins, and small toys, are radiopaque and are easily visualized on radiographs or during fluoroscopy. Objects made of aluminum and some light alloys may be impossible to detect radiographically because the density of these metals is almost equal to that of soft tissue.

It is essential that any suspected foreign body be evaluated on two projections to be certain that the object projected over the esophagus truly lies within it.

Radiographic Appearance

Nonopaque foreign bodies in the esophagus, especially pieces of poorly chewed meat (masticated food bolus), can be demonstrated only after the ingestion of barium (Figure 5-23). Such foreign bodies usually become impacted in the distal esophagus just above the level of the diaphragm and are often associated with a distal stricture. These intraluminal filling defects usually have an irregular surface and may resemble a completely obstructing carcinoma.

Treatment

Medications are the first line of treatment to relax the esophagus and allow the foreign body to move naturally into the stomach. In some instances, especially for sharper-pointed objects, retrieval of the foreign body using endoscopy may be appropriate. Interventional approaches are attempted before taking the patient to surgery to remove the obstruction. If the esophageal foreign body causes obstruction for more than 12 hours, there is an increased risk of perforation.

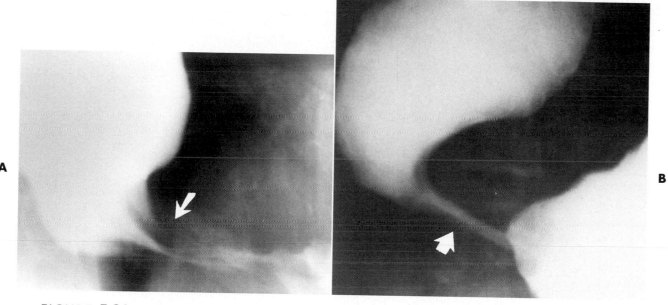

FIGURE 5-21 Achalasia. **A,** Rat-tail narrowing of distal part of the esophagus *(arrow)*. **B,** Small spurt of barium *(arrow)* enters stomach through narrowed distal segment (the jet effect).

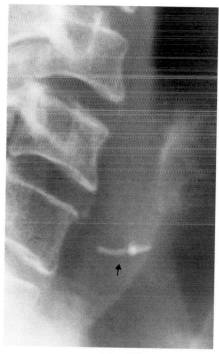

FIGURE 5-22 Fish bone *(arrow)* impacted in the lower cervical portion of the esophagus.

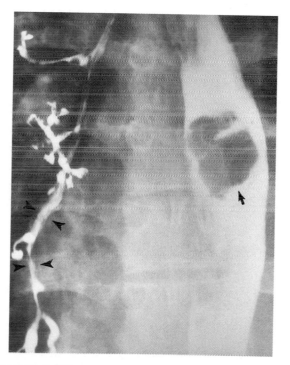

FIGURE 5-23 Meat impaction in the esophagus. Large bolus of hot dog *(arrow)* is trapped in the midesophagus of a patient with quadriplegia. Note barium in the bronchial tree *(arrowheads)* caused by aspiration.

SUMMARY of FINDINGS for the Esophagus

disorder	location	radiographic appearance	treatment
Tracheoesophageal atresia or fistula—congenital	Blind pouch superiorly Blind pouch distally or tracheal fistula	Blind pouch filled with contrast or NG tube Fistula track (if one exists), NG tube injection	Surgical repair—connect esophagus (anastomosis), fistula repair
Tracheoesophageal fistula—acquired	Usually at level of the carina or more proximal	Demonstration of connection between esophagus and tracheobronchial tree	Palliative—interventional stent placement Surgical—fistula repair
Reflux esophagitis	Distal esophagus	Streaks or dots superimposed on flat mucosa	Lifestyle modifications Weight-reduction diet Medication
Barrett's esophagitis	Mid to lower esophagus	Smooth tapered stricture(s)	Photodynamic therapy and thermal ablation Surgery—fundoplication
Candida (fungal) and herpesvirus esophagitis	Entire esophagus	Cobblestone pattern Shaggy marginal contour Small mucosal ulcers or plaques	Same treatment as for Barrett's, adding antifungal or antiviral medication
Ingestion of corrosive agents	Alkaline ingestion	Deeper ulceration Stricture formation	Call poison control
	Acidic ingestion	Superficial minimal ulceration Stricture formation	Water or milk dilution—alkaline
Esophageal cancer	Distal esophagus, esophagogastric junction	Double-contrast barium swallow: • Flat plaquelike lesion • Infiltrating lesion (irregular wall) • Polypoid mass (deep ulceration) CT with contrast enhancement—wall thickening of greater than 3-5 mm	Surgical resection—possible cure Palliative therapy—chemotherapy or radiation Laser-activated chemical photodynamic therapy
Esophageal diverticula	Traction—all layers of wall Pulsion—mucosal and submucosal layers	Esophagram—appears as an outpouching or pocket filling with barium CT—illustrates an outpouching at the pharyngoesophageal junction	Usually no treatment Surgery if diverticulum interferes with swallowing
Esophageal varices	Distal esophagus and stomach	Esophagram—Serpiginous thickening of folds—resembles rosary beads Endoscopic ultrasound—compressible hypoechoic mass in the outer or submucosal layer	Medication—vasoconstrictor drugs Active bleeding—interventional balloon tamponade or surgery to tie off collateral vessels
Hiatal hernia	Esophagogastric region	GI series—numerous thicker folds of the stomach above the diaphragm	No treatment in most instances Surgical intervention includes tightening the hiatus
Achalasia—functional obstruction	Distal esophagus with proximal dilation	Chest film—dilated esophagus GI series—narrowing of distal esophageal segment	Medication to relax sphincter Endoscopic balloon dilation Surgical myotomy

SUMMARY of FINDINGS for the Esophagus—cont'd

disorder	location	radiographic appearance	treatment
Foreign bodies—food bolus or nonopaque objects Foreign bodies—non-food-related (coin) or opaque	Any region of the esophagus	Barium swallow to demonstrate the level of impaction causing the obstruction Intraluminal filling defect with an irregular surface	Medication to relax esophagus Endoscopy to retrieve foreign body Surgical retrieval if all interventional approaches fail
Esophageal perforation—inflammatory, neoplastic, or traumatic	Any region of the esophagus	Perforation through entire wall—air in the mediastinum Contrast material extravasation through perforation	Interventional—expandable stent Treat complications Surgical band ligation

GI, Gastrointestinal; *NG,* nasogastric.

Perforation of the Esophagus

Perforation of the esophagus may be a complication of esophagitis, peptic ulcer, neoplasm, external trauma, or instrumentation. At times, perforation of a previously healthy esophagus can result from severe vomiting (the most common cause) or coughing, often from dietary or alcoholic indiscretion. Complete rupture of the wall of the esophagus may cause the sudden development of severe upper gastric pain simulating myocardial infarction. In the **Mallory-Weiss syndrome,** an increase in intraluminal and intramural pressure associated with vomiting (severe retching) after an alcoholic bout causes superficial mucosal laceration or fissures near the esophagogastric junction that produce severe hemorrhage. Endoscopy is required to best demonstrate lacerations, especially those close to the sphincter.

Radiographic Appearance

A perforation that extends throughout the entire esophageal wall can lead to free air in the mediastinum or periesophageal soft tissues. The administration of radiopaque contrast material may demonstrate extravasation through the perforation (Figure 5-24) or an intramural dissection channel separated by an intervening lucent line from the normal esophageal lumen. CT is the preferred modality to define the extent of the process.

Treatment

Place an expandable stent and then treat the complications (chest tube for pneumothorax; antibiotics to prevent infection). A surgical procedure (band ligation) can be performed to close the perforation.

Stomach

Gastritis

Inflammation of the stomach can be the result of a variety of irritants including alcohol, corrosive agents, and infection. Gastritis changes the normal surface pattern of the gastric mucosa. *Helicobacter pylori* can cause chronic gastritis that may lead to peptic ulcer disease.

Radiographic Appearance

Alcoholic gastritis may produce thickening of gastric folds (Figure 5-25), multiple superficial gastric erosions, or both. In **corrosive gastritis,** the acute inflammatory reaction heals by fibrosis and scarring, which results in severe narrowing of the antrum and may cause gastric outlet obstruction. In **bacterial (phlegmonous) gastritis,** inflammatory thickening of the gastric wall causes narrowing of the stomach that may mimic gastric cancer. The diagnosis of **infectious gastritis** can be made if there is evidence of gas bubbles (produced by the bacteria) in the stomach wall (Figure 5-26). These types of gastritis are known as erosive or acute gastritis.

Chronic atrophic gastritis (nonerosive) refers to severe mucosal atrophy (wasting) that causes thinning and a relative absence of mucosal folds, with the fundus or entire stomach having a bald appearance. This is a nonspecific radiographic pattern that can be related to such factors as age, malnutrition, medication, and complications of alcoholism. Chronic atrophic gastritis also occurs in patients with pernicious anemia, who cannot absorb vitamin B_{12} because of an inability of the stomach to secrete intrinsic factor (or hydrochloric acid).

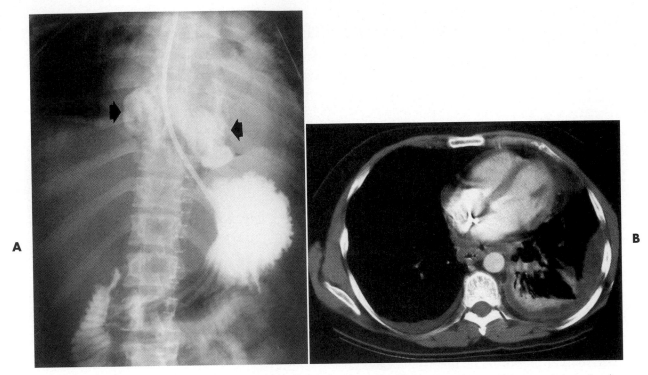

FIGURE 5-24 A, Esophageal perforation. Extravasation of contrast material *(arrows)* is seen in previously healthy patient who experienced severe vomiting after excessive ingestion of alcohol. **B,** CT scan of the chest of a 41-year-old man illustrates perforation of the esophagus with drainage into the thoracic cavity.

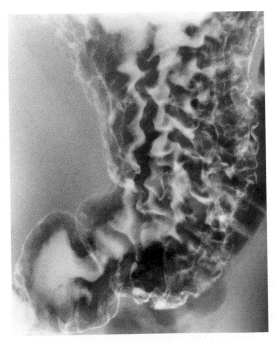

FIGURE 5-25 Gastritis. Note pronounced thickening of rugal folds throughout the stomach.

Treatment

The causative agent in erosive gastritis determines treatment. Eliminating the causative agent, such as alcohol, reduces the changes in the mucosal lining as well as the symptoms. If overproduction of stomach acid produces the changes, acid-reduction medications are used to help maintain the mucous defense barrier. Antibiotics are the appropriate medication for bacterial or infectious gastritis. Patients with *H. pylori* gastritis receive a regimen of multiple antibiotics because this infection may be antibiotic resistant. Using a combination of antibiotics has resulted in an 80% to 90% cure rate.

Peptic Ulcer Disease

Peptic ulcer disease is a group of inflammatory processes involving the stomach and duodenum. It is caused by the action of acid and the enzyme pepsin secreted by the stomach and occurs most frequently on the lesser curvature. The spectrum of peptic ulcer disease varies from small and shallow superficial erosions to huge ulcers that may perforate through the bowel wall.

The major complications of peptic ulcer disease are hemorrhage (20%), gastric outlet obstruction (5% to 10%), and perforation (less than 5%). Peptic ulcer disease is the most common cause of acute upper

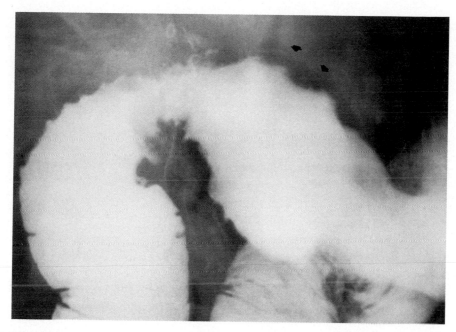

FIGURE 5-26 Phlegmonous emphysematous gastritis. Note severe, irregular ulceration of the distal stomach, with air in the wall *(arrows)*.

gastrointestinal bleeding. Free perforation of a peptic ulcer located in the anterior wall of the stomach or duodenum is the most common cause of pneumoperitoneum with peritonitis (see Pneumoperitoneum, later). Narrowing of the lumen of the distal stomach or duodenal bulb caused by peptic ulcer disease is by far the most common cause of gastric outlet obstruction.

Duodenal Ulcer

Duodenal ulcer is the most common manifestation of peptic ulcer disease. More than 95% of duodenal ulcers occur in the first portion of the duodenum (the duodenal bulb).

Radiographic Appearance

An unequivocal diagnosis of active duodenal ulcer requires the demonstration of an ulcer crater, which appears in profile as a small collection of barium projecting from the lumen. When seen en face (face on), the ulcer niche appears as a rounded or linear collection of contrast material surrounded by lucent folds that often radiate toward the crater (Figure 5-27). Secondary signs of duodenal ulcer disease include thickening of the mucosal folds and a deformity of the duodenal bulb. Acute ulcers incite muscular spasm, leading to deformity of the margins of the duodenal bulb that may be inconsistent and varied during the examination. With chronic ulceration, fibrosis and scarring cause a fixed deformity that persists even though the ulcer heals. Symmetric narrowing of the duodenal bulb in its midportion may

produce the typical cloverleaf deformity of chronic duodenal ulcer disease (Figure 5-28). CT demonstrates an irregularity or collection of contrast material in the gastric wall; however, as with barium studies, the appearance may be difficult to differentiate from malignancy.

Gastric Ulcer

Gastric ulcers, another form of peptic ulcer disease, usually occur on the lesser curvature of the stomach. Unlike duodenal ulcers, which are virtually always benign, up to 5% of gastric ulcers are malignant.

Radiographic Appearance

Radiographic signs that indicate whether a gastric ulcer is more likely to be benign or malignant have been described. The classic sign of a benign gastric ulcer in profile is penetration, with clear projection of the ulcer outside the normal barium-filled gastric lumen because the ulcer represents an excavation in the wall of the stomach (Figure 5-29). A thin lucency at the base of the ulcer, reflecting mucosal edema caused by inflammatory exudate, is another sign of benignancy. When viewed en face, a gastric ulcer appears as a persistent collection of barium surrounded by a halo of edema (the ulcer collar) (Figure 5-30).

A hallmark of benign gastric ulcer is radiation of mucosal folds to the edge of the crater. However, because radiating folds can be identified in both malignant and benign ulcers, the character of the folds must be carefully assessed. If the folds are smooth and slender and appear to extend into the edge of the

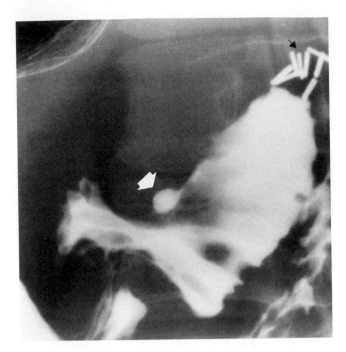

FIGURE 5-27 Duodenal ulcer. An ulcer niche appears as a rounded collection of barium *(white arrow)* surrounded by lucent edema. Multiple surgical clips are noted incidentally *(black arrow)*.

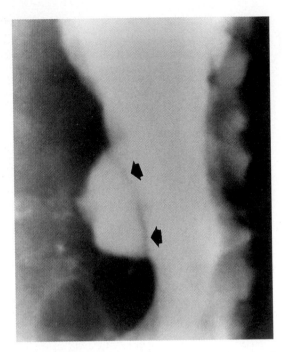

FIGURE 5-29 Benign gastric ulcer. Penetration of contrast material outside normal, barium-filled gastric lumen associated with thin, sharply demarcated, lucent line with parallel straight margins *(arrows)*, representing edema at the base of the ulcer crater.

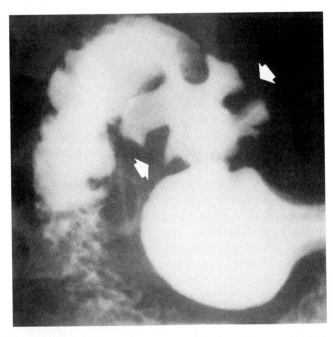

FIGURE 5-28 Chronic duodenal ulcer disease. Typical cloverleaf deformity is visible *(arrows)*.

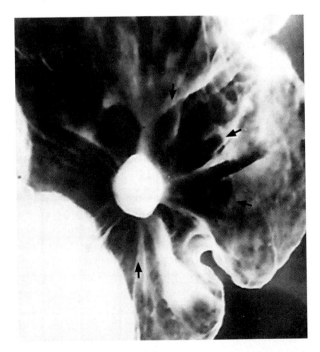

FIGURE 5-30 Benign gastric ulcer. On en face projection, prominent radiating folds extend directly to the ulcer. Lucency around the ulcer *(arrows)* represents inflammatory mass effect.

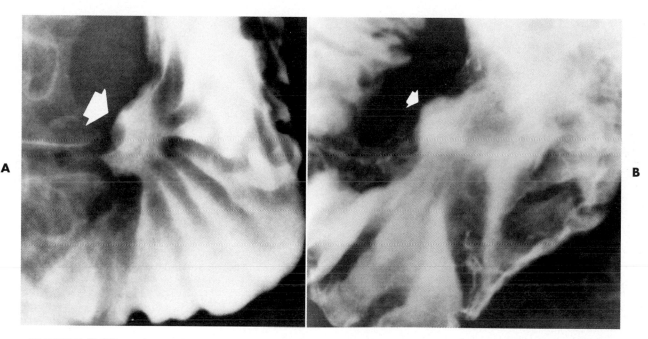

FIGURE 5-31 Radiating folds in gastric ulcers. **A,** Small, slender folds extending to edge of crater *(arrow)* indicate the benign nature of this ulcer. **B,** In this malignant gastric ulcer, thick folds radiate to an irregular mound of tissue around the ulcer *(arrow).*

crater, the ulcer is most likely benign (Figure 5-31, *A*). In contrast, irregular folds that merge into a mound of polypoid tissue around the crater are suggestive of malignancy (Figure 5-31, *B*).

Although the size, shape, number, and location of gastric ulcers have been suggested as criteria for distinguishing between benign and malignant lesions, these findings are of little practical value. One exception is ulcers in the gastric fundus above the level of the esophagogastric junction: essentially all of these are malignant.

An abrupt transition between the normal mucosa and the abnormal tissues surrounding a gastric ulcer is characteristic of a malignant lesion (Figure 5-32), in contrast to the diffuse and almost imperceptible transition between the normal gastric mucosa and the mound of edema surrounding a benign ulcer. Neoplastic tissue surrounding a malignant ulcer is usually nodular, unlike the smooth contour of the edematous mound around a benign ulcer. A malignant ulcer does not penetrate beyond the normal gastric lumen but remains within it because the ulcer merely represents a necrotic area within an intramural or intraluminal mass.

Most benign gastric ulcers heal completely with medical therapy (see Treatment of Ulcers) (Figure 5-33). Complete healing does not necessarily mean that the stomach returns to an absolutely normal radiographic appearance; bizarre deformities can result because of fibrotic retraction and stiffening of the stomach wall.

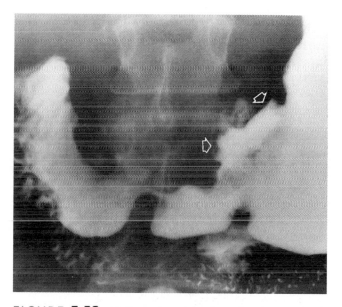

FIGURE 5-32 Malignant gastric ulcer. An abrupt transition occurs between normal mucosa and abnormal tissue surrounding an irregular gastric ulcer *(arrows).*

Although many malignant ulcers show significant healing, there is almost never complete disappearance of the ulcer crater.

The role of endoscopy in evaluating patients with gastric ulcers is controversial. At present, endoscopy is indicated only when the radiographic findings are not typical for a benign ulcer, if healing of the ulcer does not progress at the expected rate, or if the mucosa

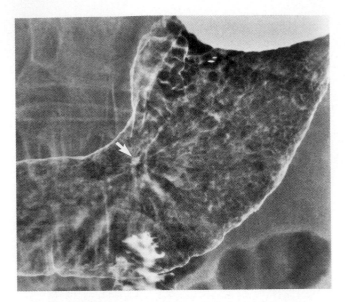

FIGURE 5-33 A healing gastric ulcer. Folds converge to a residual central depression *(arrow)*.

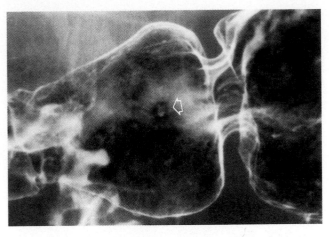

FIGURE 5-34 Superficial gastric erosions in patient with gastritis. Collection of barium represents shallow erosion surrounded by a radiolucent halo *(arrow)*.

surrounding a healed ulcer crater has a nodular surface or any other feature suggestive of an underlying early gastric cancer.

Superficial Gastric Erosions

Superficial gastric erosions are ulcerations that are so small and shallow that they are rarely demonstrated on conventional single-contrast upper gastrointestinal examinations. With the increasing use of double-contrast techniques, a superficial gastric erosion typically appears radiographically as a tiny fleck of barium, which represents the erosion, surrounded by a radiolucent halo, which represents a mound of edematous mucosa (Figure 5-34). Possible factors implicated in the production of superficial gastric erosions include alcohol, antiinflammatory drugs (aspirin, steroids), Crohn's disease (see Crohn's Disease [Regional Enteritis], later), and candidiasis (see *Candida* and Herpesvirus, earlier).

Treatment of Ulcers

Lifestyle modifications are the first line of treatment for ulcers. First, the patient should avoid foods that cause an increase in the acid secretions (i.e., alcohol and caffeine). Antacids aid in neutralizing stomach acid. If stress is the cause of the increase in acidic secretions, stress management is appropriate. When the ulceration is caused by an infection (*H. pylori*), antibiotics are given to kill the bacteria. If the acidic secretions cannot be controlled by these methods, histamine H_2 antagonists help in reducing stomach acids and protecting the stomach lining. When more aggressive treatment is required, proton-pump

inhibitors may be used. Surgical treatment for management of complications may be necessary when patients do not respond to other treatments.

Cancer of the Stomach

Because pain is infrequently an early symptom, carcinoma of the stomach is rarely noted until the disease is far advanced and thus has a dismal prognosis (survival rate, 10%). The incidence of gastric cancer varies widely throughout the world. It is very high in Japan, Chile, and parts of Eastern Europe. It is low in the United States, where for reasons unknown it has been decreasing.

Several conditions appear to predispose persons to the development of carcinoma of the stomach. There is an increased risk of gastric cancer in patients with atrophic gastric mucosa, as in pernicious anemia, and in persons 10 to 20 years after a partial gastrectomy for peptic ulcer disease. A suggestive laboratory sign is achlorhydria, the absence of hydrochloric acid in gastric secretions obtained by means of a stomach tube. Most carcinomas occur in the distal stomach and are adenomatous in nature.

Radiographic Appearance

Gastric carcinoma can present a broad spectrum of radiographic appearances. Tumor infiltration of the gastric wall may stimulate intense fibrosis, which produces diffuse thickening, narrowing, and fixation of the stomach wall (a linitis plastica pattern) (Figure 5-35). The stomach is contracted into a tubular structure without normal pliability. This fibrotic process usually begins near the pylorus and progresses slowly upward; the fundus is the area least involved.

SUMMARY of FINDINGS for the Stomach

disorder	location	radiographic appearance	treatment
Gastritis	Alcohol—gastric folds Corrosive—narrowing of antrum	Thickened gastric folds Gastric outlet obstruction	Depends on cause: Avoid long-term irritants Acid-reduction medications Antibiotics for infections Treat cause
	Bacterial or infectious—gastric wall Chronic atrophic	Thickened gastric wall causing narrowing of stomach and gas in the stomach wall Thinning and absence of mucosal folds ("bald")	
Peptic ulcer	Inflammatory process Duodenal ulcer	Small shallow erosions to perforations—bleeding ulcer CT—irregular collection of contrast material in the gastric wall Rounded or linear collection of contrast material surrounded by lucent folds that often radiate toward the crater	Avoid foods causing increased acid secretion (alcohol, caffeine) Antibiotics for infectious process Histamine H_2 antagonist to reduce acidic secretions Proton-pump inhibitors
	Gastric ulcer	Benign—mucosal folds are smooth and slender and appear to extend into the edge of the crater Malignant—irregular folds merge into a mound of polypoid tissue around the crater	
	Superficial gastric erosions	Fleck of barium with radiolucent halo	
Cancer	Gastric wall infiltration Polypoid mass	Diffuse thickening, narrowing, and fixation of stomach wall Irregularity and ulceration suggest malignancy CT—intraluminal mass without wall thickening—Stage I; wall thickening < 1 cm without invasion outside the organ—Stage II; thickened wall with extension into adjacent organs—Stage III; wall thickening and obliteration of perigastric fat planes—Stage IV Endoscopic ultrasound—increased echogenicity of gastric mucosa with vertical invasion through the wall	Surgical resection of all or part of stomach

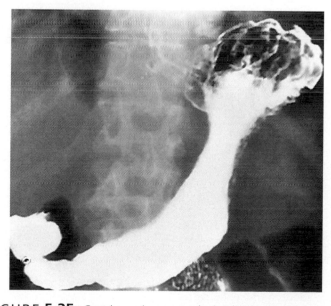

FIGURE 5-35 Gastric carcinoma producing linitis plastica pattern.

Another major form of gastric carcinoma is a large irregular polypoid mass (about one third of cancers). Irregularity and ulceration within the mass are suggestive of malignancy, whereas the presence of a stalk or normal-appearing gastric folds extending to the tumor are signs of benignancy. Ulceration can develop in any gastric carcinoma and occurs in approximately one third. This varies from shallow erosions in relatively superficial mucosal lesions to huge excavations within fungating polypoid masses (Figure 5-36).

CT is of major value in the staging of gastric carcinoma, in planning its treatment, in assessing the response to therapy, and in detecting tumor recurrence (Figure 5-37). Carcinoma of the stomach may appear as thickening of the gastric wall or as an intraluminal mass. The earliest stage demonstrates as an intraluminal mass without wall thickening. Stage II presents with wall thickening of greater than 1 cm without invasion of other tissue or organs. As the disease progresses, the stomach wall thickens and invades adjacent organs (Stage III). Obliteration of the fat planes (the covering layers of fat) around the stomach is a reliable indicator of the extragastric spread of tumor (Stage IV). CT can demonstrate direct tumor extension to intraabdominal organs, and distant metastases, especially to the liver.

Gastric carcinoma may also be demonstrated using endoscopic ultrasound. The gastric mucosa produces an increased echogenicity and demonstrates vertical invasion through the gastric wall. If diagnosed at a late stage, the lesion may extend into the perigastric lymph nodes.

Treatment
In most cases, treatment consists of surgical resection of all or part of the stomach.

Lymphoma of the Stomach
See Lymphoma in Chapter 9.

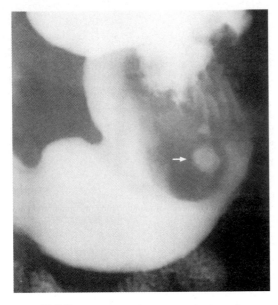

FIGURE 5-36 Gastric carcinoma producing a large polypoid mass with associated ulceration *(arrow)*.

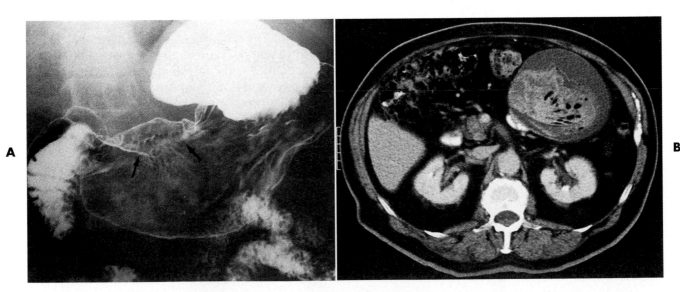

FIGURE 5-37 CT staging of gastric carcinoma. **A,** Double-contrast study demonstrates large lesser-curvature mass *(arrows)*. **B,** CT image shows a thickened gastric wall; the contrast agent demonstrates the lumen of the stomach.

Small Bowel

Crohn's Disease (Regional Enteritis)

Crohn's disease is a chronic inflammatory disorder of unknown cause that most often involves the terminal area of the ileum, but can affect any part of the gastrointestinal tract. Although it can occur at any age, Crohn's disease is most common in young adults. The underlying cause is unknown, although there appears to be some psychogenic element; stress or emotional upsets are frequently related to the onset or relapse of the disease.

The granulomatous inflammatory process in Crohn's disease is frequently discontinuous, with diseased segments of bowel separated by apparently healthy portions (skip areas). Diffuse inflammation with edema involves all layers of the intestinal wall. Ulceration is common, and fistulas running in the bowel wall or extending to other organs are not infrequent.

The clinical spectrum of Crohn's disease is broad, ranging from a relatively benign course with unpredictable acute attacks and remissions to severe diarrhea and an acute condition in the abdomen. Although acute Crohn's disease may produce right lower quadrant pain simulating appendicitis, there is often blood in the stools that has come from the intensely congested mucous membranes. Small bowel obstruction and fistula formation occur in up to half of patients. Rectal fissures and perirectal abscesses occur in about one third.

Radiographic Appearance

In the small bowel, the earliest radiographic changes of Crohn's disease include irregular thickening and distortion of mucosal folds caused by submucosal inflammation and edema. Transverse and longitudinal ulcerations can separate islands of thickened mucosa and submucosa, leading to a characteristic rough cobblestone appearance (Figure 5-38). Rigid thickening of the entire bowel wall produces pipelike narrowing. Continued inflammation and fibrosis can result in a severely narrowed, rigid segment of small bowel in which the mucosal pattern is lost (string sign) (Figure 5-39). When several areas of small bowel are diseased, involved segments of varying length are often sharply separated from radiographically normal segments (skip lesions). On CT images, there is thickening of the wall of the small bowel, and the mesentery has an appearance that is described as "dirty fat." The new technology of CT enterography demonstrates subtle findings of mild wall thickening and mucosal vascular changes. CT is recommended for patients with active Crohn's disease to determine the nature of the mass.

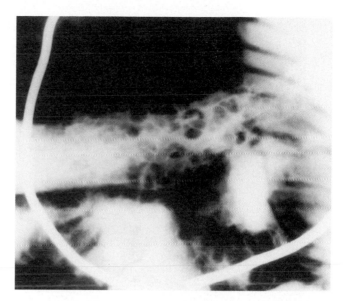

FIGURE 5-38 Crohn's disease. Cobblestone appearance is produced by transverse and longitudinal ulcerations separating islands of thickened mucosa and submucosa.

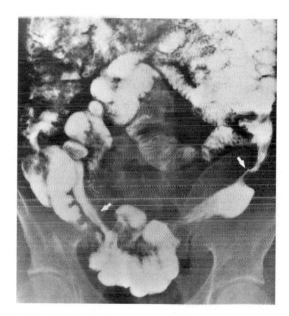

FIGURE 5-39 Crohn's disease. Arrows point to widely separated areas of disease (skip lesions). The lesions are greatly narrowed segments of small bowel (string sign).

Fistula formation, a hallmark of chronic Crohn's disease, is found in at least half of all patients with this condition (Figure 5-40). The diffuse inflammation of the serosa and mesentery in Crohn's disease causes involved loops of bowel to be firmly matted together by fibrous peritoneal and mesenteric bands. Fistulas apparently begin as ulcerations that burrow through the bowel wall into adjacent loops of small bowel and colon. In addition to fistulas between loops of bowel, a characteristic finding in Crohn's disease is

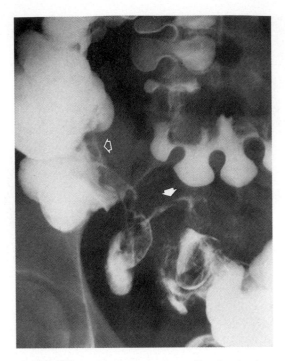

FIGURE 5-40 Crohn's disease. Note fistulization between the terminal ileum and the sigmoid colon *(solid arrow)* and along the cecum *(open arrow)*.

the appearance of fistulous tracts ending blindly in abscess cavities surrounded by dense inflammatory tissue. These abscess cavities can produce palpable masses, persistent fever, or pain. Although less common than bowel-to-bowel fistulas, internal fistulas extending from the bowel to the bladder or vagina can occur. A common complication is the development of external gastrointestinal fistulas, which usually extend to the perianal area and may be associated with fissures and perirectal abscesses.

Treatment
Whenever possible, Crohn's disease is treated with medications, and surgery is performed only if complications require it. Surgical resection of an involved segment of small bowel is associated with a high incidence of recurrence of Crohn's disease adjacent to the anastomosis.

Small Bowel Obstruction
Fibrous adhesions caused by previous surgery or peritonitis account for almost 75% of all small bowel obstructions. External hernias (inguinal, femoral, umbilical, incisional) are the second most common cause. Other general causes of mechanical small bowel obstruction include luminal occlusion (gallstone, intussusception) and intrinsic lesions of the bowel wall (neoplastic or inflammatory strictures, vascular insufficiency).

Radiographic Appearance
Distended loops of small bowel containing gas and fluid can usually be recognized within 3 to 5 hours of the onset of complete obstruction. Almost all gas proximal to a small bowel obstruction represents swallowed air. On upright or lateral decubitus projections, the interface between gas and fluid forms a straight horizontal margin (Figure 5-41). Although the presence of gas-fluid levels at different heights in the same loop has traditionally been considered evidence for mechanical obstruction, an identical pattern can also be demonstrated in some patients with adynamic ileus (see next section). The caliber of the air-filled bowel appears as a dilated proximal bowel and a collapsed distal bowel. On upright films, a string-of-beads sign appears. In adynamic ileus, the bowel has no caliber change.

As time passes, the small bowel may become so distended as to be almost indistinguishable from the colon. To make the critical differentiation between small and large bowel obstruction, it is essential to determine which loops of bowel contain abnormally large amounts of air. Small bowel loops generally occupy the more central portion of the abdomen, whereas colonic loops are positioned laterally around the periphery of the abdomen or inferiorly in the pelvis (Figure 5-42). Gas within the lumen of the small bowel outlines the thin valvulae conniventes, which completely encircle the bowel. In contrast, colonic haustral markings are thicker and farther apart and occupy only a portion of the transverse diameter of the bowel.

The site of obstruction can usually be predicted with considerable accuracy if the number and position of dilated bowel loops are analyzed. The presence of a few dilated loops of small bowel located high in the abdomen (in the center or slightly to the left) indicates an obstruction in the distal duodenum or jejunum. The involvement of additional small bowel loops is suggestive of a lower obstruction. As more loops are affected, they appear to be placed one above the other upward and to the left, producing a characteristic stepladder appearance (Figure 5-43). The point of obstruction is always distal to the lowest loop of dilated bowel.

Patients with complete mechanical small bowel obstruction demonstrate little or no gas in the colon. This is a valuable point in the differentiation between mechanical obstruction and adynamic ileus, in which gas is seen within distended loops throughout the bowel. Although a small amount of gas or fecal accumulation may be present at an early stage of a small bowel obstruction (see Figure 5-42), the detection of a large amount of gas in the colon effectively eliminates this diagnosis.

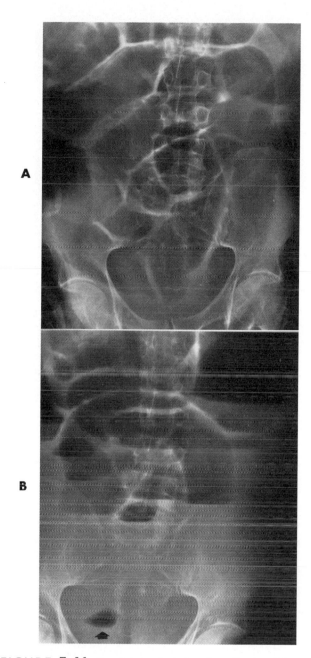

FIGURE 5-41 Small bowel obstruction. Supine **(A)** and upright **(B)** projections demonstrate large amounts of gas in dilated loops of small bowel with multiple prominent air-fluid levels. Single, small collection of gas (*arrow*) remains in colon.

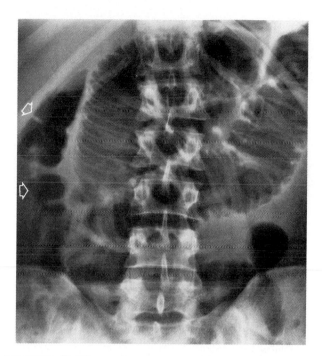

FIGURE 5-42 Small bowel obstruction. Dilated loops of small bowel occupy the central portion of the abdomen, with the nondilated cecum and ascending colon positioned laterally around the periphery of the abdomen (*arrows*).

The bowel proximal to an obstruction can contain no gas, but be completely filled with fluid. This may produce a confusing picture of a normal-appearing abdomen or a large soft tissue abdominal mass.

Plain abdominal radiographs are occasionally insufficient for a distinction to be made between small and large bowel obstruction. In these instances, a carefully performed barium enema examination will document or eliminate the possibility of large

bowel obstruction. If it is necessary to determine the precise site of small bowel obstruction, barium can be administered in either a retrograde (by means of an enema) or an antegrade (by way of the mouth) manner. Orally administered barium (*not* water-soluble agents) is the most effective contrast material for demonstrating the site of small bowel obstruction (Figure 5-44). The large amount of fluid proximal to a small bowel obstruction prevents any trapped barium from hardening or increasing the degree of obstruction. The density of barium permits excellent visualization far into the intestine; water-soluble agents, however, are lost to sight because of dilution and absorption. It must be emphasized that if plain radiographs clearly demonstrate a mechanical small bowel obstruction, *any* contrast examination is unnecessary.

Strangulation of bowel caused by interference with the blood supply is a serious complication of small bowel obstruction. In a closed-loop obstruction (e.g., volvulus and incarcerated hernia) (Figure 5-45), the loops going both toward (afferent) and away from (efferent) the area of narrowing become obstructed. The involved segments usually fill with fluid and appear radiographically as a tumorlike soft tissue mass. A closed loop is a clinically dangerous form of obstruction, since the continuing outpouring of fluid into the enclosed space can raise intraluminal pressure and rapidly lead to occlusion of the blood supply to that segment of bowel. Because venous pressure

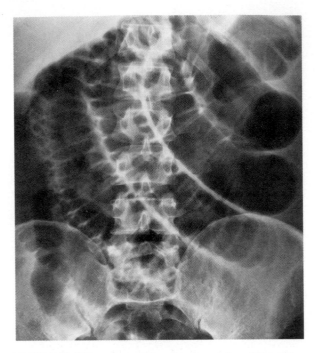

FIGURE 5-43 Low small bowel obstruction. Dilated loops of gas-filled bowel appear to be placed one above the other, upward and to the left, producing the characteristic stepladder appearance.

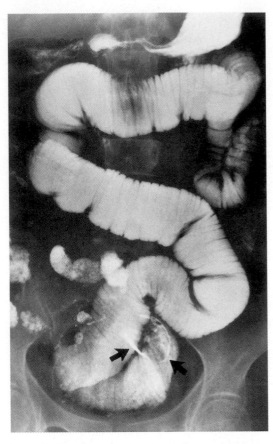

FIGURE 5-44 Barium upper gastrointestinal series demonstrates an impacted bezoar *(arrows)* to be the cause of a small bowel obstruction.

is normally lower than arterial pressure, blockage of venous outflow from the strangulated segment occurs before obstruction of the mesenteric arterial supply. Ischemia can rapidly cause necrosis of the bowel with sepsis, peritonitis, and a potentially fatal outcome.

CT may aid in demonstrating small bowel obstruction when the plain abdominal radiographs are normal or nonspecific. In addition to showing the site, level, and cause of the obstruction, this modality may indicate whether there is strangulation of the involved loops of bowel. Specifically, herniation causes slight wall thickening that appears as a "target sign" as a result of engorgement of the superior and inferior mesenteric vessels. CT appears to be the most valuable modality for patients with a history of abdominal malignancy and for those who have signs of infection, bowel infarction, or a palpable abdominal mass (Figure 5-46).

Treatment
Surgery is usually required to decompress the bowel as soon as possible to prevent necrosis or bowel perforation from occurring.

Adynamic Ileus
Adynamic ileus is a common disorder of intestinal motor activity in which fluid and gas do not progress normally through a nonobstructed small and large

bowel. A variety of neural, hormonal, and metabolic factors can precipitate reflexes that inhibit intestinal motility. Adynamic ileus occurs to some extent in almost every patient who undergoes abdominal surgery. Other causes of adynamic ileus include peritonitis, medications that decrease intestinal peristalsis (those with an atropine-like effect), electrolyte and metabolic disorders, and trauma. Adynamic ileus (or paralytic ileus) occurs more often than mechanical bowel obstruction. The clinical findings in patients with adynamic ileus vary from minimal symptoms to generalized abdominal distention with a sharp decrease in the frequency and intensity of bowel sounds.

Radiographic Appearance
The radiographic hallmark of adynamic ileus is the retention of large amounts of gas and fluid in dilated small and large bowel. The entire small and large bowel in adynamic ileus, unlike in mechanical small bowel obstruction, appears almost uniformly dilated with no demonstrable point of obstruction (Figure 5-47).

There are two major variants of adynamic ileus. **Localized ileus** refers to an isolated distended loop

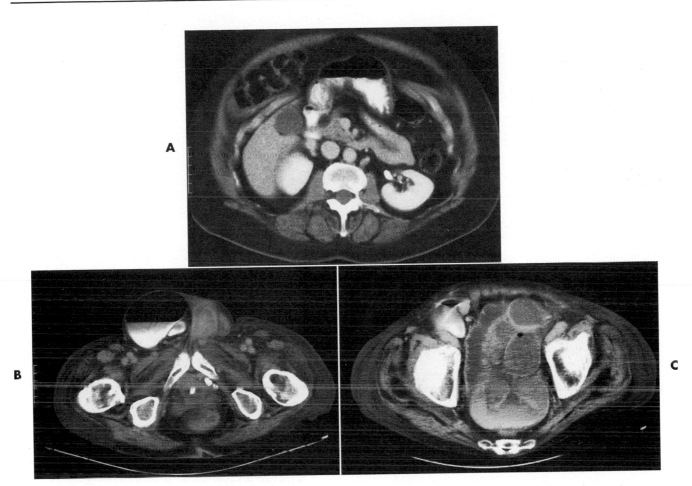

FIGURE 5-45 CT scan of bowel obstructions. **A,** Herniation of small bowel and stomach through anterior abdominal wall. **B,** Scrotal herniation of large bowel causing bowel obstruction. **C,** Dilated sigmoid colon caused by obstruction.

of small or large bowel (the sentinel loop), which is often associated with an adjacent acute inflammatory process. The portion of the involved bowel can offer a clue to the underlying disease. Localized segments of the jejunum or transverse colon are frequently dilated in patients with acute pancreatitis. Similarly the hepatic flexure of the colon can be distended in acute cholecystitis, the terminal ileum can be dilated in acute appendicitis, the descending colon can be distended in acute diverticulitis, and dilated loops can be seen along the course of the ureter in acute ureteral colic (Figure 5-48). Unfortunately, isolated segments of distended small bowel are commonly seen in patients with abdominal pain and thus the sentinel loop may be found "guarding" the wrong area.

Colonic ileus refers to selective or disproportionate gaseous distention of the large bowel without an obstruction (Figure 5-49). Massive distention of the cecum, which is often horizontally oriented, characteristically dominates the radiographic appearance. Colonic ileus usually accompanies or follows an acute abdominal inflammatory process or abdominal surgery. The clinical presentation and the findings on plain abdominal radiographs simulate those of mechanical obstruction of the colon. A barium enema examination is usually necessary to exclude an obstructing lesion.

Treatment

Adynamic ileus caused by surgery usually resolves itself spontaneously in 36 to 48 hours if no complications are involved. Treatment includes insertion of a nasogastric tube to aspirate the stomach, decompress the bowel, and allow the intestine to rest. Electrolyte and fluid imbalances are corrected by intravenous (IV) injection.

Intussusception

Intussusception is a major cause of bowel obstruction in children; it is much less common in adults. Intussusception is the telescoping of one part of the intestinal tract into another because of peristalsis, which forces the proximal segment of bowel to move

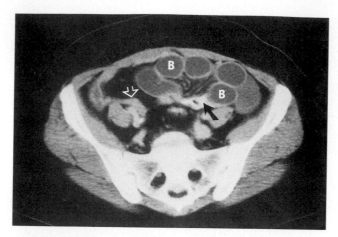

FIGURE 5-46 CT diagnosis of clinically unsuspected small bowel obstruction caused by adhesions. Note transition point between the dilated loops of small bowel *(B)* and the collapsed ileum *(black arrow)*. Note also the collapsed terminal ileum *(open arrow)*.

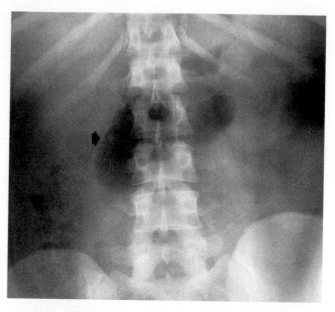

FIGURE 5-48 Localized ileus in patient with acute ureteral colic. Arrow points to impacted ureteral stone.

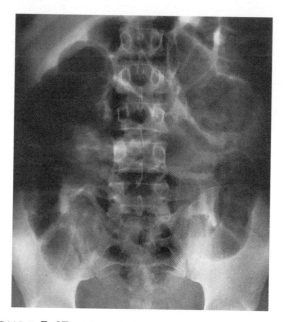

FIGURE 5-47 Adynamic ileus. Large amounts of gas and fluid are retained in loops of dilated small and large bowel. The entire bowel, small and large, appears almost uniformly dilated with no demonstrable point of obstruction.

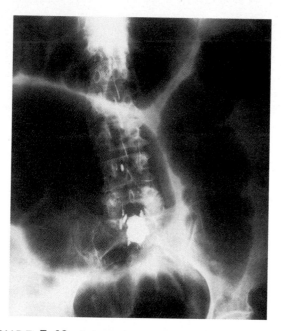

FIGURE 5-49 Colonic ileus. Massive distention of large bowel without obstruction in a patient with severe diabetes and electrolyte abnormalities.

distally within the ensheathing outer portion. Once such a lead point has been established, it gradually progresses forward and causes increased obstruction. This can compromise the vascular supply and produce ischemic necrosis of the intussuscepted bowel.

In children, intussusception is most common in the region of the ileocecal valve. The clinical onset tends to be abrupt, with severe abdominal pain, blood in the stool ("currant jelly"), and often a palpable right-sided mass. If the diagnosis is made early and therapy instituted promptly, the mortality of intussusception in children is less than 1%. However, if treatment is delayed more than 48 hours after the onset of symptoms, the mortality increases dramatically. In adults, intussusception is

SUMMARY *of* FINDINGS *for* the Small Bowel

disorder	location	radiographic appearance	treatment
Crohn's disease (regional enteritis)	Most often in terminal ileum	Small bowel series • Irregular thickened mucosal folds • Cobblestone appearance • String sign and skip lesions CT—thick mucosal walls and "dirty fat" mesenteric appearance CT enterography—subtle wall thickening and mucosal vascular changes Ulcerations—fistula formation	Medications Surgery if complications occur
Small bowel obstruction	Mechanical	Abdomen • Caliber of the air-filled bowel appears as a dilated proximal bowel and a collapsed distal bowel • Stepladder appearance CT—herniation illustrates as a "target sign" as a result of slight wall thickening with mesenteric engorgement	Decompression as soon as possible Usually surgery
Adynamic ileus	Motility loss in small bowel	Large amounts of gas and fluid in small and large bowel	Usually resolves itself in 36–48 hr Place NG tube and balance fluids
Intussusception	Children—ileocecal valve	Radiograph—coiled spring appearance on contrast enema CT—three concentric circles forming a soft tissue mass US—doughnut-shaped lesion	Reduction of telescoping bowel (rectal insufflation) Therapeutic enema of air or barium
Malabsorption disorders	Throughout small bowel	Dilatation with normal folds Irregular distorted folds	Medications to increase nutrient absorption

NG, Nasogastric; *US,* ultrasound.

often chronic or subacute and is characterized by irregular recurrent episodes of colicky pain, nausea, and vomiting. A specific cause of intussusception often cannot be detected in children. In adults, however, the leading edge is frequently a polypoid tumor with a stalk (pedunculated) or an inflammatory mass.

Radiographic Appearance

Radiographically, an intussusception produces the classic coiled-spring appearance of barium trapped between the intussusceptum and the surrounding portions of bowel (Figure 5-50, *A*). Reduction of a colonic intussusception can sometimes be accomplished by a barium enema examination (Figure 5-50, *B* and *C*), although great care must be exercised to prevent excessive intraluminal pressure, which may lead to perforation of the colon. On CT images, intussusception appears as three concentric circles forming a soft tissue mass.

Ultrasound, used especially in children, demonstrates the obstructive mass as a doughnut-shaped lesion on the transverse scan and as a "pseudokidney" on the longitudinal scan (Figure 5-51).

Treatment

Reduction of intussusceptions by rectal insufflation of air (instead of barium) has been reported to be an effective technique in children. In older children and adults, a repeat barium enema after reduction is necessary to determine whether an underlying polyp or a tumor caused the intussusception.

Malabsorption Disorders

The term **malabsorption disorder** refers to a multitude of conditions in which there is defective absorption of carbohydrates, proteins, and fats from the small bowel. Regardless of the cause, malabsorption results in steatorrhea—the passage of bulky, foul-smelling, high-fat-content stools that float.

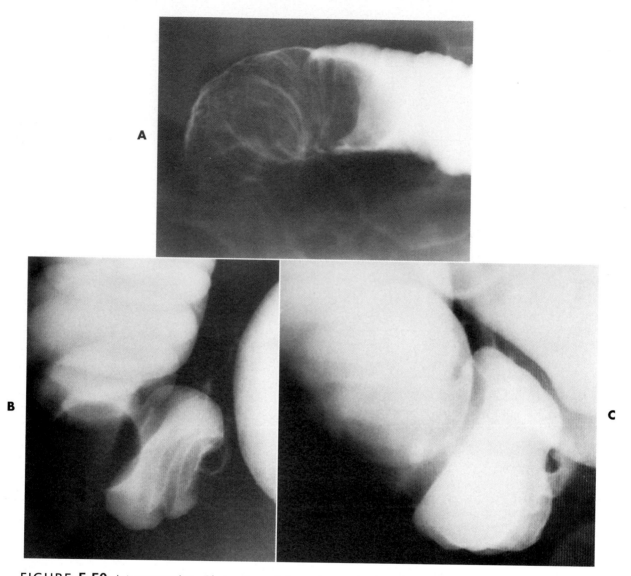

FIGURE 5-50 Intussusception. Obstruction of the colon at the hepatic flexure produces the characteristic coiled-spring appearance of intussuscepted bowel **(A)**. Partial **(B)** and complete **(C)** reduction of intussusception by careful barium enema examination.

Radiographic Appearance

Many of the diseases that cause malabsorption produce radiographic abnormalities in the small bowel, although malabsorption can exist without any detectable small bowel changes. The two major radiographic appearances are (1) small bowel dilatation with normal folds (Figure 5-52) and (2) a pattern of generalized, irregular, distorted small bowel folds (Figure 5-53).

Treatment

Patients afflicted with malabsorption disorders take medications to assist in absorbing key nutrients to keep the body's systems in good health. Probiotics are live microbial food supplements that aid in improving the intestinal microbial balance. These supplements enhance the bioavailability of nutrients to the body.

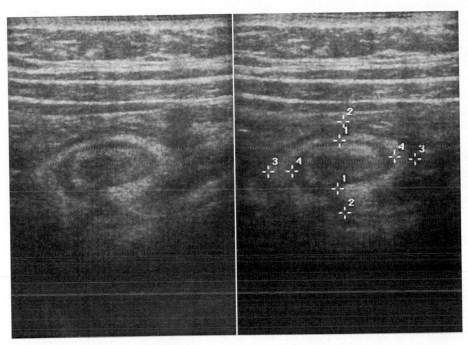

FIGURE 5-51 Intussusception. Ultrasound image illustrates doughnut-shaped lesion marked for measurement.

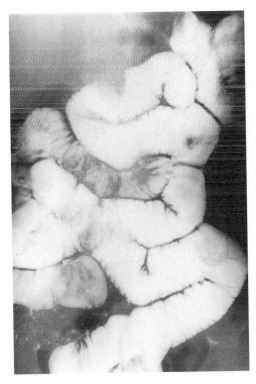

FIGURE 5-52 Diffuse dilatation of entire small bowel with excessive intraluminal fluid in a patient with malabsorption caused by sprue.

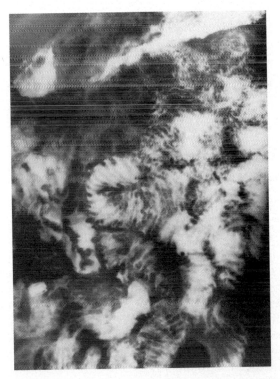

FIGURE 5-53 Diffuse, irregular thickening of small bowel folds in a patient with malabsorption secondary to Whipple's disease.

Colon

Appendicitis

Acute appendicitis develops when the neck of the appendix becomes blocked by a fecalith or by post-inflammatory scarring that creates a closed-loop obstruction within the organ. Because of inadequate drainage, fluid accumulates in the obstructed portion and serves as a breeding ground for bacteria. High intraluminal pressure causes distention and thinning of the appendix distal to the obstruction, which interferes with the circulation and may lead to gangrene and perforation. If the process evolves slowly, adjacent organs (terminal ileum, cecum, omentum) may wall off the appendiceal area so that a localized abscess develops; rapid vascular compromise may permit free perforation with the spilling of fecal material into the peritoneal cavity and the development of generalized peritonitis. Appendicitis occurs in all age groups, but is more common in children and adolescents.

The clinical symptoms (and lab results) of acute appendicitis are usually so characteristic that there is no need for routine radiographs to make the correct diagnosis. The presence of severe right lower quadrant pain, low-grade fever, and slight leukocytosis, especially in younger adults, is presumed to be evidence of appendicitis. However, in some patients, especially the elderly, the clinical findings may be obscure or minimal. In addition, because the appendix is mobile and may be in an unusual location, the pain of acute appendicitis may mimic cholecystitis, diverticulitis, or pelvic inflammatory disease. When the symptoms are confusing, an imaging examination may be necessary for prompt diagnosis and surgical intervention before perforation occurs.

Radiographic Appearance

Plain abdominal radiographs may demonstrate a round or oval, laminated calcified fecalith in the appendix (appendicolith) (Figure 5-54) in about one third of patients. Surgical experience indicates that the presence of an appendicolith in combination with symptoms of acute appendicitis usually implies that the appendix is gangrenous (necrotic) and likely to perforate. Most appendicoliths are located in the right lower quadrant overlying the iliac fossa. Depending on the length and position of the appendix, however, an appendicolith can also be seen in the pelvis or in the right upper quadrant (retrocecal appendix), where it can simulate a gallstone.

Because of the danger of perforation, barium enema examination is usually avoided in acute appendicitis. If it is performed, an irregular impression of the base

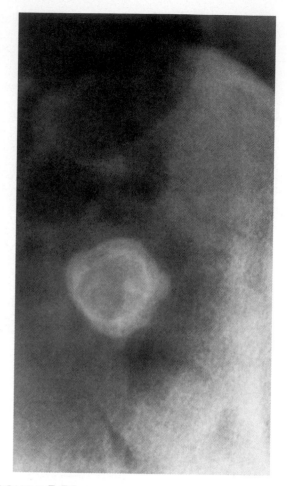

FIGURE 5-54 Laminated calcification in appendicolith.

of the cecum (caused by inflammatory edema), in association with failure of barium to enter the appendix, is a characteristic finding. Nevertheless, failure of barium to fill the appendix is not a reliable sign of appendicitis, because the appendix does not fill in about 20% of normal patients. Partial filling of the appendix with distortion of its shape or caliber strongly suggests acute appendicitis (Figure 5-55), especially if there is a cecal impression. In contrast, a patent (open) appendiceal lumen effectively excludes the diagnosis of acute appendicitis, especially when barium extends to fill the rounded appendiceal tip.

When the clinical presentation is unclear, high-resolution ultrasound with graded compression is the imaging modality of choice for diagnosing acute appendicitis, especially when ionizing radiation is contraindicated in the patient. A noncompressible appendix measuring 7 mm or more in maximal outer diameter is considered virtually pathognomonic of acute appendicitis (Figure 5-56).

CT, the gold standard, shows an appendiceal abscess as a round or oval mass of soft tissue–density that may contain gas. After administration of IV contrast material, the appendix appears as a dilated structure with a thickened, circumferentially enhancing wall (Figure 5-57). This modality provides a more precise evaluation of the nature, extent, and location of the pathologic process and can detect intraabdominal disease unrelated to appendicitis, which may explain the patient's clinical presentation.

Treatment

When a patient is diagnosed with appendicitis, an immediate appendectomy should be performed before perforation occurs to prevent complications (e.g., peritonitis, gangrene, and abscess formation). If perforation occurs, a regimen of antibiotics helps to reduce the risk of peritonitis and sepsis.

Diverticulosis

Colonic diverticula are outpouchings that represent acquired herniations of mucosa and submucosa through the muscular layers at points of weakness in the bowel wall. The incidence of colonic diverticulosis increases with age. Rare in persons less than 30 years of age, diverticula can be demonstrated in up to half of persons over 60 years of age. Diverticular disease is presumed to occur in individuals who frequently exert high pressures in the lumen while straining to pass a large bulk of stool. Those consuming low-fiber and low-bulk meals are more susceptible. Diverticula occur most commonly in the sigmoid colon and decrease in frequency in the proximal colon. Although most patients with diverticulosis have no symptoms, a substantial number have chronic or intermittent lower abdominal pain, frequently related to meals or emotional stress, and alternating bouts of diarrhea and constipation.

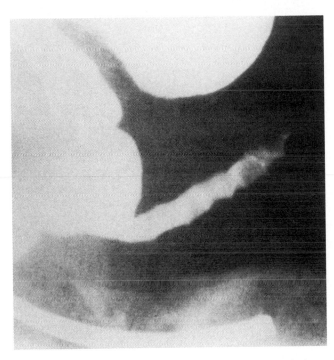

FIGURE 5-55 Acute appendicitis. Spot radiograph from barium enema examination shows incomplete filling of appendix.

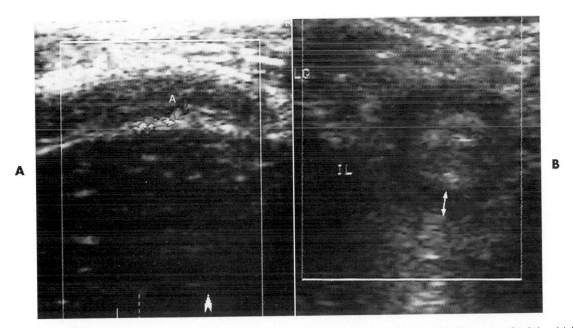

FIGURE 5-56 Ultrasound images of appendicitis. **A,** Sagittal sonogram shows inflamed appendix *(A)*, which is elongated and hypoechoic. **B,** Transverse scan shows appendiceal lumen surrounded by hypoechoic inflamed tissue *(arrows)*.

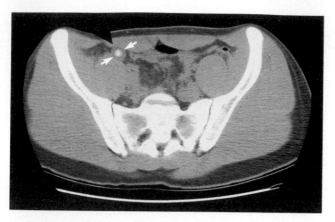

FIGURE 5-57 CT scan of the abdomen shows an appendix with an enlarged thickened wall indicating inflammation. An appendicolith can be seen in the appendix *(arrows)*.

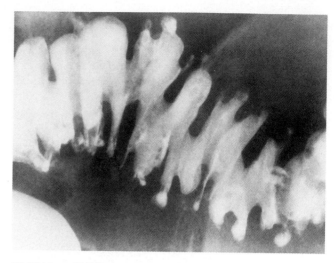

FIGURE 5-58 Diverticulosis. The typical saw-toothed configuration is produced by thickened circular muscle and is associated with multiple diverticula.

Bleeding may be caused by inflammatory erosion of penetrating blood vessels at the base of the diverticulum. The leading cause of massive lower gastrointestinal bleeding in adults and guaiac-positive (indicating occult blood) stools in the elderly is diverticular disease.

Radiographic Appearance

Colonic diverticula appear radiographically as round or oval outpouchings of barium projecting beyond the confines of the lumen. They vary in size from barely visible dimples to saclike structures 2 cm or more in diameter. Giant sigmoid diverticula up to 25 cm in diameter, which probably represent slowly progressing chronic diverticular abscesses, may appear as large, well-circumscribed, lucent cystic structures in the lower abdomen.

Diverticula are usually multiple and tend to occur in clusters, although a solitary diverticulum is occasionally found. When diverticula are multiple, deep crisscrossing ridges of thickened circular muscle (saw-toothed configuration) can produce a characteristic series of sacculations (Figure 5-58).

Diverticula also commonly occur in the esophagus and duodenum and infrequently may develop in the jejunum and ileum.

Diverticulitis

Diverticulitis is a complication of diverticular disease of the colon (necrosing inflammation in the diverticula), especially in the sigmoid region, in which perforation of a diverticulum leads to the development of a peridiverticular abscess. It is estimated that up to 20% of patients with diverticulosis eventually develop acute diverticulitis. Retained fecal material trapped in a diverticulum by the narrow opening

of the diverticular neck causes inflammation of the mucosal lining, which then leads to perforation of the diverticulum. This usually results in a localized peridiverticular abscess that is walled off by fibrous adhesions. The inflammatory process may localize within the wall of the colon and produce an intramural mass, or it may dissect around the colon, causing segmental narrowing of the lumen. Extension of the inflammatory process along the colon wall can involve adjacent diverticula, resulting in a longitudinal sinus tract along the bowel wall. A common complication of diverticulitis is the development of fistulas to adjacent organs (bladder, vagina, ureter, small bowel).

Radiographic Appearance

The radiographic diagnosis of diverticulitis requires direct or indirect evidence of diverticular perforation. The most specific sign is extravasation, which can appear either as a tiny projection of contrast material from the tip of a diverticulum (Figure 5-59, *A*) or as an obvious filling of a pericolic abscess (Figure 5-59, *B*). A more common, although somewhat less specific, sign of diverticulitis is the demonstration of a pericolic soft tissue mass that is attributable to a localized abscess and represents a walled-off perforation. This extraluminal mass appears as a filling defect causing eccentric narrowing of the bowel lumen. The adjacent diverticula are spastic, irritable, and attenuated and frequently seem to drape over the mass. It is important to remember, however, that a peridiverticular abscess caused by diverticulitis can occur without radiographically detectable diverticula (Figure 5-60).

Severe spasm or fibrotic healing of diverticulitis can cause a rigidity and progressive narrowing of

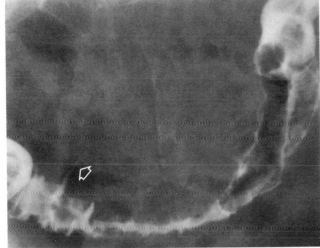

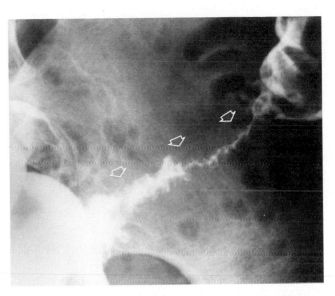

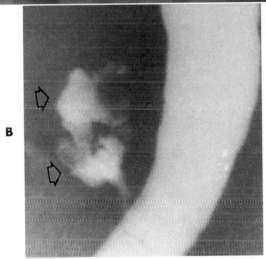

FIGURE 5-60 Sigmoid diverticulitis. Severe narrowing of the long involved portion of the sigmoid colon *(arrows)* in a patient with no radiographically detectable diverticula.

FIGURE 5-59 Diverticulitis. **A,** Thin projection of contrast material *(arrow)* implies extravasation from colonic lumen. Note severe spasm of the sigmoid colon caused by intense adjacent inflammation. **B,** The pericolic abscess is clearly filled with contrast material *(arrows).*

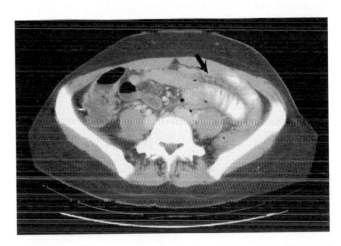

FIGURE 5-61 Diverticulitis. CT scan illustrates thickened small bowel wall. The tissue has a "dirty" appearance *(arrow).*

the colon that simulates annular carcinoma. Although radiographic distinction from carcinoma may be impossible, findings favoring the diagnosis of diverticulitis include the involvement of a relatively long segment, a gradual transition from diseased to normal colon, a relative preservation of mucosal detail, and fistulous tracts and intramural abscesses. At times, colonoscopy or surgery may be required to make a definitive diagnosis.

Acute diverticulitis on ultrasound appears as a hypoechoic projection that arises from the wall of the bowel and is surrounded by inflamed fat. CT demonstrates pericolic fluids or gas collections, usually with nonspecific colonic wall thickening that produces narrowing of the bowel lumen (Figure 5-61). Inflammatory stranding may appear in the adjacent fat.

Treatment of Diverticulosis and Diverticulitis

Noninvasive treatment is the first choice, using dietary modifications (nothing with seeds, nuts, popcorn, etc.) and exercise (to increase peristalsis). If diverticulitis has developed, antibiotics and diet adjustments (liquids) are given until the bowel heals. Perforation requires surgical repair and a regimen of antibiotics.

Ulcerative Colitis

Ulcerative colitis is one of the two major inflammatory bowel diseases (the other is Crohn's colitis; see later). It primarily affects young adults and is highly variable in severity, clinical course, and ultimate prognosis. The cause is unknown, although an auto-immune cause has been suggested and a psychogenic factor may be involved because the condition is often aggravated by stress. The onset of the disease and subsequent exacerbations can be insidious or abrupt. The main symptoms include bloody diarrhea, abdominal pain, fever, and weight loss. A characteristic feature of ulcerative colitis is alternating periods of remission and relapse. Most patients have intermittent episodes of symptoms, with complete remission between attacks. In fewer than 15% of patients, ulcerative colitis is an acute severe process with a far higher incidence of serious complications, such as toxic megacolon (extreme dilatation of a segment of colon with systemic toxicity) and free perforation into the peritoneal cavity. Usually, ulcerative colitis involves only the mucosal layer of the colon.

Radiographic Appearance

In the radiographic evaluation of a patient with known or suspected ulcerative colitis, plain abdominal radiographs are essential. Large nodular protrusions of hyperplastic mucosa, deep ulcers outlined by intraluminal gas, or polypoid changes along with a loss of haustral markings (normal indentations in the wall of the colon) may indicate the diagnosis. Plain abdominal radiographs can also demonstrate evidence of toxic megacolon, a dramatic and ominous complication of ulcerative colitis that is characterized by extreme dilatation of a segment of colon (Figure 5-62), or evidence of an entire diseased colon, combined

with systemic toxicity (abdominal pain and tenderness, tachycardia, fever, and leukocytosis). Toxic megacolon can lead to spontaneous perforation of the colon, which can be dramatic and sudden and can cause irreversible shock. Because there is such a high danger of spontaneous perforation, barium enema examination is absolutely contraindicated during a recognized attack of toxic megacolon.

Ulcerative colitis has a strong tendency to begin in the rectosigmoid area. Although by radiographic criteria alone the rectum appears normal in about 20% of patients with ulcerative colitis, true rectal sparing is infrequent, and there is usually evidence of disease on sigmoidoscopy or rectal biopsy. Isolated right colon disease with a normal left colon does not occur, and ulcerative colitis may spread to involve the entire colon (pancolitis). The disease is almost always continuous, without evidence of the skip areas seen in Crohn's disease. Except for "backwash ileitis" (minimal inflammatory changes involving a short segment of terminal ileum), ulcerative colitis does not involve the small bowel, a feature distinguishing it from Crohn's disease, which may involve both the large and the small intestines.

On double-contrast studies, the earliest detectable radiographic abnormality in ulcerative colitis is fine granularity of the mucosa corresponding to the hyperemia and edema seen endoscopically (Figure 5-63). Once superficial ulcers develop, small flecks of adherent barium produce a stippled mucosal pattern. As the disease progresses, the ulcerations become deeper. Extension into the submucosa may

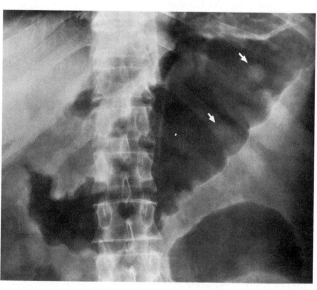

FIGURE 5-62 Toxic megacolon in ulcerative colitis. Note dilatation of the transverse colon with multiple pseudopolypoid projections extending into the lumen *(arrows)*.

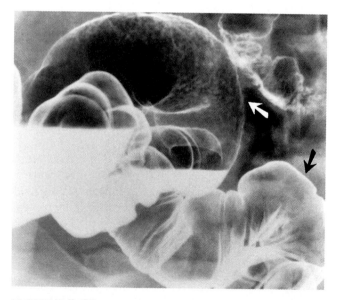

FIGURE 5-63 Ulcerative colitis involving primarily the rectosigmoid. Distal rectosigmoid mucosa *(white arrow)* is finely granular compared with the normal-appearing mucosa *(black arrow)* in the more proximal colon.

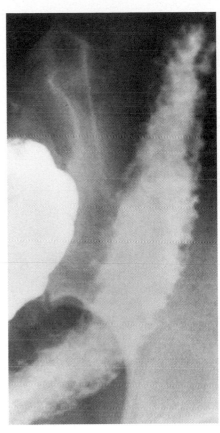

FIGURE 5-64 Ulcerative colitis. Progression of disease results in deep ulcerations (collar-button ulcers) extending into the submucosal layer.

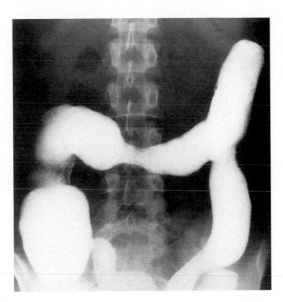

FIGURE 5-65 Chronic ulcerative colitis (lead-pipe colon). Muscular hypertrophy and spasm cause shortening and rigidity of the colon with loss of haustral markings.

produce broad-based ulcers with a collar-button appearance (Figure 5-64). Perirectal inflammation can cause widening of the soft tissue space between the anterior sacrum and the posterior rectum (retrorectal space).

When the disease is chronic, fibrosis and muscular spasm cause progressive shortening and rigidity of the colon (Figure 5-65). The haustral pattern is absent, and the bowel contour is relatively smooth because of ulcer healing and subsequent reepithelization. Eventually, the colon may appear as a symmetric, rigid, tubular structure (lead-pipe colon).

Carcinoma of the colon is about 10 times more frequent in patients with ulcerative colitis than in the general population. During the first 10 years of disease, there is only a small risk of malignancy. Thereafter, it is estimated that there is a 20% chance per decade that a patient with ulcerative colitis will develop carcinoma. Malignant lesions in ulcerative colitis generally occur at a much younger age than they occur in the general population, and they tend to be extremely virulent. Carcinoma of the colon in patients with chronic ulcerative colitis often appears as a bizarre stricture rather than with the more

characteristic polypoid or apple-core appearance of a primary colonic malignancy (Figure 5-66). The tumor typically produces a narrowed segment with an eccentric lumen, irregular contours, and margins that are rigid and tapered. Because it is frequently difficult to distinguish carcinoma from benign stricture in patients with ulcerative colitis, colonoscopy or surgery is often required for an unequivocal diagnosis.

Crohn's Colitis

Crohn's disease of the colon, the second major cause of inflammatory bowel disease, is identical to Crohn's disease in the small bowel and must be distinguished from ulcerative colitis. The proximal portion of the colon is most frequently involved in Crohn's disease; associated disease of the terminal ileum is seen in up to 80% of these patients. Unlike in ulcerative colitis, in Crohn's colitis the rectum is often spared, and isolated rectal disease very rarely occurs. Crohn's disease usually has a patchy distribution, with involvement of multiple noncontiguous segments of colon (skip lesions), unlike the continuous colonic involvement in ulcerative colitis. Perirectal abnormalities (fissures, abscesses, fistulas) occur at some point during the course of disease in half of patients with Crohn's colitis, but are rare in ulcerative colitis. Crohn's disease involves all layers of the gastrointestinal tract.

Radiographic Appearance

The earliest radiographic findings of Crohn's disease of the colon are seen on double-contrast examinations. Isolated tiny, discrete erosions (aphthous ulcers)

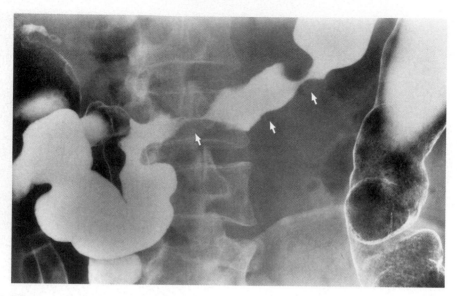

FIGURE 5-66 Carcinoma of the colon developing in a patient with long-standing chronic ulcerative colitis. A long, irregular lesion with a bizarre pattern is visible in the transverse colon *(arrows)*.

appear as punctate collections of barium with a thin halo of edema around them (Figure 5-67). Aphthous ulcers in Crohn's disease have a patchy distribution against a background of normal mucosa, unlike the blanket of abnormal granular mucosa seen in ulcerative colitis.

As Crohn's colitis progresses, the ulcers become deeper and more irregular, with a great variation in size, shape, and overall appearance. Deep linear, transverse, and longitudinal ulcers often separate intervening mounds of edematous but nonulcerating mucosa, producing a characteristic cobblestone appearance (see Figure 5-38). If the penetrating ulcers extend beyond the contour of the bowel, they can coalesce (grow together) to form long tracts running parallel to the long axis of the colon (Figure 5-68). The penetration of ulcers into adjacent loops of bowel or into the bladder, vagina, or abdominal wall causes fistulas, which can often be demonstrated radiographically. Inflammatory and fibrotic thickening of the bowel wall leads to narrowing of the lumen and stricture formation. Occasionally an eccentric stricture with a suggestion of overhanging edges can be difficult to distinguish from annular carcinoma (Figure 5-69). In most instances, however, characteristic features of Crohn's disease elsewhere in the colon (deep ulcerations, pseudopolyps, skip lesions, sinus tracts, fistulas) clearly indicate the correct diagnosis.

CT demonstrates the mesenteric and extraintestinal extent of the disease, and any abscess formation or colonic wall thickening. Magnetic resonance (MR) spectroscopy is currently under investigation to help distinguish ulcerative colitis from Crohn's. Preliminary results indicate that this technique is able

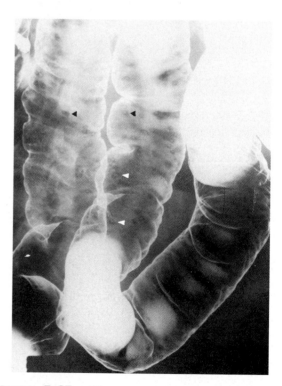

FIGURE 5-67 Diffuse aphthous ulcers *(arrowheads)* in early Crohn's colitis.

to differentiate between the two inflammatory bowel diseases in more than 90% of cases.

Patients with Crohn's colitis appear to have a higher incidence of developing colon cancer than the general population, although this association is less striking than that between colon cancer and ulcerative colitis. Carcinoma complicating Crohn's

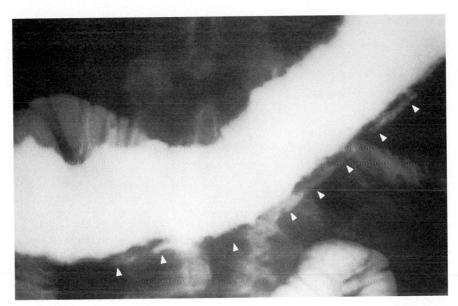

FIGURE 5-68 Crohn's colitis. Note long intramural fistula *(arrowheads)* in transverse colon.

colitis is most common in the proximal portion of the colon and usually appears radiographically as a fungating mass with typical malignant features, unlike the mildly irregular stricture characteristic of colon cancer in patients with ulcerative colitis. A small bowel examination may be necessary to demonstrate the terminal ileum.

Treatment of Ulcerative Colitis and Crohn's Colitis

The initial treatments for ulcerative colitis and Crohn's disease are identical, as both are inflammatory bowel diseases. First, nutritional supplements and dietary modifications (decrease bulk to reduce stool frequency) begin to decrease the inflammatory process. A regimen of antiinflammatory drugs interrupts the inflammatory cycle. Stress-related conditions require psychological support to control episodes. For ulcerative colitis, surgical resection may be necessary to prevent the spread of the condition. With proper treatment or spontaneous remission, many of the radiographic changes in this disease are reversible. In Crohn's, surgery is usually ineffective because the area adjacent to the anastomosis becomes involved as a result of the resection. For severe cases of Crohn's, parenteral (IV) nutrition allows the intestine time to heal.

Ischemic Colitis

Ischemic colitis is characterized by the abrupt onset of lower abdominal pain and rectal bleeding. Diarrhea is common, as is abdominal tenderness on physical examination. Most patients are older than 50 years, and many have a history of prior cardiovascular disease.

Radiographic Appearance

The initial radiographic appearance of ischemic colitis is fine superficial ulceration caused by inflammatory edema of the mucosa. As the disease progresses, deep penetrating ulcers, pseudopolyps, and characteristic "thumbprinting" can be demonstrated. Thumbprinting refers to sharply defined, fingerlike indentations along the margins of the colon wall (Figure 5-70). In most cases, the radiographic appearance of the colon returns to normal within 1 month if good collateral circulation is established. Extensive fibrosis during the healing phase can cause tubular narrowing and a smooth stricture. If blood flow is insufficient, acute bowel necrosis and perforation may result.

Treatment

In some cases, no intervention is needed, as the bowel heals itself. Patients taking vasoconstricting drugs are most susceptible, and when the diagnosis is ischemic colitis, these medications are discontinued and supportive care is given. Immediate surgical intervention is required for bowel infarctions and other complications.

Irritable Bowel Syndrome

The term **irritable bowel syndrome** refers to several conditions that have an alteration in intestinal motility as the underlying pathophysiologic abnormality. Most consider these conditions to be functional disorders because there is a disruption of the food sequence breakdown in the stomach and intestines. Patients with irritable bowel syndrome may complain primarily of chronic abdominal pain and constipation

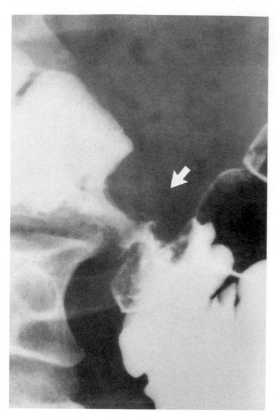

FIGURE 5-69 Chronic Crohn's colitis. Benign stricture with overhanging edges in transverse colon simulates carcinoma *(arrow)*.

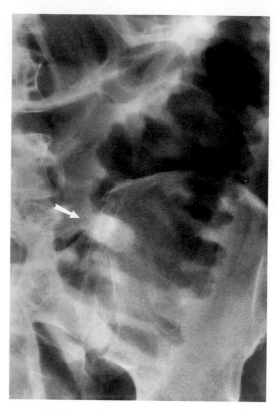

FIGURE 5-70 Ischemic colitis. Soft-tissue polypoid densities *(arrow)* protrude into lumen of descending colon in a patient with acute abdominal pain and rectal bleeding.

(spastic colitis), chronic intermittent watery diarrhea, often without pain, or alternating bouts of constipation and diarrhea.

Radiographic Appearance

Although there are no specific radiographic findings in irritable bowel syndrome, patients with this condition usually undergo a barium enema examination to exclude another chronic disorder as the cause of the symptoms. When the patient is symptomatic, a barium enema may demonstrate areas of irritability and spasticity and accentuated haustration, although similar radiographic findings may be observed in normal asymptomatic persons, especially those who have received laxatives and enemas.

Treatment

No cure exists for irritable bowel syndrome. As the precise cause of this functional disorder has not been determined, symptomatic relief is provided. It is necessary to identify trigger foods so that they can be avoided, thus decreasing the spasms and pain. Alternative therapies, relaxation, meditation, and physical exercise have value if the patient can use them to help ease some of the spasms and pain.

Cancer of the Colon

Carcinoma of the colon and rectum is the leading cause of death from cancer in the United States, even though it can be more easily diagnosed than most other malignant neoplasms. About half of colon carcinomas occur in the rectum and sigmoid, where they can be felt by rectal examination or seen with a sigmoidoscope. Carcinoma of the colon and rectum is primarily a disease of older persons, with a peak incidence in the 50- to 70-year range, and twice as common in men. Two diseases predispose to the development of cancer of the colon: long-standing ulcerative colitis and familial polyposis, a hereditary disease in which innumerable polyps develop in the colon and elsewhere in the intestinal tract.

Radiographic Appearance

Because cancer of the colon is curable if discovered early in the course, delay in diagnosis is the most significant factor in the poor prognosis. There is considerable evidence to indicate that many, if not most, carcinomas of the colon arise in preexisting polyps. Therefore the early diagnosis of colonic cancer depends on polyp detection. Malignant polyps (Figure 5-71) tend to be sessile lesions (without stalks)

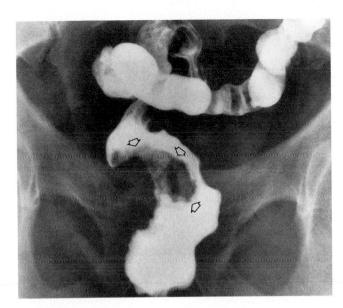

FIGURE 5-71 Carcinoma of rectum. Bulky lesion *(arrows)* could be felt on rectal examination.

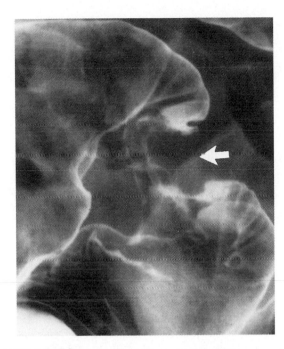

FIGURE 5-72 Annular carcinoma of sigmoid colon. Note sharply defined proximal and distal margins of this relatively short, apple-core lesion *(arrow)*.

with an irregular or lobulated surface, unlike benign polyps that are usually smooth and often have a stalk (are pedunculated). Other radiographic criteria suggestive that a polyp is malignant include large size (especially if greater than 2 cm in diameter), retraction or indentation (puckering) of the colon wall seen on profile view at the site of origin of a sessile polyp, and evidence of interval growth of a polyp on sequential examinations.

Annular carcinoma (described as apple-core or napkin-ring carcinoma) is one of the most typical forms of primary colonic malignancy (Figure 5-72). Annular carcinomas appear to arise from flat plaques of tumor (saddle lesions) that involve only a portion of the circumference of the colon wall. Unless meticulous care is taken to search for an area of minimal straightening or slight contour defects, the small and subtle, but lethal, saddle carcinomas can be easily overlooked. As the tumor grows, it characteristically infiltrates the bowel wall rather than forming a bulky intraluminal mass. This produces a classic bilateral contour defect with ulcerated mucosa, eccentric and irregular lumen, and overhanging margins. Progressive constriction of the bowel can cause complete colonic obstruction, most commonly in the sigmoid region.

Ulceration is common in carcinoma of the colon. It can vary from an excavation within a large fungating mass to mucosal destruction within an annular apple-core tumor.

A patient with carcinoma of the colon has a 1% risk of having multiple synchronous (occurring simultaneously) colon cancers. Therefore it is essential to

carefully examine the rest of the colon once an obviously malignant lesion has been detected. In addition, such a patient has a 3% risk of developing additional metachronous cancers later.

CT virtual colonoscopy has become more frequently used as a screening tool for colon cancer. Today, 2-D or 3-D CT colonoscopy can demonstrate lesions of 8 to 10 mm with an accuracy similar to that obtained with traditional colonoscopy. CT virtual colonoscopy is an alternative for incomplete or equivocal studies performed by traditional colonoscopy. CT is also the modality of choice for staging carcinoma of the colon and for assessing tumor recurrence (Figure 5-73). Carcinoma causes asymmetric or circumferential thickening of the bowel wall with narrowing and deformity of the lumen. CT can demonstrate local extension of tumor to the pelvic organs and lymphadenopathy and metastases to the adrenal glands or liver (Figure 5-74).

Transrectal ultrasound produces the most accurate images for staging local rectal cancer by demonstrating the depth of invasion within the bowel wall. Ultrasound also may determine the presence of a tumor in adjacent, normal-size lymph nodes.

Positron emission tomography (PET) with 18-fluorodeoxyglucose (FDG-PET), although less specific than CT and ultrasound, has a higher accuracy for detecting distant nodular metastases. Fusion imaging, which superimposes the functional (PET) and anatomic (CT) studies, provides more specific detail

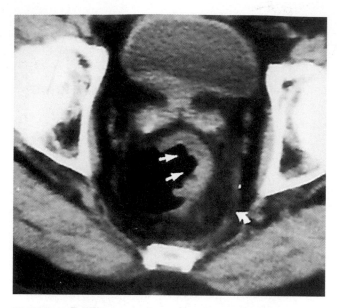

FIGURE 5-73 CT scan of a patient with rectal carcinoma shows a soft tissue mass on the lateral wall of the rectum containing a central ulceration *(straight arrows)*. Thickening of the perirectal fascia *(curved arrow)*, the presence of multiple lymph nodes (on the more cephalic images), and increased soft tissue density of perirectal fat were suggestive of tumor extension beyond the bowel wall, which was confirmed at surgery.

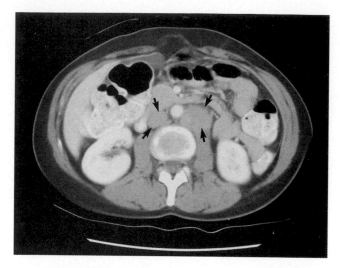

FIGURE 5-74 CT scan. Retroperitoneal and periaortic lymphadenopathy *(arrows)* in a 51-year-old woman with colon cancer.

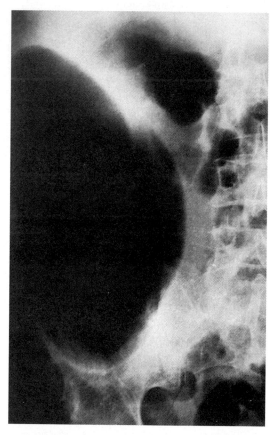

FIGURE 5-75 Large bowel obstruction. Huge dilatation of cecum (up to 13 cm in diameter) without perforation.

to localize and evaluate the severity of the disease process.

Treatment

Surgical resection is required to remove a solitary carcinoma. Postoperative treatment may include chemotherapy or radiation therapy. Following resection, FDG-PET in combination with a CT scan helps rule out recurrence. FDG-PET images can differentiate recurrence of the tumor from adhesions or scar tissue resulting from the resection. The presence of multiple lesions requires radiation and chemotherapy.

Large Bowel Obstruction

About 70% of large bowel obstructions result from primary colonic carcinoma. Diverticulitis and volvulus account for most other cases. Colonic obstructions tend to be less acute than small bowel obstructions; the symptoms develop more slowly, and fewer fluid and electrolyte disturbances are produced.

Radiographic Appearance

The radiographic appearance of colonic obstruction depends on the competency of the ileocecal valve. If the ileocecal valve is competent, obstruction causes a large, dilated colon with a greatly distended, thin-walled cecum and little small bowel gas (Figure 5-75).

The colon distal to the obstruction is usually collapsed and free of gas. If the ileocecal valve is incompetent, there is distention of gas-filled loops of both colon and small bowel, which may simulate an adynamic ileus.

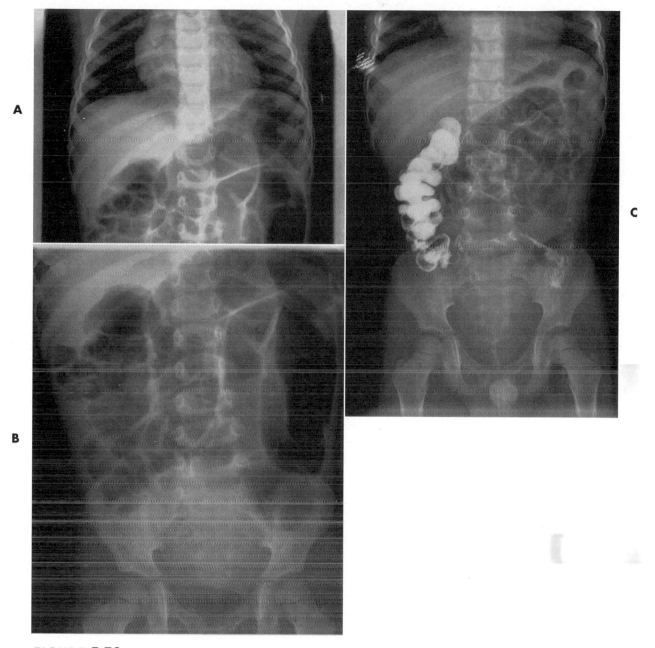

FIGURE 5-76 Abdominal images, **A** (upper) and **B** (lower), on a 4-year-old illustrate a gas pattern indicating a large bowel obstruction. A low pressure barium enema was performed to relieve the obstruction as seen on the post evac. **C,** As barium is seen in the cecum.

The major danger in colonic obstruction is perforation. If the ileocecal valve is competent, the colon behaves like a closed loop, and the increased pressure caused by the obstruction cannot be relieved. Because the cecum is spherical and has a large diameter, it is the most likely site for perforation. In acute colonic obstruction, perforation is very likely if the cecum distends to more than 10 cm; in intermittent or chronic obstruction, however, the cecal wall can become hypertrophied, and the diameter of the cecum can greatly exceed 10 cm without perforation (see Figure 5-75). In the patient with suspected large bowel obstruction, a low-pressure barium enema can be safely performed (Figure 5-76) and will demonstrate the site and often the cause of the obstruction (Figure 5-77).

Some professionals recommend an abdominal/pelvic CT scan as an initial examination, especially for patients without a surgical history who have symptomatic signs suggesting infection, bowel infarction,

SUMMARY of FINDINGS for the Colon

disorder	location	radiographic appearance	treatment
Appendicitis	Appendix	KUB—appendicolith US—noncompressible 7 mm or more outer diameter CT—round or oval mass, possibly containing gas; dilated lumen with thickened circumferentially enhancing wall	Appendectomy should be performed before perforation
Diverticulosis	Most common in sigmoid	Round or oval out-pouching projecting beyond lumen; usually multiple	Noninvasive: —Dietary modifications and exercise —Antibiotics for diverticulitis Invasive: —Surgery for perforated diverticula
Diverticulitis	Inflammation of diverticula	Diverticular perforation with possible abscess US—hypoechoic projection surrounded by inflamed fat CT—nonspecific wall thickening with a narrowed bowel lumen	
Ulcerative colitis	Superficial and acute; beginning in rectosigmoid area with continuous involvement throughout colon	KUB—deep ulcers with intraluminal gas or polypoid changes, loss of haustral markings BE (double contrast)—fine granularity of mucosa; submucosa with broad-based ulcers have a collar-button appearance	Nutritional supplements Dietary modifications (to decrease bulk) Antiinflammatory drugs Surgical resection for severe ulcerative colitis
Crohn's disease	Terminal ileum and proximal colon most often	BE (double contrast)—patchy distribution, noncontiguous segments (skip lesions) CT—colonic wall thickening and abscess formation	Nutritional supplements Dietary modifications (to decrease bulk) Antiinflammatory drugs
Ischemic colitis	Entire colon	Fine superficial ulceration Characteristic "thumbprinting" Tubular narrowing and a smooth stricture	Many cases resolve spontaneously Restrict vasoconstrictor drugs and give supportive care Immediate surgery for infarctions and complications
Irritable bowel syndrome	Alteration of intestinal motility	No specific findings Rule out other disorders	No cure exists; treatments aid in alleviating the symptoms Identify and avoid trigger foods to reduce pain Alternative therapies: relaxation, meditation to reduce stress
Cancer	50% in rectum and sigmoid region	Sessile lesion: irregular, lobulated surface Larger than 2 cm: "apple-core" or "napkin-ring" appearance CT • Circumferential bowel wall thickening, metastasis, lymphadenopathy • Virtual colonoscopy demonstrates 8-10 mm lesions US—transrectal; depth of tumor invasion into bowel wall PET—detection of distant nodular metastasis Fusion—PET/CT provides the most specific detail	Solitary lesion: surgical resection, with or without chemotherapy Multiple or distant lesions: chemotherapy and/or radiation therapy

SUMMARY of FINDINGS for the Colon—cont'd

disorder	location	radiographic appearance	treatment
Large bowel obstruction	Large bowel	Ileocecal valve competent: large dilated colon, thin-walled cecum, little small-bowel gas Ileocecal valve incompetent: gas-filled loops of colon and of small bowel	Surgical detorsion Water-soluble enema may be therapeutic
Volvulus	Cecal or sigmoid colon	Distended cecum, displaced upward and to the left Distended rectum, devoid of haustral markings, and a sausage or balloon shape Bird's-beak appearance	
Hemorrhoids	Distal rectum	Single or multiple rectal filling defects simulating polyps	Nonsurgical—rubber-band ligations Surgical—circumferential mucosectomy

KUB, Kidney–ureter–bladder radiograph; *US*, ultrasound; *BE*, barium enema.

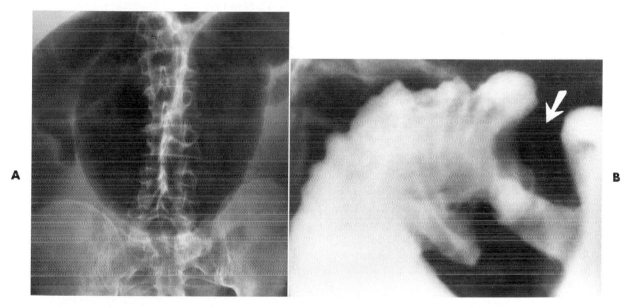

FIGURE 5-77 Large bowel obstruction caused by annular carcinoma of the sigmoid. **A,** Plain abdominal radiograph demonstrates pronounced dilatation of gas-filled transverse and ascending colon. **B,** Barium enema demonstrates typical apple-core lesion *(arrow)* producing the colonic obstruction.

or palpable mass. CT can demonstrate causes of an obstruction, such as diverticulitis or appendicitis.

Volvulus of the Colon

Volvulus refers to a twisting of the bowel on itself that may lead to intestinal obstruction. Because twisting of the bowel usually requires a long, movable mesentery, volvulus of the large bowel most frequently involves the cecum and sigmoid colon. The transverse colon, which has a short mesentery, is rarely affected by volvulus. A sigmoid volvulus, more commonly

found in the elderly, results from a bulky high-residue diet causing constipation.

Cecal Volvulus

The ascending colon and the cecum may have a long mesentery as a fault of rotation and fixation during the embryonic development of the gut. This situation predisposes to volvulus, with the cecum twisting on its long axis. It should be stressed, however, that only a few patients with an extremely mobile cecum ever develop cecal volvulus.

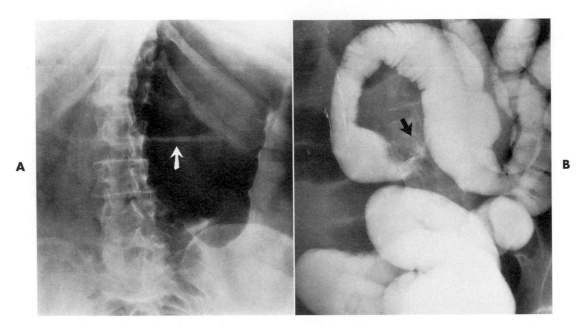

FIGURE 5-78 Cecal volvulus. **A,** Dilated, gas-filled cecum appears as a kidney-shaped mass with twisted and thickening mesentery *(arrow)* mimicking the renal pelvis. **B,** Barium enema examination demonstrates obstruction of the contrast column at the level of stenosis *(arrow);* tapered edge of column points toward the torsion site.

Radiographic Appearance

In cecal volvulus, the distended cecum tends to be displaced upward and to the left, although it can be found anywhere within the abdomen. A pathognomonic sign of cecal volvulus is a kidney-shaped mass (representing the twisted cecum) with the twisted and thickening mesentery mimicking the renal pelvis (Figure 5-78, *A*). A barium enema examination is usually required for definite confirmation of the diagnosis. This study demonstrates obstruction of the contrast column at the level of the stenosis, with the tapered edge of the column pointing toward the site of the twist (Figure 5-78, *B*).

Sigmoid Volvulus

A long, redundant loop of sigmoid colon can undergo a twist on its mesenteric axis and form a closed-loop obstruction. In sigmoid volvulus, the greatly inflated sigmoid loop appears as an inverted U-shaped shadow that rises out of the pelvis in a vertical or oblique direction and can even reach the level of the diaphragm. The affected loop appears devoid of haustral markings and has a sausage or balloon shape.

Radiographic Appearance

A barium enema examination demonstrates an obstruction to the flow of contrast material at the site of volvulus and considerable distention of the rectum. The lumen of the sigmoid tapers toward the site of stenosis, and a pathognomonic bird's-beak appearance is produced (Figure 5-79).

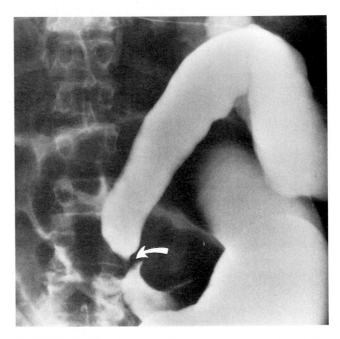

FIGURE 5-79 Sigmoid volvulus. Luminal tapering at site of stenosis produces characteristic bird's-beak configuration.

Treatment for Large Bowel Obstruction or Volvulus

Surgical detorsion is usually required, although a water-soluble enema may be therapeutic and resolve the obstruction.

Hemorrhoids

Hemorrhoids are varicose veins of the lower end of the rectum that cause pain, itching, and bleeding. Like varicose veins in the leg, hemorrhoids are caused by increased venous pressure. The most common cause of increased pressure is chronic constipation with resulting excessive muscular straining needed to empty the bowel. Increased venous pressure can also be produced by a pelvic tumor or a pregnant uterus.

Radiographic Appearance

On barium enema examinations, hemorrhoids occasionally can produce single or multiple rectal filling defects that simulate polyps (Figure 5-80). The proper diagnosis can easily be made by inspection, digital examination, or direct vision through the anoscope.

Treatment

Hemorrhoids may be treated nonsurgically and surgically. The nonsurgical approach consists of rubber band ligation. The surgical intervention consists of circumferential mucosectomy, which is a stapled hemorrhoidectomy, a safe and effective procedure for advanced stages (third- and fourth-degree hemorrhoidal prolapse).

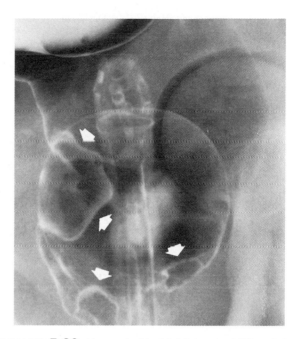

FIGURE 5-80 Hemorrhoids. Multiple rectal filling defects *(arrows)* simulate polyps.

Gallbladder

Gallstones (Cholelithiasis)

Gallstones consist of two major types: cholesterol stones and pigment stones. Cholesterol stones are predominant (75%) in the United States, whereas pigment stones occur more frequently in the tropics and the Orient. Genetic predispositions associated with higher incidence include family history of the disorder, age over 40 years, excess weight, and female sex. Gallstones can develop whenever bile contains insufficient bile salts and lecithin in proportion to cholesterol to maintain the cholesterol in solution. This situation can result from a decrease in the amount of bile salts present (because of decreased reabsorption in the terminal ileum as a result of inflammatory disease or surgical resection), or it can be caused by increased hepatic synthesis of cholesterol.

Radiographic Appearance

Because cholesterol is not radiopaque, most gallstones are radiolucent and visible only on contrast examinations or ultrasound. In up to 20% of patients, however, gallstones contain sufficient calcium to be detectable on plain abdominal radiographs (Figure 5-81). Gallstones can have a central nidus (or focus) of calcification, a laminated appearance (with

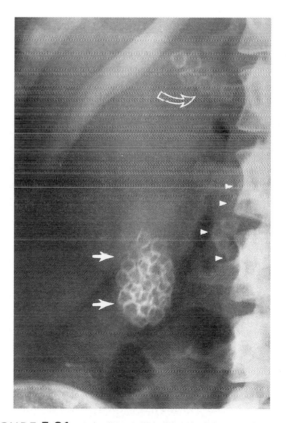

FIGURE 5-81 Calculi in gallbladder *(solid arrows)* and bile ducts *(open arrow)*. Calculi *(arrowheads)* lie in common bile duct, some of which overlie spine and are difficult to detect.

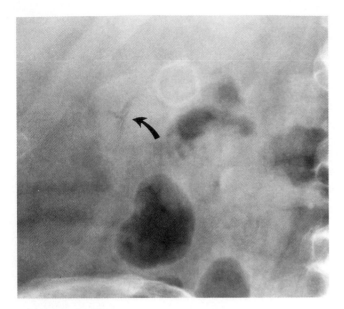

FIGURE 5-82 Mercedes-Benz sign of fissuring in gallstone *(arrow)*. Note adjacent gallstone with radiopaque rim.

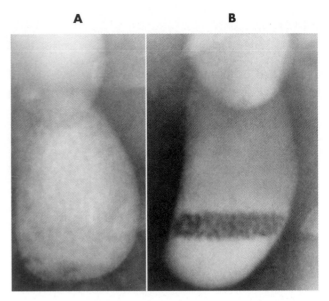

FIGURE 5-83 Oral cholecystogram showing multiple gallstones. **A,** With the patient supine, the stones are poorly defined and have a gravel-like consistency. **B,** On an erect film taken with a horizontal beam, the innumerable gallstones layer out and are easily seen.

alternating opaque and lucent rings), or calcification around the periphery. Occasionally a nonopaque stone may contain gas-filled fissures that produce the Mercedes-Benz sign, a characteristic triradiate pattern similar to the German automobile trademark (Figure 5-82).

Oral cholecystography (OCG) was the traditional technique for the diagnosis of gallstones. It is rarely used today as it has been replaced in most institutions by ultrasound (see later). Gallstones appear as freely movable filling defects in the opacified gallbladder. They fall by gravity to the dependent portion of the gallbladder and frequently layer out at a level that depends on the relationship of the specific gravity of the stone to that of the surrounding bile (Figure 5-83). Solitary gallstones are usually rounded; multiple stones are generally faceted. Large numbers of stones can have a sandlike or gravel-like consistency and be visible only when they layer out on radiographs obtained using a horizontal beam and with the patient in an erect or lateral decubitus position. Infrequently a gallstone is coated with tenacious mucus and adheres to the gallbladder wall.

Malabsorption of the radiopaque contrast material, hepatocellular dysfunction (serum bilirubin ≥2 mg/dl), and intrinsic disease of the gallbladder (cystic duct obstruction, chronic cholecystitis) can lead to nonvisualization of the gallbladder on OCG. If these causes can be excluded, failure of the gallbladder to opacify after the administration of two doses of orally administered cholecystographic contrast material is highly reliable evidence of gallbladder disease.

Ultrasound is now the imaging modality of choice for demonstrating gallstones. This noninvasive technique is as accurate as OCG, is independent of hepatic function, and does not rely on patient compliance in taking oral contrast agents. In addition to imaging the gallbladder, ultrasound can provide important additional information by effectively demonstrating the biliary tree and hepatic parenchyma. Gallstones appear on ultrasound as foci of high-amplitude echoes associated with posterior acoustic shadowing (Figure 5-84). The mobility of free-floating gallstones may be demonstrated by performing the examination with the patient in various positions.

Acute Cholecystitis

Acute cholecystitis (inflammation of the gallbladder) usually (in 95% of cases) occurs after obstruction of the cystic duct by an impacted gallstone. Gallstones may injure the mucosal wall, allowing bacteria to enter.

Radiographic Appearance

Either ultrasound or radionuclide scanning can be used. The sonographic diagnosis of acute cholecystitis requires the demonstration of a distended gallbladder containing gallstones. Important additional findings include edema of the gallbladder wall and focal tenderness elicited directly over the gallbladder.

SUMMARY *of* FINDINGS *for* the Gallbladder

disorder	location	radiographic appearance	treatment
Gallstones	Gallbladder and biliary tree	KUB—cholelithiasis evident if calcified US—foci of high-amplitude echoes associated with acoustic shadowing	Asymptomatic—no treatment Noninvasive: lithotripsy; chemical dissolution Invasive: ERCP for stone retrieval; laparoscopic cholecystectomy
Acute cholecystitis	Gallbladder and biliary tree	US—demonstrates distended gallbladder containing gallstones and possibly edema of the gallbladder wall NM cholescintigram—failure to accumulate radioactivity after 4 hr MR cholangiopancreatography—demonstrates the cystic duct and obstructing calculi located in gallbladder neck	
Emphysematous cholecystitis	Gallbladder	KUB—demonstrates gas in the gallbladder lumen that dissects into the wall to produce appearance of a rim of lucent bubbles or streaks of gas outside of and roughly parallel to the gallbladder lumen	
Porcelain gallbladder	Extensive calcification in the wall	Broad continuous band of calcification in the muscular layers, or multiple and punctate calcifications in the glandular spaces of mucosa	Prophylactic cholecystectomy

KUB, Kidney–ureter–bladder radiograph; *ERCP,* endoscopic retrograde cholangiopancreatography; *US,* ultrasound; *NM,* nuclear medicine.

A normal gallbladder ultrasound image virtually excludes the diagnosis of acute cholecystitis. Because many disorders may mimic acute cholecystitis, ultrasound can also be used to evaluate the remainder of the right upper quadrant to detect any other acute abnormality.

When the results of a radionuclide cholescintigram are normal, they demonstrate the bile ducts, the gallbladder, and early excretion of radionuclide into the duodenum and proximal jejunum within 30 minutes after the IV injection of the radionuclide (technetium-99m) (Figure 5-85). Failure to accumulate radioactivity (after 4 hours) in the gallbladder is highly sensitive (98%) and specific for cystic duct obstruction. If associated with appropriate symptoms, this finding is virtually diagnostic of acute cholecystitis.

When ultrasound is inconclusive, MR cholangiopancreatography can demonstrate the cystic duct and any obstructing calculi located in the gallbladder neck. MR does not, however, evaluate the gallbladder wall thickness as well as ultrasound.

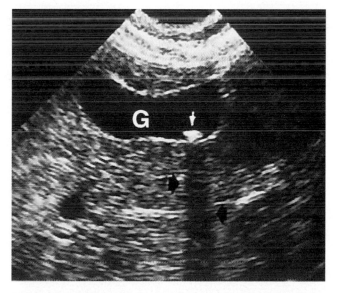

FIGURE 5-84 Ultrasound scan of gallstones. Echogenic focus *(white arrow)* in otherwise sonolucent gallbladder *(G)* represents large gallstone. Notice acoustic shadowing immediately inferior to the stone *(black arrows).*

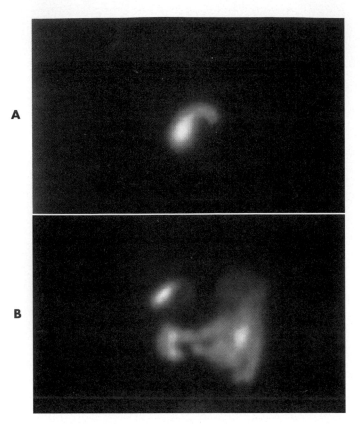

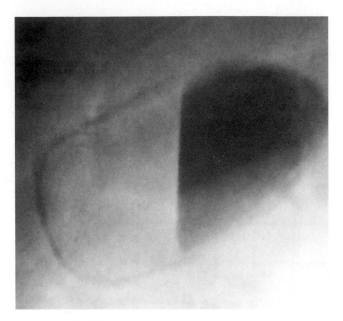

FIGURE 5-86 Emphysematous cholecystitis. Gas is found in both lumen and wall of gallbladder.

FIGURE 5-85 Acute cholecystitis. **A,** Radionuclide hepatobiliary study using technetium-99m Hepatolite in a 51-year-old woman with right upper quadrant pain demonstrates an engorged gallbladder at 1 hour after injection. **B,** At 28 minutes after injection of cholecystokinin (CCK), the gallbladder empties into the small bowel with an ejection fraction of 83%, which is normal.

Emphysematous Cholecystitis

Emphysematous cholecystitis is a rare condition in which the growth of gas-forming organisms in the gallbladder is facilitated by stasis and ischemia caused by cystic duct obstruction (most often by stones). Emphysematous cholecystitis occurs most frequently in elderly men and in patients with poorly controlled diabetes mellitus.

Radiographic Appearance

Plain abdominal radiographs demonstrate gas in the gallbladder lumen that dissects into the wall or pericholecystic tissues. This produces the pathognomonic appearance of a rim of lucent bubbles or streaks of gas outside of and roughly parallel to the gallbladder lumen (Figure 5-86).

Treatment for Cholecystitis

No treatment is necessary for asymptomatic patients. For acute impaction and biliary colic, prompt treatment using an antispasmodic and an analgesic helps

alleviate symptoms. Interventional treatments available today include extracorporeal shock wave therapy (lithotripsy), stone removal by endoscopic retrograde cholangiopancreatography (ERCP), and chemical dissolution. The most common surgical approach used currently is the laparoscopic cholecystectomy. The radiographer may be requested to obtain images during operative cholangiography to determine ductal blockage and identify remaining stones. Imaging must be performed at the appropriate medium-to-low kVp (70 to 80) at the completion of contrast injection. The contrast agent should be free of air bubbles because this artifact simulates stones.

Porcelain Gallbladder

Porcelain gallbladder refers to extensive calcification in the wall of the gallbladder, which forms an oval density that corresponds to the size and shape of the organ (Figure 5-87). Because chronic cholecystitis produces a loss of wall function, the gallbladder becomes fibrotic and calcified. The term reflects the blue discoloration and brittle consistency of the gallbladder wall.

Radiographic Appearance

The calcification in a porcelain gallbladder can appear as a broad continuous band in the muscular layers, or it may be multiple and punctate and occur in the glandular spaces of the mucosa.

The detection of extensive calcification in the wall of the gallbladder should indicate the possibility of

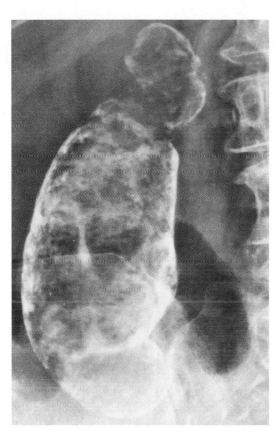

FIGURE 5-87 Porcelain gallbladder. Note extensive mural calcification around perimeter of gallbladder.

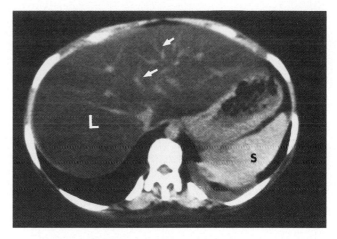

FIGURE 5-88 Fatty infiltration of the liver in cirrhosis. CT scan shows generalized decrease in attenuation value of liver *(I)*, which is far less than that of spleen *(S)*. Portal veins appear as high-density structures *(arrows)* surrounded by a background of low-density hepatic fat.

carcinoma. Although a porcelain gallbladder is uncommon in cases of carcinoma of the gallbladder, there is a striking incidence of carcinoma in patients with porcelain gallbladder (up to 60% of the cases).

Treatment

Because of this high incidence, patients with porcelain gallbladder are usually subjected to prophylactic cholecystectomy even if they are asymptomatic.

Liver

Cirrhosis of the Liver

Cirrhosis refers to the chronic destruction of liver cells and structure, with nodular regeneration of liver parenchyma and fibrosis; it is an end-stage liver disease. The major cause of cirrhosis is chronic alcoholism (i.e., 10 to 20 years of alcohol abuse), in which damage to the liver is related either to the toxic effect of alcohol or to the malnutrition that frequently accompanies chronic alcoholism. Other causes of liver destruction leading to cirrhosis include postnecrotic viral hepatitis, hepatotoxic drugs and chemicals that destroy liver cells, disease of the bile ducts (primary and

secondary biliary cirrhosis), and excessive deposition of iron pigment within the liver (hemochromatosis).

Regardless of the cause, fibrous connective tissue replaces the destroyed liver cells with cells that have no liver cell function. Initially the liver enlarges because of regeneration, but it eventually becomes smaller as the fibrous connective tissue contracts, and the surface becomes bumpy and nodular.

Radiographic Appearance

Cirrhosis causes many physiologic changes that can be detected clinically or radiographically. In alcoholic cirrhosis, a large amount of fat accumulates within the liver. This fatty infiltration is beautifully demonstrated on CT. In normal individuals, the liver always appears brighter than the spleen, whereas in patients with cirrhosis the liver is much darker because of the large amount of fat (Figure 5-88). The portal veins appear as high-density structures surrounded by a background of low density caused by hepatic fat; this is the opposite of the normal pattern of portal veins, which are low-density channels on noncontrast scans. Ultrasound images of the liver demonstrate coarse echogenicity, which results from diffuse liver disease. Multiple hyperechoic micronodules (0.1 to 1 cm) or macronodules (varying up to 5 cm) cause a nodular surface pattern.

Nodular regeneration of the liver combined with fibrosis causes obstruction of the portal vein, which drains blood from the gastrointestinal tract through the liver before emptying into the inferior vena cava near the heart. Increased pressure within this vessel causes pronounced enlargement of the spleen (splenomegaly). Because blood cannot flow through the obstructed portal vein, it must find an alternative route to bypass the liver. This leads to the development of collateral circulation, with large dilated veins becoming prominent on the abdominal wall in the area of the umbilicus. Another alternative route for blood to take in its return to the heart is the periesophageal veins, which dilate to become esophageal varices, which then can rupture and result in fatal hemorrhage (see Figure 5-17). Destruction of liver cells substantially decreases the ability of the organ to synthesize proteins, such as albumin and several of the factors required for blood clotting. A deficiency of albumin (hypoalbuminemia) results in fluid leaking out of the circulation and the development of generalized edema, which is evidenced by swelling of the lower extremities. When edema involves the wall of the intestinal tract, it can produce regular, uniform thickening of small bowel folds.

One of the most characteristic symptoms of cirrhosis is the accumulation of fluid in the peritoneal cavity (ascites), which causes characteristic abdominal distention. The abdomen is tight and quite hard, and an increase in exposure factors is required if a large amount of fluid has accumulated. Ascites develops because of a combination of albumin deficiency and increased pressure within obstructed veins, which permits fluid to leak into the abdominal cavity. Large amounts of ascitic fluid are easily detectable on plain abdominal radiographs as a general abdominal haziness (ground-glass appearance) (Figure 5-89, *A*). With the patient in a supine position, the peritoneal fluid tends to gravitate to dependent portions of the pelvis and accumulate within the pelvic peritoneal reflections, thus filling the recesses on both sides of the bladder and producing a symmetric density resembling a dog's ears. Smaller amounts of fluid (300 to 1000 ml) may widen the flank stripe and obliterate the right lateral inferior margin of the liver (the hepatic angle). Ascites is exquisitely shown on ultrasound as a mobile, echo-free fluid region shaped by adjacent structures (Figure 5-89, *B*), or on CT as an extravisceral collection of fluid with a low attenuation value (Figure 5-89, *C*).

Cirrhosis may lead to the development of jaundice, either from destruction of liver cells or from obstruction of bile ducts. Because the liver cannot perform its usual task of inactivating the small amounts of female sex hormones secreted by the adrenal glands in both men and women, men with cirrhosis often develop breast enlargement (gynecomastia). The inability of necrotic liver cells to detoxify harmful substances leads to an accumulation of ammonia and other poisonous material in the circulation. The patient becomes confused and disoriented, develops a typical flapping tremor or shaking, becomes abnormally sleepy (exhibits somnolence), and may lapse into a potentially fatal hepatic coma. Ascites occurs in advance stages of cirrhosis; of those afflicted, only 20% survive 5 years.

Treatment
The damage caused by cirrhosis is irreversible and incurable except by liver transplant. Most patients without a liver transplant die within 15 years of diagnosis. The patient may control the process by choosing a nutritional diet that decreases the metabolic load on the liver, stopping alcohol consumption, resting, and managing the complications of liver failure.

Hepatocellular Carcinoma
In the United States, primary liver cell carcinoma most commonly occurs in patients with underlying diffuse hepatocellular disease, especially alcoholic or postnecrotic cirrhosis. The clinical presentation varies from mild right upper quadrant discomfort and weight loss, to hemorrhagic shock from massive intraperitoneal bleeding, which reflects rupture of the tumor into the peritoneal cavity. Invasion of the biliary tree may produce obstructive jaundice.

Radiographic Appearance
CT is the modality of choice in the diagnosis of hepatocellular carcinoma. The tumor appears as a large mass, with an attenuation value close to that of normal parenchyma, that tends to alter the contour of the liver by projecting beyond its outer margin (Figure 5-90). After the rapid administration of IV contrast material, there is usually dense, diffuse, and nonuniform enhancement of the tumor. Unlike metastases, hepatocellular carcinoma tends to be a solitary mass or to produce a small number of lesions (thus appearing multinodular). Hepatocellular carcinoma tends to invade the hepatic and portal venous systems, and tumor thrombi within these veins are well demonstrated on CT.

Currently a three-phase contrast helical study is performed to image the arterial phase, the portal circulation, and the contrast-staining tumor in the venous or excretory phase (Figure 5-91). Sonography is used to screen chronic hepatitis B virus carriers. With the use of microbubble contrast agents, Doppler ultrasound demonstrates lesion vascularity using phasing techniques similar to those used in CT. MRI may permit a specific diagnosis by demonstrating (during the arterial phase, after gadolinium injection) a characteristic capsule of compressed liver tissue, an accumulation of fat within the tumor, and the propensity of the tumor to spread into the hepatic and portal venous system.

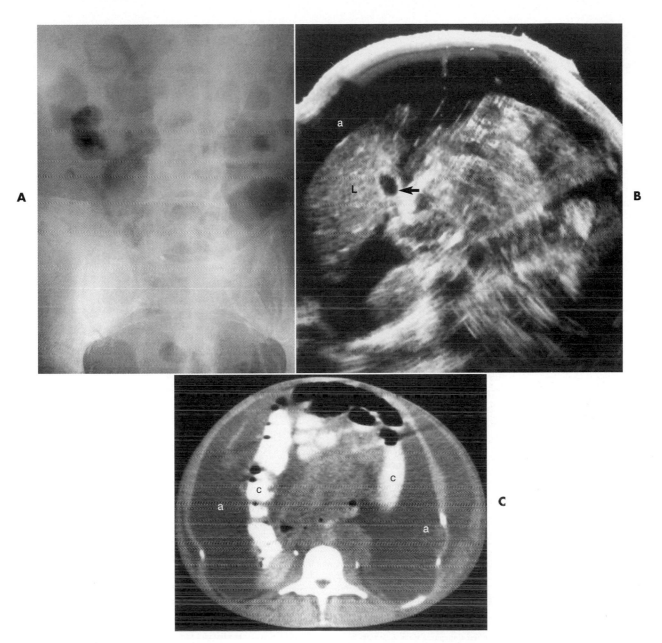

FIGURE 5-89 Ascites. **A,** Plain radiograph shows general abdominal haziness (ground-glass appearance). **B,** On an ultrasound image, a large amount of sonolucent ascitic fluid *(a)* separates liver *(L)* and other soft tissue structures from the anterior abdominal wall. Note the relative thickness of the gallbladder wall *(arrow)*. **C,** CT scan through the lower abdomen shows a huge amount of low-density ascitic fluid *(a)* with medial displacement of ascending and descending colon *(c)*.

Treatment

Although the overall prognosis for patients with hepatocellular carcinoma remains bleak, radiographic studies can determine whether the tumor can be successfully removed surgically. If the tumor is confined to one lobe of the liver and there is no evidence of metastases, arteriography is usually indicated to demonstrate the precise surgical anatomy and to detect small, staining tumor nodules that cannot be identified with noninvasive imaging techniques. Surgery and chemotherapy are the treatments of choice. Metastases occur late and are usually not the cause of death. A common cause of death is catastrophic bleeding into the peritoneal cavity from hepatic failure or esophageal varices.

Hepatic Metastases

Metastases are by far the most common malignant tumors involving the liver. Although some types of metastases (especially mucinous carcinoma of the colon or rectum) may produce diffuse, finely granular

SUMMARY of FINDINGS for the Liver

disorder	location	radiographic appearance	treatment
Cirrhosis	Liver cells and structure	KUB—haziness in ascites US—coarse echogenicity, multiple nodules of varying size and a nodular liver surface CT—fatty infiltration in liver, portal vein involvement/ obstruction, ascites, extravisceral fluid collection	Dietary modifications Stop alcohol consumption Irreversible—curable only by liver transplant
Hepatocellular carcinoma	Previously injured liver cells are most susceptible	CT—diffuse infiltrate, solitary multinodular mass	Poor prognosis Surgery and chemotherapy are treatments of choice
Hepatic metastases	Liver	CT—increased density adjacent to normal parenchyma when IV contrast administered MRI—low signal intensity on T1-weighted, high signal intensity on T2-weighted images	Terminal Treatment palliative only

KUB, Kidney–ureter–bladder radiograph; *US,* ultrasound.

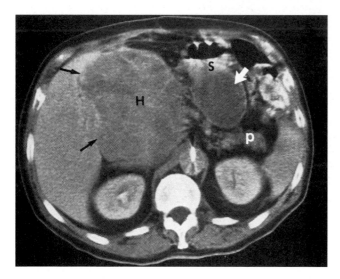

FIGURE 5-90 Hepatocellular carcinoma. CT scan shows huge mass *(H)* with attenuation value slightly less than that of normal liver. Black arrows point to interface between tumor and normal liver. Incidentally noted is a pancreatic pseudocyst *(white arrow)* in the lesser sac between stomach *(S)* and pancreas *(p).*

calcifications that can be seen on plain radiographs, the diagnosis of hepatic metastases usually requires CT, ultrasound, MRI, or radionuclide studies.

Radiographic Appearance

CT and MRI are probably the most sensitive techniques for detecting hepatic metastases. On CT, most metastases are relatively well marginated and appear less dense than normal liver parenchyma (Figure 5-92, *A*). Although frequently detectable on noncontrast scans, most metastatic lesions are best seen as areas of increased density adjacent to normally enhancing hepatic parenchyma after the administration of IV contrast material. CT-guided fine-needle aspiration biopsy can be used to obtain cells that can be studied for a definitive diagnosis. MRI demonstrates liver metastases as areas of low signal intensity on T1-weighted sequences and bright lesions on T2-weighted sequences. This modality is especially important for patients who cannot receive IV iodinated contrast agents.

Ultrasound (Figure 5-92, *B*) and radionuclide scans can demonstrate hepatic metastases, but these modalities are slightly less sensitive than CT. CT has the additional advantage of being able to detect extrahepatic metastases, such as those to abdominal lymph nodes.

Treatment

Once diagnosed with hepatic metastases, most patients face imminent death (within months).

Pancreas

Acute Pancreatitis

Acute **pancreatitis** is an inflammatory process in which protein- and lipid-digesting enzymes become activated within the pancreas and begin to digest the organ itself. Occasionally, this necrotic

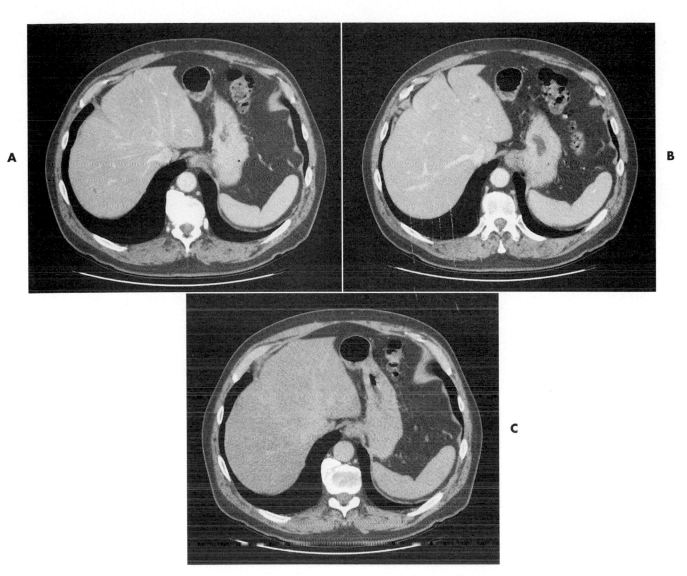

FIGURE 5-91 Three-phase CT imaging of the normal liver. **A,** Hepatic arteries. The bolus of contrast material is in the abdominal aorta. **B,** The inferior vena cava and the portal system are visible. **C,** The liver parenchyma is homogeneous, which indicates a normal study.

process extends into blood vessels, causing bleeding (acute hemorrhagic pancreatitis), which may be life threatening.

The most common cause of acute pancreatitis is excessive alcohol consumption. Less frequently, acute pancreatitis is related to gallstones, which may enter the common bile duct and obstruct the ampulla of Vater, forcing bile to reflux into the pancreas and causing an inflammatory reaction.

The first symptoms of acute pancreatitis usually include the sudden onset of severe, steady abdominal pain that radiates to the back; this may indicate a perforated ulcer. Nausea and vomiting are common, and jaundice may develop if inflammatory edema of the head of the pancreas sufficiently obstructs the common bile duct. If a large area of the pancreas is affected, the absence of lipid enzymes from the pancreas prevents the proper absorption of fat, leading to the malabsorption syndrome. Blood tests and urinalysis typically show a high level of the pancreatic enzyme amylase, which confirms the diagnosis of acute pancreatitis.

Radiographic Appearance

The findings on plain abdominal radiographs are often normal in the patient with acute pancreatitis; even when abnormal, they are usually nonspecific and consistent with any intraabdominal inflammatory disease. The most common abnormalities include a localized adynamic ileus, usually involving the jejunum (the "sentinel loop"); generalized ileus with diffuse gas-fluid levels; isolated distention of the duodenal sweep (C-loop); and localized distention

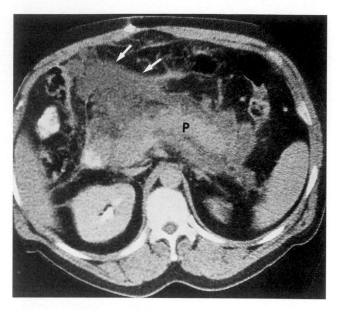

FIGURE 5-93 Acute pancreatitis. CT scan demonstrates diffuse enlargement of the pancreas *(P)* with obliteration of peripancreatic fat planes by an inflammatory process. Extension of the inflammatory reaction into the transverse mesocolon *(arrows)* is shown.

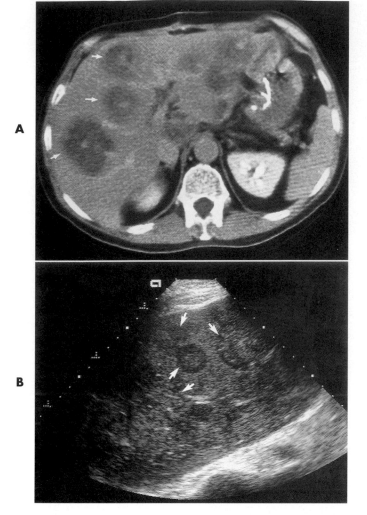

FIGURE 5-92 Hepatic metastases. **A,** CT scan shows multiple low-density metastases with high-density centers *(arrows)*. **B,** Ultrasound image of the liver demonstrates a diffuse, patchy, nodular appearance *(arrows)*.

of the transverse colon to the level of the left colonic flexure (the colon cutoff sign). Pancreatic calcifications indicate that the patient has chronic pancreatitis, and moreover they may indicate an exacerbation of the inflammatory disease.

Ultrasound and CT are the imaging modalities that most precisely define the degree of pancreatic inflammation and the pathways of its spread throughout the abdomen. They are also of great clinical importance in the early diagnosis of complications of acute pancreatitis, such as abscess, hemorrhage, and pseudocyst formation.

CT in acute pancreatitis demonstrates diffuse or focal enlargement of the gland. The margins of a normal pancreas are sharply delineated by surrounding peripancreatic fat. Spread of inflammation and edema beyond the confines of the pancreas obscures

the peripancreatic soft tissues and often thickens the surrounding fascial planes (Figure 5-93), which makes CT superior to ultrasound.

Acute pancreatitis may alter both the size and the parenchymal echogenicity of the gland on ultrasound examination. Although the pancreas usually enlarges symmetrically and retains its initial shape, nonspecific enlargement of the pancreatic head or tail can simulate focal pancreatic carcinoma. Gallstones causing pancreatitis can be demonstrated. The accompanying interstitial inflammatory edema causes the pancreas to appear relatively sonolucent when compared with the adjacent liver (Figure 5-94). One limitation of ultrasound in patients with acute pancreatitis is the frequent occurrence of adynamic ileus with excessive intestinal gas, which may prevent adequate visualization of the gland.

Chronic Pancreatitis

Chronic pancreatitis results when frequent intermittent injury to the pancreas causes increasing damage that produces scar tissue. Recurring episodes usually result from chronic alcohol abuse, which may cause the gland to lose its ability to produce digestive enzymes, insulin, and glucagon. Three symptoms that help identify chronic pancreatitis are pain, malabsorption causing weight loss (exocrine failure–digestive enzymes), and diabetes (endocrine failure–insulin and glucagon).

Radiographic Appearance

Pancreatic calcifications are a pathognomonic finding in chronic pancreatitis, developing in about one third of patients with this disease (Figure 5-95). The small, irregular calcifications are seen most frequently in the head of the pancreas and can extend upward and to the left to involve the body and tail of the organ.

On ultrasound examination, the major feature of chronic pancreatitis is an alteration of the intrinsic echo pattern caused by calcification and fibrosis (Figure 5-96). The pancreas may be atrophic as a result of fibrous scarring or appear significantly enlarged during recurrences of acute inflammation. Dilatation of the pancreatic duct as a result of gland atrophy and obstruction can be seen, although a similar pattern can be produced by the ductal obstruction in pancreatic cancer. CT can also demonstrate ductal dilatation, calcification, and atrophy of the gland in patients with chronic pancreatitis. However, since similar information can be obtained less expensively and without ionizing radiation by ultrasound, CT is usually reserved for patients with chronic pancreatitis in whom technical factors make ultrasound suboptimal.

Enlargement of the pancreatic head can cause widening and pressure changes on the inner aspect of the duodenal sweep on barium studies. This produces narrowing of the lumen (the double-contour effect) and spiny protrusions of mucosal folds (spiculation) that can be indistinguishable from those of pancreatic carcinoma.

Treatment of Acute and Chronic Pancreatitis

Most cases of acute pancreatitis require supportive treatment only (e.g., IV fluids, pain and nausea medications) because the pancreas will self-heal. If acute pancreatitis is caused by stone blockage, procedures to remove the stone (e.g., ERCP) or possibly surgery to remove the gallbladder should be done. In some cases, IV antibiotics are given to help reduce the inflammatory process and prevent infection.

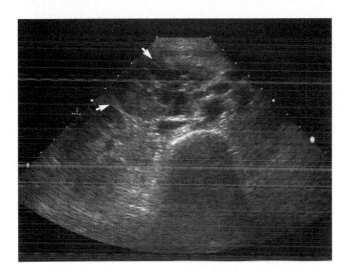

FIGURE 5-94 Acute pancreatitis. Transverse sonogram illustrates multiple hypoechoic areas in the head of the pancreas *(arrows)*, causing biliary tree dilation.

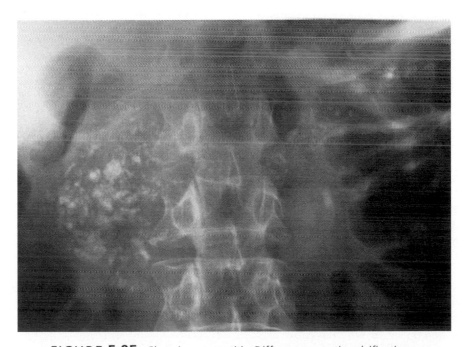

FIGURE 5-95 Chronic pancreatitis. Diffuse pancreatic calcifications.

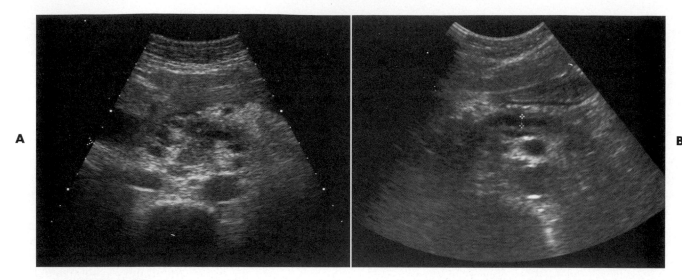

FIGURE 5-96 Chronic pancreatitis in a 40-year-old man with abdominal pain; he has a history of chronic alcoholism. **A,** In April, an ultrasound image shows the pancreas to be inhomogeneous with a patchy appearance. **B,** On the follow-up scan in May, the pancreatic ducts are considerably dilated *(cursors).*

In chronic pancreatitis, treatment is directed toward controlling pain and managing nutritional and metabolic problems. Consumption of alcohol must cease. Dietary changes reduce fat and protein intake; supplements containing pancreatic enzymes are taken to aid in digestion. If the blood sugar becomes uncontrolled, insulin is prescribed. Most patients who follow their prescribed treatment do well.

Pancreatic Pseudocyst

Pancreatic pseudocysts are loculated (walled-off) fluid collections arising from inflammation, necrosis, or hemorrhage associated with acute pancreatitis or trauma (Figure 5-97). When the infected or traumatized pancreas continues to release enzymes, pseudocysts are commonly formed. The pseudocyst has a shaggy lining surrounded by dense white scar tissue and may or may not connect with the pancreatic duct.

Radiographic Appearance

On ultrasound examination, a pseudocyst typically appears as an echo-free cystic structure with a sharp posterior wall (Figure 5-98). Hemorrhage into the pseudocyst produces a complex fluid collection containing septations of echogenic areas. CT demonstrates pseudocysts as sharply marginated, fluid-filled collections that are often best delineated after the administration of IV contrast material (Figure 5-99).

Large pseudocysts are visible on plain radiographs of the abdomen when they displace the gas-filled stomach and bowel. Similarly, pseudocysts in the head of the pancreas can cause pressure defects and widening of the duodenal sweep, whereas those arising from the body or tail of the pancreas can displace

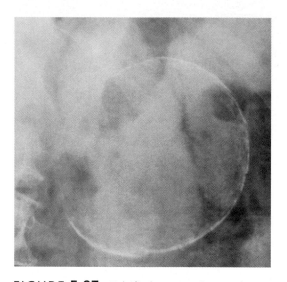

FIGURE 5-97 Calcified pancreatic pseudocyst.

and deform the stomach, proximal jejunum, or colon. However, because ultrasound is highly accurate in diagnosing pancreatic pseudocysts, it has completely replaced plain abdominal radiographs and barium studies, which display only indirect signs.

Treatment

Pseudocysts may undergo spontaneous resolution or persist as chronic collections that may require surgical intervention. Because ultrasound is relatively inexpensive and does not involve ionizing radiation, serial sonograms are usually used to monitor the progression of a pancreatic pseudocyst. Percutaneous drainage of a pseudocyst and endoscopic drainage of cysts extending into the stomach are interventional therapies used today.

Cancer of the Pancreas

The most common pancreatic malignancy is adenocarcinoma (90%), which often is far advanced and has metastasized before it is detected and thus has an extremely poor survival rate. Of these malignancies, 60% occur in the head of the pancreas. Less common pancreatic tumors include hormone-secreting neoplasms of the islet cells of the islets of Langerhans. Production of insulin by an **insulinoma** can lower blood glucose, leading to attacks of weakness, unconsciousness, and insulin shock. This tumor occurs most frequently in the tail and is usually benign. **Ulcerogenic islet cell tumors (gastrinomas—usually malignant)** produce the Zollinger-Ellison syndrome, which is characterized by intractable ulcer symptoms, hypersecretion of gastric acid, and diarrhea. **Diarrheogenic islet cell tumors** produce the WDHA syndrome; this acronym stands for watery diarrhea, hypokalemia (low serum potassium),

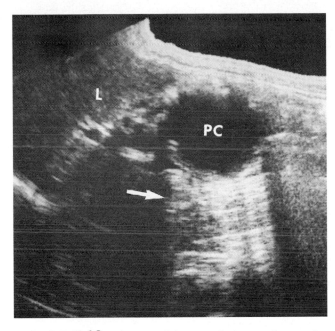

FIGURE 5-98 Ultrasound image of pancreatic pseudocyst. Longitudinal sonogram of right upper quadrant demonstrates irregularly marginated pseudocyst (PC) with acoustic shadowing (arrow). L, Liver.

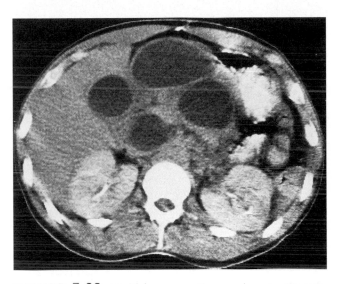

FIGURE 5-99 Multiple pancreatic pseudocysts. CT scan after IV administration of contrast material demonstrates four sharply marginated, fluid-filled collections.

SUMMARY FINDINGS for the Pancreas

disorder	location	radiographic appearance	treatment
Pancreatitis	Acute—pancreatic ducts	US—altered echogenicity CT—diffuse or focal enlargement	Supportive treatment IV antibiotics
	Chronic—pancreatic parenchyma	KUB—pancreatic calcifications US—intrinsic echo pattern, alteration by calcification and fibrosis CT—ductal dilatation, calcification, atrophy, and pseudocyst formation	Reduce fat/protein intake Pancreatic enzyme supplements Insulin for uncontrolled blood sugar levels
Pseudocyst	Cyst walled off from ductal system	US—echo-free cyst with sharp posterior wall CT—sharply marginated fluid-filled collection(s) best seen with IV contrast	Spontaneous resolution Drainage (percutaneous or endoscopic) Surgical correction
Cancer	Adenocarcinoma Head of pancreas in 60% of cases	US—tumor 2 cm or greater, irregular contour, and semi-solid pattern of intrinsic echoes CT (most effective)—tumor mass, ductal dilatation, and invasiveness	Survival, 2% Surgery Radiation therapy Chemotherapy Biologic therapy

US, Ultrasound.

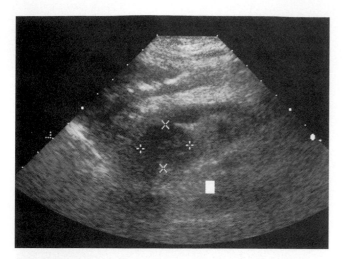

FIGURE 5-100 Pancreatic adenocarcinoma in a 66-year-old man with a 10-day history of painless jaundice and weight loss. Ultrasound image demonstrates a heterogeneous hypoechoic mass (dark area with measurements) in the pancreatic head and uncinate process; the mass is producing an obstruction of the pancreatic and common bile ducts.

and achlorhydria (low serum chloride), which are major features of the clinical picture. Adrenocorticotropic hormone (ACTH) production by pancreatic islet cell tumors causes Cushing's syndrome; the release of serotonin by pancreatic tumors may cause the carcinoid syndrome. Because these functional islet cell tumors usually become apparent by their hormonal effects rather than by the consequences of tumor bulk, they are often small and difficult to detect.

Radiographic Appearance
Because it is noninvasive and relatively inexpensive, ultrasound is often the initial screening modality for a patient with suspected pancreatic carcinoma. Ultrasound can demonstrate most tumors greater than 2 cm in diameter that lie in the head of the pancreas, but lesions in the body and tail of the pancreas are more difficult to detect. Pancreatic carcinoma typically causes the gland to have an irregular contour and a semisolid pattern of intrinsic echoes (Figure 5-100).

CT is the most effective modality for detecting pancreatic cancer in any portion of the gland and for defining its extent. CT can demonstrate the mass of the tumor, ductal dilatation, and invasion of neighboring structures. After the administration of IV contrast material, the relatively avascular tumor appears as an area of decreased attenuation when compared with the normal pancreas (Figure 5-101). CT is the best procedure for staging pancreatic carcinoma and may prevent needless surgery in patients with nonresectable lesions. This technique may permit detection of

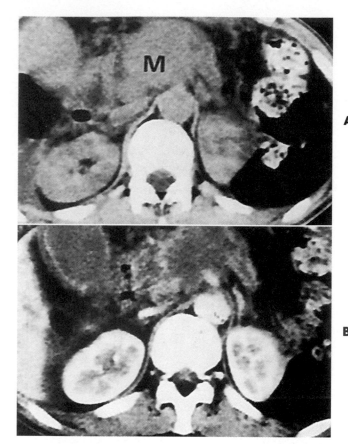

FIGURE 5-101 Carcinoma of the pancreas. **A,** Noncontrast CT scan demonstrates homogeneous mass *(M)* in the body of the pancreas. **B,** After IV injection of a bolus of contrast material, there is enhancement of the normal pancreatic parenchyma and the surrounding vascular structures. The pancreatic carcinoma remains unchanged and thus appears as a low-density mass.

hepatic metastases or involvement of regional vessels and adjacent retroperitoneal lymph nodes.

Cytologic examination of tissue obtained by percutaneous fine-needle aspiration under ultrasound or CT guidance can often provide the precise histologic diagnosis of a neoplastic mass, thus making surgical intervention unnecessary.

Carcinoma of the head of the pancreas often causes obstructive jaundice and the appearance of narrowing of the distal common bile duct on transhepatic cholangiography (Figure 5-102) or ERCP. Percutaneous biliary drainage may represent an alternative to surgical intervention for relieving biliary obstruction in patients with pancreatic carcinoma who cannot be cured. Although the transhepatic insertion of biliary drainage tubes does not alter the dismal prognosis, it can reduce patient morbidity and the need for hospitalization.

Barium upper gastrointestinal series demonstrate distortion of the mucosal pattern and configuration of the duodenal sweep in about half of patients with carcinoma of the head of the pancreas. Early or small lesions, however, rarely produce detectable radiographic abnormalities; tumors of the body or tail of the pancreas must be quite large to be visible on barium examinations.

Treatment

Finding pancreatic cancer in the earliest stages can result in a cure (2%, 5-year survival rate). In most cases, the diagnosis of the disease occurs after metastasis and most patients die within 12 to 24 months of diagnosis. Nevertheless, treatment can improve the quality of life. Surgical resection, radiation therapy, chemotherapy, and biologic therapy help alleviate the patient's symptoms.

Surgical resection (total pancreatectomy) includes the removal of the entire pancreas, duodenum, common bile duct, gallbladder, spleen, and surrounding lymph nodes. The Whipple procedure consists of removing only the head of the pancreas, the duodenum, a portion of the stomach, and other nearby tissue. If a distal pancreatectomy is performed, only the body and tail of the pancreas are removed. In most cases, the purpose of the surgery is to alleviate biliary and

small bowel obstruction. Surgery and chemotherapy are most effective for islet cell cancers.

Pneumoperitoneum

Free air in the peritoneal cavity associated with significant abdominal pain and tenderness is often caused by perforation of a gas-containing viscus and indicates a surgical emergency. Less frequently, pneumoperitoneum results from abdominal, gynecologic, intrathoracic, or iatrogenic causes and does not require operative intervention.

Radiographic Appearance

The radiographic demonstration of free air in the peritoneal cavity is a valuable sign in the diagnosis of perforation of the gastrointestinal tract. As little as 1 cc of free intraperitoneal gas can be identified. Free air is best demonstrated by examination of the patient in the upright position with a horizontal beam (Figure 5-103). Because the gas rises to the highest point in the peritoneal cavity, it accumulates beneath the domes of the diaphragm. Free intraperitoneal gas appears as a sickle-shaped lucency that is easiest to recognize on the right side between the diaphragm and the homogeneous density of the liver. On the left side, the normal gas and fluid shadows present in the fundus of the stomach can be confusing. The free air is shown to best advantage if the patient remains in an upright (or lateral decubitus) position for 10 minutes before a radiograph is obtained.

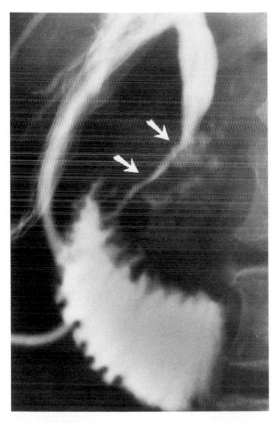

FIGURE 5-102 Carcinoma of the head of the pancreas. Transhepatic cholangiogram shows irregular narrowing of the common bile duct (arrows). Calcifications reflect underlying chronic pancreatitis.

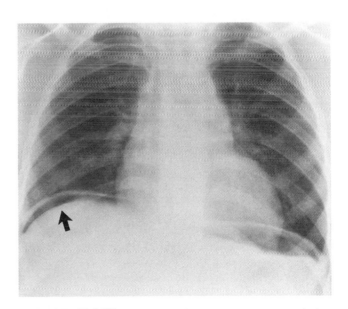

FIGURE 5-103 Pneumoperitoneum. Gas accumulating beneath dome of right hemidiaphragm (arrow) appears as a sickle-shaped lucency on this erect chest film obtained with a horizontal beam.

If the patient is too ill to sit or stand, a lateral decubitus view (preferably with the patient on the left side) can be used. In this position, free air moves to the right side and collects between the lateral margin of the liver and the abdominal wall (Figure 5-104). Some gas also collects in the right iliac fossa and, when large amounts are involved, can be seen along the flank down to the pelvis.

When the patient is in the supine position, free intraperitoneal gas accumulates between the intestinal loops and is much more difficult to demonstrate. However, a large quantity of gas can be diagnosed indirectly because the outer margins of the intestinal wall can be visualized (Figure 5-105). The demonstration of distinct inner and outer contours of the bowel wall is often the only sign of pneumoperitoneum in patients who are in such poor condition that they cannot be turned on their side or be examined upright.

In children, pneumoperitoneum can be manifest as a generalized greater-than-normal lucency of the entire abdomen. An important sign of pneumoperitoneum

on the supine radiograph is demonstration of the falciform ligament. This almost vertical, curvilinear, water-density shadow in the upper abdomen to the right of the spine is outlined only when there is gas on both sides of it, as in pneumoperitoneum (Figure 5-106).

The most common cause of pneumoperitoneum with associated inflammation is perforation of a peptic ulcer, either gastric or duodenal. Colonic perforations, especially those involving the cecum, give the most abundant quantities of free intraperitoneal gas. Septic infection of the peritoneal cavity by gas-forming organisms can result in the production of a substantial amount of gas and the radiographic appearance of pneumoperitoneum. Pneumoperitoneum can also develop after penetrating injuries of the abdominal wall and after blunt trauma causing rupture of a hollow viscus.

Iatrogenic pneumoperitoneum is generally asymptomatic and usually follows abdominal surgery. Postoperative pneumoperitoneum can be radiographically detectable for up to 3 weeks after surgery, but usually it can no longer be demonstrated after

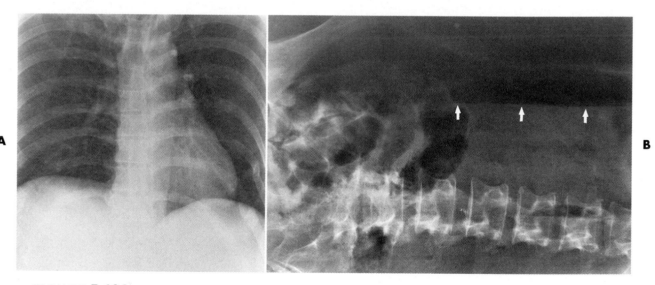

FIGURE 5-104 Pneumoperitoneum. **A,** Semierect projection obtained without a horizontal beam shows no evidence of free intraperitoneal gas beneath the domes of the diaphragm. **B,** On a lateral decubitus projection obtained with a horizontal beam on the same patient, free intraperitoneal gas is clearly seen collecting under the right side of the abdominal wall *(arrows).* Gas can even be seen extending down the flank to the region of the pelvis.

SUMMARY of FINDINGS for Pneumoperitoneum

disorder	location	radiographic appearance	treatment
Pneumoperitoneum	Abdominal cavity	Upright abdominal film (1st choice) shows 1 cc free intraperitoneal gas (air) under diaphragm Left lateral decubitus (2nd choice) shows air collection between lateral margin of liver and outer abdominal wall	Immediate surgery for visceral perforation, IV antibiotics

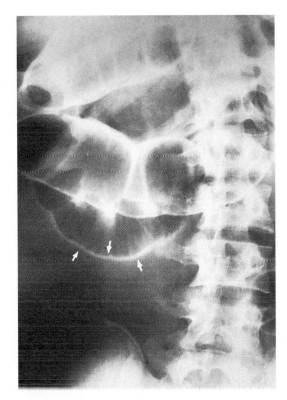

FIGURE 5-105 Double-wall sign of pneumoperitoneum demonstrated on supine projection. Large quantities of free intraperitoneal gas may be diagnosed indirectly because gas permits visualization of both inner and outer margins of the intestinal wall *(arrows)*.

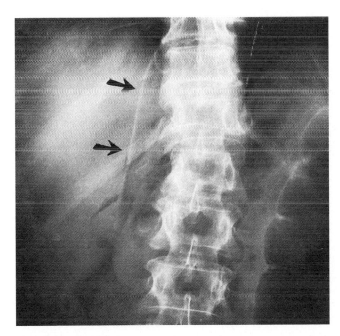

FIGURE 5-106 Falciform ligament sign of pneumoperitoneum. On supine projection, falciform ligament appears as a curvilinear water-density shadow *(arrows)* in the upper abdomen to the right of the spine. This finding implies that pneumoperitoneum with gas is on both sides of the ligament.

the first postoperative week. Rarely, free air in the peritoneal cavity may be the result of perforation during an endoscopic procedure.

Treatment

Immediate surgical repair of a perforation is required to reduce the risk of peritonitis and sepsis. IV antibiotics help control infection.

Spleen

Enlargement

Enlargement of the spleen (splenomegaly) is associated with numerous conditions, including infections (subacute bacterial endocarditis, tuberculosis, infectious mononucleosis, malaria), connective tissue disorders, neoplastic hematologic disorders (lymphoma, leukemia), hemolytic anemia and hemoglobinopathies, and portal hypertension (cirrhosis).

Radiographic Appearance

Plain abdominal radiographs can demonstrate the inferior border of the enlarged spleen well below the costal margin. An enlarged spleen can elevate the left hemidiaphragm, impress the greater curvature of the barium-filled stomach, and displace the entire stomach toward the midline. Splenomegaly can also cause downward displacement of the left kidney and the splenic flexure of the colon.

CT is of value when it is unclear whether a mass palpated in the left upper quadrant represents an enlarged spleen or a separate abdominal mass. When splenomegaly is present (Figure 5-107), CT findings

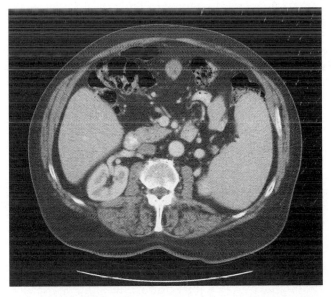

FIGURE 5-107 Splenomegaly. CT demonstrates a homogeneous and extremely enlarged spleen.

SUMMARY *of* FINDINGS *for* Splenic Disorders

disorder	location	radiographic appearance	treatment
Splenomegaly	Enlarged spleen	Abdominal film—elevated left diaphragm, stomach displacement CT—demonstrates tumor, abscess, or cyst causing splenomegaly	Treat cause Limited physical activity to prevent traumatic rupture
Splenic rupture	Fracture by trauma	CT—subcapsular hematoma appears as a crescentic fluid collection; splenic laceration appears as enlargement with an irregular splenic border	Aggressive treatment Embolization of splenic artery Laparoscopic splenectomy

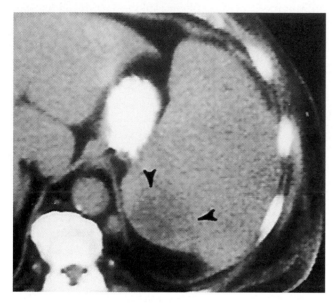

FIGURE 5-108 Lymphoma of spleen. CT scan shows focal low-attenuation lesion *(arrowheads)* posteriorly in this greatly enlarged spleen.

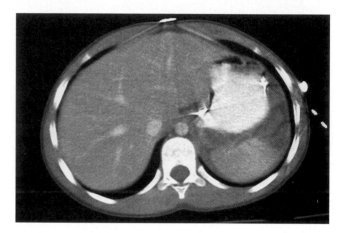

FIGURE 5-109 CT image from a patient who was ejected from a motor vehicle. Traumatic splenic rupture and hematoma are illustrated by decreased attenuation surrounding spleen.

may indicate the cause of the splenic enlargement by demonstrating a tumor (Figure 5-108), abscess, or cyst. Associated abdominal lymph node enlargement is suggestive of lymphoma; characteristic alterations in the size and shape of the liver and prominence of collateral venous structures in the splenic hilum indicate that splenomegaly may be a result of cirrhosis and portal hypertension.

Rupture

Rupture of the spleen is usually caused by trauma. Infrequently, it may be a complication of the palpation of a spleen enlarged by infection (especially infectious mononucleosis) or leukemia. In many patients suffering traumatic rupture of the spleen, the severity of clinical symptoms and the rapid loss of blood into the abdominal cavity require immediate surgery without radiographic investigation. However, in patients in whom bleeding stops temporarily or in whom there is slow bleeding over several days, radiographic studies may be of diagnostic value.

Radiographic Appearance

CT is the best imaging procedure for screening patients with blunt abdominal trauma for the presence of splenic injury. Indeed, its almost 100% sensitivity in detecting splenic injury has substantially decreased the need for abdominal arteriography and exploratory surgery. Subcapsular hematomas appear on CT as crescentic collections of fluid that flatten or indent the lateral margin of the spleen (Figure 5-109). Splenic lacerations, which may occur with or without an accompanying subcapsular hematoma, produce a CT appearance of splenic enlargement, an irregular cleft or defect in the splenic border, and free blood in the peritoneal cavity.

Before the advent of CT, splenic arteriography was the procedure of choice for demonstrating splenic rupture. Major positive findings include extravasation of contrast material into the splenic parenchyma, obstruction of a major splenic artery, and—in an enlarged spleen—vascular defects that indicate sites of rupture and hematoma.

Treatment of Splenic Disorders

Treatment depends on the causative factors. Very enlarged spleens have a higher incidence of rupture and thus the patient should limit physical activity to avoid trauma. In most cases, splenomegaly does well with conservative treatment. Aggressive treatment would include possible embolization of the splenic artery to stop the bleeding in a splenic rupture. Surgical procedures include laparoscopic splenectomy and distal pancreatectomy, if necessary.

REVIEW QUESTIONS

1. Visualization of which of the following structures indicates that the correct contrast scale has been used for a plain abdominal radiograph?
   I. Liver, kidneys, and psoas muscle shadows
   II. Lumbar spine and transverse processes
   III. Kidneys and psoas muscle shadows
   IV. Lumbar spine and psoas shadows
   A. both I and IV
   B. both I and II
   C. I only
   D. IV only

2. The rhythmic smooth muscle contractions found in the upper gastrointestinal system are called
   A. chyme
   B. digestion
   C. peristalsis
   D. mastication

3. The greatest amount of digestion occurs in which portion of the intestines?
   A. duodenum
   B. jejunum
   C. ileum
   D. colon

4. Detoxification of poisonous substances takes place in which organ?
   A. kidneys
   B. liver
   C. pancreas
   D. spleen

5. Which organ controls the level of glucose in the circulating blood?
   A. kidneys
   B. liver
   C. pancreas
   D. spleen

6. The telescoping of one part of the intestinal tract into another is termed _____.
   A. intussusception
   B. volvulus
   C. Crohn's disease
   D. ileus

7. Twisting of the bowel upon itself is termed

   _____.
   A. intussusception
   B. volvulus
   C. Crohn's disease
   D. ileus

8. What is now considered to be the major imaging modality for the demonstration of gallstones?
   A. OCG
   B. MRI
   C. CT
   D. ultrasound

9. What is the major cause of cirrhosis in the United States and Europe?
   A. hepatitis
   B. elevated cholesterol
   C. alcoholism
   D. cholecystitis

10. Rupture of the spleen as a result of blunt abdominal trauma can be best demonstrated by what imaging procedure?
    A. OCG
    B. MRI
    C. CT
    D. ultrasound

11. If a patient is too ill to stand, what projection can be used to demonstrate pneumoperitoneum?
    A. right lateral decubitus, patient on left side
    B. right lateral decubitus, patient on right side
    C. left lateral decubitus, patient on left side
    D. left lateral decubitus, patient on right side

12. Extensive calcification in the wall of the gallbladder is termed _____.
    A. cholelithiasis
    B. porcelain gallbladder
    C. cholecystitis
    D. A or B

13. Varicose veins of the rectum are termed

    _____.
    A. polyps
    B. hemorrhoids
    C. ulcerations
    D. carcinomas

14. *Apple-core* and *napkin-ring* are common descriptive terms for annular carcinoma of the

    _____.
    A. small intestine
    B. stomach
    C. jejunum
    D. colon

15. Crohn's disease occurs in what organ(s)?
    - A. colon
    - B. small bowel
    - C. stomach
    - D. all of the above

16. The presence of large amounts of gas and fluid in uniformly dilated loops of small and large bowel, often seen after abdominal surgery, is termed _____.
    - A. adynamic ileus
    - B. localized ileus
    - C. colonic ileus
    - D. ileus

17. What medical term is used to denote difficulty in swallowing?
    - A. mastication
    - B. dysphagia
    - C. deglutition
    - D. B and C

18. Gastric contents that are mixed with hydrochloric acid and pepsin are called _____.
    - A. chyme
    - B. digest
    - C. enzyme
    - D. emulsifier

19. To demonstrate esophageal reflux, the patient is often asked to perform the _____.
    - A. Trendelenburg maneuver
    - B. Sims maneuver
    - C. Fowler maneuver
    - D. Valsalva maneuver

20. An abnormal connection between the esophagus and trachea is termed _____.
    - A. intussusception
    - B. volvulus
    - C. fistula
    - D. abscess

21. An abnormal accumulation of fluid in the peritoneal cavity is termed _____.
    - A. pneumoperitoneum
    - B. ascites
    - C. volvulus
    - D. hydroperitoneum

22. Herniations, or outpouchings, of the walls of a hollow organ are termed _____.
    - A. ulcers
    - B. diverticula
    - C. hemorrhoids
    - D. polyps

23. A colonic intussusception can sometimes be reduced by what radiographic procedure?
    - A. upper gastrointestinal series
    - B. small bowel series
    - C. enteroclysis series
    - D. barium enema

24. Patients older than 40 years with a history of difficulty in swallowing are usually assumed, until proven otherwise, to have what pathologic condition?
    - A. esophageal fistula
    - B. esophageal hernia
    - C. esophageal varices
    - D. esophageal carcinoma

25. What is the most common manifestation of peptic ulcer disease?
    - A. gastric ulcer
    - B. esophageal ulcer
    - C. duodenal ulcer
    - D. peritoneal ulcer

26. If loops of bowel are distended by abnormally large amounts of air and are occupying the central portion of the abdomen, the patient most likely has a _____.
    - A. small bowel obstruction
    - B. large bowel obstruction
    - C. gastric obstruction
    - D. A and B

BIBLIOGRAPHY

Burgener FA, Kormano M: *Differential diagnosis in computed tomography,* New York, 1996, Thieme.

Eisenberg RL: *Gastrointestinal radiology: a pattern approach,* Philadelphia, 1990, Lippincott.

Farman J: *Gastrointestinal radiology,* New York, 1989, Gower Medical.

Gore RM, Levine MS, Laufer I: *Textbook of gastrointestinal radiology,* Philadelphia, 1993, Saunders.

Jones B, Braver JM: *Essentials of gastrointestinal radiology,* Philadelphia, 1982, Saunders.

Margulis AR, Burhenne HJ: *Alimentary tract radiology,* ed 4, St Louis, 1989, Mosby.

Meyers MA: *Dynamic radiology of the abdomen,* New York, 1994, Springer-Verlag.

Rumack CM, Wilson SR, Charbonneau JW: *Diagnostic ultrasound,* ed 3, St Louis, 2005, Mosby.

URINARY *System*

Chapter Outline

Key Terms

acid-base balance
Bowman's capsule
collecting tubules
complete fusion
crossed ectopia
duplication
ectopic kidney
electrolyte balance
glomerulus
horseshoe kidney
hydronephrosis
hydroureter
hypernephroma
hypoplastic kidney
incontinence
intrathoracic kidney

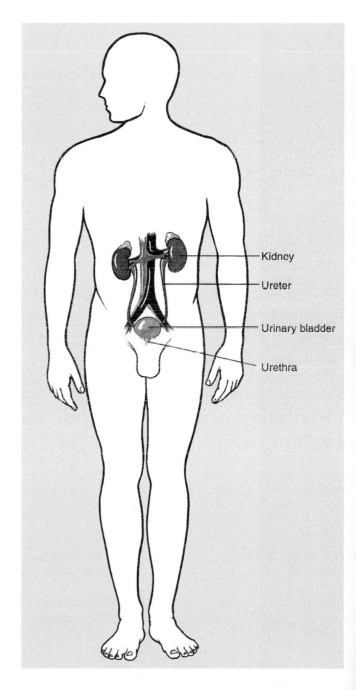

Kidney

Ureter

Urinary bladder

Urethra

loop of Henle
micturate
nephrocalcinosis
pelvic kidney

proximal convoluted tubule
staghorn calculus
supernumerary kidney
trigone

unilateral renal agenesis
uremia
ureterocele

Prerequisite Knowledge

The student should have a basic knowledge of the anatomy and physiology of the urinary system. In addition, proper learning and understanding of the material will be facilitated if the student has some clinical experience in urinary radiography and image evaluation.

Goals

To acquaint the student radiographer with the pathophysiology and radiographic manifestations of all of the common and some of the unusual disorders of the urinary system.

Objectives

After reading this chapter, the reader will be able to:
1. Classify the more common diseases in terms of their attenuation of x-rays
2. Explain the changes in technical factors required for obtaining optimal-quality radiographs in patients with various underlying pathologic conditions
3. Define all key terms in this chapter
4. Describe the physiology of the urinary system
5. Identify anatomic structures on both diagrams and radiographs of the urinary system
6. Differentiate the various pathologic conditions affecting the urinary system and their radiographic manifestations

Physiology of the Urinary System

The urinary system consists of the kidneys, ureters, and bladder. The functional unit of the kidney is the nephron. Each kidney contains more than a million nephrons, which filter waste products from the blood, reabsorb water and nutrients (e.g., glucose and amino acids) from the tubular fluid, and secrete excess substances in the form of urine. In an average person, the nephron filters about 190 L of water out of glomerular blood each day. This enormous amount is many times the total volume of blood in the body. However, only a small proportion of this water (1 to 2 L) is excreted in the urine. Therefore more than 99% of water is reabsorbed into tubular blood.

The formation of urine begins in the **glomerulus**, a tuft of capillaries with very thin walls and a large surface area. The blood pressure within the glomerulus is higher than that in **Bowman's capsule**, which surrounds it. This causes the filtration of fluid into Bowman's capsule that is equivalent to plasma containing neither protein nor red blood cells (if the nephron is healthy). The initial urine proceeds into the **proximal convoluted tubule**, where a large amount of water and virtually all nutrients are reabsorbed into the blood capillaries surrounding the tubules. The amount of sodium and chloride reabsorbed is determined by the concentration of these substances in the body, and it occurs at a variable rate designed to keep the osmotic pressure of the body constant. This process is greatly influenced by two hormones: antidiuretic hormone (ADH), secreted by the posterior pituitary gland, and aldosterone, secreted by the adrenal glands.

After passing through the proximal tubule, the fluid flows through the **loop of Henle**, a complex structure consisting of a descending limb, a loop, and an ascending limb. Following the reabsorption of salt and water in the loop of Henle, the distal convoluted tubules permit the excretion of concentrated urine by actively secreting substances such as potassium (K^+) and hydrogen (H^+) ions and some drugs. In this way the kidney plays an essential role in maintaining salt or **electrolyte balance** and **acid-base balance** of blood and body fluids.

To maintain a healthy metabolism, the pH must be maintained in the very limited range of 7.35 to 7.45. If the pH of blood is lower than this (i.e., too acidic), the kidney excretes an acid urine to remove H^+; if the pH of blood is higher than 7.5 (i.e., too alkaline), the kidney preserves H^+ and secretes an alkaline urine.

Eventually, urine passes from the **collecting tubules**, whose openings are in the papillae, into the calyces, and on to the funnel-shaped renal pelvis and tubular ureters. Peristaltic waves (about 1 to 5 per minute) force the urine down the ureters and into the bladder. The ureters enter the bladder through an oblique tunnel that functions as a valve to prevent back flow of urine into the ureters (vesicoureteral reflux) during bladder contraction.

The bladder acts as a reservoir for the urine before it leaves the body. The openings of the two ureters lie at the posterior corners of the triangle-shaped floor (the **trigone**), and the urethral opening is situated at

RADIOGRAPHER *Notes*

Ultrasound and computed tomography (CT) are being used with increasing frequency, and plain radiography with contrast material introduced intravenously or by means of a catheter has become a less frequently used technique for imaging the urinary system. For excretory urography, the radiographer is responsible for preparing sterile injections of contrast material, and for operating the equipment properly and positioning the patient. In some instances, the radiographer may have to perform these functions in an operating room using sterile technique.

All radiographic studies begin with a "scout" image that is obtained before the injection of any contrast material. The radiographer should evaluate this image for proper technique and positioning so that any required alterations can be made on subsequent radiographs during the procedure. An image with correct density and contrast should demonstrate the kidney and psoas muscle shadows, and the lumbar vertebrae and their transverse processes. A correctly positioned image should demonstrate all of both kidneys down to the superior portion of the pubic bones (to ensure that the entire bladder is included). The radiograph must be in a true anteroposterior position with the pelvis appearing symmetric and the spinous processes of the lumbar vertebrae projected over the central portions of the vertebral bodies. The radiologist evaluates the scout radiograph to make certain that the technique and positioning are appropriate for the clinical history and to evaluate proper patient preparation. The radiograph is also checked for any radiopaque calculi or other abnormality that might be obscured after the injection of contrast material.

The radiographer must be alert to the possibility of an allergic reaction whenever contrast agents are used. It is essential that the radiographer be aware of the proper procedures to follow in the event of an allergic reaction and be able to initiate and maintain basic life support until advanced life-support personnel have arrived. Depending on departmental policy, it is usually the radiographer's responsibility to assist during resuscitation procedures. Therefore, it is essential that the radiographer be familiar with the contents of the emergency cart and take responsibility for ensuring that the cart is completely stocked with appropriate medications.

All radiographs of the urinary system must be made with the patient in full exhalation so that the diaphragm assumes its highest position and does not compress the abdominal contents. Depending on the specific area being evaluated, the radiographer may have to perform oblique or erect projections, coned-down views of the kidneys or bladder, tomograms, or images made with abdominal compression. In certain pathologic conditions, radiographs must be obtained at precisely timed intervals, and delayed images may be necessary.

---

the anterior and lower corner. Filling of the bladder (about 250 ml in the average person) stimulates autonomic nerve endings in the wall that are perceived as a distended sensation and the desire to void (**micturate**). A complicated sequence of bladder contractions and relaxation of the sphincter muscles permits the bladder to expel urine from the body through the urethra. Voluntary contraction of the external sphincter to prevent or terminate micturition is learned and is possible only if the motor system is intact. Nervous system injury (cerebral hemorrhage, spinal cord injury) results in involuntary emptying of the bladder at intervals (**incontinence**).

The kidney is also important in the production of red blood cells and in the control of blood pressure. Erythropoietin, a substance produced by the kidney, stimulates the rate of production of red blood cells. Therefore renal failure is often associated with a severe anemia. The juxtaglomerular apparatus refers to specialized cells within renal arterioles that secrete renin, an enzyme that acts with one of the plasma proteins to produce angiotensin. Decreased blood flow through these arterioles increases the secretion of renin and thus the blood level of angiotensin, which constricts peripheral arterioles throughout the body and elevates the blood pressure.

Congenital/Hereditary Diseases

Anomalies of Number and Size

Unilateral renal agenesis (solitary kidney) is a rare anomaly that may be associated with a variety of other congenital malformations (Figure 6-1). Before the diagnosis can be made, it is essential to exclude a nonfunctioning, diseased kidney or a prior nephrectomy. Unilateral renal agenesis results from a failure of the embryonic renal bud or renal vascular system

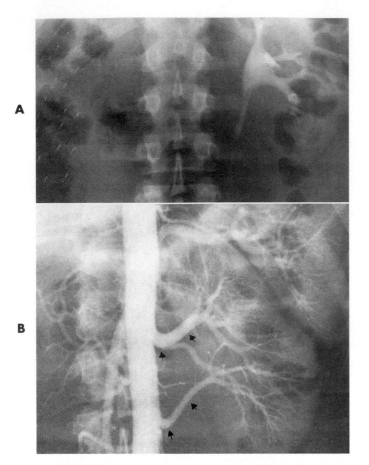

FIGURE 6-1 Solitary kidney. **A,** Excretory urogram demonstrates normal left kidney with no evidence of right renal tissue. **B,** Aortogram shows two renal arteries leading to the left kidney *(arrows)* and no evidence of a right renal artery, thus confirming the diagnosis of unilateral renal agenesis.

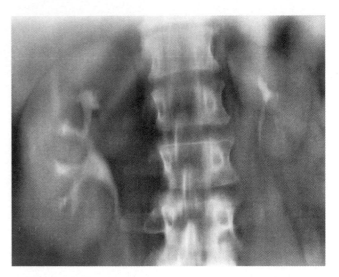

FIGURE 6-2 Hypoplastic kidney with compensatory hypertrophy. Small left kidney (miniature replica of a normal kidney) has good function and normal relationship between amount of parenchyma and size of the collecting system. Greatly enlarged right kidney represents compensatory hypertrophy.

to form. In true renal agenesis, the ureter and corresponding half of the trigone are missing also. Ultrasound or CT can demonstrate the absence of renal tissue. A solitary kidney tends to be larger than expected, reflecting compensatory hypertrophy.

A **supernumerary kidney** is also a rare anomaly. The third kidney is usually small and rudimentary and possesses a separate pelvis, ureter, and blood supply. Although these kidneys function normally, they tend to lead to secondary infections that eventually may require their removal.

A small, **hypoplastic kidney** often appears as a miniature replica of a normal kidney, with good function and a normal relationship between the amount of parenchyma and the size of the collecting system (Figure 6-2). Renal hypoplasia must be differentiated from an acquired atrophic kidney, which is small and contracted because of vascular or inflammatory disease that has reduced the volume of renal parenchyma.

Compensatory hypertrophy is an acquired condition that develops when one kidney is forced to perform the function normally carried out by two kidneys (see Figure 6-2). This phenomenon may follow unilateral renal agenesis, hypoplasia, atrophy, or nephrectomy. The ability of the kidney to undergo compensatory hypertrophy is greatest in children and diminishes in adulthood. Sonography demonstrates the size of the renal parenchyma, calyces, and pelvis without using a contrast agent or ionizing radiation to provide a diagnosis.

Anomalies of Rotation, Position, and Fusion

Malrotation of one or both kidneys may produce a bizarre appearance of the renal parenchyma, calyces, and pelvis that suggests a pathologic condition when in reality the kidney is otherwise entirely normal (Figure 6-3). Abnormally positioned kidneys **(ectopic kidney)** may be found in various locations, from the true pelvis **(pelvic kidney)** (Figure 6-4) to above the diaphragm **(intrathoracic kidney)** (Figure 6-5). Pelvic kidneys occur much more frequently than intrathoracic kidneys. Whenever only one kidney is seen on excretory urography, a full view of the abdomen is essential to search for an ectopic kidney. Although the ectopic kidney usually functions, the nephrogram and the pelvicalyceal system may be obscured by overlying bone and fecal contents. Patient history can distinguish a true pelvic kidney from a kidney transplant, which typically is located in the right pelvis. **Crossed ectopia** refers to a situation in which an ectopic kidney lies on the same side as the normal kidney and is very commonly fused with it.

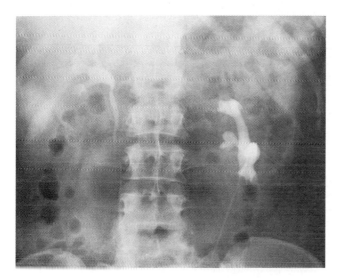

FIGURE **6-3** Malrotation of left kidney. Note apparent lateral displacement of upper ureter and elongation of pelvis.

Horseshoe kidney is the most common type of fusion anomaly. In this condition, both kidneys are malrotated and their lower poles are joined by a band of normal renal parenchyma (isthmus) or connective tissue (Figure 6-6). The ureters arise from the kidneys anteriorly instead of medially, and the lower pole calyces point medially rather than laterally. The pelves are often large and flabby and may simulate obstruction. Obstruction at the ureteropelvic junction may occur because of the anterior position of the ureters. **Complete fusion** of the kidneys is a rare anomaly that produces a single irregular mass that has no resemblance to a renal structure. The resulting bizarre appearance has been given such varied names as disk, cake, lump, and doughnut kidney.

Anomalies of Renal Pelvis and Ureter

Duplication (duplex kidney) is a common anomaly that may vary from a simple bifid pelvis to a completely double pelvis, ureter, and ureterovesical orifice. The ureter draining the upper renal segment enters the bladder below the ureter draining the lower renal segment. Complete duplication can be complicated by obstruction or by vesicoureteral reflux with infection.

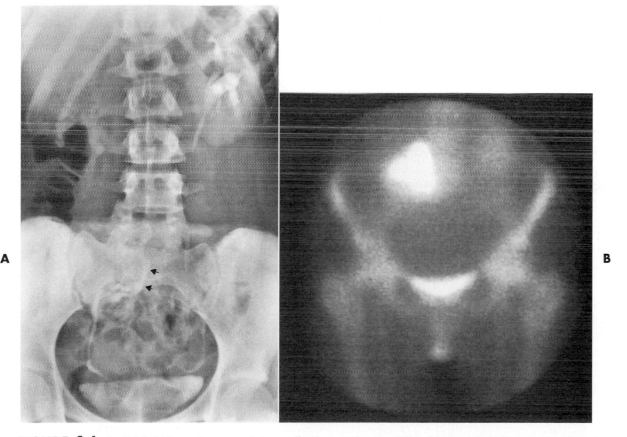

FIGURE **6-4** **A,** Pelvic kidney. Arrows point to collecting system. **B,** Right-sided pelvic kidney, an incidental finding on a bone scan.

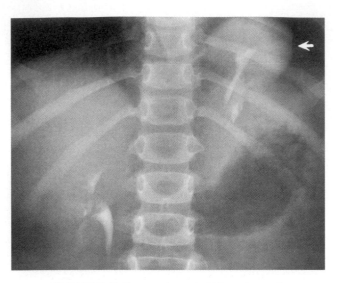

FIGURE 6-5   Intrathoracic kidney *(arrow)*.

Vesicoureteral reflux and infection more commonly involve the ureter draining the lower renal segment; obstruction more frequently affects the upper pole, where it can cause a hydronephrotic mass that displaces and compresses the lower calyces.

Treatment of Congenital/Hereditary Anomalies

Most cases of congenital/hereditary anomalies of the urinary tract require no treatment. If obstruction occurs as a result of the anomaly (because of twisting or angulation of the ureter), therapy (stent placement or surgery) is necessary to maintain normal urine flow. In cases of infection, which occur more frequently in renal or ureteral duplication because of vesicoureteral reflux, antibiotics are required and it is necessary to determine if there is an anatomic cause that can be corrected surgically. The large pelvis in a horseshoe kidney makes this anomaly more prone to infection.

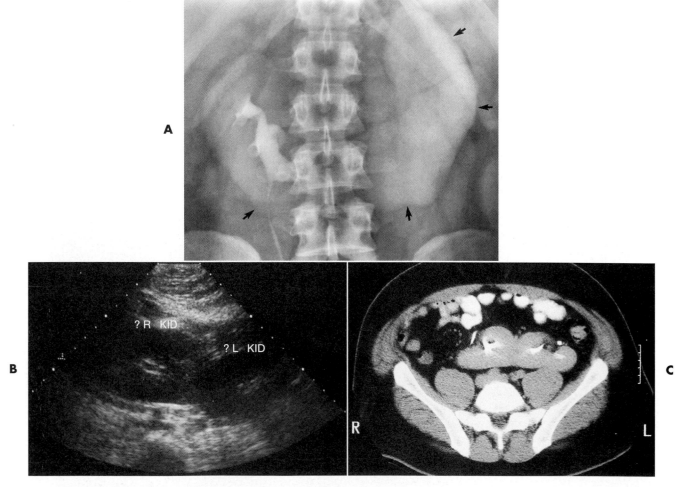

FIGURE 6-6   **A,** Horseshoe kidney *(arrows)*. Prolonged nephrogram and delayed calyceal filling on left are caused by obstructing stone at ureteropelvic junction on that side. **B,** Ultrasound shows fused lower poles of a horseshoe kidney in a 51-year-old woman. She had right flank pain and symptoms of a urinary tract infection for 1 week. **C,** CT image shows the lower pole connection.

Ureterocele

A **ureterocele** is a cystic dilatation of the distal ureter near its insertion into the bladder. In the simple (adult) type, the opening in the ureter is situated at or near the normal position in the bladder, usually with stenosis of the ureteral orifice and with varying degrees of dilatation of the proximal ureter. The stenosis leads to prolapse of the distal ureter into the bladder and dilatation of the lumen of the prolapsed segment. Ectopic ureteroceles are found almost exclusively in infants and children; most are associated with ureteral duplication.

Radiographic Appearance

The appearance on excretory urography depends on whether opaque medium fills the ureterocele. If it is filled, the lesion appears as a round or oval density surrounded by a thin radiolucent halo representing the wall of the prolapsed ureter and the mucosa of the bladder (cobra head sign) (Figure 6-7, *A*). When the ureterocele is not filled with contrast material, it appears as a radiolucent mass within the opacified bladder in the region of the ureteral orifice (Figure 6-7, *B*). Ultrasound is the modality of choice to evaluate infants and children. Children with ureteral duplication have an 80% incidence of an associated ureterocele. On ultrasound images, a ureterocele appears as a round cystlike structure within the bladder (Figure 6-7, *C*).

On excretory urography, an ectopic ureterocele typically appears as a large, eccentric filling defect impressing the floor of the bladder (Figure 6-8). The ureterocele arises from the ureter draining the upper segment of the duplicated collecting system. A mass effect, representing hydronephrosis, often involves

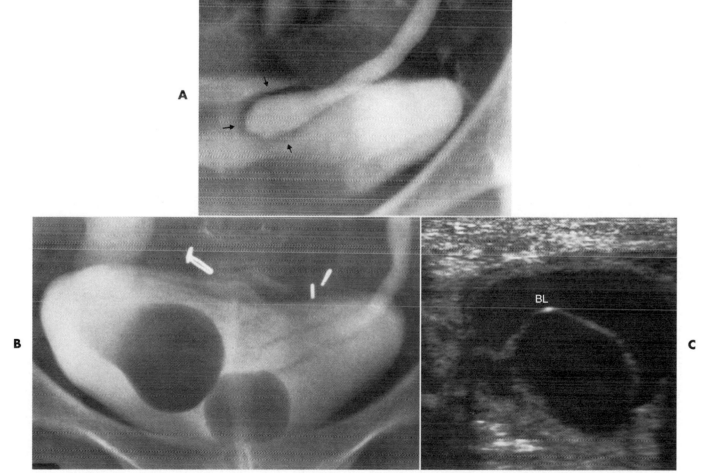

FIGURE 6-7 Simple ureteroceles. **A,** Unilateral ureterocele *(arrows)* filled with contrast material. **B,** Bilateral ureteroceles without contrast material appear as radiolucent masses in the bladder. **C,** Ultrasound of a 1-day-old infant boy. Left ureter exhibits massive dilatation.

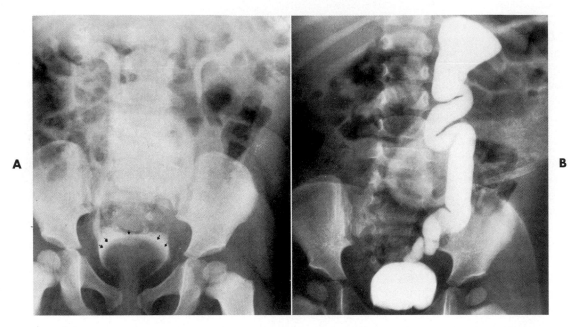

FIGURE 6-8 Ectopic ureteroceles. **A,** Excretory urogram demonstrates large lucency *(arrows)* filling much of the bladder. A slight downward and lateral displacement of the pelvicalyceal system can be seen on the left. **B,** Cystogram shows contrast material undergoing reflux to fill the greatly dilated collecting system draining the upper pole of left kidney. Note the severe dilatation and tortuosity of the ureter.

the upper pole of the kidney and causes downward and lateral displacement of the lower portion of the collecting system.

Treatment

Ureteroceles may need to be treated to preserve kidney function and to reduce the risk of infection. An endoscopic incision of the ureterocele (at the vesicoureteral junction) allows normal urine drainage into the bladder. More aggressive treatment includes surgical resection of the ureterocele with bladder reconstruction.

Posterior Urethral Valves

Posterior urethral valves are thin transverse membranes, found almost exclusively in males, that cause bladder outlet obstruction and may lead to severe hydronephrosis, hydroureter, and renal damage. The thin transverse membranes work as a reverse valve, meaning that catheterization is normal but the valve prevents antegrade flow. They are best demonstrated on a voiding cystourethrogram (Figure 6-9). The proximal urethra is dilated and the thin, lucent transverse membrane of the valve can be identified.

Treatment

Surgical intervention to correct the anatomic relationships and allow normal urine flow is required to prevent any kidney or ureteral destruction.

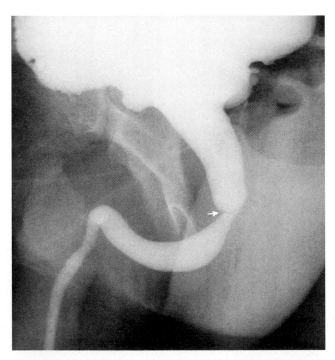

FIGURE 6-9 Posterior urethral valve. Voiding cystourethrogram shows characteristic thin transverse membrane of the valve *(arrow).* Distally the caliber of the bulbous urethra is normal.

SUMMARY of FINDINGS for Congenital/Hereditary Diseases

disorder	location/description	radiographic appearance	treatment
Renal agenesis	Solitary kidney	IVU—hypertrophic single functioning kidney US—size of renal parenchyma, calyces, and pelves	Usually no treatment Obstruction: alleviate cause of obstruction Infection: antibiotics, and determine cause, if any
Supernumerary kidney	More than two kidneys	IVU—hypoplastic 3rd kidney, may or may not be fused	
Malrotation	Abnormal position of kidney	Bizarre appearance of renal parenchyma, calyces, and pelvis	
Ectopic kidney		Solitary kidney—2nd kidney seen in another location (pelvis or thorax)	
Horseshoe kidney	Lower-pole parenchymal fusion	IVU—kidney malrotation and possible nephrogram demonstrating parenchymal fusion US/CT—demonstration of renal fusion	
Duplication	More than one renal pelvis or ureter	IVU—double renal pelvis in single kidney; two ureters exiting kidney and emptying into bladder	
Ureterocele	Distal ureter (vesicoureteral junction)	Round or oval dilated ureter with radiolucent halo US—round cyst-like structure within the bladder	Endoscopic incision of vesicoureteral junction Surgical resection with bladder reconstruction
Posterior urethral valves	Transverse membranes in urethra	VCUG—stricture or narrowing of urethra and a thin radiolucency representing the membrane	Surgical intervention to correct anatomic function

IVU, Intravenous urography; *US,* ultrasound; *VCUG,* voiding cystourethrography.

Inflammatory Disorders

Glomerulonephritis

Glomerulonephritis is a nonsuppurative inflammatory process involving the tufts of capillaries (glomeruli) that filter the blood within the kidney. It represents an antigen-antibody reaction that most commonly occurs several weeks after an acute upper respiratory or middle ear infection with certain strains of hemolytic streptococci. In recent years, western countries have seen a decrease in acute glomerulonephritis caused by streptococci. More frequently, the inflammatory process is caused by a chronic autoimmune disorder. The inflammatory process causes the glomeruli to be extremely permeable, allowing albumin and red blood cells to leak into the urine (resulting in proteinuria or hematuria). Decreased glomerular filtration rate causes oliguria, a smaller-than-normal amount of urine.

Radiographic Appearance

The excretory urographic findings in glomerulonephritis depend on the duration and severity of the disease process and on the level of renal function. In patients with acute glomerulonephritis, the kidneys may be normal or diffusely increased in size with smooth contours and normal calyces. A loss of renal substance in chronic glomerulonephritis produces bilateral small kidneys (Figure 6-10). The renal outline remains smooth and the collecting system is normal, unlike the irregular contours and blunted calyces seen in chronic pyelonephritis. Ultrasound may

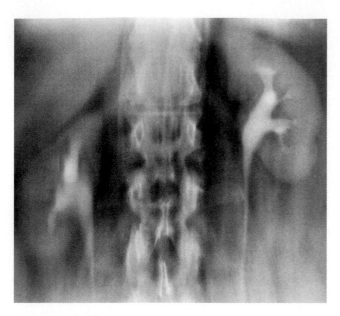

FIGURE 6-10 Chronic glomerulonephritis. Nephrotomogram shows bilateral small smooth kidneys. Uniform reduction in parenchymal thickness is particularly apparent in right kidney. Notice that the pelvicalyceal system is well opacified and without the irregular contours and blunted calyces seen in chronic pyelonephritis.

demonstrate these findings more efficiently without contrast enhancement or radiation exposure.

Treatment

Most cases of acute glomerulonephritis resolve completely, and the kidney returns to normal. In some patients, however, chronic inflammation with periods of remission and exacerbation (increased seriousness) leads to a fibrotic reaction that results in shrinkage of the kidneys with loss of renal function and the development of uremia. Before therapy is implemented, a renal biopsy may be required to determine the specific cause. If there is an underlying antigen-antibody reaction, corticosteroids for immunosuppression would be appropriate. Infectious processes are treated with antibiotics.

Pyelonephritis

Pyelonephritis is a suppurative inflammation of the kidney and renal pelvis caused by pyogenic (pus-forming) bacteria. Unlike glomerulonephritis, which primarily involves the parenchyma (glomeruli and tubules) of the kidney, the inflammatory process of pyelonephritis affects the interstitial tissue between the tubules. The infection is patchy in distribution, often involves only one kidney, and is asymmetric if both kidneys are involved. Although the infection may spread from the bloodstream or lymphatics, the infection usually originates in the bladder and

ascends by means of the ureter to involve the kidneys. Pyelonephritis often occurs in women and children. The disease frequently develops in patients with obstruction of the urinary tract (enlarged prostate gland, kidney stone, congenital defect), which causes stagnation of the urine and provides a breeding ground for infection. Instrumentation or catheterization of the ureter is also an important contributing factor to the development of pyelonephritis.

Patients with pyelonephritis have high fever, chills, and sudden back pain that spreads over the abdomen. Painful urination (dysuria) usually occurs. Large amounts of pus may be detected in the urine (pyuria), and bacteria can be cultured from the urine or observed in the urinary sediment.

Radiographic Appearance

In most patients with acute pyelonephritis, the excretory urogram is normal. Occasional abnormalities include generalized enlargement of the kidney on the symptomatic side, delayed calyceal opacification, and decreased density of the contrast material. A characteristic finding is linear striation in the renal pelvis, which probably represents mucosal edema.

The urographic hallmark of chronic pyelonephritis is patchy calyceal clubbing with overlying parenchymal scarring (Figure 6-11). Initially, there is blunting of the calyces, which then become rounded or clubbed. Fibrotic scarring causes a cortical depression overlying the dilated calyx. Progressive cortical atrophy and thinning may be so extensive that the tip of the blunted calyx appears to lie directly beneath the renal capsule. The urographic findings may be unilateral or bilateral and are often most pronounced at the poles. If calyceal changes are minimal, the overlying cortical depressions may simulate lobar infarctions or normal kidney lobulations. However, in chronic pyelonephritis, the cortical depression lies directly over a calyx rather than between calyces as in lobar infarctions or congenital lobulation. Chronic pyelonephritis may progress to end-stage renal disease with small, usually irregular, poorly functioning kidneys.

CT has become the modality of choice. Contrast-enhanced CT demonstrates the cortical changes and may show an associated abscess. Sonography also can demonstrate the abscess, but is less sensitive. Both CT and sonography can detect hydronephrosis, indicating that urinary tract obstruction is a predisposing factor. In chronic nephritis, ultrasound shows loss of renal parenchyma as an increase in echogenicity in the area of the scar and extension of the central renal sinus echoes to the periphery of the affected area. Dimercaptosuccinic acid scintigraphy (nuclear medicine study) can demonstrate inflammation and scarring of the kidney and determine the distribution

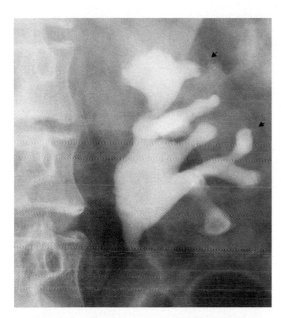

FIGURE 6-11 Chronic pyelonephritis. Diffuse rounded clubbing of multiple calyces with atrophy and thinning of overlying renal parenchyma. Arrows indicate outer margin of kidney.

of function in the renal cortex. Some clinicians select this modality as the preferred study rather than CT because of the lower radiation dose.

Treatment

With the availability of antibiotic therapy, pyelonephritis generally heals without complication. However, fibrous scarring can cause irregular contraction of the kidney. Severe infection can destroy large amounts of renal tissue, leading to uremia or septicemia as a result of diffuse spread of infection throughout the body. In cases of chronic pyelonephritis, a long-term regimen of antibiotics is appropriate. If this is ineffective, more aggressive therapy may be required. Some consider percutaneous drain placement an acceptable alternative to surgery in such cases.

Emphysematous Pyelonephritis

Emphysematous pyelonephritis is a severe form of acute parenchymal and perirenal infection with gas-forming bacteria that occurs virtually only in diabetic patients and causes an acute necrosis of the entire kidney. The presence of radiolucent gas shadows within and around the kidney is pathognomonic of emphysematous pyelonephritis (Figure 6-12). CT is the preferred modality for localizing the gas patterns within and around (perinephric) the kidney. The affected region appears as mottled areas of low attenuation.

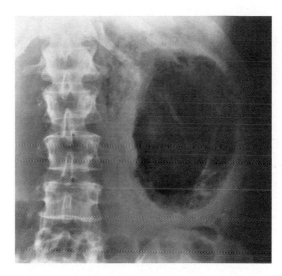

FIGURE 6-12 Emphysematous pyelonephritis.

Treatment

When the gas pattern is within the kidney—a finding associated with a mortality rate of 60%—antibiotics and drainage are necessary. This condition is a surgical emergency, requiring nephrectomy, which lowers the mortality rate to 20%. In most cases this disease process is fatal if the patient is treated with just medications.

Tuberculosis

The hematogenous spread of tuberculosis may lead to the development of small granulomas scattered in the cortical portion of the kidneys. Renal tuberculosis usually occurs as a secondary infection from lung involvement, but can evolve from other sites. It typically becomes manifest 5 to 10 years following the primary infection.

Radiographic Appearance

Spread of infection to the renal pyramid causes an ulcerative, destructive process in the tips of the papillae with irregularity and enlargement of the calyces (Figure 6-13). Fibrosis and stricture formation lead to cortical scarring and parenchymal atrophy, which may simulate the appearance of chronic bacterial pyelonephritis. Flecks of calcification may develop in multiple tuberculous granulomas. With progressive disease, gross amorphous and irregular calcifications can form. Eventually the entire nonfunctioning renal parenchyma may be replaced by massive calcification (autonephrectomy) (Figure 6-14).

Tuberculosis can also involve the ureter and bladder. Initially, there are multiple ulcerations that result in a ragged, irregular appearance of the ureteral wall. As the disease heals, there are usually multiple areas in

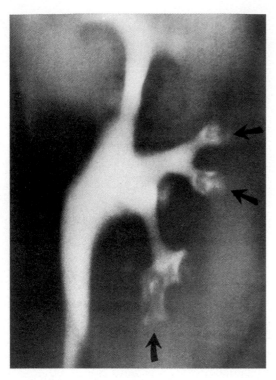

FIGURE 6-13 Tuberculosis. Early stage of papillary destruction *(arrows)*.

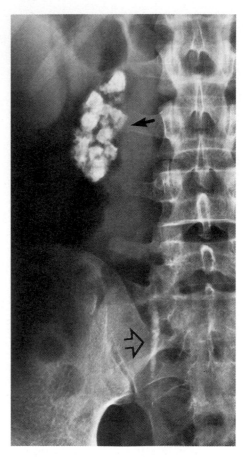

FIGURE 6-14 Tuberculous autonephrectomy. Plain film shows coarse, irregular calcification that retains a kidney-like shape *(solid arrow)*. Notice also the tuberculous calcification of the right distal ureter *(open arrow)*.

which the ureteral strictures alternate with dilated segments, producing a beaded or corkscrew appearance. In advanced cases, the wall of the ureter may become thickened and fixed with no peristalsis; this results in a pipestem ureter that runs a direct course toward the bladder (Figure 6-15). Tuberculous involvement of the urinary bladder may produce mural irregularities simulating carcinoma or, more commonly, a small, contracted bladder with a thickened wall.

Treatment
A regimen (6 to 8 months) of a combination of powerful tuberculostatic drugs is required for a cure. If the tuberculostatic drugs are not used in combination, a drug resistance can develop, making the treatment ineffective.

Papillary Necrosis
Papillary necrosis refers to a destructive process involving a varying amount of the medullary papillae and the terminal portion of the renal pyramids. Common predisposing factors include diabetes, pyelonephritis, urinary tract infection or obstruction, sickle cell disease, and phenacetin abuse.

Radiographic Appearance
The necrotic process causes cavitation of the central portion of the papillae or complete sloughing of the papillary tip (Figure 6-16). When a piece of medullary

tissue has been completely separated from the rest of the renal parenchyma, an excretory urogram shows a characteristic ring of contrast material surrounding a triangular lucent filling defect representing the sloughed necrotic tissue. The remaining calyx has a round, saccular, or club-shaped configuration. The sloughed papilla may stay in place and become calcified, or it may pass down the ureter, where it may simulate a stone and even cause obstruction. Ultrasound images show sloughing as an echogenic, nonshadowing structure in the collecting system.

Treatment
In most cases the treatment is supportive. If the condition is induced by medication, the offending agent must be discontinued. Any predisposing condition (diabetes or sickle cell anemia) should be controlled. If obstruction occurs as a result of medullary tissue separation, removal of the obstruction endoscopically or surgically is necessary to prevent renal failure. Ureteral tamponade placement can control papillary bleeding caused by the separation.

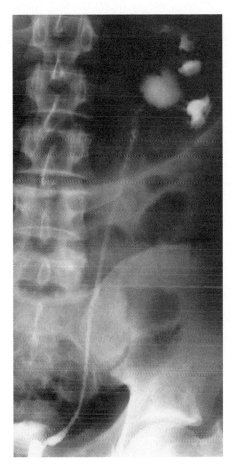

FIGURE 6-15 Ureteral tuberculosis.

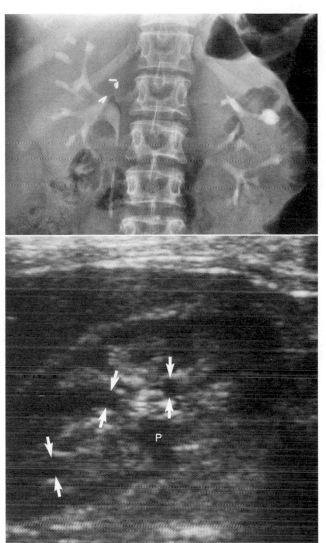

FIGURE 6-16 **A,** Papillary necrosis. Generalized saccular or club-shaped configuration of most calyces bilaterally in patient with sickle cell disease. Note surgical clips. **B,** Ultrasound illustrates sloughed papilla causing shadowing and swollen pyramids *(arrows).* P, Renal pelvis.

Cystitis

Inflammation of the urinary bladder is most common in women because the urethra is shorter. The major cause is the inadvertent spread of bacteria present in fecal material, which reaches the urinary opening and travels upward to the bladder. Instrumentation or catheterization of the bladder is another important cause of cystitis, which is the most common infection in hospitalized patients (nosocomial infection). The radiographer needs to keep the urine bag below the patient to prevent retrograde flow that may cause cystitis. Cystitis can also develop from sexual intercourse, with the spread of infecting organisms from around the vaginal opening. Urinary frequency, urgency, and a burning sensation during urination are typical clinical findings.

Radiographic Appearance

Although acute inflammation of the bladder generally does not produce changes detectable on excretory urography, chronic cystitis causes a decrease in bladder size that is often associated with irregularity of the bladder wall (Figure 6-17). In candidal cystitis,

fungus balls may produce lucent filling defects in the opacified bladder. Similar lucent filling defects in the bladder may reflect blood clots in patients with hemorrhagic cystitis and may complicate chemotherapy in the treatment of leukemia and lymphoma. Sonographic images demonstrate a thickened bladder wall.

A dramatic radiographic appearance is produced by emphysematous cystitis, an inflammatory disease of the bladder that most often occurs in diabetic patients and is caused by gas-forming bacteria. Characteristic plain film findings are a ring of lucent gas outlining all or a part of the bladder wall and the presence of gas within the bladder lumen

SUMMARY of FINDINGS for Inflammatory Disorders

disorder	location	radiographic appearance	treatment
Glomerulonephritis (nonsuppurative)	Parenchyma (glomeruli and tubules)	Normal contour Acute—normal to increased kidney size Chronic—small kidney	Most cases resolve completely Corticosteroids for immunosuppression Antibiotics for infection
Pyelonephritis (suppurative)	Interstitial tissue between tubules	IVU—Acute produces striation in renal pelvis; chronic blunting to clubbing of calyces CT—changes in cortex and associated abscesses US—large pelvis with loss of parenchyma NM—inflammation, scarring and renal distribution function	Conservative: antibiotics, fluid management Aggressive: percutaneous drainage, antibiotics, surgery
Emphysematous pyelonephritis	Parenchymal and perirenal	Radiolucent gas CT—mottled areas of low attenuation	Acute medical emergency—nephrectomy
Tuberculosis	Cortex	Irregularity and enlargement of calyces, calcifications	Regimen of combination of tuberculostatic drugs
Papillary necrosis	Medullary papillae and terminal portion of renal pyramids	Cavitation of central portion of papillae US—sloughing appears as an echogenic nonshadowing structure in the collecting system	Medication induced—discontinue offending agent Predisposing conditions—control to reduce risk Obstruction—remove endoscopically or surgically
Cystitis	Bladder	Irregularity of bladder wall US—thickened bladder wall CT—bladder wall filled with gaseous material	Antibiotics or sulfa drugs

IVU, Intravenous urography; *NM*, nuclear medicine; *US*, ultrasound.

(Figure 6-18). The CT demonstration of gas within the bladder wall aids in determining the extent of the inflammation.

Treatment

Using antibiotic and sulfa drug therapy, cystitis generally heals without complication.

Kidney Stones

Urinary calculi most commonly form in the kidney. They are asymptomatic until they lodge in the ureter and cause partial obstruction, resulting in extreme pain that radiates from the area of the kidney to the groin (Figure 6-19). The cause of kidney stones varies and often reflects an underlying metabolic abnormality, such as hypercalcemia (resulting from hyperparathyroidism) or any cause of increased calcium excretion in the urine. Urinary stasis and infection are also important factors in promoting stone formation.

Radiographic Appearance

More than 80% of symptomatic renal stones contain enough calcium to be radiopaque and detectable on plain abdominal radiographs (Figure 6-20). Completely radiolucent calculi contain no calcium and are composed of a variety of substances (e.g., oxalates, mineral magnesium, or uric acid) that are in excessive concentration in the urine. Plain abdominal radiographs miss approximately 34% of the stones because of their size or location, or because they are obscured by bowel or bone. Noncontrast helical CT is used most frequently to best demonstrate the stone without anatomically obscuring the area (Figure 6-21, *A*). This modality is safer, easier, and more accurate (95%) than excretory urography. CT demonstrates the

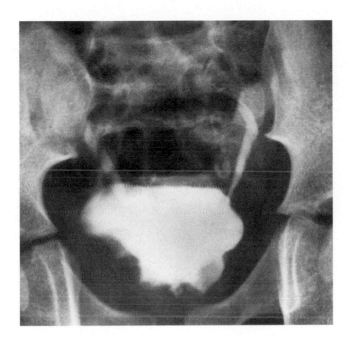

FIGURE **6-17** Cystitis. Excretory urogram shows irregular, lobulated filling defects (representing intense mucosal edema) at base of bladder.

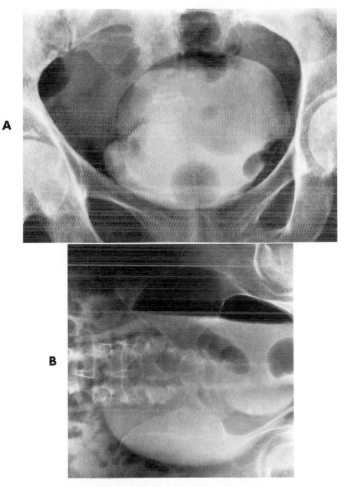

A

B

FIGURE **6-18** Emphysematous cystitis. **A,** Film from cystogram shows thin rim of lucency surrounding much of the bladder, which is filled with contrast material. **B,** Right lateral decubitus view clearly shows long air-fluid level.

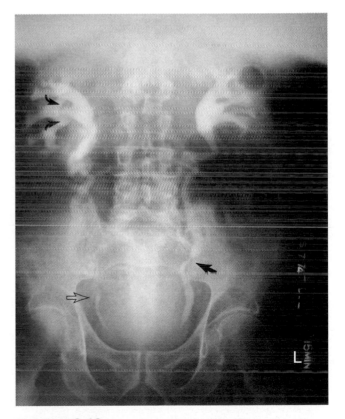

FIGURE **6-19** Contrast extravasation. Fifteen minute excretory urogram demonstrates a stricture on the left ureter *(straight black arrow)* and a filling defect in the right ureter *(white arrow)*. Both renal pelves are dilated and the right demonstrates extravasation of contrast material *(curved black arrows)*.

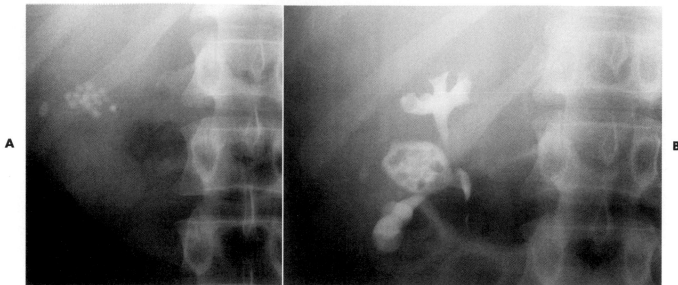

FIGURE 6-20 Cystine stones. **A,** Plain film shows multiple radiopaque calculi. **B,** Excretory urogram demonstrates stones as lucent filling defects in opacified renal pelvis.

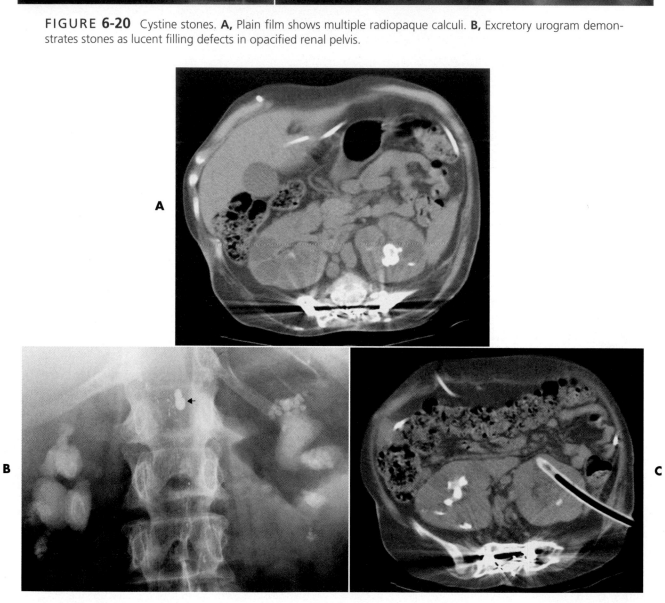

FIGURE 6-21 **A,** Spiral CT image done at 5-mm intervals on an 11-year-old boy, demonstrating bilateral renal calculi with caliectasis (dilated calyces) and kidney enlargement. **B,** Staghorn calculi fill renal pelves bilaterally. Of incidental note is residual contrast material *(arrow)* from prior myelogram. **C,** Nephrostomy tube placement in the left renal pelvis to drain the kidney.

hydroureter or hydronephrosis that results from the obstruction, and density readings help determine the type of stone.

Sonography demonstrates an echogenic region with acoustic shadowing of the stone with hydroureter or hydronephrosis; however, stones smaller than 3 mm may not produce a detectable acoustic shadow. This modality is used when ionizing radiation is contraindicated.

When CT is unavailable, excretory urography is used to detect these otherwise invisible, nonopaque stones that appear as filling defects in the contrast-filled collecting system. In patients with acute renal colic caused by an obstructing stone in the ureter, excretory urography may demonstrate the point of cutoff and dilatation of the proximal ureter and pelvicalyceal system. With acute obstruction, the intrapelvic pressure may increase to such an extent that there is little or no glomerular filtration, resulting in a delayed and prolonged nephrogram and a lack of calyceal filling on the affected side.

Small renal stones (3 mm or less) may pass spontaneously in the urine. At times, a stone may completely fill the renal pelvis (**staghorn calculus**) (see Figure 6-21, *B*), blocking the flow of urine. Figure 6-21, *C* shows nephrostomy placement to drain the kidney.

Calcium can also deposit within the renal parenchyma **(nephrocalcinosis)** (Figure 6-22). This calcification varies from a few scattered punctate densities to very dense and extensive calcifications throughout both kidneys. The most common causes of nephrocalcinosis include hyperparathyroidism, increased intestinal absorption of calcium (sarcoidosis, hypervitaminosis D, milk-alkali syndrome), and renal tubular acidosis, a disorder in which the kidney is unable to excrete an acid urine (below pH 5.4).

Stones can also form in other portions of the genitourinary tract. Ureteral calculi almost invariably result from the downward movement of kidney stones (Figure 6-23). They are usually small, irregular, and poorly calcified and are therefore easily missed on abdominal radiographs that are not of good quality. Calculi most commonly lodge in the lower portion of the ureter, especially at the ureterovesical junction and at the pelvic brim (Figure 6-24). They are often oval, with their long axes paralleling the course of the ureter. Ureteral calculi must be differentiated from the far more common phleboliths, which are spherical and located in the lateral portion of the pelvis below a line joining the ischial spines. In contrast, ureteral stones are situated medially above the interspinous line.

Stone formation in the bladder is a disorder primarily of elderly men with obstruction or infection of the lower urinary tract (Figure 6-25, *A*). Frequently

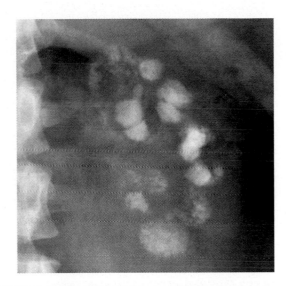

FIGURE 6-22 Nephrolithiasis. Multiple deposits are scattered throughout parenchyma of left kidney.

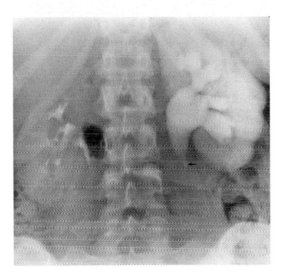

FIGURE 6-23 Obstructing ureteral calculus. Excretory urogram demonstrates prolonged nephrogram and pronounced dilatation of collecting system and pelvis proximal to obstructing stone *(arrow)*.

associated lesions include bladder-outlet obstruction, urethral strictures, neurogenic bladder, and bladder diverticula (Figure 6-25, *B*). At times, upper urinary tract stones migrate down the ureter and are retained in the bladder. Bladder calculi can be single or multiple. They vary in size from tiny concretions, each the size of a grain of sand, to an enormous single calculus occupying the entire bladder lumen. Most bladder calculi are circular or oval; however, almost any shape can be encountered. They can be amorphous, laminated (layered), or even spiculated. One unusual type with a characteristic radiographic appearance is the hard burr, or jackstone, variety, which gets its

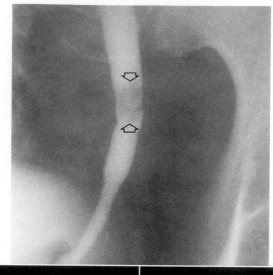

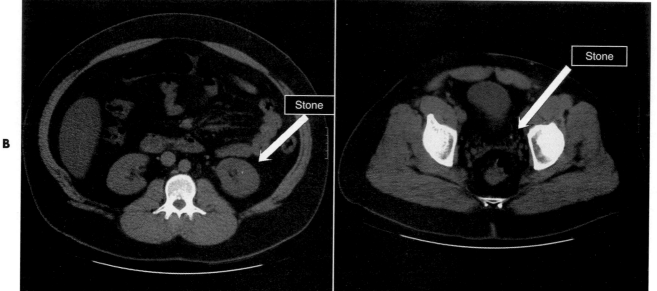

FIGURE 6-24 Ureteral calculus. **A,** Stone appears as nonopaque filling defect *(arrows)* in distal portion of ureter. **B,** CT image done at 5-mm intervals without contrast material demonstrates a stone in the right kidney. **C,** A scan of the lower pelvis demonstrates a second stone in the distal portion of the ureter.

name from the many irregular prongs that project from its surface and simulate the child's toy.

Treatment

Preventive measures include increasing fluid intake and decreasing the intake of the stone-forming substances. In the past, surgery was frequently necessary to remove large kidney stones. More recently, medication introduced into the upper urinary tract by means of a percutaneous catheter has been used to dissolve large kidney stones into smaller pieces that pass easily (chemolysis). Lithotripsy is a technique to break up the stone using an external source of shock waves that shatter the hard stones into sand-sized particles, which are then excreted in the urine. This technique

works well for stones in the kidney or the upper ureter (above the pelvic brim). For stones in the lower ureter (in the pelvis), cystoscopic retrieval (ureteroscopy basket) or laser destruction is an option. The last resort is performing surgery because this traumatizes the patient and requires a longer recovery period.

Urinary Tract Obstruction

Urinary tract obstruction produces anatomic and functional changes that vary with regard to rapidity of onset, degree of occlusion, and distance between the kidney and the obstructing lesion. In adults, urinary calculi, pelvic tumors, urethral strictures, and enlargement of the prostate gland are the major

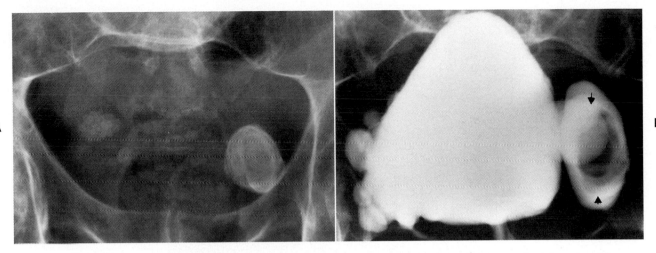

FIGURE 6-25 Bladder calculi. **A,** Plain radiograph of pelvis shows large laminated stone on the left and multiple smaller calculi on the right. **B,** Excretory urogram demonstrates large stone *(arrows)* in the bladder diverticulum on the left side. Multiple smaller calculi on the right have been obscured by overlying contrast material.

causes. In children, congenital malformations (ureteropelvic junction narrowing, ureterocele, retrocaval ureter, posterior urethral valve) are usually responsible for mechanical obstruction. Normal points of narrowing, such as the ureteropelvic and ureterovesical junctions, the bladder neck, and the urethral meatus, are common sites of obstruction. Blockage above the level of the bladder causes unilateral dilatation of the ureter **(hydroureter)** and renal pelvicalyceal system **(hydronephrosis);** if the lesion is at or below the level of the bladder, as in prostatic hypertrophy or tumor, bilateral involvement is the rule.

Radiographic Appearance

Noncontrast helical CT scanning detects mass effects, stones, or other causes of obstruction better than excretory urography. A contrast agent may be used to demonstrate renal function and the renal vascular structures if needed. In acute urinary tract obstruction, diminished filtration of urographic contrast material results in parenchymal opacification that is delayed compared with that of the nonobstructed kidney. The nephrogram eventually becomes more dense than normal because of a decreased rate of flow of fluid through the tubules, which results in enhanced water reabsorption by the nephrons and greater concentration of the contrast material (Figure 6-26). There is delayed and decreased pelvicalyceal filling because of dilatation and elevated pressure in the collecting system. The radiographic study may have to be prolonged for up to 48 hours after the administration of contrast material to determine the precise site of obstruction.

In the patient with acute urinary tract obstruction, the kidney is generally enlarged, and the calyces are moderately dilated. An uncommon but pathognomonic urographic finding in acute unilateral obstruction (usually caused by a ureteral stone) is opacification of the gallbladder 8 to 24 hours after the injection of contrast material. This "vicarious excretion" is related to increased liver excretion of contrast material that cannot be promptly excreted by the kidneys.

As an obstruction becomes more chronic, the predominant urographic finding is a greatly dilated pelvicalyceal system and ureter proximal to the obstruction (Figure 6-27). Prolonged increased pressure causes progressive papillary atrophy, leading to calyceal clubbing. Gradual enlargement of the calyces and renal pelvis with progressive destruction of renal parenchyma may continue until the kidney becomes a nonfunctioning hydronephrotic sac in which its normal anatomy is obliterated.

Whenever possible, the site of obstruction should be demonstrated. Although excretory urography with delayed films may accomplish this purpose, antegrade pyelography is often required. In this procedure, a catheter or needle is placed percutaneously into the dilated collecting system under ultrasound or fluoroscopic guidance, and contrast material is then introduced. This approach has the added advantage of providing immediate and certain decompression of a unilateral obstructing lesion.

Ultrasound is of particular value in detecting hydronephrosis in patients with such severe urinary tract obstruction and renal dysfunction that there is no opacification of the kidneys and collecting systems on excretory urograms. The dilated calyces and pelvis become large, hydronephrotic, echo-free sacs separated by septa of compressed tissue and vessels (Figure 6-28, *A*). With increased duration and severity

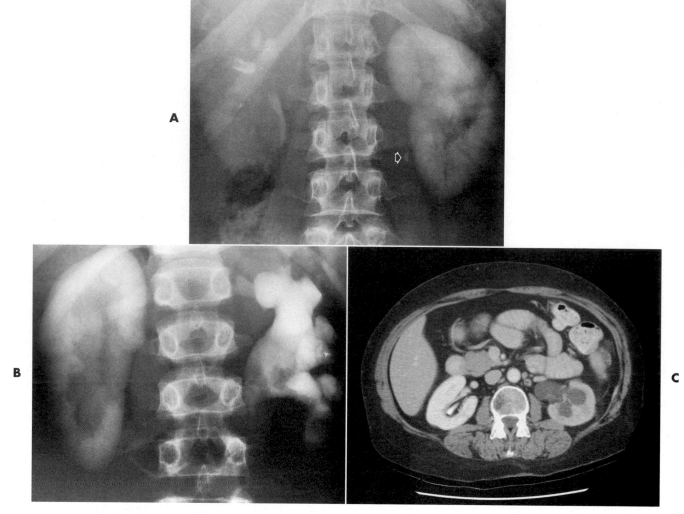

FIGURE 6-26 Urinary tract obstruction. **A,** Excretory urogram demonstrates prolonged nephrogram on the left and no calyceal filling. Arrow points to obstructing stone in the proximal left ureter. **B,** In another patient, there is a prolonged and intensified obstructive nephrogram of right kidney. On the left, there is pronounced dilatation of the pelvicalyceal system but no persistent nephrogram, reflecting intermittent chronic obstruction on this side. **C,** CT scan on a different patient shows large renal calyces, hydronephrosis, and a hydroureter on the left.

of hydronephrosis, the intervening septa may disappear, leaving a large fluid-filled sac with no evidence of internal structure and no normal parenchyma apparent at its margins (Figure 6-28, *B*).

A physiologic form of hydronephrosis often develops during pregnancy. The enlarging uterine mass and physiologic hormonal changes cause extrinsic pressure on the ureter, leading to progressive dilatation of the proximal collecting systems (Figure 6-29). Often bilateral, the dilatation usually is more prominent and develops earlier on the right side. After delivery, the urinary tract returns to normal within several weeks. In some women, however, persistent dilatation of the ovarian vein can compress the ureter and result in prolonged postpartum hydronephrosis.

Treatment

Appropriate treatment requires decompressing the urinary tract to prevent parenchymal damage and possible ureteral rupture because of the blockage. Percutaneous nephrostomy provides drainage and may help demonstrate the site of obstruction (see Figure 6-21, *C*). Once the cause of the obstruction is determined, therapy for that specific cause can be initiated.

Cysts and Tumors

Renal Cyst

Simple renal cysts are the most common unifocal masses of the kidney. They are fluid filled and usually unilocular, although septa sometimes divide the

SUMMARY of FINDINGS for Urinary Obstructions

disorder	location	radiographic appearance	treatment
Calculi	Most commonly form in the kidney	KUB—radiopaque calcium renal stones CT—demonstrates location of stone IVU—noncalcium stones cause filling defects US—demonstrates an echogenic region with acoustic shadowing	Medications to dissolve stone Lithotripsy to break up the stone Cystoscopy for retrieval or laser destruction Surgery
Obstruction	Internal or external pressure prevents normal urine flow	CT—demonstrates mass effects, stones, or other causes of obstruction IVU—dense nephrogram, delayed or decreased pelvicalyceal filling Chronic shows calyceal clubbing US—chronic hydronephrosis with echo-free sacs	Decompress urinary tract to prevent damage Percutaneous nephrostomy to demonstrate obstruction and provide drainage Treat cause of obstruction

IVU, Intravenous urography; *KUB,* kidney–ureter–bladder radiograph; *US,* ultrasound.

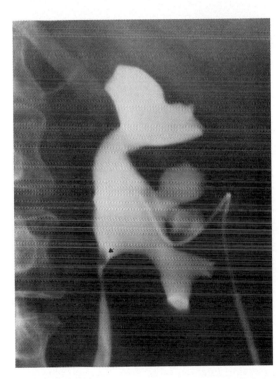

FIGURE 6-27 Hydronephrosis. Dilatation of the entire pelvicalyceal system proximal to an obstructing *Cryptococcus* fungus ball *(arrow)* at the ureteropelvic junction.

cyst into chambers, which may or may not communicate with each other. Cysts vary in size, and they may occur at single or multiple sites in one or both kidneys. Thin curvilinear calcifications can be demonstrated in the wall of about 3% of simple cysts. However, this peripheral type of calcification is not pathognomonic

of a benign process because malignant kidney lesions can produce a similar pattern.

Radiographic Appearance

As a simple renal cyst slowly increases in size, its protruding portion elevates the adjacent edges of the cortex. The cortical margin appears on nephrotomography as a very thin, smooth, radiopaque rim about the bulging lucent cyst (beak sign) (Figure 6-30). Although the beak sign is generally considered characteristic of benign renal cysts, it merely reflects a slow expansion of a mass and thus may occasionally be seen in slow-growing solid lesions, including carcinoma. Thickening of the rim about a lucent mass is suggestive of bleeding into a cyst, cyst infection, or a malignant lesion. Renal cysts cause focal displacement of adjacent portions of the pelvicalyceal system. The displaced, attenuated collecting structures remain smooth, unlike the shagginess and obliteration that often occur when focal displacement is caused by a malignant neoplasm.

Ultrasound is the modality of choice for distinguishing fluid-filled simple cysts from solid mass lesions. Fluid-filled cysts classically appear as echo-free structures with strongly enhanced posterior walls (Figure 6-31), in contrast to solid or complex lesions, such as tumors, that appear as echo-filled masses without posterior wall enhancement. CT is also highly accurate in detecting and characterizing simple renal cysts. On unenhanced scans, the cyst has a uniform attenuation value near that of water. After the injection of contrast material, a simple cyst becomes more apparent as the contrast material is concentrated by

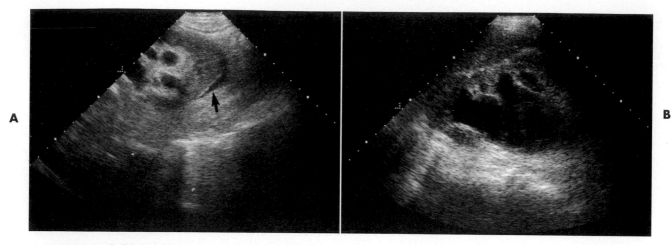

FIGURE 6-28 Hydronephrosis. Longitudinal ultrasound images demonstrating dilatation of renal collecting system appearing as echo-free sacs *(dark areas)* in this 73-year-old patient. **A,** Left kidney with perirenal fluid *(arrow)*. **B,** Right kidney demonstrates more severe dilatation.

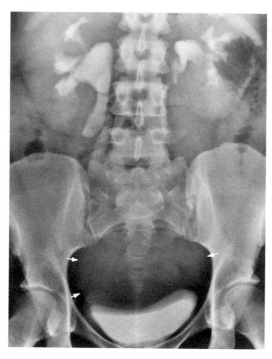

FIGURE 6-29 Hydronephrosis of pregnancy. Excretory urogram performed 3 days postpartum demonstrates bilateral large kidneys with dilatation of ureters and pelvicalyceal systems, especially on the right. The large pelvic mass *(arrows)* indenting the superior surface of the bladder represents the uterus, which is still causing extrinsic pressure on the ureters.

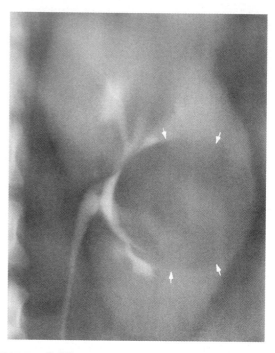

FIGURE 6-30 Renal cyst. Nephrotomogram shows smooth-walled, fluid-filled mass "beak sign" *(arrows)*.

the normal surrounding parenchyma (Figure 6-32). The cyst itself shows no change in attenuation value, unlike a solid renal neoplasm, which always shows a small but definite increase in density. Because of the accuracy of CT and ultrasound, percutaneous cyst puncture is rarely necessary if these modalities provide unequivocal evidence of a simple cyst.

However, because abscesses, cystic or necrotic tumors, and inflammatory or hemorrhagic cysts can mimic simple cysts, cyst puncture should be performed if there is an atypical appearance or a strong clinical suspicion of abscess, or if the patient has hematuria or hypertension. Fluid aspirated from a renal cyst can be clearly differentiated from that obtained from an abscess or a renal tumor. The introduction of contrast material or air after the cyst fluid has been removed demonstrates the smooth inner wall of the cyst and further decreases the possibility of missing a malignant neoplasm (Figure 6-33).

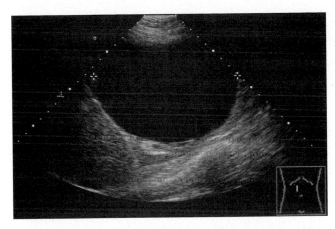

FIGURE 6-31 Huge renal cyst. Anechoic lesion (*dark round area*) with a well-defined posterior wall.

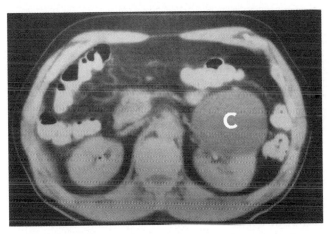

FIGURE 6-32 Renal cyst appears as a nonenhancing left renal mass (*C*) with sharply marginated border and thin wall.

Treatment
Following needle puncture, a catheter can be placed for drainage if needed. An injection of iodine or alcohol may obliterate the cyst.

Polycystic Kidney Disease
Polycystic kidney disease is an inherited disorder in which multiple cysts of varying size cause lobulated enlargement of the kidneys and progressive renal impairment, which presumably results from cystic compression of nephrons, which in turn causes localized intrarenal obstruction. One third of patients with this condition have associated cysts of the liver, which do not interfere with hepatic function. About 10% have one or more saccular (berry) aneurysms of cerebral arteries, which may rupture and produce a fatal subarachnoid hemorrhage. Many patients with polycystic disease are hypertensive, a condition that may cause further deterioration of renal function and increase the likelihood that a cerebral aneurysm will

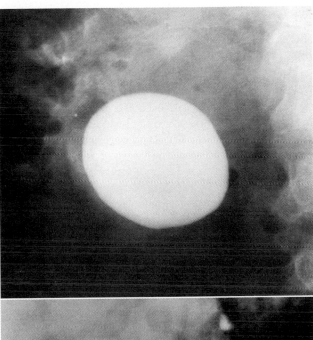

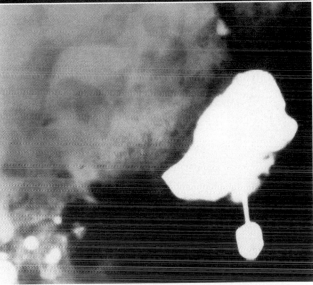

FIGURE 6-33 Renal cyst puncture. **A,** Instillation of contrast material shows a smooth inner wall characteristic of a benign cyst. **B,** In another patient, injection of contrast material reveals a highly irregular inner border of a necrotic renal cell carcinoma.

rupture. Because patients tend to be asymptomatic during the first three decades of life, early diagnosis is made either by chance or as a result of a specific search prompted by the discovery of findings in the family history.

Radiographic Appearance
Excretory urography demonstrates enlarged kidneys with a multilobulated contour. The pelvic and infundibular structures are elongated, effaced, and often displaced around larger cysts, producing a crescentic outline. The nephrogram typically has a

distinctive mottled or Swiss cheese pattern caused by the presence of innumerable lucent cysts of varying size throughout the kidneys (Figure 6-34). Plaques of calcification occasionally occur in cyst walls.

Ultrasound demonstrates grossly enlarged kidneys containing multiple cysts that vary considerably in size and are randomly distributed throughout the kidney (Figure 6-35). The renal parenchyma becomes hyperechoic because of small cysts that do not appear as fluid filled, but are large enough to cause echoes. The demonstration of similar hepatic cysts further strengthens the diagnosis. Ultrasound is also of value in screening family members of a patient known to have this hereditary disorder. In patients with bilateral kidney enlargement and poor renal function, ultrasound permits the differentiation of polycystic kidney disease from multiple solid masses.

The multiple cysts in polycystic kidney disease can also be detected on CT scans (Figure 6-36) and magnetic resonance imaging (MRI). Although most individual cysts are histologically identical to simple

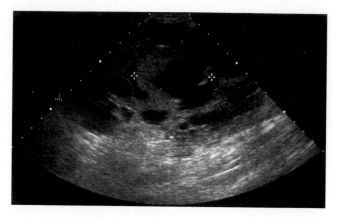

FIGURE 6-35 Polycystic kidney disease. Right kidney longitudinal ultrasound scan demonstrating multiple cysts *(dark areas)*.

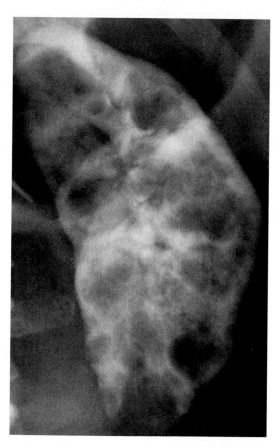

FIGURE 6-34 Polycystic kidney disease. Nephrogram phase from selective arteriography of left kidney demonstrates innumerable cysts ranging from pinhead size to 2 cm. The opposite kidney had an identical appearance.

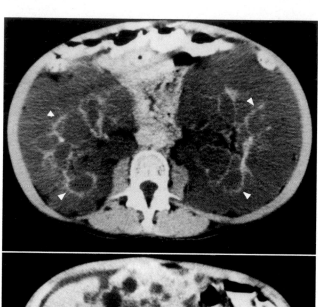

A

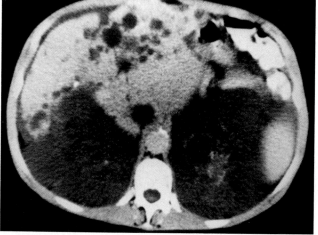

B

FIGURE 6-36 Polycystic kidney disease. **A,** CT scan shows contrast-enhancing rims *(arrowheads)* in severely thinned renal parenchyma about innumerable large renal cysts. **B,** CT scan at higher level also shows diffuse cystic involvement of liver.

cysts, intracystic hemorrhage is common. Unlike simple renal cysts, which demonstrate low attenuation on CT scan, hemorrhagic cysts have high attenuation values. On MRI, a hemorrhagic cyst has high signal intensity on both T1- and T2-weighted images, unlike simple renal cysts, which have low signal intensity on T1-weighted images.

A rare, usually fatal form of polycystic disease can present at birth; it involves diffusely enlarged kidneys, renal failure, and maldevelopment of intrahepatic bile ducts. The margins of the kidneys are smooth in infantile polycystic disease, unlike the irregular renal contours in the adult form of polycystic disease that are attributable to the protrusion of innumerable cysts from the kidney surface. When renal function is sufficient, excretory urography results in a striking nephrogram in which a streaky pattern of alternating dense and lucent bands reflects contrast material puddling in elongated cystic spaces that radiate perpendicularly to the cortical surface (Figure 6-37). Ultrasound shows distortion of the intraparenchymal architecture, although the individual cysts are too small to be visualized.

Treatment

No cure is available. Medications are prescribed to control pain, high blood pressure, and infection related to the disease. Renal failure due to the loss of functioning kidney tissue requires dialysis, and renal transplantation may be considered.

Renal Carcinoma

Renal cell carcinoma **(hypernephroma)** is the most common renal neoplasm, occurring predominantly in patients older than 40 years and often with painless hematuria. The tumor usually originates in the tubular epithelium of the renal cortex. About 10% of hypernephromas involve calcification, usually located in reactive fibrous zones about areas of tumor necrosis. In the differentiation of a solid tumor from fluid-filled benign cysts, the location of calcium within the mass is more important than the pattern of calcification. Of all masses containing calcium in a nonperipheral location, almost 90% are malignant. The classic triad of symptoms (seen in about 10% of cases) includes hematuria, flank pain, and possibly a palpable abdominal mass. Although peripheral curvilinear calcification is much more suggestive of a benign cyst, hypernephromas can have a calcified fibrous pseudocapsule that results in an identical radiographic appearance.

Radiographic Appearance

Hypernephromas typically produce urographic evidence of localized bulging or generalized renal enlargement. The tumor initially causes elongation of adjacent calyces; progressive enlargement and infiltration lead to distortion, narrowing, or obliteration of part or all of the collecting system (Figure 6-38). Large tumors may partially obstruct the pelvis or

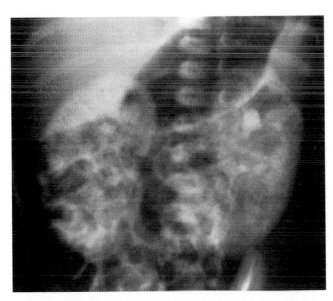

FIGURE 6-37 Infantile polycystic kidney disease. Excretory urogram in a young boy with large, palpable abdominal masses demonstrates renal enlargement with characteristic streaky densities leading to calyceal tips. There is only minimal distortion of the calyces.

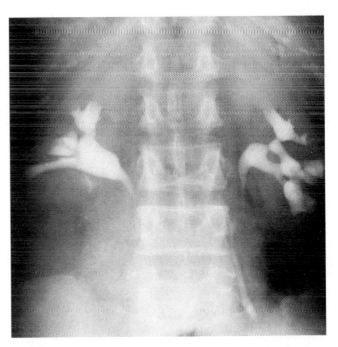

FIGURE 6-38 Renal cell carcinoma. Upward displacement of right kidney and distortion of collecting system by a large lower pole mass.

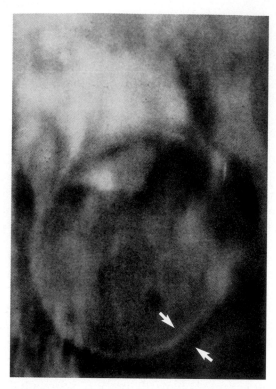

FIGURE 6-39 Renal cell carcinoma. Nephrotomogram demonstrates lucent, well-demarcated renal mass with thick wall *(arrows)*.

upper ureter and cause proximal dilatation. Complete loss of function on excretory urography usually indicates tumor invasion of the renal vein.

On nephrotomography, a hypernephroma generally appears as a mass with indistinct outlines and a density similar to that of normal parenchyma, unlike the classic radiolucent mass with sharp margins and a thin wall that represents a benign cyst. Necrotic neoplasms can also appear cystic, although they are usually surrounded by thick, irregular walls (Figure 6-39).

Ultrasound reveals a renal carcinoma as a solid mass with numerous internal echoes and no evidence of the acoustic enhancement seen with renal cysts (Figure 6-40). On unenhanced CT scans, a hypernephroma appears as a solid neoplasm that is often not homogeneous and has an attenuation value near that of normal renal parenchyma, unlike a simple cyst, which has a uniform attenuation value near that of water. After the injection of contrast material, a simple cyst shows no change in attenuation value, whereas a solid renal neoplasm demonstrates a small but definite increase in density that is probably attributable primarily to vascular perfusion. However, this increased density is much less than that of surrounding normal parenchyma, which also tends to concentrate the contrast material, and thus renal neoplasms become more apparent on contrast-enhanced scans

(Figure 6-41). Helical 3-phase CT aids in evaluation of arterial anatomy, which is of value in determining the type of treatment.

Currently, CT is considered the most accurate method for detecting local and regional spread of hypernephroma. It can usually distinguish between neoplasms confined to the renal capsule and those that have extended beyond it. CT is also the most accurate method for detecting enlargement of para-aortic, paracaval, and retrocrural lymph nodes and spread to the ipsilateral renal vein and inferior vena cava (Figure 6-42). When CT is equivocal or contrast enhancement is contraindicated, MRI can be useful.

MRI allows detailed demonstration of the renal anatomy and approaches the accuracy of CT in staging the abdominal extent of tumor in the patient with renal cell carcinoma (Figure 6-43, *A*). Advantages of MRI include its ability to determine the origin of the mass, to detect perihilar and perivascular lymph node metastases, and to demonstrate tumor invasion of adjacent organs. On T1-weighted images, the tumor appears isointense or hypointense compared with normal kidney tissue; on T2-weighted images, the tumor is usually hyperintense and heterogeneous. The superb delineation of blood vessels with MRI permits evaluation of tumor thrombus extension into the renal veins (a common occurrence) and into the inferior vena cava without the need for intravenous contrast material (Figure 6-43, *B*). MRI is only more definitive than CT if contrast enhancement cannot be used.

The most common sites of metastasis from renal cell carcinoma include the lungs, liver, bones, and brain.

Treatment
Nephrectomy, the most common treatment, is associated with a 40% survival rate. Radiation and chemotherapy are ineffective in treating renal cell carcinoma. Radiofrequency ablation is suggested for patients with bilateral lesions and those at high surgical risk.

Wilms' Tumor (Nephroblastoma)
Wilms' tumor is the most common abdominal neoplasm of infancy and childhood. The lesion arises from embryonic renal tissue, it may be bilateral, and it tends to become very large and appear as a palpable mass.

Wilms' tumor (highly malignant) must be differentiated from neuroblastoma, a tumor of adrenal medullary origin that is the second most common malignancy in children. Peripheral cystic calcification occurs in about 10% of Wilms' tumors, in contrast to the fine, granular, or stippled calcification seen in about half of the cases of neuroblastoma.

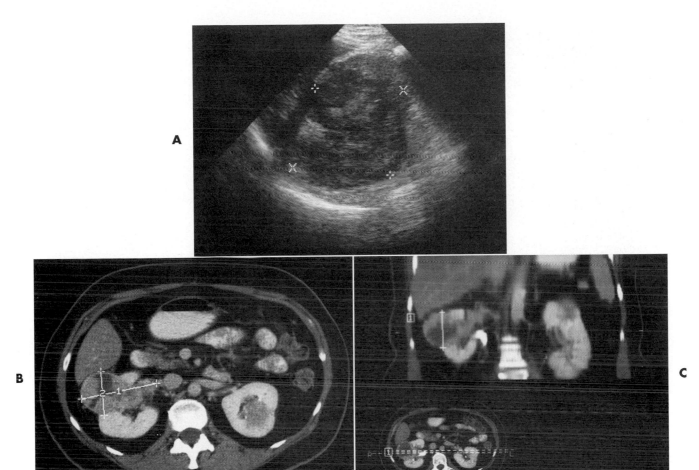

FIGURE 6-40 Renal cell carcinoma. Ultrasound image **(A)** shows a solid echo-filled mass measuring approximately 10 × 9 cm in a 55-year-old woman with hematuria. Axial **(B)** and coronal **(C)** CT images demonstrate an inhomogeneous mass in the middle pole of the right kidney. The left kidney mass in the superior pole exhibits inhomogeneous attenuation and a decreased central density, indicating areas of necrosis.

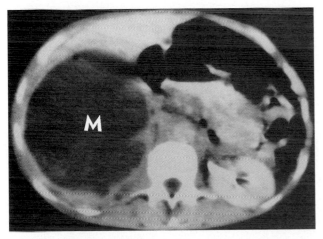

FIGURE 6-41 Necrotic renal cell carcinoma. CT image shows huge, nonenhancing, cystlike mass *(M)* with irregular margins (especially on its medial and posterior aspects).

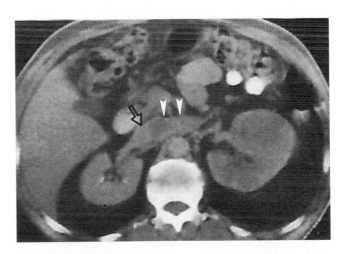

FIGURE 6-42 Renal cell carcinoma with left renal vein invasion. CT scan after administration of contrast shows dilated left renal vein filled with tumor thrombus *(arrowheads)*. The thrombus extends to the inferior vena cava *(arrow)*.

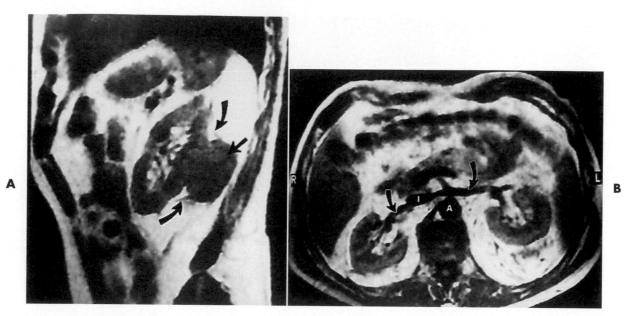

FIGURE 6-43 Renal cell carcinoma. **A,** Sagittal T1-weighted MR image through the left kidney demonstrates a large renal cell carcinoma *(straight arrow)* arising from the posterior aspect of the kidney and displacing Gerota's fascia outward *(curved arrows)*. **B,** Transverse MR image at the level of the renal veins *(arrows)* and inferior vena cava *(I)* demonstrates normal signal from flowing blood without evidence of a tumor thrombus. This modality is especially useful for staging renal cell carcinoma because of its multiplanar capability and its ability to allow assessment of vascular invasion. *A,* Aorta.

Radiographic Appearance

At excretory urography, the intrarenal Wilms' tumor causes pronounced distortion and displacement of the pelvicalyceal system (Figure 6-44). The major effect of the extrarenal neuroblastoma is to displace the entire kidney downward and laterally. Because the kidney itself is usually not invaded, there is no distortion of the pelvicalyceal system.

Ultrasound is of value in distinguishing Wilms' tumor from hydronephrosis, another major cause of a palpable renal mass in a child. Wilms' tumors typically have a solid appearance with gross distortion of the renal structure (Figure 6-45), which is not like the precise organization of symmetrically positioned fluid-filled spaces in hydronephrosis. Ultrasound can also demonstrate the intrarenal location of Wilms' tumor, which is different from the extrarenal origin of a neuroblastoma.

Although it entails the use of ionizing radiation, CT can demonstrate the full extent of the tumor (including invasion of the inferior vena cava) and can detect any recurrence of the neoplasm after surgical removal (Figure 6-46). Coronal T1-weighted MR images can accurately differentiate Wilms' tumor from renal or hepatic lesions (Figure 6-47). This is also extremely useful in defining the extent of the lesion and showing possible tumor thrombus within the renal vein or the inferior vena cava. Because MRI

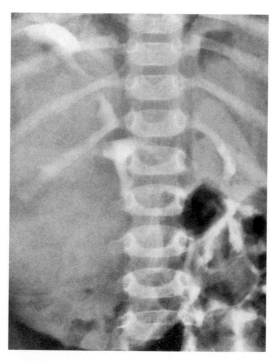

FIGURE 6-44 Wilms' tumor. Huge mass in right kidney distorts and displaces pelvicalyceal system.

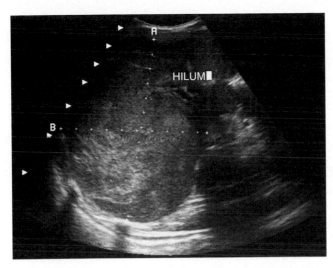

FIGURE **6-45** Wilms' tumor. Ultrasound image of the right kidney shows a large, complex mass measuring 12.6 × 9.95 cm. The kidney hilum is pushed medially.

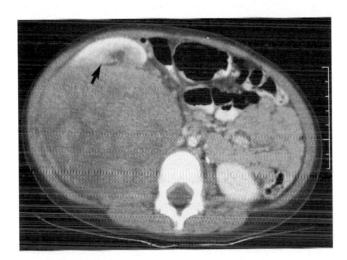

FIGURE **6-46** Wilms' tumor. CT scan of a 3-year-old child with a large nonfunctioning mass pushing the functioning right kidney anteriorly (arrow).

has no ionizing radiation, it is an ideal modality for follow-up evaluation after surgical removal of the tumor.

Treatment

Surgery, radiation therapy, and chemotherapy result in an 85% cure rate in patients with Wilms' tumor.

Carcinoma of the Bladder

Bladder carcinoma most commonly originates in the epithelium and is called urothelial carcinoma (previously known as transitional cell carcinoma). Bladder

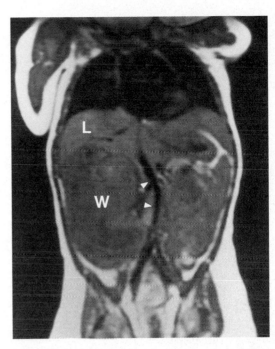

FIGURE **6-47** T1-weighted coronal MR scan shows sharply marginated infrahepatic mass (W) that is clearly distinct from the liver. The inferior vena cava (arrowheads), although displaced by the mass, shows no evidence of tumor extension into it. L, Liver.

carcinoma is usually seen in men more than 50 years of age and is the fourth most common cancer in men. Many industrial chemicals have been implicated as factors in the development of carcinoma of the bladder. Cigarette smoking has also been associated with bladder tumors, presumably because of carcinogenic metabolites being excreted in the urine. Internationally, the incidence of bladder cancer is especially high in Egypt, most likely related to the high prevalence of the parasitic infection schistosomiasis in that country.

Radiographic Appearance

Carcinoma of the bladder may produce fingerlike projections into the lumen or it may infiltrate the bladder wall. Plain radiographs may demonstrate punctate, coarse, or linear calcifications that are usually encrusted on the surface of the tumor, but occasionally lie within it. On excretory urograms, bladder cancer appears as one or more polypoid defects arising from the bladder wall or as focal bladder wall thickening (Figure 6-48). However, urography can detect only about 60% of bladder carcinomas because most are small when first symptomatic and are located on the trigone, where they can be difficult to visualize. Therefore all patients with lower urinary tract hematuria should undergo cystoscopy to exclude a bladder neoplasm.

SUMMARY of FINDINGS for Cysts and Tumors

disorder	location	radiographic appearance	treatment
Renal cyst	Renal parenchyma	US—fluid-filled cyst, echo free with enhanced posterior wall CT—region with lack of contrast enhancement IVU—radiopaque rim surrounding lucent cyst "beak sign"	Percutaneous drainage; if indicated, an injection to collapse the cyst
Polycystic kidney	Renal parenchyma	IVU—mottled presence of multiple lucent lesions US—enlarged and hyperechoic kidneys, multiple anechoic lesions CT—hemorrhagic cyst with increased attenuation MRI—hemorrhagic cyst with increased signal intensity on both T1- and T2-weighted images	No cure Loss of kidney function—dialysis and renal transplantation
Renal carcinoma	Kidney	Nephrotomogram—indistinct outlines; tumor density similar to that of normal tissue; cystic type surrounded by thick irregular walls US—solid mass with numerous internal echoes CT—solid mass with heterogeneous attenuation values that increase with contrast MRI—determines extent of involvement and staging of tumor; T1-weighted—tumor appears isointense or hypointense; the tumor is usually hyperintense and most often heterogeneous on T2-weighted images	Nephrectomy Radiofrequency ablation
Wilms' tumor	Embryonic renal tissue	IVU—kidney displacement inferiorly and laterally US—solid structure with gross distortion of the renal structure CT—tumor and extent of invasion MRI—differentiates Wilms' from other renal or hepatic tumors; demonstrates vascular involvement	Surgical removal, with chemotherapy and radiation therapy
Bladder carcinoma	Wall of bladder (epithelium)	KUB—punctate, coarse, or linear calcifications IVU—polypoid defects with wall thickening CT—mass projecting into bladder lumen, focal thickening of bladder wall MRI—predicts depth of wall invasion	Surgical removal of tumor Surgical removal of bladder and redirection of ureters into the ileum

IVU, Intravenous urography; *KUB,* kidney–ureter–bladder radiograph; *US,* ultrasound.

CT with full distention of the bladder demonstrates a neoplasm as a mass projecting into the bladder lumen or as focal thickening of the bladder wall (Figure 6-49, *A*). This modality is excellent when MRI is not available for preoperative staging because it can determine the presence and degree of extravesical extension, involvement of the pelvic sidewalls (Figure 6-49, *B*), and enlargement of pelvic or para-aortic lymph nodes.

MRI can demonstrate the depth of bladder wall invasion by showing a high signal intensity tumor disruption on T2-weighted images. The extension in the perivesical fat appears as a low signal intensity on T1-weighted images. MRI is equal to or better than CT for this purpose.

Treatment

Many carcinomas of the bladder have a low grade of malignancy, although they tend to recur repeatedly after surgical removal. More invasive tumors require removal of the entire bladder with transplantation of the ureters into a loop of ileum.

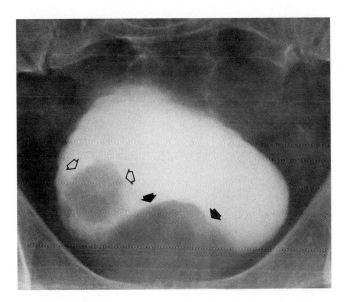

FIGURE **6-48** Bladder carcinoma. An irregular tumor *(open arrows)* is associated with a large filling defect *(solid arrows)*, representing benign prostatic hypertrophy, at the base of the bladder.

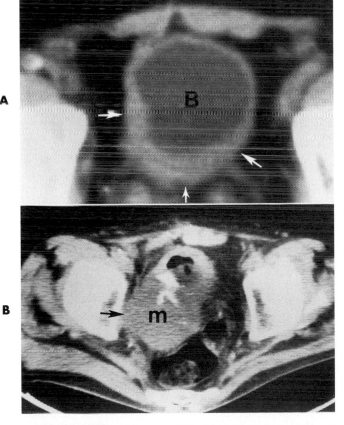

FIGURE **6-49** CT scan of bladder carcinoma. **A,** Focal thickening of the posterior wall *(arrows).* **B,** Extensive bladder cancer *(m)* has extended to involve the sidewall of the pelvis *(arrow).*

Renal Vein Thrombosis

Renal vein thrombosis occurs most frequently in children who are severely dehydrated. In the adult, thrombosis is most often a complication of another renal disease (e.g., chronic glomerulonephritis, amyloidosis, or pyelonephritis), trauma, the extension of a thrombus from the inferior vena cava, or direct invasion or extrinsic pressure resulting from renal tumors.

Radiographic Appearance

Renal vein thrombosis may be unilateral or bilateral. The clinical and radiographic findings are greatly influenced by the rapidity with which venous occlusion occurs. Sudden total occlusion causes striking kidney enlargement with minimal or no opacification on excretory urograms (Figure 6-50). If unresolved, this acute venous occlusion leads to the urographic appearance of a small, atrophic, nonfunctioning kidney.

When venous occlusion is partial or accompanied by adequate collateral formation, the kidney enlarges and appears smooth, and there is some degree of contrast excretion. The collecting system is stretched and thinned as a result of surrounding interstitial edema. Enlargement of collateral pathways (e.g., gonadal and ureteric veins) for renal venous outflow produces characteristic notching of the upper ureter.

Diagnostic ultrasound, currently the initial modality of choice, shows enlarged kidneys that have decreased echogenicity because of diffuse edema in acute renal vein thrombosis; the kidneys become increasingly atrophic as the disease slowly progresses. Doppler sonography may permit direct visualization of the clot within the renal vein. CT does not allow visualization of a clot-filled renal vein on

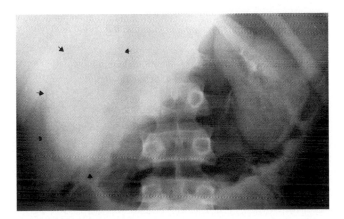

FIGURE **6-50** Acute renal vein thrombosis. Radiograph of the right kidney taken 5 minutes after injection of contrast material shows a dense nephrogram *(arrows)* and an absence of calyceal filling.

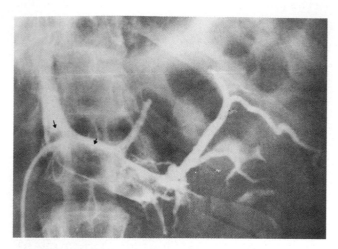

FIGURE **6-51** Renal vein thrombosis. Renal venogram demonstrates a large filling defect in the left renal vein *(arrows)* that extends into the vena cava.

contrast-enhanced images. Magnetic resonance angiography (MRA) can detect an abnormally strong signal from the renal veins, suggesting stasis (no flow) of blood. A renal vein with a slow flow caused by partial obstruction by a clot produces a lower signal. Ultrasound and MRI are the modalities used more frequently because they do not require an iodinated contrast agent to demonstrate the anatomy.

The confirmation of renal vein thrombosis requires venographic demonstration of vessel occlusion or a localized filling defect (Figure 6-51). An examination of the inferior vena cava with a catheter placed well below the renal veins is often performed initially to exclude caval thrombosis with proximal extension before the renal veins are catheterized directly.

Treatment

Anticoagulants are generally given to prevent new clots from forming. To reduce the possibility of emboli, the patient assumes bed rest and limited activity. Medications can be given intravenously or can be directly injected into the clot to lyse it. Renal vein thrombosis usually resolves without permanent damage to the kidneys.

Acute Renal Failure

Acute renal failure refers to a rapid deterioration in kidney function that is sufficient to result in the accumulation of nitrogen-containing wastes in the blood and a characteristic odor of ammonia on the breath. In prerenal failure, there is decreased blood flow to the kidneys caused by low blood volume (e.g., because of hemorrhage, dehydration, or surgical shock), cardiac failure, or obstruction of both renal arteries. Postrenal failure is caused by obstruction of the urine outflow

from both kidneys, most commonly a result of prostatic disease or functional obstruction of the bladder neck. Acute renal failure may also be the result of specific kidney diseases, such as glomerulonephritis, bilateral acute pyelonephritis, and malignant (severe) hypertension. Other causes of acute renal failure include nephrotoxic agents (antibiotics, radiographic contrast material, anesthetic agents, heavy metals, organic solvents), intravascular hemolysis, and large amounts of myoglobin (muscle protein) in the circulation resulting from muscle trauma or ischemia. Urine output may decrease to less than 400 ml per 24-hour period (oliguria).

Radiographic Appearance

Because it is independent of renal function, ultrasound is especially useful in the evaluation of patients with acute renal failure. In addition to demonstrating dilatation of the ureters and pelves caused by postobstructive hypernephrosis, ultrasound can assess renal size and the presence of focal kidney lesions or diffuse renal cystic disease. In the patient with prerenal failure, ultrasound can aid in distinguishing low blood volume from right-sided heart failure. In the latter, there is dilatation of the inferior vena cava and hepatic veins that does not occur in patients with low circulating blood volume.

Conventional tomography can often demonstrate renal size and contours. Bilaterally enlarged, smooth kidneys are suggestive of acute renal parenchymal dysfunction; small kidneys usually indicate chronic, preexisting renal disease. Plain film tomograms can also demonstrate bilateral renal calcification, which may indicate either secondary hyperparathyroidism caused by chronic renal disease or bilateral stones that have obstructed both ureters to produce postrenal failure.

Excretory urography in the patient with acute renal failure demonstrates bilateral renal enlargement with a delayed and prolonged nephrogram (Figure 6-52); vicarious excretion of contrast material by the liver occasionally results in opacification of the gallbladder. However, in most instances excretory urography is unnecessary in the patient with acute renal failure, especially as many authors believe that intravenous contrast material can cause further damage to the kidneys in this condition.

Sonography is the modality of choice because it does not require the use of intravenous contrast agents. Ultrasound can assess renal size, identify renal parenchymal disease, and exclude hydronephrosis. Renal parenchymal disease appears as a diffuse increase in echogenicity, with loss of corticomedullary differentiation. If a vascular cause is suggested clinically, color Doppler studies allow visualization of

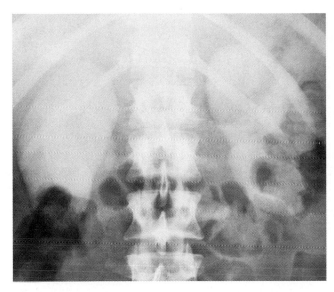

FIGURE **6-52** Acute renal failure. Excretory urogram 20 minutes after injection of contrast material shows bilateral persistent nephrograms with no calyceal filling.

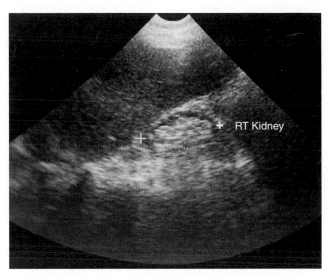

FIGURE **6-53** Ultrasound of patient with chronic renal failure. The right kidney is very small, measuring less than 6 cm, which suggests irreversible end-stage renal disease.

patency or occlusion. If this is unsuccessful, a radionuclide scan or an MRI study may show these vessels without the use of an intravenous contrast agent.

Treatment

Treatment of predisposing conditions reduces the risk of acute renal failure becoming chronic or continued. Some physicians use diuretics to increase urine flow, and vasodilators to increase renal blood flow to help prevent the likelihood of more severe renal failure. Dietary modifications, including decreasing potassium and protein intake and increasing carbohydrates, can decrease the load on the kidneys. Antibiotics may be used to prevent or treat infections because of the high associated risk of sepsis with renal failure. In some cases, renal dialysis provides time for the kidneys to recover.

Chronic Renal Failure

Like acute renal failure, chronic kidney dysfunction may reflect prerenal, postrenal, or intrinsic kidney disease. Therefore, underlying causes of chronic renal failure include bilateral renal artery stenosis, bilateral ureteral obstruction, and intrinsic renal disorders, such as chronic glomerulonephritis, pyelonephritis, and familial cystic diseases.

A failure to clear nitrogen-containing wastes adequately from the circulation leads to the accumulation of excessive blood levels of urea and creatinine (waste products of protein metabolism) in the blood. This condition, called **uremia,** produces toxic effects on many body systems. Irritation of the gastrointestinal tract produces nausea, vomiting, and diarrhea. In the nervous system, uremia causes drowsiness, dim vision, decreased mental ability, convulsions, and eventually coma. A decreased ability of the kidney to synthesize erythropoietin, which helps regulate the production of red blood cells, leads to the development of anemia. In the skin, uremia causes intense itching (pruritus) and a sallow (yellowish) coloring resulting from the combined effects of anemia and retention of a variety of pigmented metabolites (urochromes).

Because of the kidney's role in maintaining water balance and regulating acid-base balance and electrolyte levels, chronic renal failure causes abnormalities involving all these vital functions. Retention of sodium leads to increased water retention and the development of generalized edema and congestive heart failure. An elevated serum potassium level is potentially life threatening because of its direct effect on cardiac muscle contractility and the possibility of causing an arrhythmia or cardiac arrest. A reduction of serum calcium can produce the muscle twitching commonly seen in uremic patients. Low calcium levels also lead to increased activity of the parathyroid glands, which results in the removal of calcium from bones and a high incidence of renal stones.

Radiographic Appearance

Because it is independent of renal function, ultrasound is most often the initial procedure in the evaluation of patients with chronic renal failure and demonstrates a small echogenic kidney (Figure 6-53). It is of special value in diagnosing treatable diseases,

SUMMARY of FINDINGS for Renal Disorders

disorder	location	radiographic appearance	treatment
Renal vein thrombosis	Renal vein	IVU—kidney enlarged, appearing smooth with some contrast excretion; collecting system stretches and thins; notching of upper ureter US—acute: enlarged kidneys; chronic: atrophic kidneys with increased echogenicity Doppler—visualization of clot MRA—abnormally high signal intensity, suggesting stasis	Prevention of new clots—anticoagulants Bed rest and limited activity to reduce risk of clot travel Medications to lyse clot Usually resolves without permanent injury
Acute renal failure	Nephron function	Tomography—acute: enlarged smooth kidneys; chronic: small kidneys IVU—delayed and prolonged nephrogram US—renal size, identify parenchymal disease, and exclude hydronephrosis	Prevention—treat predisposing conditions Drug and dietary intervention Short-term dialysis
Chronic renal failure	Renal parenchyma	US—small echogenic kidney size, lesions, and cysts; hydronephrosis, intrarenal or perirenal infections	Slow destructive process Correct fluid imbalances Dialysis and transplantation

IVU, Intravenous urography; *US*, ultrasound.

such as hydronephrosis and intrarenal or perirenal infections. This modality can also allow assessment of renal size and the presence of focal kidney lesions or diffuse renal cystic disease, and it can be used to localize the kidneys for percutaneous renal biopsy.

Even in patients with chronic renal failure and uremia, excretory urography with tomography may produce sufficient opacification of the kidneys to be of diagnostic value. However, excretory urography is infrequently required because similar information can be provided by ultrasound or retrograde pyelography. An initial plain abdominal radiograph may demonstrate bilateral renal calcifications (nephrocalcinosis) or obstructing ureteral stones (see Figure 6-23). Small kidneys with smooth contours are suggestive of chronic glomerulonephritis (see Figure 6-10), nephrosclerosis, or bilateral renal artery stenosis. Small kidneys with irregular contours, thin cortices, and typical clubbing of the calyces are consistent with chronic pyelonephritis (see Figure 6-11). Large kidneys are suggestive of obstructive disease, infiltrative processes (lymphoma, myeloma, amyloidosis), renal vein thrombosis (see Figure 6-50), or polycystic kidney disease (see Figure 6-35).

Treatment

The initial goal of treatment is to slow the nephron loss and minimize complications. Antihypertensive drugs assist in preventing the continuation of this process. It is essential to properly balance intake and output of fluids and electrolyte levels. The inevitable occurrence of kidney failure requires dialysis to maintain the balance of body fluids. At this point, kidney transplant may be suggested.

REVIEW QUESTIONS

1. The imaging criteria for pyelography are the same as for an abdominal radiograph, but must include the area from the _____ to include the _____.
   A. diaphragm; kidneys
   B. kidneys; pelvis
   C. kidneys; superior pubis
   D. diaphragm; inferior bladder

2. What organ of the body plays an essential role in maintaining the acid-base balance of the blood and body fluids, and also the electrolyte balance?
   A. nephron
   B. glomerulus
   C. bladder
   D. kidney

3. A bacterial inflammation of the kidney and renal pelvis is termed _____.
   A. renitis
   B. pyelonephritis
   C. glomerulitis
   D. none of the above

4. The medical term used to describe dilated calyces and renal pelvis is _____.
   A. hydronephrosis
   B. pyelonephritis
   C. nephrosis
   D. none of the above

5. What is the name for the most common abdominal neoplasm of infants and children?
   A. polycystic disease
   B. pyelonephritis
   C. Wilms' tumor
   D. hypernephroma

6. What is the name of the most common fusion anomaly of the kidneys?
   A. complete fusion
   B. crossed ectopia
   C. pelvic kidney
   D. horseshoe kidney

7. What is the name for a cystic dilatation of the distal ureter near the bladder?
   A. compensatory hypertrophy
   B. renal agenesis
   C. ureterocele
   D. hypoplasty

8. Name the first portion of the kidney to become visible after injection of a contrast agent.
   A. nephron
   B. glomerulus
   C. Bowman's capsule
   D. calyces

9. What term is used to describe a kidney not in the normal area of the abdomen?
   A. horseshoe
   B. duplex
   C. ectopic
   D. ectopic ureterocele

10. The medical term for painful urination is _____.
    A. dysuria
    B. anuria
    C. micturition
    D. exacerbation

BIBLIOGRAPHY

Burgener FA, Kormano M: *Differential diagnosis in computed tomography*, New York, 1996, Thieme.

Davidson AJ: *Radiology of the kidney*, Philadelphia, 1985, Saunders.

eMedicine Specialties>Radiology>Genitourinary: emedicine.com

Pollack HM: *Clinical urography: an atlas and textbook of urological imaging*, Philadelphia, 1990, Saunders.

Rumack CM, Wilson SR, Charborneau JW: *Diagnostic ultrasound*, St Louis, 2005, Mosby.

CARDIOVASCULAR
System

Chapter Outline

Key Terms

aortic valve
atrial septal defect
coeur en sabot
diastole
ectopic pacemakers
Eisenmenger's syndrome
embolus
fibromuscular dysplasia
fusiform aneurysm
insufficiency
intrinsic rhythm
left-to-right shunts
mitral valve (bicuspid valve)
myocardial infarction

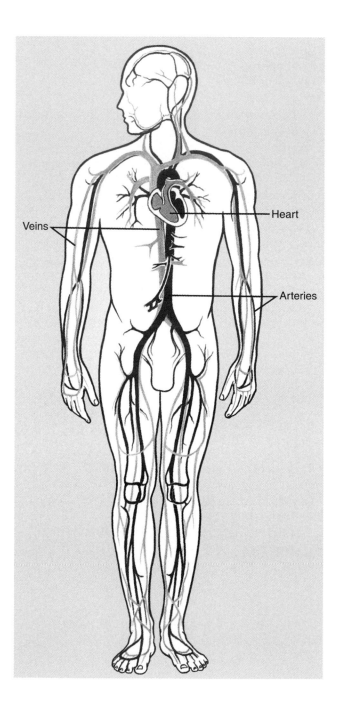

Veins — Heart

Arteries

patent ductus arteriosus	saccular aneurysm	thrombus
pericardium	stenosis	tricuspid valve
pulmonary valve	systemic circulation	vegetations
right-to-left shunting	systole	ventricular septal defect

Prerequisite Knowledge

The student should have a basic knowledge of the anatomy and physiology of the cardiovascular system. In addition, proper learning and understanding of the material will be facilitated if the student has some clinical experience in chest radiography and image evaluation, including a concept of the changes in technique required to compensate for density differences produced by the underlying pathologic conditions. Experience in a cardiac or a vascular catheterization laboratory would be beneficial.

Goals

To acquaint the student radiographer with the pathophysiology and radiographic manifestations of all of the common and some of the unusual disorders of the cardiovascular system.

Objectives

After reading this chapter, the reader will be able to:
1. Define all key terms in this chapter
2. Describe the physiology of the cardiovascular system
3. Identify anatomic structures on both diagrams and radiographs of the cardiovascular system
4. Differentiate the various pathologic conditions affecting the cardiovascular system and their radiographic manifestations
5. Provide a description of the special procedures that are used when imaging particular pathologic conditions

Physiology of the Cardiovascular System

The function of the cardiovascular system is to maintain an adequate supply of blood to all the tissues of the body. This is accomplished by the rhythmic contractions of the heart, the rate of which is controlled by the autonomic nervous system. The vagus nerve slows heart action by transmitting the chemical acetylcholine, whereas the sympathetic nervous system stimulates the release of epinephrine that accelerates the heart rate and increases the force of its contractions.

The heart consists of four chambers whose walls are composed of striated muscle (myocardium), and it is lined with a smooth delicate membrane (endocardium), which is continuous with the inner surface of the blood vessels. The heart consists of two atria and two ventricles, with a partition (the septum) separating the right and left sides of the heart. The ventricles are considerably larger and thicker walled than the atria because they have a substantially heavier pumping load. Between each atrium and its associated ventricle are the atrioventricular valves (one on the right and one on the left side of the heart), which permit blood to flow in only one direction. These valves consist of flaps (or cusps) of endocardium that are anchored to the papillary muscles of the ventricles by cordlike structures called the chordae tendineae. The **mitral valve (bicuspid valve)** (left atrioventricular) between the left atrium and the left ventricle has two cusps, whereas the **tricuspid valve** (right atrioventricular) between the right atrium and the right ventricle has three cusps. The semilunar valves separate the ventricles from the great vessels leaving the heart. The **pulmonary valve** lies between the right ventricle and the pulmonary artery, whereas the **aortic valve** separates the aorta from the left ventricle.

Deoxygenated venous blood is returned to the heart from the body through the superior and inferior venae cavae, which empty into the right atrium. Blood flows from the right atrium across the tricuspid valve into the right ventricle, which then pumps blood through the pulmonary valve into the pulmonary artery. Within the capillaries of the lungs, the red blood cells take up oxygen and release carbon dioxide. The freshly oxygenated blood then passes through the pulmonary veins into the left atrium, from which it flows across the mitral valve into the left ventricle. Contraction of the left ventricle forces oxygenated blood through the aortic valve into the aorta and the rest of the arterial tree to provide oxygen and nourishment to tissues throughout the body. The general circulation of the body is termed the **systemic circulation,** whereas the circulation of blood through the lungs is the pulmonary circulation. Because greater pressure is needed to pump blood through the systemic circulation than through the pulmonary circulation, the wall of the left ventricle is considerably thicker than that of the right ventricle.

RADIOGRAPHER *Notes*

Plain chest radiography and fluoroscopy of the cardiovascular system are used to identify abnormalities in the size and shape of the heart and to detect calcification of heart valves, coronary arteries, or the pericardium. The presence and extent of functional disorders are better demonstrated using angiography, computed tomography (CT), ultrasound, radionuclide imaging, and magnetic resonance imaging (MRI).

As for all chest radiographs, it is essential that the radiographer perform cardiovascular studies with the patient positioned correctly and using proper technical factors. To this end, it would be helpful for the reader to review the radiographer notes at the beginning of the chapter on the respiratory system. An abnormality identified on a chest radiograph may be the first evidence of cardiovascular disease in an asymptomatic patient.

Radiographers can specialize in invasive diagnostic and therapeutic cardiovascular procedures, gain advanced certification in cardiovascular interventional technology, and be employed by cardiac or vascular catheterization laboratories. Angiocardiography is a diagnostic procedure performed to identify the exact anatomic location of an intracardiac disorder. Coronary angioplasty is a therapeutic procedure in which a narrowed coronary artery is dilated by inflation of a balloon, which is attached to a catheter and manipulated fluoroscopically to the site of the stenosis. Because both angiocardiography and angioplasty involve the use of contrast material in patients who often have severe preexisting medical conditions, it is essential that the radiographer be always alert to the possibility of cardiac or respiratory arrest and be prepared to immediately assist with basic and advanced life support.

The injection of contrast material into arteries (arteriograms) and veins (venograms) can be performed in almost any portion of the body. As in the heart, these invasive studies use potentially dangerous substances, so the radiographer must be alert for possible complications and be prepared to assist in cardiorespiratory emergencies. In addition, these examinations require that the radiographer be trained in sterile technique, be able to use specialty equipment, and be familiar with the various types of catheters that are inserted into the vascular system for the delivery of contrast material.

Ultrasound, Doppler ultrasound, CT, and MRI are quickly becoming preferred initial modalities in imaging the vascular system.

The atria and ventricles alternately contract and relax. The contraction phase is called **systole;** the heart chambers relax and fill with blood during **diastole** (the relaxation phase). The normal cardiac impulse that stimulates mechanical contraction of the heart arises in the sinoatrial (SA) node, or pacemaker, which is situated in the right atrial wall near the opening of the superior vena cava. The impulse passes slowly through the atrioventricular (AV) node, which is located in the right atrium along the lower portion of the interatrial septum, and then spreads quickly throughout the ventricles by way of the fibrous bundle of His. The bundle of His terminates in Purkinje's fibers that can conduct impulses throughout the muscle of both ventricles and stimulate them to contract almost simultaneously. Specialized pacemaker cells in the SA node possess an **intrinsic rhythm,** so that even without any stimulation by the autonomic nervous system the node itself initiates impulses at regular intervals (about 70 to 75 beats per minute).

If the SA node for some reason is unable to generate an impulse, pacemaker activity shifts to another excitable component of the conduction system. These **ectopic pacemakers** also generate impulses rhythmically, although at a much slower rate. For example, if the AV node were to control pacemaker activity, the heart would beat 40 to 60 times per minute. If the conduction system of the heart is unable to maintain an adequate rhythm, the patient may receive an artificial pacemaker that electrically stimulates the heart, either at a set rhythm or only when the heart rate decreases below a preset minimum.

The heart muscle is supplied with oxygenated arterial blood by way of the right and left coronary arteries. These small vessels arise from the aorta just above the aortic valve. Unoxygenated blood from the myocardium drains into the coronary veins, which lead into the coronary sinus before opening into the right atrium.

The heart is surrounded by a double membranous sac termed the **pericardium**. The pericardium has a well-lubricated lining that protects against friction and permits the heart to move easily during contraction.

Congenital Heart Disease

Left-to-Right Shunts

The most common congenital cardiac lesions are **left-to-right shunts**, which permit mixing of blood in the systemic and pulmonary circulations. Because blood is preferentially shunted from the high-pressure systemic circulation to the relatively low-pressure pulmonary circulation, the lungs become overloaded with blood. The magnitude of the shunt depends on the size of the defect and the differences in pressure on both sides. An increased load on the heart produces enlargement of specific cardiac chambers, depending on the location of the shunt. The size of the defect will determine the hemodynamic consequence on the systemic cardiac output.

The most common congenital cardiac lesion is **atrial septal defect,** which permits free communication between the two atria as a result of the lack of closure of the foramen ovale after birth or of improper closure during gestation. Because the left atrial pressure is usually higher than the pressure in the right atrium, the resulting shunt is from left to right and causes increased pulmonary blood flow and overloading of the right ventricle. This produces the radiographic appearance of enlargement of the right ventricle, the right atrium, and the pulmonary outflow tract (Figure 7-1).

In a patient with a **ventricular septal defect,** the resulting shunt is also from left to right because the left ventricular pressure is usually higher than the pressure in the right ventricle. The shunt causes increased pulmonary blood flow and consequently increased pulmonary venous return (Figure 7-2). This leads to diastolic overloading and enlargement of the left atrium and left ventricle. Because shunting occurs primarily in systole and any blood directed to the right ventricle immediately goes into the pulmonary artery, there is no overloading of the right ventricle and radiographically no right ventricular enlargement is seen.

The third major type of left-to-right shunt is **patent ductus arteriosus.** The ductus arteriosus is a vessel that extends from the bifurcation of the pulmonary artery to join the aorta just distal to the left subclavian artery. It serves to shunt blood from the pulmonary artery into the systemic circulation during intrauterine life. Persistence of the ductus arteriosus, which normally closes soon after birth, results in a left-to-right shunt. The flow of blood from the higher pressure aorta to the lower pressure pulmonary artery causes increased pulmonary blood flow, and an excess volume of blood is returned to the left atrium and left ventricle. Radiographically, there is enlargement of the left atrium, the left ventricle, and the central pulmonary arteries,

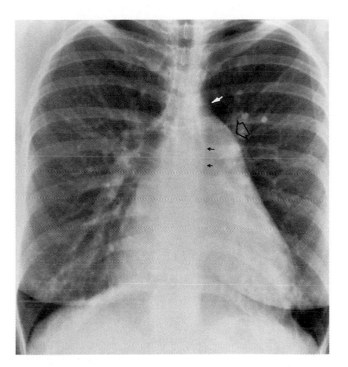

FIGURE 7-1 Atrial septal defect. Frontal projection of the chest demonstrates cardiomegaly along with an increase in pulmonary vascularity reflecting a left-to-right shunt. Small aortic knob *(white arrow)* and descending aorta *(small arrows)* are dwarfed by enlarged pulmonary outflow tract *(open arrow).*

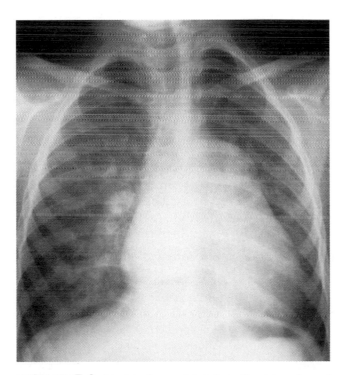

FIGURE 7-2 Ventricular septal defect. Heart is enlarged and somewhat triangular, and there is increased pulmonary vascular volume. Pulmonary trunk is very large and overshadows normal-sized aorta, which seems small by comparison.

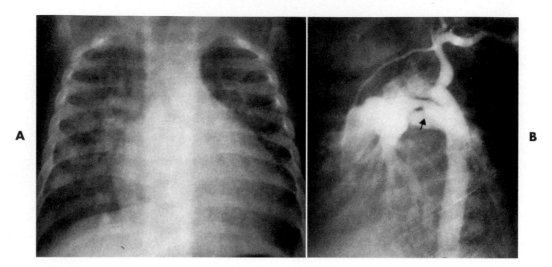

FIGURE 7-3 Patent ductus arteriosus. **A,** Frontal chest radiograph demonstrates cardiomegaly with enlargement of left atrium, left ventricle, and central pulmonary arteries. There is diffuse increase in pulmonary vascularity. **B,** In another patient, aortogram shows patency of ductus arteriosus *(arrow)*.

along with a diffuse increase in pulmonary vascularity (Figure 7-3). The increased blood flow through the aorta proximal to the shunt produces a prominent aortic knob in contrast to the small- or normal-size aorta seen in atrial and ventricular septal defects.

All left-to-right shunts can be complicated by the development of pulmonary hypertension **(Eisenmenger's syndrome)**. This is caused by increased vascular resistance within the pulmonary arteries related to chronic increased flow through the pulmonary circulation. Pulmonary hypertension appears radiographically as an increased fullness of the central pulmonary arteries with abrupt narrowing and pruning of peripheral vessels (Figure 7-4). The elevation of pulmonary arterial pressure tends to balance or even reverse the left-to-right shunt, thus easing the volume overloading of the heart.

Radiographic Appearance

Chest radiographs provide an initial assessment of pulmonary vasculature, size of the main pulmonary arteries, size and position of the aorta, and size and contour of the cardiac silhouette. In the preceding paragraphs, specific descriptions appear with each septal defect.

Doppler echocardiography can identify atrial and ventricular defects and extent of blood flow to determine the severity of the left-to-right shunting (Figure 7-5). Pressures can be measured to determine cardiac output from both the atria and ventricles. Dilatation of the ventricles implies patent ductus arteriosus.

Spin-echo MRI breath-hold magnetic resonance angiography (MRA), and cine studies are being used for imaging in cases in which sonography is not diagnostic or feasible to demonstrate the congenital heart disease. MRI demonstrates both the morphologic

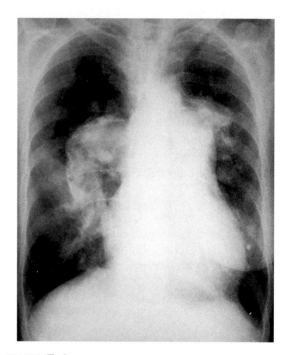

FIGURE 7-4 Eisenmenger's syndrome in atrial septal defect. There is slight but definite cardiomegaly and great increase in size of the pulmonary trunk. Right and left pulmonary artery branches are huge, but peripheral pulmonary vasculature is relatively sparse. Long-standing pulmonary hypertension has produced degenerative changes in the walls of the pulmonary arteries, which have become densely calcified.

and the functional anomalies in multiple planes. Patent ductus arteriosus appears as a signal loss on cine MRA images.

Angiocardiography is the most definitive imaging technique for demonstrating the atria and ventricles of the heart, but it is also the most invasive.

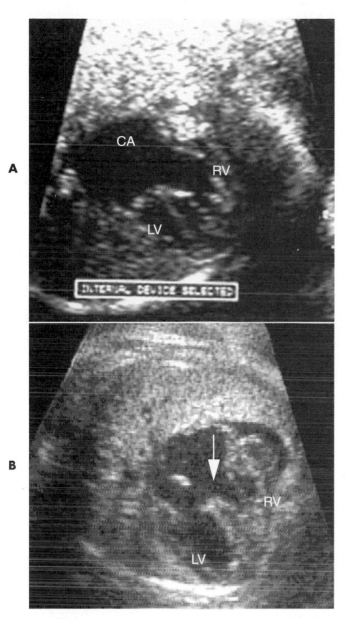

FIGURE 7-5 Atrial septal defect and ventricular septal defect. **A,** Right (RV) and left (LV) ventricles are demonstrated with a common atrium (CA). **B,** Right (RV) and left (LV) ventricle is seen without septal closure (arrow), allowing shunting of the blood.

Treatment

Small defects may not require treatment and may spontaneously close. The use of prostaglandin synthetase inhibitors may achieve closure. Surgery may be necessary to correct a large defect.

Tetralogy of Fallot

Tetralogy of Fallot is the most common cause of cyanotic congenital heart disease. It consists of four (thus "tetra") abnormalities: (1) high ventricular septal defect, (2) pulmonary stenosis, (3) overriding of

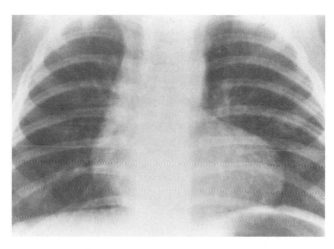

FIGURE 7-6 Tetralogy of Fallot. Plain chest radiograph demonstrates characteristic lateral displacement and upward tilting of prominent cardiac apex. There is also decreased pulmonary vascularity and flat pulmonary outflow tract.

the aortic orifice above the ventricular defect, and (4) right ventricular hypertrophy. Pulmonary stenosis causes an elevation of pressure in the right ventricle and hypertrophy of that chamber. Because of the narrow opening of the pulmonary valve, an inadequate amount of blood reaches the lungs to be oxygenated. The ventricular septal defect and the overriding of the aorta produce **right-to-left shunting** of unoxygenated venous blood into the left ventricle and then into the systemic circulation, thus increasing the degree of cyanosis.

Radiographic Appearance

Enlargement of the right ventricle causes upward and lateral displacement of the apex of the heart (Figure 7-6). This results in the classic **coeur en sabot** appearance resembling the curved-toe portion of a wooden shoe. In about one fourth of patients with tetralogy of Fallot, the aorta is on the right side.

Currently, echocardiography is the modality of choice to demonstrate the four abnormalities comprising tetralogy of Fallot. Spin-echo MRI best demonstrates the ventricular septal defect, right ventricular outflow (pulmonary stenosis), overriding aorta, and right ventricular hypertrophy. Cine MRI demonstrates pulmonary stenosis as a flow void. For this type of lesion, cine MRI demonstrates it better than echocardiography.

Treatment

Without surgical repair, most patients die before reaching puberty. Although operative repair provides some chance of recovery, the outcome depends on the severity of the defect and other extenuating circumstances. In some cases, surgery provides only a palliative supportive role.

Coarctation of the Aorta

Coarctation refers to a narrowing, or constriction, of the aorta that most commonly occurs just beyond the branching of the blood vessels to the head and arms. The blood supply and the pressure to the upper extremities are higher than normal. As a result, there is decreased blood flow through the constricted area to the abdomen and legs. Classically the patient has normal blood pressure in the arms, but very low blood pressure in the legs.

The relative obstruction of aortic blood flow leads to the progressive development of collateral circulation—the enlargement of normally tiny vessels in an attempt to compensate for the inadequate blood supply to the lower portion of the body.

Radiographic Appearance

Coarctation of the aorta is often seen radiographically as rib notching (usually involving the posterior fourth to eighth ribs) resulting from pressure erosion by dilated and pulsating intercostal collateral vessels, which run along the inferior margins of these ribs (Figure 7-7, *A*). Notching of the posterior border of the sternum may be produced by dilation of mammary artery collaterals.

Coarctation of the aorta often causes two bulges in the region of the aortic knob that produce a characteristic figure-3 sign on plain chest radiographs (see Figure 7-7, *B*) and a reverse figure-3 (or figure-E)

SUMMARY *of* FINDINGS *for* Congenital Heart Disease

disorder	location	radiographic appearance	treatment
Atrial septal defect	Communication between atria	PA chest—enlarged right ventricle, right atrium, and pulmonary outflow tract	Small defects may spontaneously close and not require treatment Medical treatment to achieve closure Large defects require surgical repair
Ventricular septal defect	Communication between ventricles	PA chest—pulmonary trunk enlargement No right ventricular enlargement	
Patent ductus arteriosus	Vascular connection between pulmonary artery and aorta	PA chest—enlargement of left atrium, left ventricle, and pulmonary arteries with an increase in pulmonary vascularity MRI—spin-echo MRA breath-hold and cine—to investigate morphologic and functional anomalies when US is not feasible or not diagnostic US—atrial defect has a common atria; ventricular defect demonstrates lack of septal closure	
Tetralogy of Fallot	High ventricular septal defect Pulmonary stenosis Overriding of the aortic orifice above the ventricular defect Right ventricular hypertrophy	PA chest—enlarged right ventricle causes upward and lateral displacement of the heart apex Echocardiography—demonstrates the four abnormalities of the disease MRI—demonstrates the morphologic conditions • spin-echo scans to identify abnormalities • cine to demonstrate flow void in pulmonary stenosis	Operative repair
Coarctation of the aorta	Constriction of aorta at the distal arch	PA chest—rib notching, "figure 3" Barium-filled esophagus—"reverse figure 3" or "figure E" Echocardiography—demonstrates the severity of stricture Doppler echo—determines flow gradient and possible collateral vessels Aortography—localizes obstruction, determines length of coarctation, and identifies an associated malformation MRI—demonstrates narrowing; used for follow-up of corrective surgery	Surgical repair

US, Ultrasound.

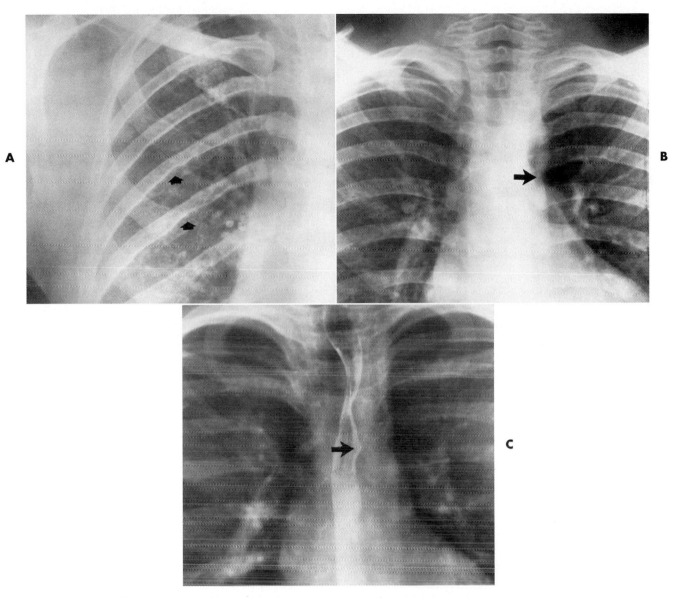

FIGURE **7-7** Coarctation of the aorta. **A,** There is notching of the fourth through eighth posterior ribs *(arrows)*. **B,** Plain chest radiograph demonstrates a figure-3 sign *(arrow pointing to its center)*. Upper bulge represents prestenotic dilatation; lower bulge represents poststenotic dilatation. **C,** Esophagram demonstrates reverse figure-3 sign *(arrow pointing to its center)*.

impression on the barium-filled esophagus (see Figure 7-7, *C*). The more cephalic bulge represents dilatation of the proximal aorta and the base of the subclavian artery (prestenotic dilatation); the lower bulge reflects poststenotic aortic dilatation.

Using echocardiography to evaluate the aortic arch, the severity of the coarctation can be determined. Doppler echocardiography measures the gradient flow at the stenosis, and the diastolic runoff can be demonstrated.

Aortography can accurately localize the site of obstruction, determine the length of the coarctation, and identify any associated cardiac malformations. More recently, MRI has been used to demonstrate aortic narrowing (Figure 7-8) and to evaluate the appearance of the aorta after corrective surgery.

Treatment

Uncorrected aortic coarctation has a dismal prognosis, and surgical repair is required for patient survival. Currently, three surgical repairs are being used: (1) end-to-end anastomosis, (2) patch aortoplasty, and (3) left subclavian flap aortoplasty (surgical reformation of the aorta).

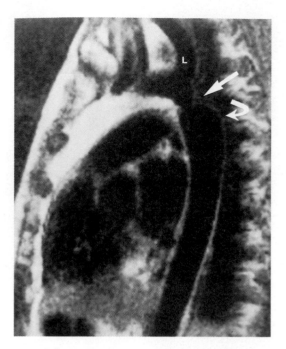

FIGURE 7-8 Coarctation of the aorta. Sagittal MR image demonstrates coarctation *(straight arrow)* of thoracic aorta with associated poststenotic dilatation of proximal descending thoracic aorta *(curved arrow). L,* Left subclavian artery.

Acquired Vascular Disease

Coronary Artery Disease

Narrowing of the coronary arteries causes oxygen deprivation of the myocardium and ischemic heart disease. In most patients, narrowing of the lumen of one or more of the coronary arteries is attributable to the deposition of fatty material on the inner arterial wall (atherosclerosis). Factors predisposing to the development of coronary artery disease include hypertension, obesity, smoking, a high-cholesterol diet, and lack of exercise.

The speed and degree of luminal narrowing determine whether an atherosclerotic lesion causes significant and clinically evident ischemia. Temporary oxygen insufficiency causes angina pectoris, a feeling of severe chest pain that may radiate to the neck, jaw, and left arm and is often associated with the sensation of chest tightness or suffocation. Attacks of angina pectoris are often related to a sudden increase in the demand of the myocardium for oxygen, as after strenuous exercise, a heavy meal, emotional stress, or exposure to severe cold. The placing of a nitroglycerin tablet under the tongue causes venous dilatation thus decreasing preload and myocardial oxygen demand.

Occlusion of a coronary artery deprives an area of myocardium of its blood supply and leads to the death of muscle cells **(myocardial infarction)** in the

area of vascular distribution. The size of the coronary artery that is occluded determines the extent of heart muscle damage. The greater the area affected, the poorer the prognosis because of the increased loss of pumping function that may result in congestive heart failure (CHF). A favorable prognostic factor is the development of collateral circulation, through which blood from surrounding vessels is channeled into the damaged tissue. If the patient survives, the infarcted region heals with fibrosis. Long-term complications include the development of thrombi on the surface of the damaged area and the production of a local bulge (ventricular aneurysm) at the site of the weakness of the myocardial wall.

Radiographic Appearance

Radionuclide thallium perfusion scanning is the major noninvasive study for assessment of regional blood flow to the myocardium. Focal decreases in thallium uptake that are observed immediately after exercise but are no longer identified on delayed scans usually indicate transient ischemia associated with significant coronary artery stenosis or spasm. After exercise, focal defects that remain unchanged on delayed scans more frequently reflect scar formation. A normal thallium exercise scan makes the diagnosis of myocardial ischemia unlikely, although in about 10% of patients with significant obstructive disease the presence of sufficient collateral vessels can prevent the radionuclide demonstration of regional ischemia.

Radionuclide scanning (single-photon emission computed tomography, or SPECT), using technetium pyrophosphate or other compounds that are taken up by acutely infarcted myocardium, is a new noninvasive technique for detecting, localizing, and classifying myocardial necrosis (Figure 7-9). On CT, areas of myocardial ischemia appear as regions of decreased attenuation because of the increased water content resulting from intramyocardial cellular edema. Multidetector helical CT images provide calcium screening for detecting hard plaque. To evaluate soft plaque, CT angiography (CTA) is required. Initial studies have indicated that MRI will also be of value in detecting early signs of muscular necrosis in myocardial infarction (Figure 7-10) and may help determine whether the infarction is acute or remote.

Plain chest radiographs are usually normal or nonspecific in most patients with ischemic heart disease. Calcification of a coronary artery, although infrequently visualized on routine chest radiographs and usually requiring cardiac fluoroscopy, strongly suggests the presence of hemodynamically significant coronary artery disease (Figure 7-11). Plain chest radiographs are also entirely normal in many, if not most, patients after myocardial infarction. They are

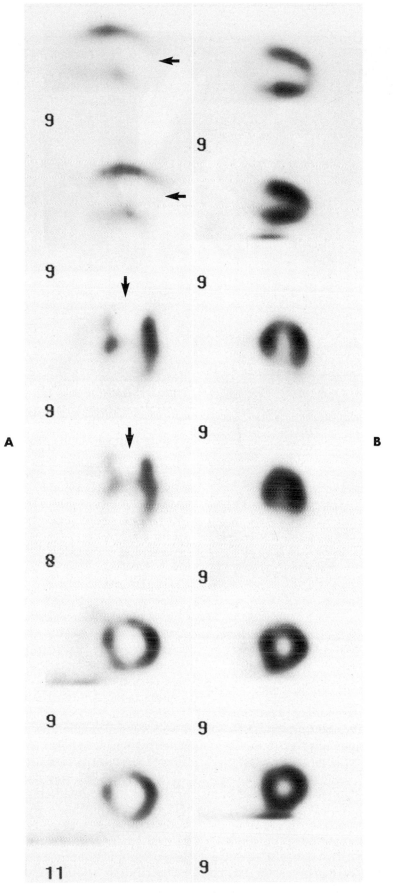

FIGURE 7-9 Myocardial stress/rest perfusion single-photon emission computed tomography scan. **A,** Apical defect is demonstrated on the stress images because of the lack of uptake in the cardiac apex *(arrows)*. **B,** The defect on rest images shows perfusion to the apex of the heart, indicating ischemia.

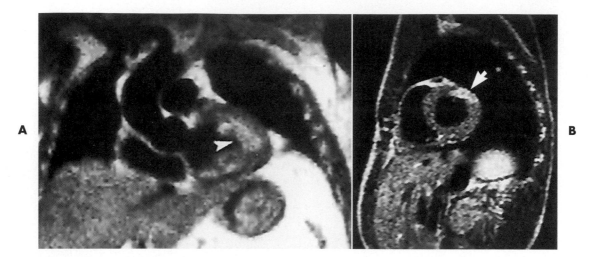

FIGURE 7-10 MR image of acute myocardial infarction. **A,** T2-weighted coronal image obtained in patient 10 days after acute myocardial infarction demonstrates area of increased signal intensity (indicating edema associated with muscle necrosis) in subendocardial regions of lateral wall *(arrowhead)*. **B,** Short-axis view of another patient shows acute transmural infarction *(arrow)* of anterolateral wall.

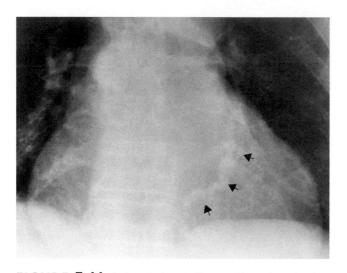

FIGURE 7-11 Ischemic heart disease. Frontal projection of chest demonstrates cardiomegaly with typical linear calcification in coronary artery *(arrows)*.

primarily of value in detecting evidence of pulmonary venous congestion in patients who develop CHF as a result of an inability of the remaining heart muscle to propel blood through the circulation adequately.

Coronary arteriography is generally considered the definitive test for determining the presence and assessing the severity of coronary artery disease. About 30% of significant stenoses involve a single vessel, most commonly the anterior descending artery. Another 30% involve two vessels, and significant stenosis of the three main vessels can be demonstrated in the remaining 40%. About 50% of coronary artery disease occurs in the left coronary

artery, 35% in the right coronary artery, and 15% in the left circumflex artery (Figure 7-12).

Intravascular ultrasound is a new technique that provides the most precise anatomic information to guide interventional procedures. The severity of arterial stenosis, measurement of lesion length, lumen dimension, and any unusual morphology can be determined. This modality is especially helpful in demonstrating the origin of the left main coronary artery, which may be obscured by the catheter in angiography. However, this equipment is not readily available because of its expense.

Treatment

Aortocoronary bypass grafting, usually using sections of saphenous vein, is an increasingly popular procedure in patients with ischemic heart disease. Arteriography has been the procedure of choice for demonstrating the patency and functional efficiency of aortocoronary bypass grafts. Patent functioning grafts demonstrate prompt clearing of contrast material and adequate filling of the grafted artery. Stenotic or malfunctioning grafts demonstrate areas of narrowing, filling defects, and slow flow with delayed washout of contrast material.

Percutaneous transluminal angioplasty (PTA) using a balloon catheter is now a recognized procedure for the treatment of patients with narrowing of one or more coronary arteries (Figure 7-13). As in other types of PTA, a catheter is placed under fluoroscopic guidance into the affected coronary artery, and an arteriogram is performed for localization. The angioplasty balloon is then positioned at the level of the stenosis and inflated. After dilation,

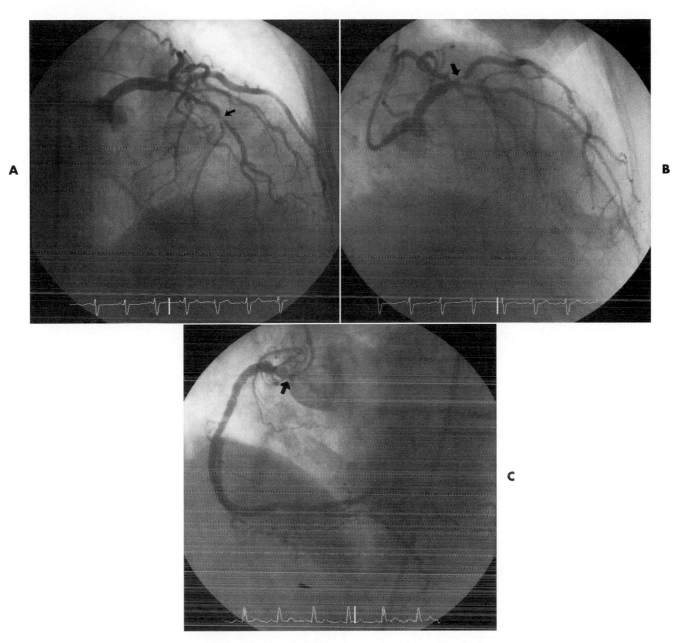

FIGURE 7-12 Coronary angiography. **A,** Posteroanterior cranial projection of the left main coronary artery shows a lesion involving the left anterior descending artery. **B,** Right anterior oblique cranial projection of left main coronary artery shows a lesion in the diagonal artery. **C,** Left anterior oblique projection of the right coronary artery demonstrates an ostial lesion at the origin.

coronary arteriography is repeated to illustrate the resulting appearance of the stenosis and to detect any complications of the procedure. Symptomatic improvement occurs in 50% to 70% of dilations. About 3% to 8% of patients who undergo PTA develop either persistent coronary insufficiency or sudden occlusion of a coronary artery at the site of dilation at the time of the procedure. Therefore the procedure should be performed at a time when an operating room, an anesthetist, and a cardiac surgeon are available so that immediate coronary bypass surgery can be performed if necessary. The percentage of deaths from coronary angioplasty is less than 1%. In conjunction with PTA, deployment of a stent helps in many cases to maintain the open lumen (Figure 7-14). Other interventional procedures include endovascular stent, atherectomy, and laser-assisted angioplasty.

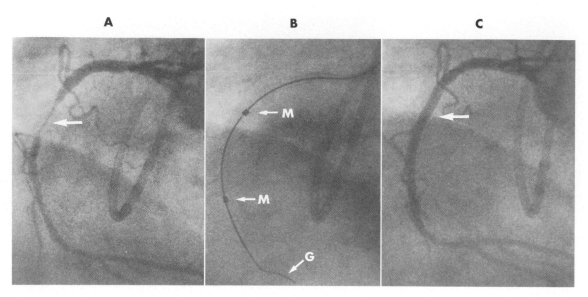

FIGURE 7-13 Percutaneous transluminal coronary angioplasty. **A,** Initial right coronary angiogram shows severe narrowing *(arrow)* of the midportion of the right coronary artery. **B,** During percutaneous transluminal coronary angioplasty, a steerable guide wire *(G)* is passed down the coronary artery and through the coronary stenosis. The tip lies within the distal right coronary artery. Radiopaque markers *(M)* identify the balloon portion of the dilating catheter that has been advanced over the guide wire through the coronary stenosis. **C,** Immediately after angioplasty, the previous site of stenosis *(arrow)* is now patent.

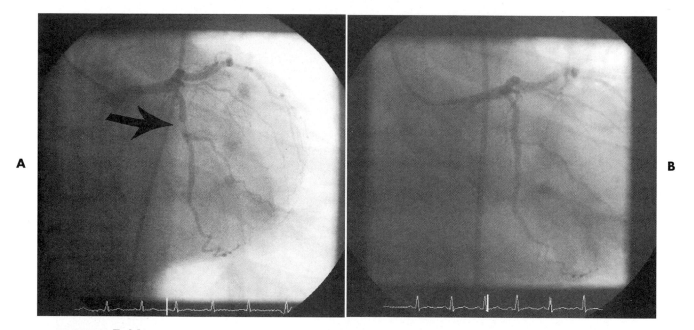

FIGURE 7-14 **A,** Angiogram of left coronary artery with a stenotic lesion in the circumflex artery *(arrow)*. **B,** Angiogram demonstrating the left circumflex artery after PTA and stent placement with no evidence of a stenotic lesion.

Congestive Heart Failure

CHF refers to the inability of the heart to propel blood at a rate and volume sufficient to provide an adequate supply to the tissues. Causes of CHF include an intrinsic cardiac abnormality, hypertension, or any obstructive process that abnormally increases the peripheral resistance to blood flow. Intrinsic cardiac abnormalities include insufficient or defective cardiac filling and/or impaired contractions for emptying.

Radiographic Appearance

Left-sided heart failure produces a classic radiographic appearance of cardiac enlargement, redistribution of pulmonary venous blood flow (enlarged superior pulmonary veins and decreased caliber of the veins draining the lower lungs), interstitial edema, alveolar edema (irregular, poorly defined patchy densities), and pleural effusions (Figure 7-15). In acute left ventricular failure resulting from coronary thrombosis, however, there may be severe pulmonary congestion and edema with very little cardiac enlargement. Pulmonary congestion and edema may require a change in technique to compensate for the increased fluid in the lungs. The major causes of left-sided heart failure include coronary heart disease, valvular disease, and hypertension.

In right-sided heart failure, dilatation of the right ventricle and right atrium is present (Figure 7-16). The transmission of increased pressure may cause dilatation of the superior vena cava, widening of the right superior mediastinum, and edema of the lower extremities. The enlargement of a congested liver may elevate the right hemidiaphragm. Common causes of right-sided heart failure include pulmonary valvular stenosis, emphysema, and pulmonary hypertension resulting from pulmonary emboli.

Many patients with CHF have cardiomegaly. A simple measurement made on a posteroanterior (PA) chest to evaluate the heart size is the cardiothoracic ratio (C/T ratio), with greater than 50% indicating cardiomegaly. In these cases, the radiologist relies on information provided by the radiographer about the images: erect versus recumbent, PA versus anteroposterior (AP), and source-to-image receptor distance, all of which influence the heart size. Lack of (or inaccurate) information can result in misdiagnosis.

Echocardiography is the modality of choice for measuring left ventricle performance, ejection fraction, and filling pressures in the pulmonary artery and ventricles.

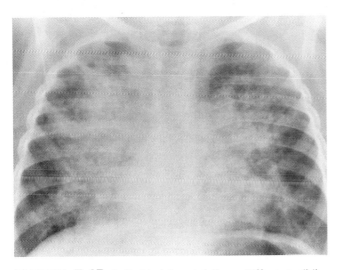

FIGURE 7-15 Left-sided heart failure. Diffuse perihilar alveolar densities.

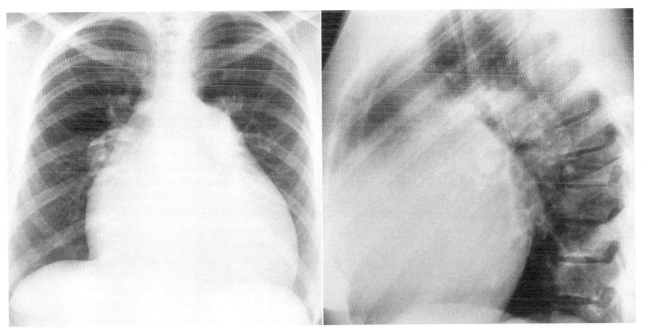

FIGURE 7-16 Right-sided heart failure. Frontal **(A)** and lateral **(B)** projections of the chest in a patient with primary pulmonary hypertension show pronounced globular cardiomegaly with prominence of the pulmonary trunk and central pulmonary arteries. Peripheral pulmonary vascularity is strikingly reduced. Right ventricular enlargement has obliterated retrosternal air space on the lateral projection.

Pulmonary Edema

Pulmonary edema refers to an abnormal accumulation of fluid in the extravascular pulmonary tissues. The most common cause of pulmonary edema is an elevation of the pulmonary venous pressure. This is most often attributable to left-sided heart failure, but may also be caused by pulmonary venous obstruction (mitral valve disease, left atrial tumor) or lymphatic blockage (fibrotic, inflammatory, or metastatic disease involving the mediastinal lymph nodes). Other causes of pulmonary edema include uremia, narcotic overdose, exposure to noxious fumes, excessive oxygen, high altitudes, fat embolism, adult respiratory distress syndrome, and various neurologic abnormalities.

Radiographic Appearance

Transudation of fluid into the interstitial spaces of the lungs is the earliest stage of pulmonary edema. However, in patients with CHF or pulmonary venous hypertension, increased pulmonary venous pressure first appears as a redistribution of blood flow from the lower to the upper lung zones. This phenomenon, probably caused by reflex venous spasm, causes prominent enlargement of the superior pulmonary veins and decreased caliber of the veins draining the inferior portions of the lung. Edema fluid in the interstitial space causes a loss of the normal sharp definition of pulmonary vascular markings (Figure 7-17). Accentuation of the vascular markings about the hila produces a perihilar haze. Fluid in the interlobular septa produces characteristic thin horizontal lines of increased density at the axillary margins of the lung inferiorly (Kerley B lines).

A further increase in pulmonary venous pressure leads to the development of alveolar or pleural transudates. Alveolar edema appears as irregular, poorly defined patchy densities scattered throughout the lungs. The classic radiographic finding of alveolar pulmonary edema is the butterfly (or bat's-wing) pattern, a diffuse, bilaterally symmetric, fan-shaped infiltration that is most prominent in the central portion of the lungs and fades toward the periphery (Figure 7-18).

Pleural effusion associated with pulmonary edema usually occurs on the right side (Figure 7-19). When bilateral, the effusion tends to be more noticeable on the right. There is often an associated thickening of the interlobar fissures. Pleural effusions are best demonstrated radiographically using a horizontal beam with the patient in a lateral decubitus position.

After adequate treatment of pulmonary edema, the interstitial, alveolar, and pleural abnormalities may

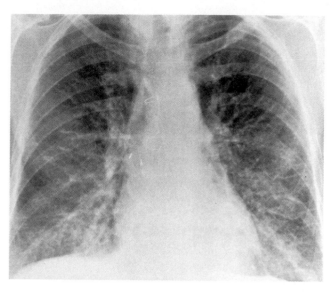

FIGURE 7-17 Interstitial pulmonary edema. Edema fluid in the interstitial space causes loss of the normal sharp definition of pulmonary vascular markings and a perihilar haze. At the bases, notice the thin horizontal lines of increased density (Kerley B lines), which represent fluid in interlobular septa.

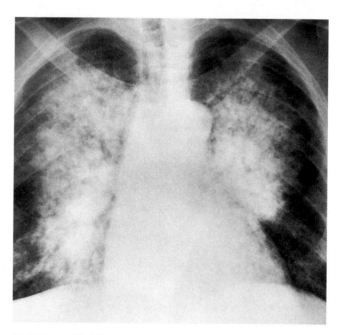

FIGURE 7-18 Butterfly pattern of severe pulmonary edema. Diffuse bilateral symmetric infiltration of the central portion of lungs along with relative sparing of the periphery produces a butterfly pattern.

disappear within several hours. Loculated pleural fluid within a fissure (especially the minor fissure) may resorb more slowly and appear as a sharply defined, elliptical, or circular density that simulates a solid parenchymal mass (Figure 7-20).

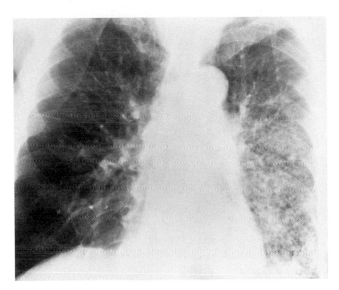

FIGURE **7-19** Unilateral pulmonary edema. Diffuse alveolar pattern limited to the left lung because of the effect of gravity on the patient lying on the left side.

Most patients with pulmonary edema caused by CHF or other heart disease have evidence of cardiomegaly. When the cause of the pulmonary edema is noncardiogenic, the heart often remains normal in size (Figure 7-21).

Treatment of Congestive Heart Failure and Pulmonary Edema

The nonpharmacologic approach includes avoiding excessive physical stress, decreasing dietary salt, and wearing compressive stockings to decrease the incidence of deep vein thrombosis (DVT). Pharmacologic therapy includes some combination of the following drugs: diuretics, angiotensin-converting enzyme inhibitors, digoxin (digitalis), parenteral inotropic agents, calcium channel blockers, beta blockers, and antithrombotic therapy.

Hypertension

Hypertension, or high blood pressure, is the leading cause of strokes and CHF. The blood pressure is a function of cardiac output (the amount of blood pumped per minute by the heart) and the total peripheral resistance, which reflects the condition of the walls of the blood vessels throughout the body. Although the peripheral resistance and cardiac output may fluctuate rapidly, depending on such factors as whether a person sits or stands and is quiet or excited, the systemic blood pressure remains remarkably constant in a healthy person.

A blood pressure reading consists of two parts. The systolic pressure is the highest pressure in the

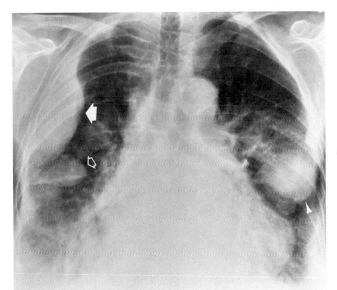

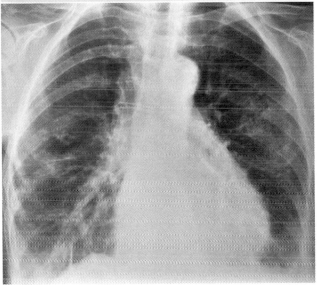

A

B

FIGURE **7-20** Loculated pleural fluid (phantom tumors). **A,** Frontal chest radiograph taken during an episode of CHF demonstrates pronounced cardiomegaly with bilateral pleural effusions. Note fluid collections along the lateral chest wall *(solid arrow),* in minor fissure *(open arrow),* and in left major fissure *(arrowhead).* **B,** With improvement in the patient's cardiac status, phantom tumors have disappeared. Bilateral small pleural effusions persist.

peripheral arteries that occurs when the left ventricle contracts. The diastolic pressure is the pressure in the peripheral arteries when the left ventricle is relaxing and filling with blood from the left atrium. High blood pressure is defined as elevation of the systolic pressure above 140 millimeters of mercury (mm Hg) and of the diastolic pressure above 90 mm Hg. In patients older than 40 years, the systolic pressure may be somewhat higher and still be considered within normal limits. As a rough rule of thumb, a person is

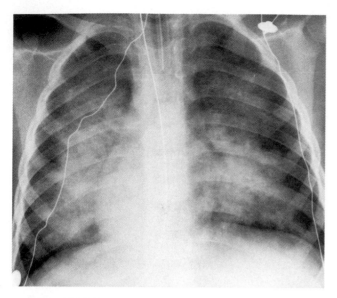

FIGURE 7-21 After a near-drowning event, the patient has a normal-size heart and a pattern of diffuse pulmonary edema.

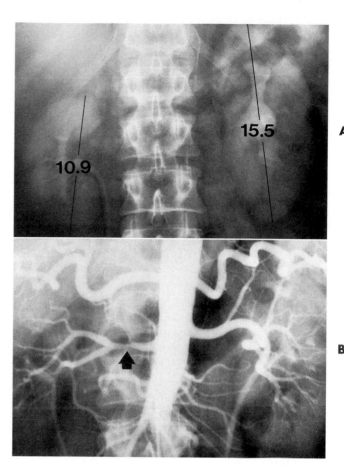

FIGURE 7-22 Renovascular hypertension. **A,** Radiograph shows diminished size of right kidney. **B,** Arteriography demonstrates that the cause is renal artery stenosis *(arrow).*

allowed an additional 10 mm Hg in systolic pressure for each decade over 40 years of age.

Most patients with elevated blood pressure have essential, or idiopathic, hypertension. The benign form of essential hypertension is characterized by a gradual onset and a prolonged course, often of many years. In the much less common malignant form, the elevated blood pressure has an abrupt onset, runs a rapid course, and often leads to renal failure or cerebral hemorrhage.

About 6% of patients have secondary hypertension resulting from another disease. Although some patients in this group have adrenal abnormalities (Cushing's syndrome, primary aldosteronism, pheochromocytoma) in which there is an abnormality of the regulation of salt and water content (and thus the blood volume), and others have an abnormality involving the secretion of a substance that increases vascular tone and peripheral arterial resistance, most have renal parenchymal or vascular disease as the underlying cause of hypertension.

Radiographic Appearance

Arteriography is the most accurate screening examination for detecting renovascular lesions. If a noninvasive screening test is desired, a radionuclide renogram with captopril is performed. The most common cause of renal artery obstruction is arteriosclerotic narrowing, which usually occurs in the proximal portion of the vessel close to its origin from the aorta (Figure 7-22). Bilateral renal artery stenoses are noted in up to one third of these patients. Oblique projections, which

demonstrate the vessel origins in profile, are often required to demonstrate renal artery stenosis. CT angiography can detect renal artery stenosis, including fibromuscular dysplasia. MR angiography (MRA) can detect stenosis, but the resolution is still inadequate to visualize segmental renal branches. One of the advantages of MRA is that iodinated contrast agents are not required to visualize the vessel anatomy.

The other major cause of renovascular hypertension is **fibromuscular dysplasia**. This disease is most common in young adult women and is often bilateral. The most common radiographic appearance of fibromuscular dysplasia is the string-of-beads pattern, in which there are alternating areas of narrowing and dilatation (Figure 7-23). Smooth, concentric stenoses occur less frequently.

The mere presence of a renovascular lesion does not mean that it is the cause of hypertension; indeed, many patients with normal blood pressure have severe renal artery disease. Therefore bilateral renal vein catheterization for the measurement of plasma renin activity is used to assess the functional significance of any stenotic lesion. A renal vein renin

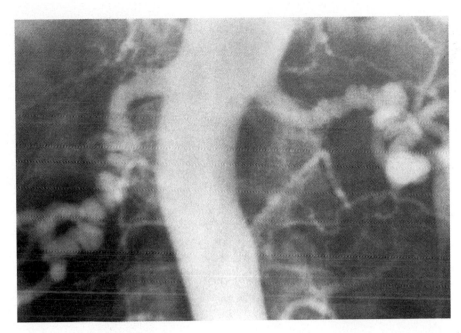

FIGURE 7-23 Renovascular hypertension. String-of-beads pattern of fibromuscular dysplasia bilaterally.

concentration on the abnormal side that is more than 50% greater than the renin level in the renal vein on the normal side indicates the functional significance of a lesion with an accuracy rate of about 85%.

Prolonged high blood pressure forces the heart to overwork, causing the left ventricle to enlarge and eventually fail. Since high blood pressure affects all arteries of the body, including the coronary and carotid vessels, this condition increases the risk of coronary occlusion, myocardial infarction, and carotid narrowing leading to a stroke.

Decreased function of the kidneys leads to the retention of water and salt, which increases the blood volume and elevates the blood pressure. Long-standing hypertension causes atherosclerosis of the renal artery, which reduces blood flow to the kidneys and causes further damage.

Treatment

Medical treatment includes some combination of diuretics and beta, alpha, and calcium blockers to control blood pressure. Surgery has traditionally been the treatment for a patient with arteriographically demonstrated renal artery lesions and confirmatory renal vein renin studies. Recently, PTA, with stent placement, has been shown to be effective in dilating renal artery stenoses (Figure 7-24). Although insufficient time has elapsed to compare the long-term results of renal transluminal angioplasty with corrective surgical procedures, initial studies demonstrate the improvement or cure of hypertension in about 80% of patients treated with angioplasty. Stenosis recurs in 10% to 20%, usually because of incomplete dilation.

Hypertensive Heart Disease

Long-standing high blood pressure causes narrowing of systemic blood vessels and an increased resistance to blood flow. The left ventricle is forced to assume an increased work load, which initially causes hypertrophy (double thickness of normal wall) and little if any change in the radiographic appearance of the cardiac silhouette.

Radiographic Appearance

Eventually, the continued strain on the heart leads to dilatation and enlargement of the left ventricle (Figure 7-25), along with downward displacement of the cardiac apex, which often projects below the left hemidiaphragm. Aortic tortuosity with prominence of the ascending portion commonly occurs (Figure 7-26). Notching of the undersurface of the ribs may become evident. Failure of the left ventricle leads to increased pulmonary venous pressure and CHF (in 40% of cases).

Treatment

Therapy includes treating the high blood pressure and complications, such as CHF.

Aneurysm

An aneurysm is a localized dilatation of an artery that most commonly involves the aorta, especially its abdominal portion. A **saccular aneurysm** involves only one side of the arterial wall, whereas bulging of the entire circumference of the vessel wall is termed a **fusiform aneurysm**. An aneurysm represents a

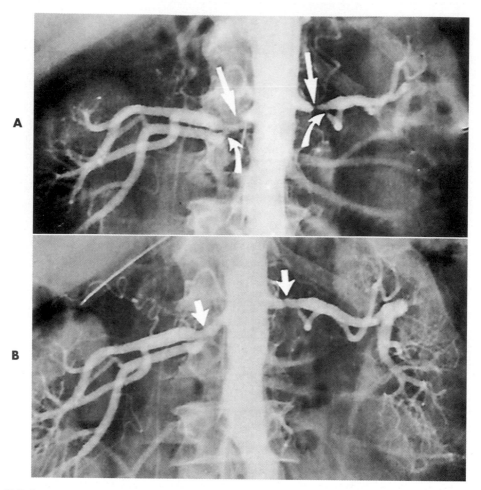

FIGURE 7-24 PTA for renovascular hypertension. **A,** Abdominal aortogram demonstrates severe bilateral stenoses of main renal arteries *(straight arrows)* and stenoses at origins of early bifurcations *(curved arrows).* **B,** Aortogram after angioplasty of both renal arteries shows irregularities in areas of previous atherosclerotic narrowing *(arrows),* but an improved residual lumen in both main renal arteries. After the procedure, the patient's previous severe hypertension was controllable to normal levels with only minimal dosages of diuretic medication.

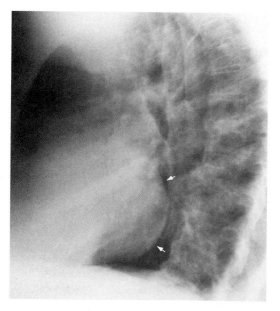

FIGURE **7-25** Hypertensive heart disease. Lateral projection of chest shows prominence of left ventricle *(arrows).*

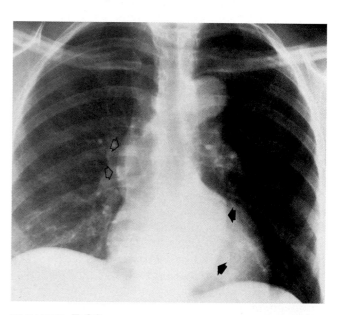

FIGURE **7-26** Hypertensive heart disease. Generalized tortuosity and elongation of ascending aorta *(open arrows)* and descending aorta *(solid arrows).*

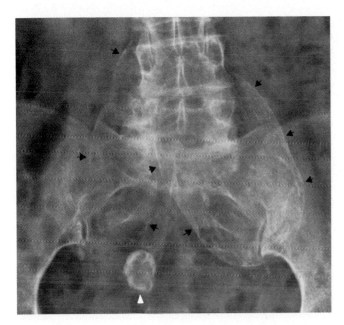

FIGURE 7-27 Calcification in walls of aneurysms of lower abdominal aorta and both common iliac arteries *(arrows)*. Of incidental note is calcified uterine fibroid *(arrowhead)* in pelvis.

weakness in the wall (decreased elastin and increased collagen production) of a blood vessel caused by atherosclerosis, syphilis or other infection, trauma, or a congenital defect, such as Marfan's syndrome. The presence of multiple small aneurysms is suggestive of a generalized arterial inflammation (arteritis). In the abdominal aorta, most aneurysms occur below the origin of the renal arteries, and thus the aneurysm can be surgically replaced by a prosthetic graft without injuring the kidneys. The danger of an aneurysm is its tendency to increase in size and rupture, leading to massive hemorrhage, which may be fatal if it involves a critical organ, such as the brain.

Radiographic Appearance

Although plain abdominal radiographs can demonstrate curvilinear calcification in the wall of an aneurysm (Figure 7-27), ultrasound is the modality of choice for detection of an abdominal aortic aneurysm. The sonographic definition of aneurysmal dilatation of the abdominal aorta is an enlargement of the structure to a diameter greater than 3 cm. Ultrasound can demonstrate an intraluminal clot as a hypoechoic or anechoic lesion (Figure 7-28, *A*), and the noninvasive nature of ultrasound permits an evaluation of the enlargement of an aneurysm on serial studies. Sonography is the best imaging modality for defining the abdominal aortic aneurysm; CTA and MRA are superior for demonstrating aortic rupture.

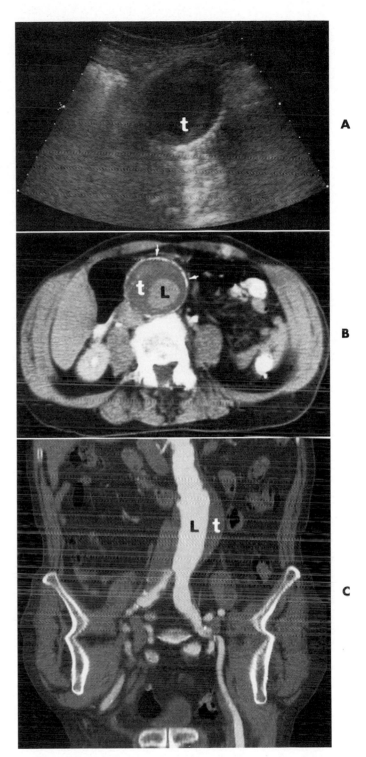

FIGURE 7-28 Abdominal aortic aneurysm. **A,** Ultrasound shows large aneurysm with echogenic thrombus *(t)* filling the outer margins of the aorta, creating a false lumen 2.25 cm in diameter. **B,** CT axial scan of an abdominal aortic aneurysm in another patient shows a low-density thrombus *(t)* surrounding a blood-filled lumen *(L)*. The wall of the aneurysm contains high-density calcification *(arrows)*. **C,** CT coronal reconstruction of third patient shows an abdominal aortic aneurysm beginning below the renal arteries and extending below the iliac bifurcation.

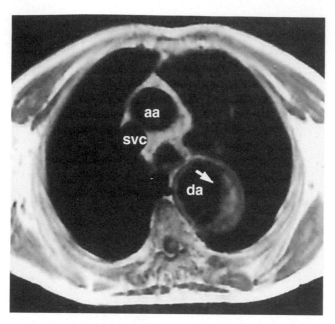

FIGURE 7-29 MR image of aortic aneurysm. Transverse scan with cardiac gating permits differentiation of large mural thrombus *(arrow)* from signal void of rapidly flowing intraluminal blood. *aa,* Ascending aorta; *da,* descending aorta; *svc,* superior vena cava.

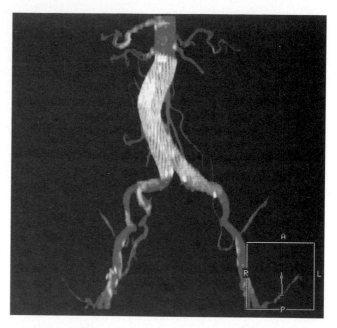

FIGURE 7-30 CTA of an abdominal aortic stent placed for an abdominal aortic aneurysm. Posterior perspective demonstrates the stent placed in the aorta and a second stent placed in the right iliac artery.

CTA and MRA also can demonstrate the location and extent of an aneurysm, and these modalities have begun to replace catheter angiography. CTA can identify a retroperitoneal hematoma secondary to leaking or acute rupture of the aneurysm. With helical CT, three-dimensional reformation permits demonstration of the abdominal aorta in multiple planes, improving visualization of the origin of the aneurysm and its relationship to the renal arteries (see Figure 7-28, *B*). When a thrombus is demonstrated on CT, the attenuation values (Hounsfield unit) can be used to determine whether the rupture and/or thrombus is fresh or weeks old. A new bleed has a high attenuation value, whereas older blood causes isoattenuation or hypoattenuation. MRA may be the better choice if the patient has depressed renal function because the contrast agent used is not nephrotoxic.

The major value of arteriography in patients with abdominal aortic aneurysm is as a presurgical road map to define the extent of the lesion and whether the renal arteries or other major branches are involved. Because the lumen of an aneurysm may be filled with clot, aortography often produces an underestimation of the extent of aneurysmal dilatation.

In the chest, CT after the intravenous injection of contrast material is the most efficient technique for demonstrating the size and extent of an aortic aneurysm and for differentiating this vascular lesion from a solid mediastinal mass. Unlike aortography, CT is relatively noninvasive and can directly identify an intraluminal thrombus (seen as a soft tissue density separating the contrast-filled portion of the lumen from the aortic wall), which can only be inferred on contrast examination (see Figure 7-28, *B* and *C*). CT can also demonstrate aortic mural calcification and effects of the aneurysm on adjacent structures, such as displacement of the mediastinum or bone erosion. Because of its ability to demonstrate flowing blood as a signal void, and clot as a heterogeneous collection of signal intensities, MRI can provide information about an aneurysm that is comparable with that obtained from CT without the need for intravenous contrast material (Figure 7-29).

Treatment

An abdominal aortic aneurysm may require surgical graft placement to maintain circulation to the inferior part of the abdomen and lower extremity. Currently a patient may be a candidate for percutaneous stent placement (Figure 7-30) to strengthen the abdominal aorta and prevent rupture and growth of the aneurysm.

Traumatic Rupture of the Aorta

Traumatic rupture of the aorta is a potentially fatal complication of closed chest trauma (rapid deceleration, blast, compression). In almost all cases, the aortic

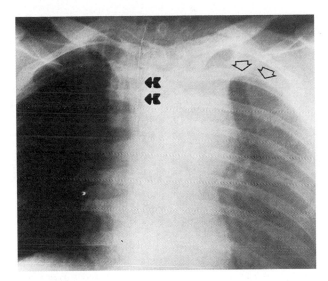

FIGURE 7-31 Traumatic aneurysm of the aorta. There is widening of the mediastinum and deviation of the nasogastric tube to the right *(solid arrows)*. Open arrows point to the collection of fluid over the left apex (apical pleural cap) in this patient who suffered severe blunt chest trauma.

tear occurs just distal to the left subclavian artery at the site of the ductus arteriosus.

Radiographic Appearance

On plain chest radiographs, hemorrhage into the mediastinum causes widening of the mediastinal silhouette and loss of a discrete aortic knob shadow. Associated rib or sternal fractures may be apparent. However, because nonspecific mediastinal widening is a frequent finding, especially on the supine AP portable radiographs taken after trauma, other plain film signs are of diagnostic importance (Figure 7-31). These include displacement of an opaque nasogastric tube to the right (because of a hematoma that displaces the esophagus), widening of the right paratracheal stripe (Figure 7-32), and a collection of blood over the apex of the left lung (apical pleural cap sign).

CT and emergency aortography are the definitive examinations for the evaluation of possible laceration or rupture of the aorta. The patient's condition and facility preferences will determine the modality of choice. CTA using multidetector helical scanners to scan in thin slices and reconstruct in multiplanar dimensions provides extremely detailed images in a very short time. If the patient has multiple traumatic injuries for which CT is needed, then CT is the modality of choice to evaluate a traumatic rupture of the aorta. In aortography, right anterior oblique and left anterior oblique projections are best to demonstrate both the contours of the aortic arch and any rupture.

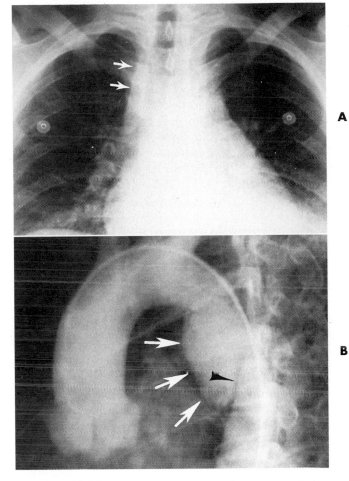

FIGURE 7-32 Traumatic aneurysm of the aorta. **A,** Supine chest radiograph in a patient with blunt chest trauma shows thickening of the right paratracheal stripe *(arrows)*, which measures 1 cm in width. **B,** Aortogram demonstrates pseudoaneurysm at the level of the aortic isthmus *(arrows)*. Arrowhead indicates intimal flap.

Treatment

Immediate surgical intervention to repair the aortic laceration or rupture is required to prevent morbidity.

Dissection of the Aorta

Dissection of the aorta is a potentially life-threatening condition in which disruption of the intima (the inner layer) permits blood to enter the wall of the aorta and separate its layers. As a result of the disruption, the aorta is divided into a true and false lumen. The false lumen may form an aneurysm as a result of the high pressure in the systemic vascular system. Most aortic dissections occur in patients with arterial hypertension. Some are a result of trauma, whereas others are attributable to a congenital defect, such as Marfan's syndrome. An acute dissection typically causes sudden sharp or excruciating pain in the chest or abdomen. Although the pain passes, death frequently occurs some days later from rupture of the aneurysm into the chest or abdominal cavity.

Most aortic dissections begin as a tear in the intima immediately above the aortic valve. In two thirds of these (type I), the dissection continues into the descending aorta, often extending as far as the level of the iliac bifurcation. In the remainder (type II), the dissection is limited to the ascending aorta and stops at the origin of the innominate artery. In type III disease, the dissection begins in the thoracic aorta distal to the subclavian artery and extends for a variable distance proximally and distally to the original site.

Radiographic Appearance

On plain chest radiographs, aortic dissection causes progressive widening of the aortic shadow, which may have an irregular or wavy outer border (Figure 7-33) that most likely represents the site of origin of the dissection. However, this is a nonspecific appearance and a definite diagnosis of dissection must be made on the basis of aortography or CT. CT, MRI, and transesophageal echocardiography (TEE) can demonstrate aortic dissection. The modality of choice will depend on the patient's status, including such factors as overall physical condition, degree of renal function, suspected complications, and equipment availability. Spiral multidetector CT has made this the modality of choice. CT, nonenhanced scans followed with enhanced images, is the protocol recommended for demonstrating acute rupture and hemorrhage. The detection of an intimal flap will identify the true and false lumens.

In the patient in whom nonacute aortic dissection is being considered in the differential diagnosis of chest pain, CT and MRI offer low-risk alternative diagnostic methods to arteriography. The emergence of spiral multidetector CT has enhanced the ability to demonstrate aortic dissection as a double channel with an intimal flap. With dynamic scanning and the rapid injection of a bolus of contrast material, differential filling of the true and false channels can be observed as with aortography (Figure 7-34). The major limitation of CT in the patient with suspected acute dissection is that only a single level can be evaluated on a given slice, as opposed to the rapid series of images covering a large portion of the aorta that can be obtained with aortography. With the development of helical CT, multiplane images are available to quickly visualize the classic double-barrel aorta and the linear filling defect within the aortic lumen. With the new technology, CT has a sensitivity of about 90% and specificity of 96%.

The high contrast between rapidly flowing blood, vessel wall, and adjacent soft tissue structures permits identification of vessels by MRI without the need for intravenous injection of contrast material. This technique can demonstrate aortic dissections and show their extent. The intimal flap is usually detected as a linear, medium signal intensity structure separating the true and false lumina (Figure 7-35). Rapidly flowing blood in these lumina appears as a signal void. If the false lumen is thrombosed, or even if it is open but the flow is slow, the intimal flap may not be visualized. In this situation, aortic dissection is difficult to differentiate from an aortic aneurysm with mural

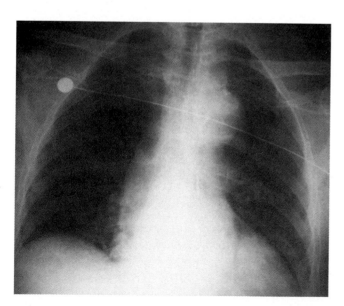

FIGURE 7-33 Aortic dissection. Plain chest radiograph shows diffuse widening of descending aorta with irregular, wavy outer border.

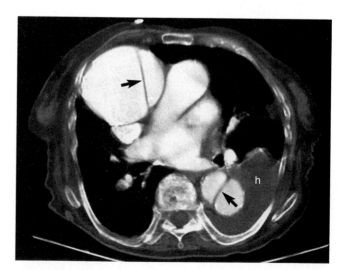

FIGURE 7-34 CT image of aortic dissection. The ascending aorta is dilated and has a radiolucent intimal flap *(arrows)*. The descending aorta demonstrates a much larger tear and hemorrhage *(h)* surrounding the aorta.

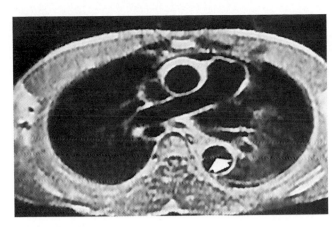

FIGURE 7-35 MR image of aortic dissection. Axial scan at level of main and right pulmonary arteries clearly shows intimal flap *(arrow)* in descending aorta.

thrombus, and aortography may be required to make this distinction. A new MR sequence is available to evaluate aortic dissection. Cardiac-gated gradient-echo sequence demonstrates the intimal flap as a dark line against the high signal intensity of flowing blood. MRA has largely replaced conventional angiography. MR is the modality of choice for follow-up and for evaluating treatment.

TEE is another modality available to provide images of the ascending aorta to demonstrate an intimal tear, the extension of the dissection, and pleural effusion.

In aortography, the diagnosis of aortic dissection depends on the demonstration of two channels separated by a thin radiolucent intimal flap (Figure 7-36). The false channel may be filled with clot and impossible to opacify with contrast material. In this case, the diagnosis can be made by demonstration of narrowing and compression of the true channel. When both true and false lumina fill with contrast material, it is important to demonstrate the distal reentry point where the false lumen joins the true lumen. If the dissection extends below the diaphragm, arteriography can provide presurgical information about which major vessel branches from the aorta are blocked and which remain patent.

Treatment

Proximal aortic dissections are fatal if not immediately treated surgically (by graft placement). Interventional treatment involves creating an opening (fenestration) between the true and false lumina to provide blood supply to the descending aortic vascular system. As an alternative, an aortic stent may be placed in the true lumen to allow blood to flow freely. The stent provides the same results as surgery; however, this is a new technique and the long-term

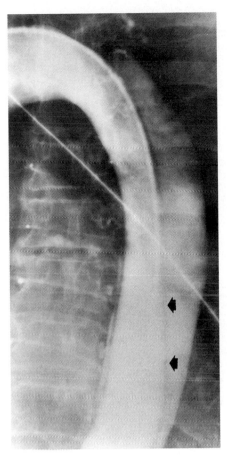

FIGURE 7-36 Aortic dissection. Aortogram demonstrates thin radiolucent intimal flap *(arrows)* separating true and false aortic channels.

effectiveness is unknown. Many other dissections require only medical management (80% survival rate).

Atherosclerosis

Arteriosclerosis occurs when arteries become marked by thickening, hardening, and loss of elasticity in the arterial wall. Atherosclerosis is one form of arteriosclerosis. The major cause of vascular disease of the extremities is atherosclerosis, in which fatty deposits called plaques develop in the intima and produce progressive narrowing and often complete occlusion of large and medium-size arteries. In the abdomen, the disease primarily involves the aorta and the common iliac arteries, often sparing the external iliac vessels. In the lower extremities, atherosclerotic narrowing most commonly affects the superficial femoral artery just above the knee. Plaque formation and luminal narrowing often involve the coronary and cerebral arteries, thus decreasing the blood flow to the heart muscle and the brain and leading to a myocardial infarction or stroke (cerebrovascular accident).

Radiographic Appearance

Atherosclerotic plaques often calcify and appear on plain radiographs as irregularly distributed densities along the course of an artery (Figure 7-37). Small vessel calcification, especially in the hands and feet, is often seen in patients with accelerated arteriosclerosis, especially those with diabetes mellitus.

Doppler ultrasound is an effective and preferred noninvasive technique for screening patients with clinically suspected peripheral arteriosclerotic disease. Color Doppler demonstrates the presence of atherosclerotic plaques and assesses the degree of luminal stenosis. Definitive diagnosis requires arteriographic demonstration of the peripheral vascular tree. Evidence of arteriosclerosis includes diffuse vascular narrowing, irregularity of the lumen, and filling defects. In patients with severe stenosis or obstruction, arteriography demonstrates the degree and source of collateral circulation and the status of the vessels distal to an area of narrowing (Figure 7-38). As MRA has evolved, 3-D MRA has become the method of choice and replaced catheter angiography. The two-dimensional time-of-flight method is preferred for evaluating the infrapopliteal vessels. MRA images illustrate areas of narrowing and occlusion as an absence of signal intensity.

Treatment

PTA using a balloon catheter is now a recognized procedure for the alleviation of symptoms of peripheral ischemia in patients with arteriosclerosis (Figure 7-39). In addition, a stent may be placed to aid in keeping the vessel open. The results of this interventional approach (95% success for the iliac artery and 50% to 60% for the thigh and calf) are similar to those of bypass grafting, but with a much lower morbidity rate. It is of special value in patients who are extremely ill

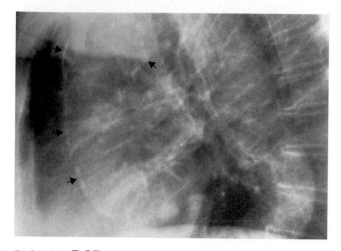

FIGURE 7-37 Atherosclerosis. Lateral projection of chest demonstrates calcification of anterior and posterior walls of ascending aorta *(arrows)*. Descending thoracic aorta is tortuous.

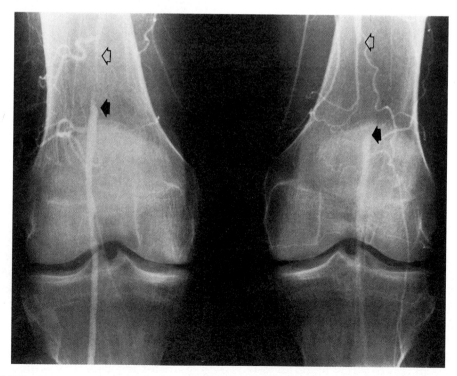

FIGURE 7-38 Bilateral atherosclerotic occlusion of superficial femoral arteries. Arteriogram demonstrates occlusion of both distal superficial femoral arteries *(open arrows)* with reconstitution by collateral vessels *(solid arrows)*.

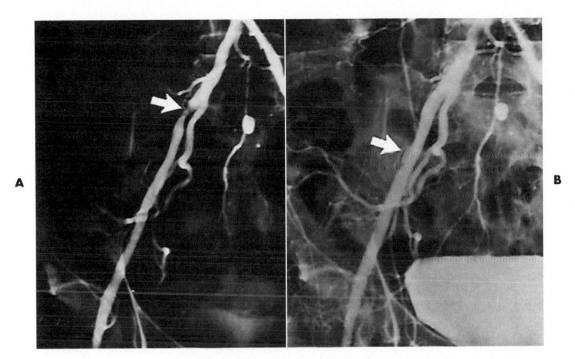

FIGURE 7-39 PTA of right external iliac artery stenosis. **A,** Initial film in patient with claudication demonstrates narrowing of proximal right external iliac artery *(arrow)*. **B,** After angioplasty, there is relief of stenosis *(arrow)* and of symptoms.

and in those who would not benefit from reconstructive arterial surgery.

Thrombosis and Embolism

The blood-clotting mechanism is the major protective device of the body in response to the escape of blood from a vessel (hemorrhage). This same mechanism can occur in intact blood vessels, leading to the development of an intravascular clot called a **thrombus**. Three factors lead to the development of intravascular thrombosis. Clots tend to form where blood flow is slow and thus develop much more commonly in veins than in arteries. Thrombi occur especially in areas of stasis (slow circulation) in patients who are inactive or immobilized, as after abdominal surgery.

The second factor is a change in the wall of blood vessels, leading to thrombosis. Normally, the inner wall of a blood vessel has a very smooth lining (endothelium), and platelets cannot stick, or adhere, to it. However, when the endothelium is destroyed by injury or inflammation, platelets rapidly adhere to the rough spot, and a clot begins to form from the blood as it flows past. Arteriosclerosis is the major cause of endothelial irregularity and subsequent thrombosis. Nodules of vegetation on heart valves caused by rheumatic heart disease are also important predisposing factors for thrombus formation.

The third factor is a change in the blood itself, which leads to thrombosis. A low level of oxygen within the blood, as in some forms of heart disease, forces the body to compensate by increasing the number of red blood cells (polycythemia). This causes the blood to become more viscous and increases the risk of thrombosis. Changes in the clotting and fibrinolytic mechanisms also may increase the risk of thrombus formation.

Once a thrombus is formed, it may follow one of three courses. The thrombus may contract or become canalized so that blood can once again flow through the lumen. The thrombus may continually enlarge or become converted into fibrous tissue, resulting in permanent occlusion of the vessel. A potentially catastrophic event is the production of an **embolus**, which refers to part or all of a thrombus that becomes detached from the vessel wall and enters the bloodstream. Embolization is especially likely to occur if there is infected tissue around the thrombus or if there is a sudden movement caused by rough handling of the involved area. An embolism may lodge at any of several points, depending on the size of the vessels through which it travels. Since veins become larger as they approach the heart, an embolism arising from a thrombus in a leg vein flows easily to the heart and typically gets stuck in a pulmonary artery (pulmonary embolism). An embolism arising from a mitral valve damaged by rheumatic heart disease

SUMMARY of FINDINGS for Acquired Vascular Disease

disorder	location	radiographic appearance	treatment
Coronary artery disease	Blood vessels supplying the heart	PA chest—vessel calcifications SPECT—classifies myocardial necrosis CT—decreased attenuation in affected myocardial tissue; calcium scoring to visualize hard plaque; CTA to visualize soft plaque MRI—increased T2-weighted signal intensity in affected myocardial tissue NM—focal defects (cold spots) after exercise with filling at rest indicates stenosis IVUS—vessel size and length of lesion Angiogram—strictures or narrowings are filling defects	Surgery—bypass graft Interventional—PTCA, PTCA with stent placement, percutaneous atherectomy
Congestive heart failure	Insufficient cardiac output	PA chest—C/T ratio greater than 50% —Left sided: cardiac enlargement, pulmonary edema, and pulmonary effusion —Right sided: widened mediastinum and elevated right hemidiaphragm Echocardiography—measuring left ventricular performance, ejection fraction, and filling pressures of the pulmonary artery and ventricles	Diuretics Digoxin
Pulmonary edema	Extravascular fluid in the lungs	PA chest—vascular markings not sharp; severe edema produces a butterfly pattern	Treat cause of edema
Hypertension	Increased pressure in the systemic vascular system	Arteriography—detects renovascular lesions Radionuclide renogram—noninvasive screening to demonstrate lesions	Drug therapy to control vascular volume and heart rates Interventional—PTA with or without stent
Hypertensive heart disease	Left ventricle enlargement	PA chest—enlarged left ventricle, inferior displacement of cardiac apex, aortic tortuosity	Therapy for high blood pressure and/or CHF
Aneurysm	Dilatation of artery; fusiform or saccular	Radiograph—calcification outlining vessel US—abdominal aortic enlargement, of a diameter greater than 3 cm CTA—aneurysm extent and size, evidence of leak or rupture by retroperitoneal hematoma MRA—same as CTA, but used when iodinated contrast agents are contraindicated	Surgical graft placement Percutaneous stent placement
Traumatic aortic rupture	Aortic tear distal to left subclavian artery	PA chest—widened mediastinum; deviation of NG tube to right; apical pleural cap CTA/aortography—demonstrates tear and hemorrhage	Surgical repair
Aortic dissection	Disruption of aortic intima	PA chest—widening of aortic shadow, which may be irregular CT—double-barrel channel with linear filling defect within lumen (intimal flap) MRI—intimal flap causes medium-intensity signal separating true and false lumina; blood flow causes signal void TEE—demonstrates intimal tear, extension of dissection and pleural effusion Aortography—extent of true and false lumina	Proximal or continuous dissection—immediate surgical repair Intervention—fenestration and stenting Other dissections—medical management

SUMMARY of FINDINGS for Acquired Vascular Disease—cont'd

disorder	location	radiographic appearance	treatment
Atherosclerosis	Plaques develop in the intima of the artery	Radiograph—calcification demonstrating "hardening" of the artery Color Doppler—demonstrates plaque and degree of luminal stenosis MRA—two dimensional time-of-flight view demonstrates narrowing and flow changes in infrapopliteal vessels; 3-D images demonstrate narrow occlusions as a signal absence	PTA with or without stent placement Surgical arterial bypass
Thrombus and embolism	Blockage of a vessel	Arteriography—extent of occlusion, degree of collateral circulation, and distal vessel condition	Surgical removal Medical treatment to reduce thrombus or emboli

SPECT, Single-photon emission computed topography; *IVUS,* intravascular ultrasound; *NG,* nasogastric; *NM,* nuclear medicine; *PTCA,* percutaneous transluminal coronary angioplasty; *US,* ultrasound.

flows through the left ventricle and aorta and lodges in a smaller artery in the brain, kidney, or other organ. A septic embolism contains infected material from pyogenic bacteria, whereas tumor emboli are groups of cancer cells that have invaded a vein, become detached, and are then carried to the lungs or other organs where they form metastases. Fat emboli are the result of trauma, especially leg fractures, in which marrow fat enters torn peripheral veins and is trapped by the pulmonary circulation. An air embolism refers to bubbles of air introduced into a vein during surgery, trauma, or an improperly administered intravenous injection.

Regardless of its type or source, an embolism blocks the vascular lumen and cuts off the blood supply to the organ or parts supplied by that artery. The effect of an embolism depends on the size of the embolus and on the extent of collateral circulation, which can bring blood to an affected part by an alternate route, and the location of the embolus.

Radiographic Appearance

Acute embolic occlusion of an artery most commonly affects the lower extremities. The success of therapy depends on the rapid recognition of the clinical problem and the institution of appropriate treatment. Arteriography is the procedure of choice to confirm the clinical diagnosis and to demonstrate the extent of occlusion, the degree of collateral circulation, and the condition of the distal vessels. Embolic occlusion typically appears as an abrupt termination of the contrast column, along with a proximal curved margin reflecting the nonopaque embolus protruding into the contrast-filled lumen (Figure 7-40). In acute occlusion, there is usually little if any evidence of collateral circulation. Further discussion is located later

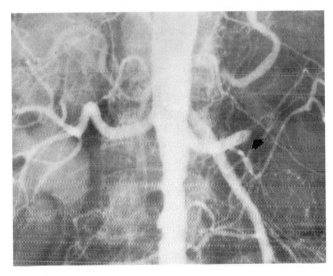

FIGURE 7-40 Acute embolic occlusion of left renal artery. There is abrupt termination of contrast column *(arrow).* Note irregular infrarenal aortic contour, which represents atherosclerotic disease.

in this chapter under Venous Disease—Deep Venous Thrombosis.

Treatment

Anticoagulants, such as heparin and Coumadin, are often used to prevent intravascular clotting. Heparin prevents platelets from sticking together and to the vessel wall, helping prevent thrombus formation. Coumadin acts by antagonizing the action of vitamin K, which is necessary for blood clotting. However, these medications also interfere with the person's normal ability to stop bleeding and may lead to severe hemorrhage from relatively minor trauma or to potentially fatal bleeding in the brain and

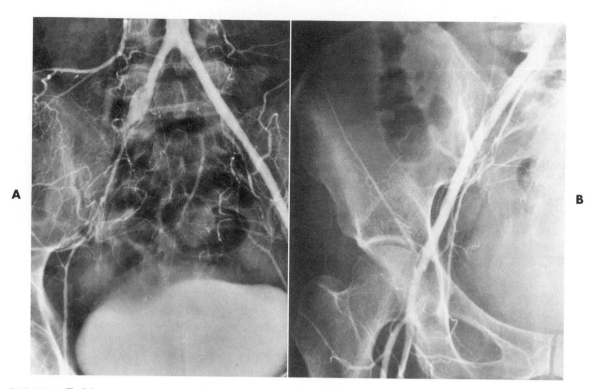

FIGURE 7-41 Streptokinase therapy for acute arterial occlusion. **A,** After angioplasty of right external iliac artery, there was loss of right common femoral pulse. Repeat arteriogram from left femoral approach shows complete occlusion of external iliac artery at its origin. **B,** After 8 hours of streptokinase administration, arteriogram demonstrates lysis of thrombus and reestablishment of lumen. One year after angioplasty, patient had normal femoral pulse and patent artery.

gastrointestinal tract. Recent reports have suggested the value of aspirin in preventing intravascular clotting because of its inhibition of platelet aggregation.

Although emergency surgery to remove the embolus (embolectomy) has been the traditional treatment for acute arterial occlusion, the intraarterial infusion of streptokinase by means of a catheter placed immediately proximal to the occlusion is becoming a more common alternative therapy, especially in patients who are poor surgical risks (Figure 7-41). The tissue plasminogen activator (TPA) Activase, produced by recombinant DNA technology, has been administered intravenously to lyse thrombi obstructing coronary arteries in the treatment of acute myocardial infarction.

Valvular Disease

The valves of the heart permit blood to flow in only one direction through the heart. When the valve is closed, a heart chamber fills with blood; when the valve opens, blood can move forward and leave the chamber. There are four heart valves. The tricuspid valve separates the right atrium and the right ventricle, and the mitral valve separates the left atrium and the left ventricle. The pulmonary valve lies between the right ventricle and the pulmonary artery, and the aortic valve is situated between the left ventricle and the aorta.

The malfunction of a heart valve alters the normal blood flow through the heart. Too small an opening (stenosis) does not permit sufficient blood flow. In contrast, too large an opening or failure of the valve to properly close permits backflow of blood (regurgitation) and the condition of valvular insufficiency. Both stenosis and insufficiency of valves cause heart murmurs with characteristic sounds that indicate the nature of the defect. Two-dimensional and Doppler echocardiography have become the modalities of choice to demonstrate valvular diseases. Although valvular heart disease once invariably forced a patient to restrict activity and was associated with a limited life span, surgical reconstruction or replacement of a diseased valve (Figure 7-42) can offer a patient the prospect of a normal life.

Rheumatic Heart Disease

Rheumatic fever is an autoimmune disease that results from a reaction of the patient's antibodies against antigens from a previous streptococcal infection. The disease is much less common today because

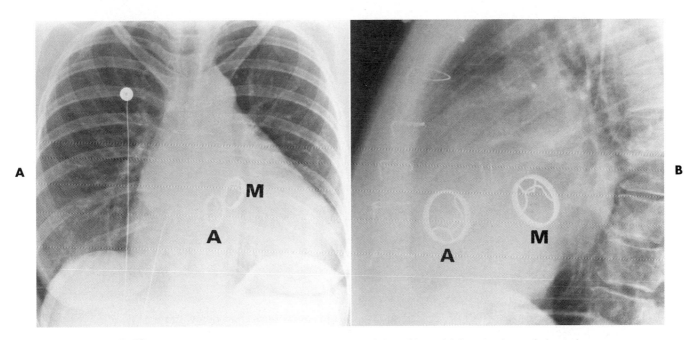

FIGURE 7-42 Prosthetic aortic and mitral valves. Frontal **(A)** and lateral **(B)** projections of chest show antero-medially located prosthetic aortic valve *(A)* and posterolaterally situated prosthetic mitral valve *(M)*.

of the frequent use of antibiotics to treat streptococcal throat or ear infections. The symptoms of rheumatic fever (fever, inflamed and painful joints, rash) typically develop several weeks after the streptococcal infection.

The major damage of rheumatic fever is to the valves of the heart, most frequently the mitral and aortic valves. Indeed, it is the major cause of acquired cardiac valve disease. The allergic response causes inflammation of the valves. Deposits of blood platelets and fibrin from blood flowing over the valve produce small nodules **(vegetations)** along the margin of the valve cusps. The thickened valves may stick together, so that the valvular opening remains permanently narrowed **(stenosis)** rather than opening properly when blood flows through. In contrast, fibrous scarring may cause retraction of the valve cusps so that the cusps are unable to meet when the valve tries to close; this is **insufficiency,** and blood leaks through the valve when it should be closed. Doppler echocardiography is used to best identify and quantify the insufficiencies and determine the degree of ventricular dysfunction.

Treatment

Prevention of rheumatic fever and subsequent heart disease by treating the streptococcal infection with a full course of antibiotic therapy is the best approach. If the infection progresses into rheumatic heart disease, antibiotics, antiinflammatory drugs, and restricted activity are the appropriate interventions.

Mitral Stenosis

Stenosis of the mitral valve, almost always a complication of rheumatic disease, results from diffuse thickening of the valve by fibrous tissue, calcific deposits, or both.

Radiographic Appearance

The obstruction of blood flow from the left atrium into the left ventricle during diastole causes increased pressure in the left atrium and enlargement of this chamber (Figure 7-43). The enlarged left atrium produces a characteristic anterior impression on and posterior displacement of the barium filled esophagus that is best seen on lateral and right anterior oblique projections. Other radiographic signs of left atrial enlargement include posterior displacement of the left mainstem bronchus, widening of the tracheal bifurcation (carina), and a characteristic "double-contour" configuration caused by the projection of the enlarged left atrium through the normal right atrial silhouette. The increased left atrial pressure is transmitted to the pulmonary veins and produces the appearance of chronic venous congestion.

Calcification of the mitral valve or left atrial wall (Figure 7-44), best demonstrated by fluoroscopy, can develop in patients with long-standing severe mitral stenosis. A thrombus may form in the dilated left atrium and be the source of emboli to the brain or elsewhere in the systemic circulation.

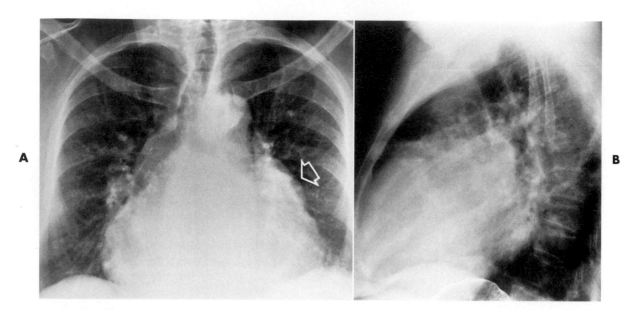

FIGURE 7-43 Mitral stenosis. Frontal **(A)** and lateral **(B)** projections of chest demonstrate cardiomegaly with enlargement of right ventricle and left atrium. Right ventricular enlargement causes obliteration of retrosternal air space, whereas left atrial enlargement produces convexity of upper left border of heart *(arrow)*.

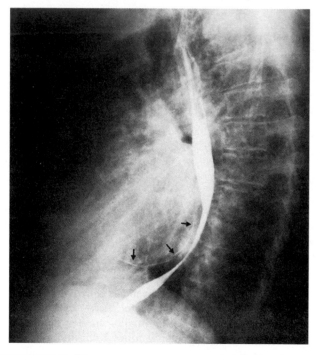

FIGURE 7-44 Left atrial calcification in mitral stenosis. Lateral projection with barium in esophagus shows enlargement of left atrium and calcification of the wall of its chamber *(arrows)*.

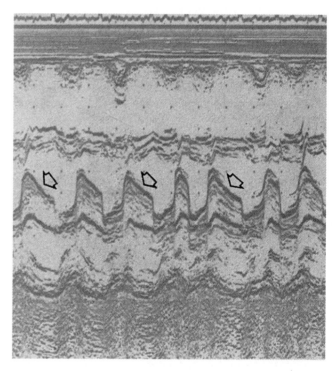

FIGURE 7-45 Echocardiogram of mitral stenosis. There is thickening of the mitral valve with decreased slope *(arrows)*.

Echocardiography is the most sensitive and most specific noninvasive method for diagnosing mitral stenosis (Figure 7-45). Echocardiography demonstrates chamber enlargement or wall thickening and permits measurement of the valvular orifices. More recently, cine MRI has been used to demonstrate and quantitate the abnormal pattern of flow between the left atrium and the left ventricle in mitral stenosis without the use of contrast agents.

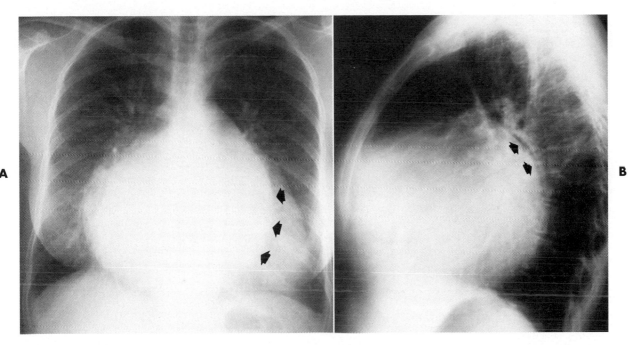

FIGURE 7-46 Mitral insufficiency. Frontal **(A)** and lateral **(B)** projections of chest demonstrate gross cardiomegaly with enlargement of left atrium and left ventricle. Note striking double-contour configuration *(arrows)* on frontal film and elevation of left mainstem bronchus *(arrows)* on lateral film, characteristic signs of left atrial enlargement.

Mitral Insufficiency

Although most often caused by rheumatic heart disease, mitral insufficiency may also be caused by the rupture of the chordae tendineae or by the dysfunction of the papillary muscles that are attached to the underside of the valve cusps and normally prevent them from swinging up into the atrium when the ventricles contract. Regurgitation of blood into the left atrium during ventricular systole causes overfilling and dilatation of this chamber, which leads to a decrease in ventricular stroke volume and cardiac output.

In most cases, the left atrium is considerably larger in mitral insufficiency than in mitral stenosis (Figure 7-46); occasionally, an enormous left atrium can form both the right and left borders of the heart on frontal projections. An increased volume of blood flowing from the dilated left atrium to the left ventricle in diastole increases the left ventricular workload and leads to dilatation and hypertrophy of this chamber. CHF, pulmonary congestion, and pulmonary hypertension may result. This causes downward displacement of the cardiac apex and rounding of the lower left border of the heart.

Treatment of Mitral Stenosis and Insufficiency

Surgical valvular replacement or correction of the stenosis may be performed to correct flow insufficiency.

CHF resulting from stenosis or insufficiency may require treatment.

Aortic Stenosis

Aortic stenosis may be caused by rheumatic heart disease, a congenital valvular deformity (especially of a bicuspid valve), or a degenerative process of aging (idiopathic calcific stenosis). The obstruction to left ventricular outflow in aortic stenosis increases the workload of the left ventricle.

Initially, this causes left ventricular hypertrophy without dilatation, which produces only some rounding of the cardiac apex on frontal chest radiographs and slight backward displacement on lateral projections. The overall size of the heart remains within normal limits until left ventricular failure develops. Significant aortic stenosis is usually associated with lateral bulging (poststenotic dilatation) of the ascending aorta caused by the jet of blood forced under high pressure through the narrowed valve (Figure 7-47). Aortic valve calcification, best demonstrated on fluoroscopic examination, is a common finding and indicates that the aortic stenosis is severe (Figure 7-48).

Aortic Insufficiency

Although most commonly caused by rheumatic heart disease, aortic insufficiency may be attributable to syphilis, infective endocarditis, dissecting aneurysm,

SUMMARY of FINDINGS for Valvular Disease

disorder	location	radiographic appearance	treatment
Rheumatic heart disease	Most frequently in mitral and aortic valves	Doppler echocardiography—quantify valvular insufficiencies	Prevention—antibiotics for streptococcal infections Therapy—antibiotics, antiinflammatory drugs, and restricted activity
Mitral stenosis	Mitral valve	PA chest—left atrium enlargement Lateral, RAO—posterior displacement of esophagus, posterior displacement of left main bronchus, calcification of valves Echocardiography—chamber enlargement, wall thickness, and size of valvular orifices Cine MRI—demonstrates and quantitates abnormal flow pattern	Surgical—valvular replacement, correction of stenosis Treat for CHF if needed
Mitral insufficiency	Valve dysfunction, rupture, or muscular dysfunction	PA chest—cardiomegaly—enlarged left atrium and left ventricle	
Aortic stenosis	Obstruction of flow exiting the heart	PA chest—enlargement of left ventricle; rounding of cardiac apex Posterior displacement of cardiac apex in lateral projection Lateral—posterior displacement of a cardiac apex; bulging of ascending aorta Aortic valve calcification	
Aortic insufficiency	Reflux of blood, causing volume overload of left ventricle	PA chest—cardiac apex—inferior, lateral, and posterior displacement	
Infective endocarditis	Nodules on heart valves	Echocardiography—shaggy echoes produced by irregular thickening of affected valves Electron-beam CT—vegetations in valve, valvular calcifications, distorted orifices	Bacterial—treat with antibiotics Surgically replace severely damaged valves

RAO, Right anterior oblique.

or Marfan's syndrome. Reflux of blood from the aorta during diastole causes volume overloading of the left ventricle and dilatation of this chamber.

Radiographic Appearance
Aortic insufficiency causes downward, lateral, and posterior displacement of the cardiac apex (Figure 7-49). Pronounced left ventricular dilatation causes relative mitral insufficiency, which leads to left atrial enlargement and signs of pulmonary edema.

Treatment of Aortic Stenosis and Aortic Insufficiency
CHF should be treated if the patient is symptomatic. Surgical valvular replacement or repair to correct stenosis can reestablish correct pressures and flow.

Infective Endocarditis
Infective endocarditis refers to the development of nodules or vegetations forming on heart valves caused by deposits of bacteria or fungi. Unlike the smaller nodules in rheumatic fever, the vegetations of infective endocarditis are filled with bacteria and tend to break apart easily (they are friable) to enter the bloodstream and form septic emboli that travel to the brain, kidney, lung, or other vital organs. Emboli lodging in the skin may cause rupture of small blood vessels and characteristic tiny hemorrhagic red spots (petechiae).

Radiographic Appearance
Plain radiography is of little value in patients with infective endocarditis. The cardiac silhouette may be normal or may demonstrate evidence of previous

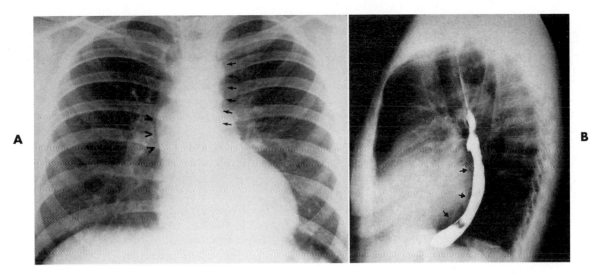

FIGURE 7-47 Aortic stenosis. **A,** Frontal projection shows downward displacement of cardiac apex with post-stenotic dilatation of ascending aorta *(arrowheads)*. Aortic knob and descending aorta *(arrows)* are normal. **B,** On lateral projection in another patient, bulging of the lower half of the posterior cardiac silhouette causes a broad indentation on the barium-filled esophagus *(arrows)*.

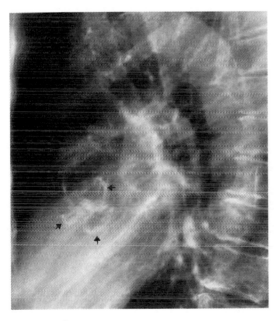

FIGURE 7-48 Aortic stenosis. Calcification in three leaflets of the aortic valve *(arrows)*.

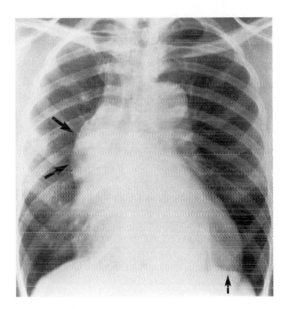

FIGURE 7-49 Aortic insufficiency. Frontal chest radiograph shows left ventricular enlargement with downward and lateral displacement of the cardiac apex. Notice that the cardiac shadow extends below the dome of the left hemidiaphragm *(small arrow)*. Ascending aorta is strikingly dilated *(large arrows)*, suggestive of some underlying aortic stenosis.

valvular heart disease or CHF. Echocardiography is the only noninvasive procedure that can detect the valvular vegetations that are the hallmark of infective endocarditis. On the echocardiogram, these vegetations appear as masses of shaggy echoes producing an irregular thickening of the affected valves (Figure 7-50). Electron-beam CT demonstrates the vegetations and the valvular calcifications, distorted orifices, and possible aneurysms.

Treatment

Antibiotics are taken until there is complete eradication of the bacterial infections. Severely damaged valves must be surgically replaced with artificial valves.

Pericardial Effusion

Pericardial effusion refers to the accumulation of fluid within the pericardial space surrounding the heart. The effusion may result from bacteria, viruses, or neoplastic involvement. In some cases, the cause cannot be determined (idiopathic pericardial effusion). Rapid accumulation of effusion interferes with cardiac function because of an increase in pericardial pressure. A slow accumulation of fluid allows the pericardium to expand, so that the pericardial pressure usually remains within the normal range.

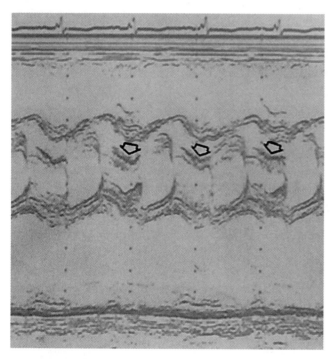

FIGURE 7-50 Infective endocarditis. Echocardiogram demonstrates vegetations as masses of shaggy echoes producing irregular thickening of the aortic valve *(arrows)*.

Radiographic Appearance

Echocardiography is the most effective imaging technique for demonstrating pericardial effusions and has largely replaced other methods. With this modality, a pericardial effusion is seen as a posterior sonolucent collection, and as little as 50 ml of fluid can be detected as an echo-free space between the visceral and parietal pericardium. Plain chest radiographs, on the other hand, which show a pericardial effusion as an enlargement of the cardiac silhouette (Figure 7-51), require at least 200 ml of fluid to be present before the effusion can be detected. Rapid enlargement of the cardiac silhouette, especially in the absence of pulmonary vascular engorgement indicating CHF, is highly suggestive of pericardial effusion.

Angiocardiography, intravenous carbon dioxide injection, and a pericardial tap with air injection have been used in the past to demonstrate pericardial effusion by showing an excessive distance (greater than 5 mm) between the contrast- or air-filled atrium and the outer border of the cardiac silhouette. CT can detect

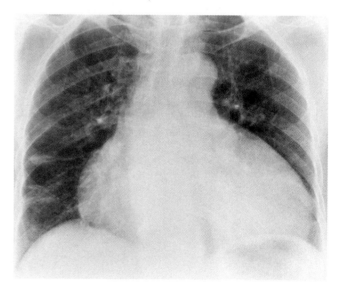

FIGURE 7-51 Pericardial effusion. Globular enlargement of cardiac silhouette.

SUMMARY of FINDINGS for Pericardial Effusion

disorder	location	radiographic appearance	treatment
Pericardial effusion	Increased fluid accumulation in pericardial sac	PA chest—enlargement of cardiac silhouette Echocardiography—posterior sonolucent fluid collection CT—loculated fluid accumulations MRI—differentiates serous from hemorrhagic fluid as a decreased signal intensity	Pericardiocentesis Pericardiectomy Administration of drugs into pericardial sac

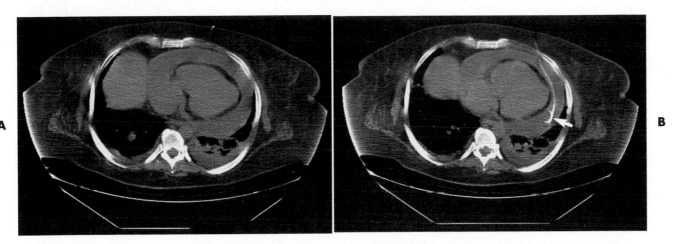

FIGURE 7-52 CT images demonstrating pericardial effusion. **A,** Heart is seen with a dark halo surrounded by fluid. **B,** A CT-guided catheter was placed in this patient for drainage *(arrow).*

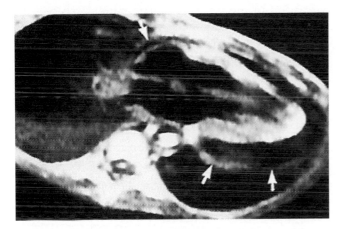

FIGURE 7-53 MR image of pericardial effusion. Pericardium *(arrows)* is displaced away from the heart by a huge pericardial effusion that has a very low signal intensity. Effect of gravity is seen in the posterior location of both pericardial and right pleural effusions.

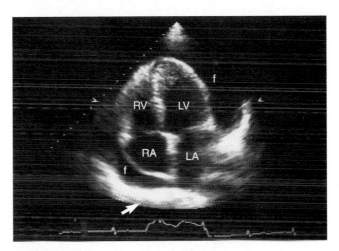

FIGURE 7-54 Pericardial effusion. Echocardiogram demonstrates an apical four-chamber heart image with fluid around the heart *(f)* producing back-wall enhancement *(arrow). LA,* Left atrium; *IV,* left ventricle; *RA,* right atrium; *RV,* right ventricle.

loculated pericardial effusions as small as 50 ml (Figure 7-52), whereas MRI may be able to characterize the fluid as serous or hemorrhagic by characteristic changes in the signal intensity and identify an accumulation of as little as 30 ml. Gated MRI (Figure 7-53) demonstrates a pericardial effusion as a region of decreased signal intensity between the myocardium and the fat on the surface of the parietal pericardium (which is usually invisible when it is in direct contact with the heart). However, echocardiography has effectively replaced these invasive techniques (Figure 7-54).

Treatment

The treatment depends on the cause. Pericardiocentesis is performed to remove fluid buildup, and insertion of a drain may be required. If the pericardial effusion recurs, a pericardiectomy may be necessary. An interventional technique includes administration of drugs into the pericardial sac.

Venous Disease

Deep Venous Thrombosis

DVT, which primarily involves the lower extremities, is the major source of potentially fatal pulmonary embolism. Precipitating factors in the development of venous thrombosis include trauma, bacterial infection, prolonged bed rest, and oral contraceptives. At times, DVT may be the earliest symptom of an unsuspected malignancy of the pancreas, lung, or gastrointestinal system.

Radiographic Appearance

A precise diagnosis of DVT requires contrast venography, which can demonstrate the major venous channels and their tributaries from the foot to the inferior vena cava. During venography, the patient's leg should not be massaged to decrease edema. If DVT exists, the pressure applied could cause a thrombus to break free, becoming an embolus. The identification of a constant filling defect, representing the actual thrombus, is conclusive evidence of DVT (Figure 7-55). Venographic findings that are highly suggestive of, although not conclusive for, the diagnosis of DVT include the abrupt ending of the opaque column in a vein, the nonfilling of one or more veins that are normally opacified, and extensive collateral venous circulation.

Because venography is an invasive technique, other modalities have been developed for detecting DVT. Duplex color Doppler ultrasound, which demonstrates changes in the velocity of venous blood flow with 95% accuracy, is now the preferred initial imaging modality. It is of special value in demonstrating thrombotic occlusion of major venous pathways in the popliteal and femoral regions. Ultrasound demonstrates lack of compressibility of the vein, an indication of the presence of a thrombus (Figure 7-56). Color Doppler allows visualization of the intraluminal thrombus itself and the characteristic changes in spontaneous flow that occur because of obstruction. However, an abnormal Doppler ultrasound examination is not specific for thrombosis because similar changes in venous blood flow may be caused by CHF, extensive leg edema, local soft tissue masses, and decreased inflow of arterial blood into the extremity.

Treatment

An anticoagulant drug is prescribed to prevent the formation of more thrombi. The patient receives an intravenous thrombolytic agent to lyse the already formed clot. If the lower extremity is involved, many recommend bed rest to prevent the possibility of emboli.

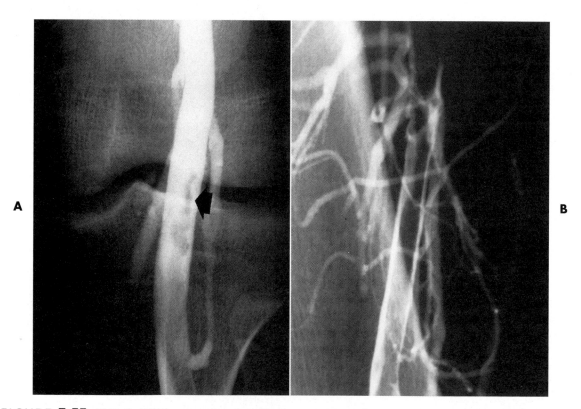

FIGURE 7-55 DVT. **A,** Initial contrast venogram demonstrates early nonocclusive thrombus extending from valve cusp. Arrow points to thrombus tail, the portion most likely to embolize. **B,** Subsequent contrast venogram demonstrates growth and proximal extension of thrombus, which has resulted in occlusion of popliteal vein at adductor hiatus.

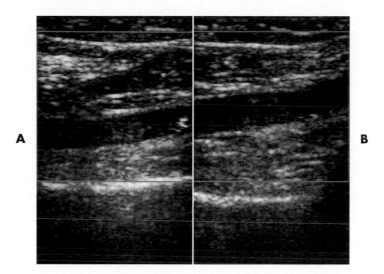

FIGURE 7-56 Doppler image of DVT. The left leg was swollen with some discoloration. The deep venous system shows abnormal intraluminal echoes involving the distal superficial femoral vein **(A)** and popliteal vein **(B)**; both areas show no compressibility, which is consistent with a diagnosis of thrombosis.

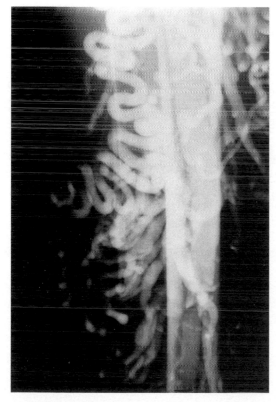

FIGURE 7-57 Varicose veins. Lower extremity venogram shows multiple tortuous, dilated venous structures.

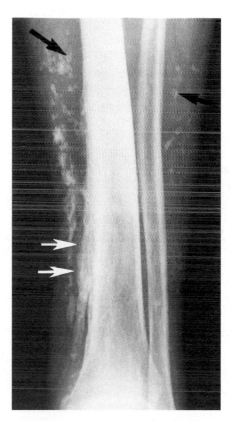

FIGURE 7-58 Varicose veins. Multiple round and oval calcifications in soft tissues (phleboliths) represent calcified thrombi, some of which have characteristic lucent centers (black arrows). Extensive new bone formation along the medial aspect of the tibial shaft (white arrows) is caused by long-standing venous stasis.

SUMMARY of FINDINGS for Venous Disease

disorder	location	radiographic appearance	treatment
Deep venous thrombosis	Primarily involves the lower extremities	Venography—constant filling defect or abrupt ending of the opaque column in a vein; nonfilling of one or more veins; extensive collateral venous circulation Color Doppler—visualization of thrombus and flow changes due to obstruction	Anticoagulants to prevent new thrombus formation Thrombolytic to lyse clot Bed rest to decrease possible emboli
Varicose veins	Commonly involve superficial veins of the leg	Venography—demonstrates patency of the deep venous system and degree of collateral circulation from the superficial to deep veins	Therapeutic—weight reduction; elevation of legs; support hose and exercise Surgical—vein stripping or cauterization; removing superficial veins

Varicose Veins

Varicose veins are dilated, elongated, and tortuous vessels that most commonly involve the superficial veins of the leg just under the skin (Figure 7-57). If the venous dilatation becomes extreme, the valves that normally prevent backflow of blood because of gravity become incompetent and cease to function, thus increasing the volume of blood in these slow-flowing vessels.

Although heredity plays some role in the development of varicose veins, the underlying cause is increased pressure in an affected vein. Varicose veins can be an occupational hazard for people who stand or sit for long periods. Normally, the action of leg muscles helps move blood upward toward the heart from one venous valve to the next. If this "milking action" of the muscles is absent, the blood puts pressure on the closed valves and the thin walls of the veins, resulting in venous dilatation, incompetence of the valves, and stasis of blood in the stagnant lower extremity veins. Increased pressure on a vein can also be attributable to a pregnant uterus or a pelvic tumor.

Stasis of blood within varicose veins may lead to the development of phleboliths, calcified clots within a vein that appear radiographically as rounded densities, which often contain lucent centers (Figure 7-58). Chronic venous stasis may also lead to periosteal new bone formation along the tibial and fibular shafts and the development of plaquelike calcifications in the chronically congested subcutaneous tissues. The poor venous flow can lead to the development of superficial ulcers, and the distended veins can rupture, causing hemorrhage into the surrounding tissues.

Radiographic Appearance

Although the diagnosis of varicose veins is primarily based on the clinical observation of the multiple bluish nodules just under the skin, venography is of value in demonstrating the patency of the deep venous system and the degree of collateral circulation from the superficial to the deep veins, especially if there is consideration of surgical intervention (tying off and removing the superficial veins). After the application of a tourniquet to occlude superficial flow, the peripheral injection of contrast material opacifies the deep venous system. Filling of the superficial veins indicates that the perforating veins above the level of the tourniquet are incompetent.

Treatment

Treatment consists of various ways to decrease the pressure in the lower extremities. If the varices are related to excess weight, weight reduction helps alleviate symptoms; if they are related to standing all day, then elevating the legs to assist blood flow return is recommended. Support hose and exercise to strengthen contractibility of the leg muscles may also aid in blood flow return. When nonsurgical treatment is not successful, vein stripping or cauterization may be performed.

REVIEW QUESTIONS

1. Heart rate is controlled by the _____ nervous system.
   A. psychogenic   C. peripheral
   B. central   D. autonomic

2. The _____ valve is located between the left atrium and the left ventricle, whereas the _____ valve is located between the right atrium and the right ventricle.
   I. tricuspid
   II. mitral
   III. pulmonary
   IV. aortic
   A. II, I   C. IV, I
   B. III, I   D. I, II

3. The general circulation of the body is termed the _____ circulation.
   A. pulmonary   C. general
   B. systemic   D. autonomic

4. The contracting phase of the heart is termed _____, whereas the relaxation phase is termed _____.
   I. autonomic
   II. diastole
   III. systemic
   IV. systole
   A. I, III   C. II, III
   B. II, IV   D. IV, II

5. Contraction of which chamber of the heart forces oxygenated blood into the aorta?
   A. right atrium   C. left atrium
   B. right ventricle   D. left ventricle

6. Oxygenated blood reaches the heart muscle by way of the _____.
   I. right coronary artery
   II. left coronary artery
   III. left coronary vein
   IV. right coronary vein
   A. I, III   C. II, I
   B. IV, I   D. II, III

7. The heart has a specialized pacemaker named the _____.
   A. bundle of His   C. Purkinje fibers
   B. sinoatrial node   D. atrioventricular node

8. Which factor(s) lead to coronary artery disease?
   A. lack of exercise   C. smoking, high-cholesterol diet
   B. obesity, hypertension   D. all of the above

9. Temporary oxygen insufficiency to the heart muscle causes severe chest pain termed _____.
   A. angina pectoris   C. myocardial pectoris
   B. myocardial occlusion   D. angina occlusion

10. Arterial disease caused by fatty deposits on the inner arterial wall is termed _____.
    A. arteriosclerosis   C. aneurysm
    B. myocardial infarction   D. myocardial ischemia

11. What radiographic procedure is used to determine the presence of coronary artery disease?
    A. angioplasty   C. coronary arteriogram
    B. chest film   D. CT

12. The procedure in which a balloon is used to dilate narrowed coronary arteries is named _____.
    A. aortocoronary bypass   C. percutaneous transluminal angioplasty
    B. coronary arteriography   D. fluoroscopy

13. Which term refers to an inability of the heart to propel blood at a sufficient rate and volume?
    A. congestive heart failure   C. valvular disease
    B. pulmonary edema   D. valvular stenosis

14. An elevation of the pulmonary venous pressure is the most common cause of _____.
    A. congestive heart failure   C. valvular disease
    B. pulmonary edema   D. valvular stenosis

15. The leading cause of strokes and CHF is _____.
    A. hypertension   C. hypotension
    B. low blood pressure   D. cor pulmonale

16. A localized bulging or dilatation of an artery is termed _____.
    A. edema
    B. effusion
    C. aneurysm
    D. fat emboli

17. What is the modality of choice for demonstration of an abdominal aortic aneurysm?
    A. MRI
    B. ultrasonography
    C. CT
    D. plain film radiography

18. A congenital narrowing or constriction of the thoracic aorta is referred to as _____.
    A. embolism
    B. plaque
    C. coarctation
    D. tetralogy

19. The _____ of the heart is/are the major site of damage from rheumatic fever.
    A. myocardium
    B. valves
    C. septum
    D. endocardium

20. The most sensitive and specific noninvasive method of diagnosing mitral stenosis is

    _____.
    A. ultrasonography
    B. echocardiography
    C. cardiac arteriography
    D. CT

21. The accumulation of fluid within the pericardial space surrounding the heart is termed

    _____.
    A. pericardial thrombosis
    B. pericardial effusion
    C. pulmonary edema
    D. pulmonary effusion

22. The invasive procedure for determining deep vein thrombosis is _____.
    A. Doppler ultrasound
    B. venography
    C. CT
    D. arteriography

23. The most accurate screening procedure for assessing renovascular lesions is _____.
    A. Doppler ultrasound
    B. venography
    C. CT
    D. arteriography

24. A potentially life-threatening condition that usually begins as a tear in the intima above the aortic valve is an _____.
    A. aortic stenosis
    B. aortic coarctation
    C. aortic thrombosis
    D. aortic dissection

BIBLIOGRAPHY

Burgener FA, Kormano M: *Differential diagnosis in computed tomography,* New York, 1996, Thieme.

Cooley RN, Schreiber MH: *Radiology of the heart and great vessels,* Baltimore, 1978, Williams & Wilkins.

eMedicine Specialties>Cardiology: emedicine.com

eMedicine Specialties>Radiology: emedicine.com

Mintz G: *Intravenous ultrasound imaging: practical considerations,* Paris Course on Revascularization, 2000, Europa Organization.

Rumack CM, Wilson SR, Charborneau JW: *Diagnostic ultrasound,* St Louis, 2005, Mosby.

Swischuk LE: *Plain film interpretation in congenital heart disease,* Baltimore, 1979, Williams & Wilkins.

CHAPTER **8**

NERVOUS *System*

Chapter Outline

Physiology of the Nervous System
Infections of the Central Nervous System
    Meningitis
    Encephalitis
    Brain Abscess
    Subdural Empyema
    Epidural Empyema
    Osteomyelitis of the Skull
Tumors of the Central Nervous System
    Glioma
    Meningioma
    Acoustic Neuroma
    Pituitary Adenoma
    Craniopharyngioma
    Pineal Tumors
    Chordoma
    Metastatic Carcinoma
Traumatic Processes of the Brain and Skull
    Skull Fracture
    Epidural Hematoma
    Subdural Hematoma
    Cerebral Contusion
    Intracerebral Hematoma
    Subarachnoid Hemorrhage
    Carotid Artery Injury
    Facial Fractures
Vascular Disease of the Central Nervous System
    Stroke Syndrome
    Transient Ischemic Attacks
    Intraparenchymal Hemorrhage
    Subarachnoid Hemorrhage
Multiple Sclerosis
Epilepsy and Convulsive Disorders
Degenerative Diseases
    Normal Aging
    Alzheimer's Disease
    Huntington's Disease
    Parkinson's Disease
    Cerebellar Atrophy
    Amyotrophic Lateral Sclerosis (Lou Gehrig's Disease)
Hydrocephalus
Sinusitis

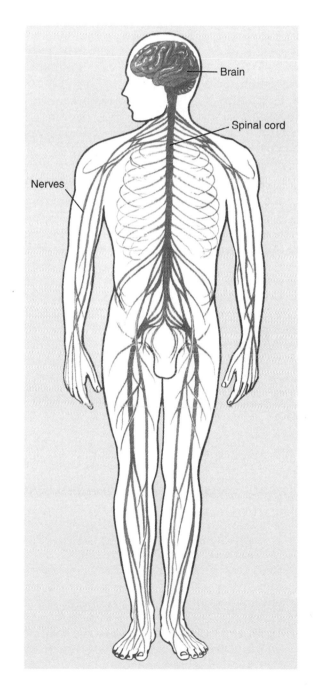

Key Terms

arachnoid membrane
arachnoid villi
astrocytomas
autonomic nervous system
bacterial meningitis
basal ganglia
blowout fracture
central nervous system (CNS)
cerebellum
cerebrovascular disease
cerebrum
choroid plexuses
chromophobe adenomas
communicating hydrocephalus
corpus callosum
cortex
depressed fractures
diastatic fracture
diencephalon
dysarthria
dura mater

ependymomas
fissures
glioblastomas
gliomas
grand mal
gyri
hemiparesis
hemiplegia
hypothalamus
linear skull fracture
mandibular fractures
medulla
medulloblastomas
meninges
meningitis
midbrain
myelin sheath
nasal bone fractures
neuron
noncommunicating (obstructive)
  hydrocephalus

normal-pressure hydrocephalus
oligodendrocytomas
peripheral nervous system (PNS)
petit mal
pia mater
pituitary adenomas
pons
reflex arc
releasing hormones
somatic nervous system
stroke
subarachnoid space
sulci
synapse
thalamus
tripod fracture
vermis
viral meningitis
zygomatic arch fractures

Prerequisite Knowledge

The student should have a basic knowledge of the anatomy and physiology of the skull and nervous system. In addition, proper learning and understanding of the material will be facilitated if the student has some clinical experience in skull radiography and image evaluation, including a concept of the newer imaging modalities: computed tomography (CT), CT angiography (CTA), magnetic resonance imaging (MRI), MR angiography (MRA), and positron emission tomography (PET).

Goals

To acquaint the student radiographer with the pathophysiology and radiographic manifestations of all of the common and some of the unusual disorders of the skull and nervous system.

Objectives

After reading this chapter, the reader will be able to:
1. Define all key terms in this chapter
2. Describe the physiology of the nervous system
3. Identify anatomic structures on both diagrams and radiographs of the skull and nervous system
4. Differentiate the various pathologic conditions affecting the skull and nervous system, and their radiographic manifestations

Physiology of the Nervous System

The divisions of the nervous system can be classified by location or by the type of tissue supplied by the nerve cells in the division. The **central nervous system (CNS)** consists of the brain and spinal cord. The remaining neural structures, including 12 pairs of cranial nerves, 31 pairs of spinal nerves, autonomic nerves, and ganglia, make up the **peripheral nervous system (PNS)**. The PNS consists of afferent and efferent neurons. Afferent (sensory) neurons conduct impulses from peripheral receptors to the CNS. Efferent (motor) neurons conduct impulses away from the CNS to the peripheral effectors. The **somatic nervous system** supplies the striated skeletal muscles, whereas the **autonomic nervous system** supplies smooth muscle, cardiac muscle, and glandular epithelial tissue.

The basic unit of the nervous system is the **neuron,** or nerve cell. A neuron consists of a cell body and two types of long, threadlike extensions. A single axon leads from the nerve cell body, and one or more dendrites lead toward it. Axons are insulated by a fatty covering called the **myelin sheath,** which increases the rate of transmission of nervous impulses. Deterioration of this fatty myelin sheath (demyelination) is a characteristic abnormality in multiple sclerosis.

RADIOGRAPHER *Notes*

Proper positioning is critical in skull and spine radiography to ensure bilateral symmetry and to permit an evaluation of the complex anatomy and structural relationships. The demonstration of asymmetry or a shift in the normal location of a structure in a patient who is positioned correctly may be indicative of an underlying pathologic condition. Proper positioning and correct angulation of the central ray may allow visualization of otherwise superimposed structures. When evaluating such anatomic areas as the sinuses or facial bones, it is often necessary to place the patient in the erect position (either standing or sitting) and to use a horizontal beam to demonstrate an air-fluid level indicative of underlying inflammatory disease or fracture. If the patient's condition prohibits placement in an erect position, air-fluid levels can be demonstrated only by obtaining a cross-table lateral projection using a horizontal beam with the patient in a dorsal decubitus position.

Exposure factors should produce a scale of contrast that provides maximal detail (definition), especially when imaging vascular structures and when looking for subtle changes in bone density, such as result from fractures of the skull or spine. Advanced stages of certain pathologic conditions may require changes in technique to maintain the proper level of density, contrast, and visibility of detail (see the Box in Chapter 1, p. 4, Relative Attenuation of X-Rays in Advanced Stages of Diseases). If contrast material is used, the kilovolts-peak level must remain in the low to mid range to provide enough radiographic contrast to properly show the contrast-filled vessels.

The administration of radiographic contrast material is an essential component of many examinations of the skull and nervous system. Therefore it is essential that the radiographer be familiar with the use of these agents and be extremely alert to the development of possible allergic reactions. Currently the radiographic scope of practice includes venous access and pharmacology of contrast agents. Some facilities may require the radiographer to inject agents, especially for computed tomography (CT) and magnetic resonance imaging (MRI). After contrast administration, the radiographer is often left alone in the room with the patient and must be able to immediately recognize an allergic reaction to contrast material and be able to initiate and maintain basic life-support techniques until advanced life-support personnel have arrived. Although departmental policy varies, it is usually the radiographer's responsibility to assist during resuscitation procedures. Therefore it is essential that the radiographer be familiar with the contents of the emergency cart and be responsible for ensuring that the cart is completely stocked with all appropriate medications.

The impulse conduction route to and from the CNS is termed a **reflex arc**. The basic reflex arc consists of an afferent, or sensory, neuron, which conducts impulses to the CNS from the periphery; and an efferent, or motor, neuron, which conducts impulses from the CNS to peripheral effectors (muscles or glandular tissue).

Impulses pass from one neuron to another at a junction called the **synapse**. Transmission at the synapse is a chemical reaction in which the termini of the axon release a neurotransmitter substance that produces an electrical impulse in the dendrites of the next axon. Once the neurotransmitter has accomplished its task, its activity rapidly terminates so that subsequent impulses can be conducted along this same route.

The largest part of the brain is the **cerebrum,** which consists of two cerebral hemispheres. The surface of the cerebrum is highly convoluted with elevations called **gyri** and shallow grooves called **sulci**. Deeper grooves called **fissures** divide each cerebral hemisphere into lobes. The outer portion of the cerebrum, termed the **cortex,** consists of a thin layer of gray matter where the nerve cell bodies are concentrated. The inner area consists of white matter, which is composed of the nerve fiber tracts.

The cerebral cortex is responsible for receiving sensory information from all parts of the body, and for triggering impulses that govern all motor activity. Just posterior to the central sulcus, the cerebral cortex has specialized areas to receive and precisely localize sensory information from the PNS. Visual impulses are transmitted to the posterior portion of the brain; olfactory (smell) and auditory impulses are received in the lateral portions. The primary motor cortex is just anterior to the central sulcus. Because efferent motor fibers cross over from one side of the body to the other at the level of the medulla and spinal cord, stimulation on one side of the cerebral cortex causes contraction of muscles on the opposite side of the body. The premotor cortex, which lies anterior to the primary motor cortex, controls movements of muscles by stimulating groups of muscles that work together. This region also contains the portion of the brain responsible for speech, which is usually on the left side in right-handed people. The cerebral cortex also is the site of all higher functions, including memory and creative thought.

The two cerebral hemispheres are connected by a mass of white matter called the **corpus callosum**. These extensive bundles of nerve fibers lie in the midline just above the roofs of the lateral ventricles.

Deep within the white matter are a few islands of gray matter that are collectively called the **basal ganglia**. These structures help control position and automatic movements and consist of the caudate nuclei, the globus pallidus, and the putamen.

Between the cerebrum and spinal cord lies the brainstem, which is composed of (from top down) the **midbrain** (mesencephalon), the **pons**, and the **medulla**. In addition to performing sensory, motor, and reflex functions, the brainstem contains the nuclei of the 12 cranial nerves and the vital centers controlling cardiac, vasomotor, and respiratory function. Centers in the medulla are responsible for such nonvital reflexes as vomiting, coughing, sneezing, hiccupping, and swallowing.

The **cerebellum,** the second largest part of the brain, is located just below the posterior portion of the cerebrum. It is composed of two large lateral masses: the cerebellar hemispheres and a central section **(vermis)** that resembles a worm coiled on itself. The cerebellum acts with the cerebral cortex to produce skilled movements by coordinating the activities of groups of muscles. It coordinates skeletal muscles used in maintaining equilibrium and posture by functioning below the level of consciousness to make movements smooth rather than jerky, steady rather than trembling, and efficient and coordinated rather than ineffective and awkward. Therefore cerebellar disease produces such characteristic symptoms as ataxia (muscle incoordination), tremors, and disturbances of gait and equilibrium.

The **diencephalon** lies between the cerebrum and the midbrain. It consists of several structures located around the third ventricle, primarily the thalamus and hypothalamus. The **thalamus** primarily functions as a relay station that receives and processes sensory information of almost all kinds of sensory impulses before sending this information on to the cerebral cortex. The tiny **hypothalamus** is an extremely complex structure that functions as a link between the mind and body and is the site of "pleasure" or "reward" centers for such primary drives as eating, drinking, and mating. It plays a major role in regulating the body's internal environment by coordinating the activities of the autonomic nervous system and secreting the **releasing hormones** that control the secretion of hormones by the anterior and posterior portions of the pituitary gland. The hypothalamus is also important in helping to maintain a normal body temperature and in keeping the individual in a waking state.

The spinal cord lies within the vertebral column and extends from its junction with the brainstem at the foramen magnum to approximately the lower border of the first lumbar vertebra. It consists of an inner core of gray matter surrounded by white matter tracts. The basic function of the spinal cord is to conduct impulses up the cord to the brain (ascending tracts) and down the cord from the brain to spinal nerves (descending tracts). It also serves as the center for spinal reflexes and involuntary responses, such as the knee jerk (patellar reflex).

The delicate, yet vital, brain and spinal cord are protected by two layers of coverings. The outer bony coverings are the cranial bones of the skull encasing the brain and the vertebrae surrounding the spinal cord. The inner coverings consist of three distinct layers of **meninges**. The innermost layer adhering to the outer surface of the brain and spinal cord is the transparent **pia mater,** and the tough outermost covering is termed the **dura mater**. Between these layers is the delicate, cobweblike **arachnoid membrane**. Inflammation of these three protective layers is called **meningitis**.

Three extensions of the dura mater separate portions of the brain. The falx cerebri projects downward into the longitudinal fissure to separate the cerebral hemispheres. Similarly, the falx cerebelli separates the two cerebellar hemispheres. The tentorium cerebelli forms a tentlike covering over the cerebellum that separates it from the occipital lobe of the cerebrum.

In addition to bony and membranous coverings, the brain and spinal cord are further protected by a cushion of fluid both around them and within them. The ventricles are four spaces within the brain that contain cerebrospinal fluid (CSF). There are two large lateral ventricles, one located in each cerebral hemisphere. The slitlike third ventricle lies between the right and left thalamus. The anterior parts of the lateral ventricles (frontal horns) are connected by a Y-shaped canal that extends downward to open into the upper part of the third ventricle at the foramen of Monro. The fourth ventricle is a diamond-shaped space between the cerebellum posteriorly and the medulla and pons anteriorly. It is continuous inferiorly with the central canal of the spinal cord. The third and fourth ventricles are connected by the aqueduct of Sylvius (cerebral aqueduct), a narrow canal that runs through the posterior part of the midbrain.

CSF is formed by the filtration of plasma from blood in the **choroid plexuses,** networks of capillaries that project from the pia mater into the lateral ventricles and into the roofs of the third and fourth ventricles. After flowing through the ventricular system, the fluid circulates in the **subarachnoid space** (between the pia mater and the arachnoid) around the brain and spinal cord before being absorbed into venous blood through **arachnoid villi.** Obstruction of CSF circulation results in hydrocephalus.

Infections of the Central Nervous System

The incidence of infectious diseases of the CNS has decreased with the widespread availability of antibiotics. Nevertheless, bacterial, fungal, viral, and protozoal organisms can infect the brain parenchyma, meningeal linings, and bones of the skull.

Meningitis

Meningitis is an acute inflammation of the pia mater and arachnoid, two of the membranes covering the brain and spinal cord. Infecting organisms can reach the meninges from a middle ear, the upper respiratory tract, or a frontal sinus infection, or they can be spread through the bloodstream (hematogenously) from an infection in the lungs or other site. **Bacterial meningitis** (pyogenic) is most commonly caused by *Haemophilus influenzae* in neonates and young children, and by meningococci and pneumococci in adolescents and adults. **Viral meningitis** may be caused by mumps, poliovirus, and occasionally by herpes simplex. A chronic form of meningitis can be caused by tuberculous infection. Bacterial meningitis is the most common form. The bacteria release toxins that destroy the meningeal cells, thus stimulating immune and inflammatory reactions.

Radiographic Appearance

Although the meninges initially demonstrate vascular congestion, edema, and minute hemorrhages, the underlying brain remains intact. MRI and CT scans are normal during most acute episodes of meningitis and remain normal if appropriate therapy is promptly instituted. If the infection extends to involve the cortex of the brain and the ependymal lining of the ventricles, contrast studies may show characteristic meningeal enhancement in the basal cisterns, interhemispheric fissure, and choroid plexus (Figure 8-1). Diffuse brain swelling may symmetrically compress the lateral and third ventricles. MRI and CT are also of value in the early detection of such complications of acute meningitis as arterial or venous vasculitis or thrombosis with infarction, hydrocephalus caused by adhesions or thickening of the arachnoid at the base of the brain, subdural effusion or empyema, and brain abscess. A spinal tap is necessary to determine the cause of meningitis. CT is the modality of choice to rule out contraindications to lumbar puncture (cerebral hemorrhage or increased ventricular pressure).

Although MRI and CT are best for evaluating acute bacterial meningitis, plain films of the sinuses and skull can demonstrate cranial osteomyelitis, paranasal sinusitis, or a skull fracture as the underlying cause of meningitis. In approximately 50% of patients, chest radiographs may show a silent area of pneumonia or a lung abscess. Contrast-enhanced MRI is the most sensitive modality for demonstrating enhancement of the two innermost layers of the meninges (pia mater and arachnoid membrane) and subarachnoid distention with interhemispheric widening that is consistent with early findings of severe meningitis. On T2-weighted images, edema produces cortical hyperintensities.

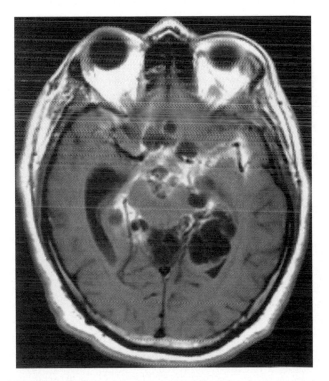

FIGURE 8-1 Meningitis. Subarachnoid enhancement in the basal cisterns and left sylvian fissure in a patient with cysticercosis.

Treatment

A sample of CSF is collected for culture, and when the organism is identified, specific antibiotics are given to eradicate the bacteria. Even before these results are available, the patient is immediately treated with a broad-spectrum antibiotic to prevent morbidity. If secondary encephalitis develops, the patient receives antiviral drugs. Any increased intracranial pressure is appropriately treated.

Encephalitis

Encephalitis, a viral inflammation of the brain and meninges (meningoencephalitis), produces symptoms ranging from mild headache and fever to severe cerebral dysfunction, seizures, and coma. About 30% of cases occur in children. Encephalitis caused by herpes simplex is an often fatal, fulminant (sudden severe infection, fever, or hemorrhage) process.

Radiographic Appearance

The earliest and predominant findings in herpetic encephalitis are poorly marginated areas (with a patchy parenchymal pattern) in the temporal lobes and inferior frontal gray matter, which have high signal intensity on T2-weighted MR images and demonstrate low density on CT scans. These changes probably represent a combination of tissue necrosis and focal brain edema. A mass effect is common and may be seen as a midline shift or as a focal mass compressing the ventricles or the sylvian cisterns. Compromise of the blood-brain barrier in areas of rapid, more progressive hemorrhagic necrosis results in a nonhomogeneous pattern of contrast enhancement. CT reveals abnormalities 3 to 5 days after the onset of symptoms, when the patient may be comatose. In toxoplasmosis, nodular lesions demonstrate ring enhancement on contrast CT. MRI is the preferred modality, even though in acute cases a contrast-enhanced scan may appear negative. Follow-up scans typically demonstrate widespread low-density encephalomalacia (sponginess) involving the temporal and frontal lobes.

Treatment

In addition to confirming the clinical diagnosis of herpes simplex encephalitis and excluding the presence of an abscess or a tumor, MRI and CT are important because they can indicate the best site for biopsy. A definitive diagnosis of herpes infection is essential before beginning treatment with adenine arabinoside, a chemotherapeutic agent that may be neurotoxic, mutagenic, and carcinogenic. Acyclovir, a new antiviral drug used in treating herpes infection, interferes with the deoxyribonucleic acid (DNA) synthesis and inhibits viral replication.

Brain Abscess

Brain abscesses are usually a result of chronic infections of the middle ear, paranasal sinuses, or mastoid air cells, or of systemic infections (pneumonia, bacterial endocarditis, osteomyelitis). The most common organisms causing brain abscesses are streptococci. In patients with acquired immunodeficiency syndrome (AIDS), unusual organisms such as toxoplasmosis and cryptococcosis often cause brain abscesses. The microorganisms lodge preferentially in the gray matter and spread to the adjacent white matter.

Radiographic Appearance

The earliest sign of brain abscess on an MR or CT image is an area of abnormal density with poorly defined borders and a mass effect reflecting vascular congestion and edema. Further progression of the inflammatory process leads to cerebral softening, which may undergo necrosis and liquefaction and result in a true abscess. MRI is considered superior for demonstrating a brain abscess, although CT can be employed when MRI is unavailable. On T1-weighted MR images, an abscess appears as a hypointense mass with an isointense capsule surrounded by low signal–intensity edema (Figure 8-2, *A*). Both the mass and the edema are hyperintense on proton density and T2-weighted images (Figure 8-2, *B*). After the intravenous administration of contrast material, an oval or circular peripheral ring of contrast enhancement outlines the abscess capsule. Although the wall is usually thin and of uniform thickness, an irregularly thick wall, resulting from the formation of granulation tissue, may mimic a malignant glioma. Diffusion MR can distinguish necrotic tumors from abscesses by demonstrating a reduced diffusion coefficient. Multiple abscesses indicate the possibility of septic emboli from a systemic infection (Figure 8-3).

Plain skull radiographs may show evidence of underlying sinusitis, mastoiditis, or osteomyelitis, although this is better evaluated by CT scanning with bone-window settings. Infection by gas-forming organisms occasionally produces an air-fluid level within the abscess cavity.

Treatment

A broad-spectrum antibiotic is given to fight the infection. A craniotomy to totally excise the abscess is most successful in cases of a multiloculated abscess. Image-directed stereotactic aspiration to provide a specimen for microbial evaluation is better because it is less invasive. In some cases, the patient may require medication to reduce increased intracranial pressure.

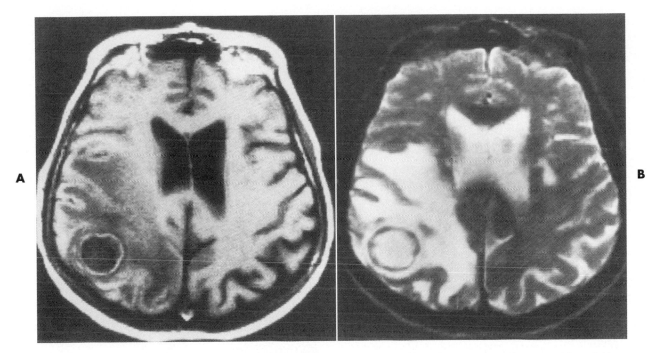

FIGURE 8-2 Brain abscess. **A,** T1-weighted MR scan shows a central hypointense necrotic mass with an isointense capsule surrounded by low signal intensity edema. **B,** On the T2-weighted image, the hypointense capsule is highlighted by increased signal centrally and peripherally.

MRI and CT can be used to assess the results of therapy for a brain abscess and to document complications. These modalities can demonstrate the often fatal intraventricular rupture of an abscess and the development of increased intracranial pressure, which may lead to brain herniation.

Subdural Empyema

Subdural empyema is a suppurative process in the space between the inner surface of the dura and the outer surface of the arachnoid. Approximately 25% of intracranial infections are subdural empyemas. The most common cause of subdural empyema is the spread of infection from the frontal or ethmoid sinuses. Less frequently, subdural empyema may result from mastoiditis, middle ear infection, purulent meningitis, penetrating wounds to the skull, craniectomy, or osteomyelitis of the skull. Subdural empyema is often bilateral and associated with a high mortality even if properly treated. The most common location of a subdural empyema is over the cerebral convexity; the base of the skull is usually spared.

Radiographic Appearance

MRI is the procedure of choice in evaluating the patient with suspected subdural empyema. Unlike CT, MRI is free from bony artifacts adjacent to the inner

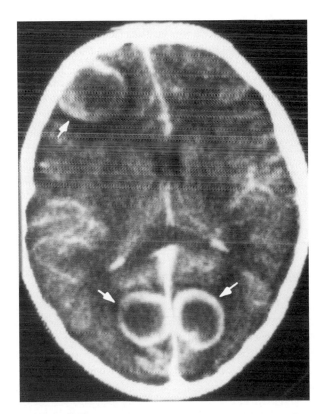

FIGURE 8-3 Pyogenic brain abscesses. CT scan shows one frontal and two occipital lesions *(arrows)* with relatively thin, uniform rings of enhancement.

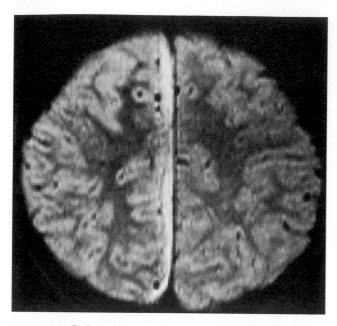

FIGURE 8-4 Subdural empyema. T2-weighted MR scan demonstrates high signal intensity of the fluid collections along the falx.

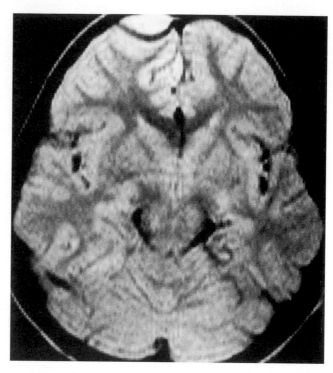

FIGURE 8-5 Epidural empyema. Black rim of dura delineates the epidural fluid collection in the right frontal region.

table of the skull. In addition, signal characteristics may permit differentiation between benign effusions and infected empyemas. Noncontrast scans demonstrate a crescentic or lentiform (lenslike), extraaxial fluid collection (representing pus) adjacent to the inner border of the skull or the falx (Figure 8-4). There is compression and displacement of the ipsilateral ventricular structures. After the intravenous administration of contrast material, a narrow zone of enhancement of relatively uniform thickness separates the extracerebral collection from the brain surface. MRI can also demonstrate involvement of the adjacent parenchyma by means of retrograde thrombophlebitis with resultant infarction or abscess formation, signs associated with a poor prognosis.

Epidural Empyema

Epidural empyema (Figure 8-5) is almost invariably associated with osteomyelitis in a cranial bone originating from an infection in the ear or paranasal sinuses. The infectious process is localized outside the dural membrane and beneath the inner table of the skull. The frontal region is most frequently affected because of its close relationship to the frontal sinuses and the ease with which the dura can be stripped from the bone.

Radiographic Appearance

Noncontrast CT scans demonstrate the epidural infection as a poorly defined area of low density adjacent to the inner table of the skull. An adjacent area of bone destruction or evidence of paranasal sinus or mastoid infection (fluid, soft tissue thickening) can often be demonstrated on CT or plain skull radiographs. After the intravenous administration of contrast material, the inflamed dural membrane appears as a thickened zone of enhancement on the convex inner side of the lesion. If the collection lies in the midline, the attachment of the falx is displaced inward and separated from the adjacent skull, thus identifying its extradural location.

Treatment of Subdural and Epidural Empyemas

Subdural and epidural empyemas should be treated as medical emergencies. Immediate surgical drainage of an empyema and the underlying sinus infection aids in preventing recurrence. Craniotomy provides the most complete evacuation. The broad-spectrum antibiotic regimen used for a brain abscess is used here also.

Osteomyelitis of the Skull

Osteomyelitis of the skull is most commonly caused by direct extension of a suppurative process from the paranasal sinuses, mastoid air cells, or scalp. As with osteomyelitis elsewhere in the skeleton, the radiographic

SUMMARY of FINDINGS for Infections of the Central Nervous System

disorder	location	radiographic appearance	treatment
Meningitis	Acute inflammation of meninges	CT/MRI—arterial or venous vasculitis or thrombosis, hydrocephalus, subdural effusion, and brain abscess MRI—enhancement of the two innermost layers of the meninges and subarachnoid distention with interhemispheric widening Radiographs—osteomyelitis, sinusitis, or fracture	Immediate broad-spectrum antibiotics followed by specific antibiotics determined by culture results
Encephalitis	Viral inflammation of brain and meninges	MRI—hyperintensity on T2-weighted images with mass effect CT—low-attenuation regions without focal enhancement; mass effect	Herpes infection—adenine arabinoside
Brain abscess	Microorganism infection of gray and white matter	MRI—T1-weighted images show hypointense mass with isointense capsule; proton density and T2-weighted images show hyperintensity of both the mass and surrounding edema; diffusion MRI distinguishes necrotic tumors from abscesses CT—contrast-enhanced scan identifies a high-attenuation capsule surrounding a hypodense necrotic center	Broad-spectrum antibiotics Craniotomy to totally excise the multiloculated abscess Image-directed stereotactic aspiration provides a specimen for microbial evaluation Medication to reduce increased intracranial pressure if symptoms occur
Subdural empyema	Infection located between the dura and the arachnoid	MRI—characteristic crescentic or lentiform extraaxial fluid collection that is mildly hyperintense to CSF on T2-weighted images	Craniotomy for immediate surgical drainage of empyema and underlying sinus empyema; aids in preventing recurrence Same broad-spectrum antibiotic regimen as for brain abscess
Epidural empyema	Infectious process above the dura and beneath the inner skull table	CT (noncontrast)—shows low-density area adjacent to the inner table of the skull, with possible bone destruction CT (contrast enhanced)—dural membrane appears as a thickened zone of enhancement on the convex inner side of the lesion	
Osteomyelitis of the skull	Cranial bones	Radiograph—multiple small poorly defined areas of lucency, 1-2 weeks after onset of symptoms	See Chapter 4

changes often develop 1 to 2 weeks after the onset of clinical symptoms and signs.

Radiographic Appearance
Acute osteomyelitis first appears radiographically as multiple small, poorly defined areas of lucency (Figure 8-6). Over the next several weeks, the lucencies enlarge and coalesce centrally with an expanding perimeter of small satellite foci. As the infection becomes more chronic (especially with syphilis, tuberculosis, or fungal infections), attempts at bone regeneration produce multiple areas of poorly defined reactive sclerosis.

Treatment
Refer to the discussion on bacterial osteomyelitis in Chapter 4.

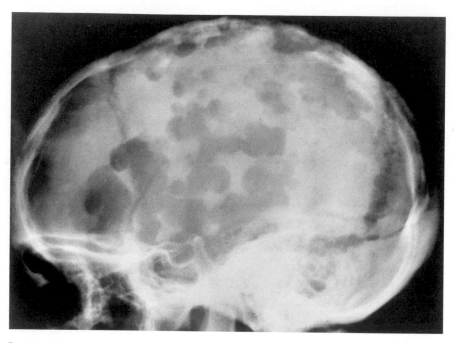

FIGURE 8-6 Osteomyelitis of skull (resulting from blastomycosis). Diffuse areas of osteolytic destruction affect most of the calvaria.

Tumors of the Central Nervous System

Intracranial neoplasms present clinically with seizure disorders or gradual neurologic deficits (difficulty thinking, slow comprehension, weakness, headache). About 50% of CNS tumors are primary lesions, and the others represent metastases.

Radiographic Appearance

The clinical presentation and radiographic appearance depend on the location of the tumor and the site of the subsequent mass effect. MRI is generally considered to be the most sensitive technique for detecting most suspected brain tumors. In general, both the tumor and its surrounding edema demonstrate high signal intensity on T2-weighted images. After the intravenous injection of contrast material, the enhancing tumor can usually be distinguished from nonenhancing edema on T1-weighted scans (Figure 8-7). In addition to its exquisite sensitivity in detecting pathologic alteration of normal tissue constituents, MRI provides excellent delineation of tumor extent and can show associated abnormalities, such as hydrocephalus. This modality is of special value in imaging neoplasms of the brainstem and posterior fossa, which may be poorly demonstrated on CT due to bone artifact. CT with contrast enhancement is an excellent examination for evaluating a patient

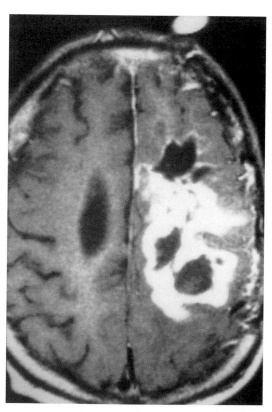

FIGURE 8-7 Glioblastoma multiforme. Axial T1-weighted MR scan shows intense contrast enhancement of this complex necrotic mass.

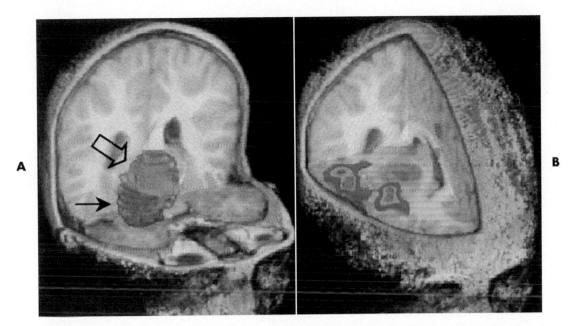

FIGURE 8-8 Low-grade brain tumor studied by three-dimensional reconstruction of a PET cerebral study using ¹¹C-methionine. **A,** Mass effect near the thalamus is evident when the increased uptake *(open arrow)* is compared with a cystic component showing lack of uptake *(solid arrow).* **B,** The greatest activity is noted in the right temporal lobe corresponding to receptive and expressive language areas.

with suspected brain tumor. It is of special value for detecting punctate or larger calcification that cannot be shown by MRI. Although skull radiographs were used in the past to demonstrate tumoral calcification, bone erosion, and displacement of the calcified pineal gland, plain films are no longer indicated because this information can be more effectively obtained on CT scans.

Before the advent of CT, cerebral arteriography was used to demonstrate evidence of brain tumors, such as mass effect, contralateral displacement of midline arteries and veins, abnormal vessels with tumor staining, and early venous filling. At present, the major use of arteriography is for precise delineation of the arterial and venous anatomy. This provides a surgical map before operative therapy and for evaluation of those cases in which a vascular anomaly is a strong consideration in the differential diagnosis of a tumor. Radionuclide brain scans have a relatively high rate of detection of cerebral tumors, but are far less specific than CT or MRI. PET scans demonstrate metabolic activity and specific location of a lesion for presurgical planning (Figure 8-8).

Treatment

Therapy depends on the location and histology of the tumor. If possible, the tumor is surgically resected, followed by radiation therapy if the tumor is not completely removed. In some cases, radiation therapy and chemotherapy are used when the tumor is inoperable.

Glioma

Gliomas, the most common primary malignant brain tumors, consist of glial cells (supporting connective tissues in the CNS) that still have the ability to multiply. They spread by direct extension and can cross from one cerebral hemisphere to the other through connecting white matter tracts, such as the corpus callosum. Gliomas have a peak incidence in middle adult life and are infrequent in persons less than 30 years of age.

Glioblastomas are highly malignant lesions that are predominantly cerebral, although similar tumors may occur in the brainstem, cerebellum, or spinal cord. **Astrocytomas** (70% of all gliomas) are slow growing tumors that have an infiltrative character and can form large cavities or pseudocysts. Favored sites are the cerebrum, cerebellum, thalamus, optic chiasm, and pons.

Less frequent types of gliomas are ependymoma, medulloblastoma, and oligodendrocytoma. **Ependymomas** most commonly arise from the walls of the fourth ventricle, especially in children, and usually from the lateral ventricles in adults. **Medulloblastomas** are rapidly growing tumors, disseminating throughout the spinal fluid, that develop in the posterior portion of the vermis in

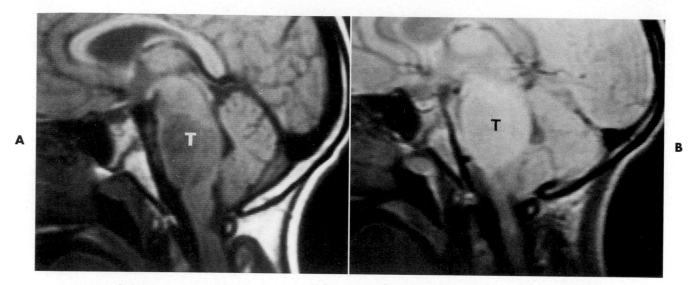

FIGURE 8-9 Brainstem glioma. Sagittal MR scans show enlargement of brainstem involving pons and midbrain. Notice that various imaging techniques alter the appearance of the tumor *(T)*. **A,** On T1-weighted image, tumor is gray (low-intensity signal). **B,** On T2-weighted image, tumor appears white (high-intensity signal).

children and rarely in the cerebellar hemisphere in adults. The tumor tends to spread through the subarachnoid space, with metastatic deposits occurring anywhere within the brain or spinal column. **Oligodendrocytomas** are slow-growing lesions that usually arise in the cerebrum and have a tendency to calcify.

Radiographic Appearance

On MR scans (Figure 8-9), gliomas typically appear as masses of high signal intensity on T2-weighted images. They may be of low intensity or isointense on T1-weighted sequences. MR spectroscopy has a typical spectral pattern with a strongly increased choline peak, which indicates myelin or the breakdown of myelin (the chemical structure that goes into making white matter). In MR spectroscopy, a highly elevated choline level, a drastically lower level of *N*-acetylaspartate (a neuronal marker), and a drastically lower creatine/phosphocreatine ratio confirm an infiltrating glioma (Figure 8-10). Ependymomas, often partially calcified and cystic, have a heterogeneous signal intensity and show enhancement.

On noncontrast CT scans, gliomas are most commonly seen as single, nonhomogeneous masses. Low-grade astrocytomas tend to be low-density lesions showing little or no enhancement (Figure 8-11); glioblastomas most frequently contain areas of both increased and decreased density, although a broad spectrum of CT appearances can occur. Edema is often seen in the adjacent subcortical white matter. After the intravenous injection of contrast material, virtually all gliomas show enhancement, with the most malignant

lesions tending to be enhanced to the greatest degree (see Figure 8-7). In MR spectroscopy, an elevated choline/creatine ratio suggests a malignant neoplasm. The most common pattern is an irregular ring of contrast enhancement, representing solid vascularized tumor, surrounding a central low-density area of necrosis. Contrast enhancement also can appear as patches of increased density distributed irregularly throughout a low-density lesion or as rounded nodules of increased density within the mass.

Treatment

Therapy depends on the location and histology of the tumor. Astrocytomas have a good 5-year survival rate after surgery and radiation therapy. For ependymomas of the filum terminale, surgical removal provides a favorable prognosis.

Meningioma

Meningioma is a benign tumor that arises from arachnoid lining cells and is attached to the dura. The most common sites of meningioma are the convexity of the calvaria, the olfactory groove, the tuberculum sellae, the parasagittal region, the sylvian fissure, the cerebellopontine angle, and the spinal canal. Of all spinal tumors, 25% are meningiomas. Seizures and neurologic defects are most often caused by mass effect.

Radiographic Appearance

Because meningiomas tend to be isointense (equal intensity) with brain on both T1- and T2-weighted images, anatomic distortion is the key to the MRI diagnosis (Figure 8-12). A thin rim of low intensity,

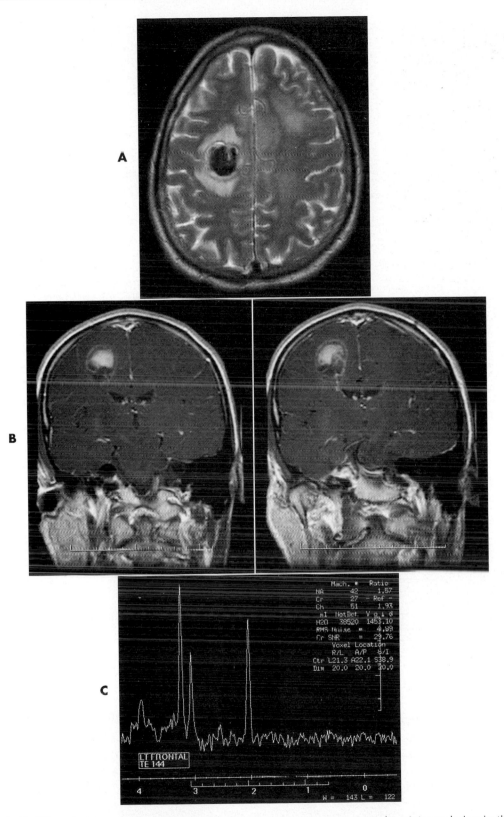

FIGURE 8-10 Infiltrating glioma. **A,** T2-weighted image demonstrates a 3-cm hypointense lesion in the deep right parietal lobe with a hyperintense peripheral rim. A poorly defined hyperintense lesion is seen within the deep white matter of the left temporal and parietal lobes. **B,** On the T1-weighted coronal image, the hyperintense periphery is seen surrounding a low signal intensity and a high signal intensity lesion. **C,** On MR spectroscopy, the left frontal lobe demonstrates an elevated choline (first) peak, a slightly lower creatine/phosphocreatine (second) peak, and a mildly depressed *N*-acetylaspartate (third) peak. These findings help confirm a low-grade, diffuse infiltrating glioma.

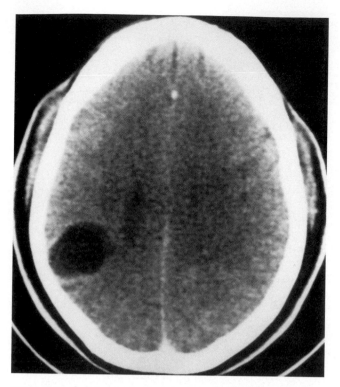

FIGURE 8-11 Cystic astrocytoma. CT scan shows hypodense mass with thin rim of contrast enhancement.

consisting of a CSF cleft, the vascular rim, or dura, may separate the tumor from the adjacent brain. Calcification within a meningioma may produce nonuniform signal or focal signal void. Surrounding edema may make the lesion easier to identify. Just as the detection of meningiomas by CT is facilitated by the use of iodinated contrast material, paramagnetic contrast agents can enhance the detection of meningiomas on MRI. MR spectroscopy has a typical spectral pattern with a strongly increased choline peak; creatine is a marker of energy metabolism. Alanine is another specific amino acid marker producing a unique peak in meningiomas. CT typically shows a meningioma as a rounded, sharply delineated, isodense (25%) or hyperdense (75%) tumor abutting a dural surface. Calcification often is seen within the mass on noncontrast scans. After the intravenous injection of contrast material, there is intense homogeneous enhancement, which reflects the highly vascular nature of the tumor (Figure 8-13).

Pronounced dilatation of meningeal and diploic vessels, which provide part of the blood supply to the tumor, may produce prominent grooves in the calvaria on plain films of the skull. Calvarial hyperostosis (increased density) may develop because of invasion of the bone by tumor cells that stimulate osteoblastic activity. Dense calcification or granular psammomatous deposits may be seen within the tumor (Figure 8-14).

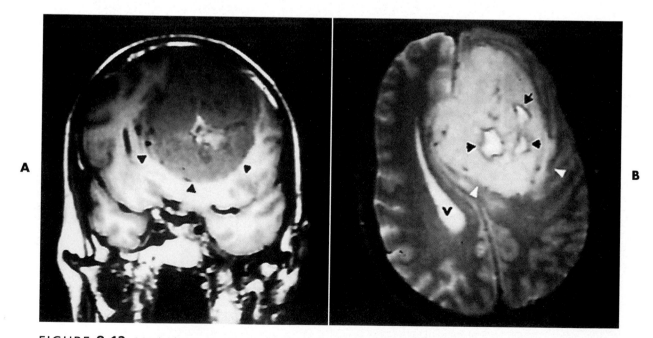

FIGURE 8-12 Meningioma. **A,** Huge mass *(arrowheads)* appears hypointense on T1-weighted coronal MR scan. **B,** The mass appears hyperintense on T2-weighted image. Notice the dramatic shift of the ventricle *(v)* caused by mass effect of tumor. *Black arrows* point to areas of hemorrhage within the neoplasm *(white arrowheads).*

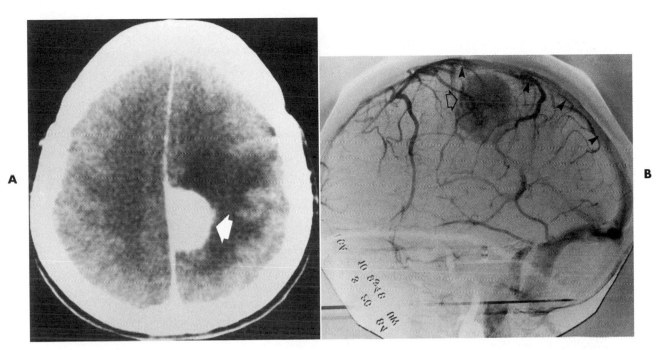

FIGURE 8-13 Meningioma. **A,** CT scan after intravenous injection of contrast material shows uniformly enhancing mass *(arrow)* with surrounding low-density edema attached to falx. **B,** Venous phase of carotid arteriogram shows characteristic prominent vascular blush *(arrow)* of meningioma. Note that the superior sagittal sinus *(arrowheads)* is patent.

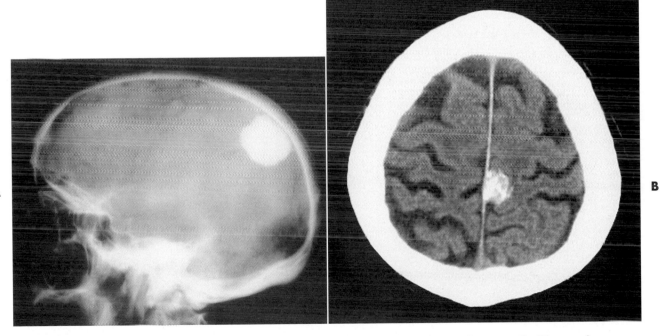

FIGURE 8-14 Parietal meningioma. **A,** Plain skull film shows dense calcification in tumor. **B,** CT scan of another patient, demonstrating a midline calcified meningioma.

Arteriography can demonstrate the feeding arteries, which most commonly arise from both the internal and the external carotid artery circulation. Preoperative embolization of the external carotid artery supply can decrease the amount of blood loss at surgery.

Spinal meningiomas are best demonstrated on T1/T2-weighted images using gadolinium enhancement as a homogeneous intense lesion. CT myelography demonstrates the location of the mass, which is usually intradural extramedullary (Figure 8-15).

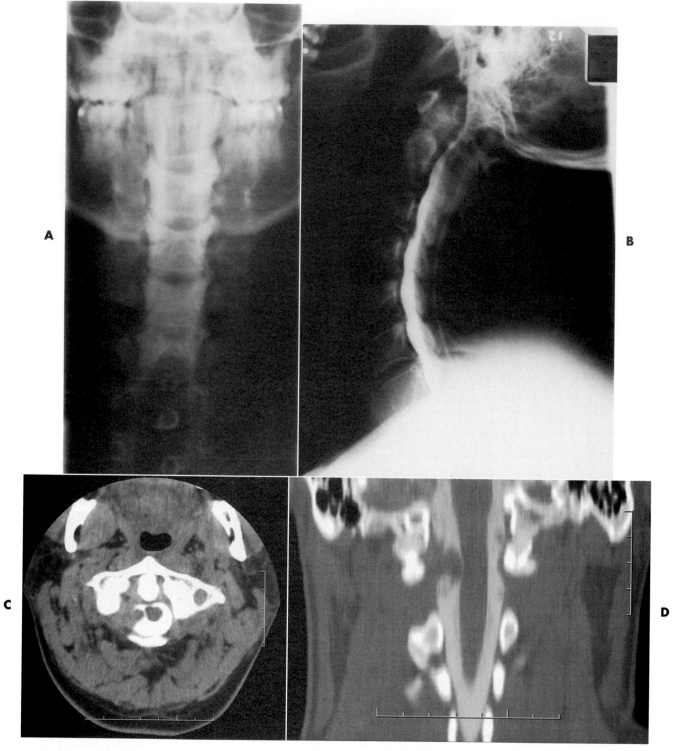

FIGURE 8-15 Spinal meningioma. **A,** Anteroposterior and, **B,** lateral myelogram images appear normal. CT scanning following the subarachnoid injection of contrast demonstrates a meningioma as a filling defect at the level of C1-2 on the right in the **C,** axial, and **D,** coronal projections.

Treatment

Surgical resection is very successful because of the superficial position of the tumor and the lack of tumor infiltration. Incomplete resection results in a lobulated and mushroom pattern of tumor growth.

Acoustic Neuroma

Acoustic neuroma is a slowly growing benign tumor that may occur as a solitary lesion or as part of the syndrome of neurofibromatosis. The tumor arises from Schwann cells in the vestibular portion of the auditory (eighth cranial) nerve. It usually originates in the internal auditory canal and extends into the cerebellopontine angle cistern.

Radiographic Appearance

MR scans (T1-weighted), the preferred modality, exquisitely show the tumor as a focal or generalized enlargement of the eighth cranial nerve (Figure 8-16). This technique can even demonstrate small intracanalicular tumors confined to the internal auditory canal, which may be impossible to show on CT unless contrast material (nonionic water-soluble material or air) is administered into the ventricular system. CT scans demonstrate enlargement and erosion of the internal auditory canal and a uniformly enhancing mass in the cerebellopontine angle (Figure 8-17). Very large tumors may compress the fourth ventricle and lead to the development of hydrocephalus.

Treatment

Surgical excision of the lesion or gamma knife radiosurgery improves symptoms

Pituitary Adenoma

Pituitary adenomas, almost all of which arise in the anterior lobe, constitute more than 10% of all intracranial tumors. Most are nonsecreting **chromophobe adenomas.** As chromophobe tumors enlarge, the adjoining secreting cells within the sella turcica are compressed, leading to diminished secretion and decreased levels of growth hormone, gonadotropins, thyrotropic hormone, and adrenocorticotropic hormone (ACTH). Large chromophobe adenomas can extend upward to distort the region of the optic chiasm, whereas lateral expansion of tumor can compress the cranial nerves passing within the cavernous sinus.

Hormone-secreting pituitary tumors can cause clinical symptoms even if too small to produce mechanical mass effect. Hypersecretion of growth hormone results in gigantism in adolescents (before the epiphyses have closed) and acromegaly in adults (after the epiphyses have closed). Excess secretion of ACTH by a pituitary tumor results in the hypersecretion of steroid hormones from the adrenal cortex and symptoms of Cushing's disease. Hypersecretion of thyroid-stimulating hormone (TSH) leads to hyperthyroidism; excess secretion of prolactin by a pituitary tumor in women causes the galactorrhea-amenorrhea syndrome.

Radiographic Appearance

Thin-section CT and MRI are the examinations of choice for evaluating a patient with a suspected pituitary tumor. After the intravenous administration of

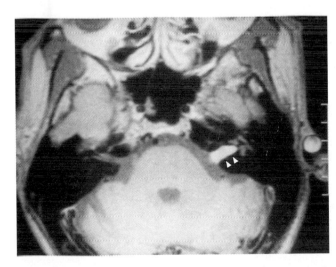

FIGURE 8-16 Acoustic neuroma. MR scan shows considerable contrast enhancement of the left-sided lesion *(arrowheads).* Notice the normal neural structures on the right.

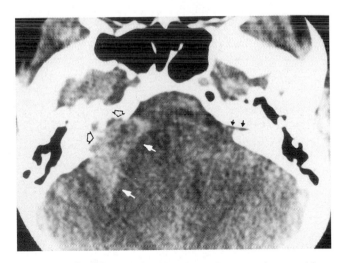

FIGURE 8-17 Acoustic neuroma. CT scan shows widening and erosion of right internal auditory canal *(open arrows)* associated with large extraaxial mass *(white arrows)* in right cerebellopontine angle. Solid black arrows point to normal internal auditory canal on left.

contrast material, large pituitary tumors are typically homogeneous and hyperdense with respect to surrounding brain tissue. Most pituitary microadenomas are of lower density than the normal pituitary gland. CT can also demonstrate adjacent bone erosion, tumor extension beyond the confines of the sella, and impression on nearby structures, such as the third ventricle, optic nerves, or optic chiasm (Figure 8-18).

The preferred modality for detecting and defining the extent of a pituitary tumor is MRI due to its superior sensitivity and multiplanar capability. Thin section coronal and sagittal T1-weighted MR scans show a microadenoma as a low signal intensity focal lesion associated with contralateral deviation of the pituitary stalk and an upwardly convex contour of the gland (Figure 8-19). The intravenous injection of paramagnetic contrast material significantly improves diagnostic sensitivity in patients with tiny secreting pituitary tumors. Immediately after injection, small microadenomas appear hypointense relative to the normally enhancing pituitary gland. On delayed scans, the neoplasm may become hyperintense relative to the normal gland.

Although plain skull radiographs can show enlargement of the sella turcica, erosion of the dorsum sellae, and a double floor resulting from the unequal downward growth of the mass, this imaging modality is now of value only in the incidental detection of sellar enlargement on films taken for other purposes.

Treatment

The size of the pituitary adenoma determines the extent of the treatment. For pituitary tumors not extending beyond the gland, surgical transsphenoidal resection has a good prognosis. Adenomas extending beyond the pituitary require surgical resection followed by radiation therapy for best results. The new gamma knife radiosurgery is another therapeutic alternative.

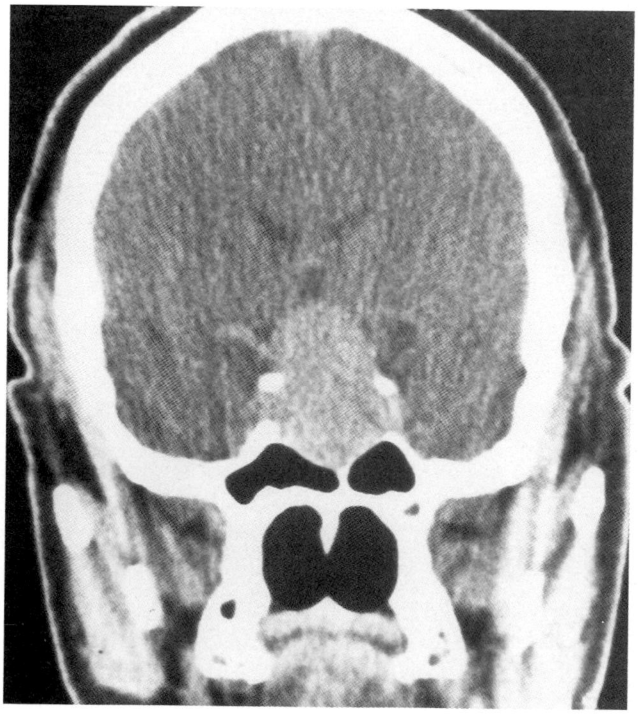

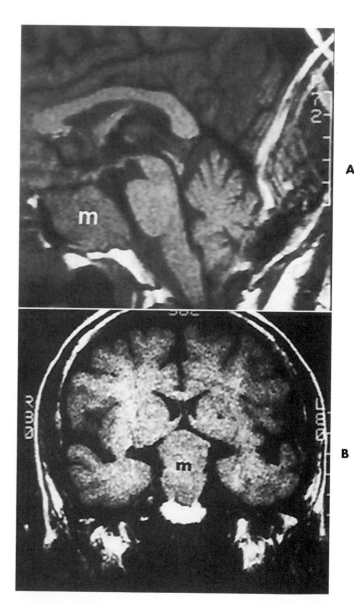

FIGURE **8-18** Pituitary adenoma. Coronal CT scan shows enhancing mass filling and extending out from pituitary fossa. Note erosion of base of sella.

FIGURE **8-19** Pituitary adenoma. Sagittal **(A)** and coronal **(B)** MR scans demonstrate large mass *(m)* that arises from sella turcica and extends upward to fill suprasellar cistern.

Craniopharyngioma

Craniopharyngioma is a benign tumor that contains both cystic and solid components and usually occurs before the age of 20 years. The lesion generally originates above the sella turcica, from embryonic remnants, depressing the optic chiasm and extending up into the third ventricle. Less commonly, a craniopharyngioma lies within the sella, where it compresses the pituitary gland and may erode adjacent bony walls.

Radiographic Appearance

Most craniopharyngiomas have calcification that can be detected on plain skull films or CT scans (Figure 8-20). In cystic lesions, the shell-like calcification lies along the periphery of the tumor; in mixed or solid lesions, the calcification is nodular, amorphous, or cloudlike. CT clearly demonstrates the cystic and solid components (isoattenuating) of the multilobulated mass. After the intravenous administration of contrast material, there is variable enhancement, depending on the type of calcification and the amount of cystic component within the tumor (Figure 8-21). CT can also demonstrate hydrocephalus if the tumor has expanded to obstruct one or both of the foramina of Monro.

The MRI appearance of craniopharyngioma depends on the tissue components of the tumor. Cystic areas have low signal intensity on T1-weighted scans and high signal intensity on T2-weighted scans; fat-containing regions have high signal intensity on T1-weighted images and show moderate signal intensity on T2-weighted scans (Figure 8-22). Large areas of calcification appear dark on all imaging sequences.

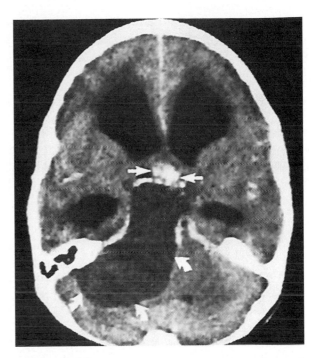

FIGURE **8-21** Craniopharyngioma. CT scan shows rim-enhancing tumor that contains dense calcification (*straight arrows*) and large cystic component (*curved arrows*) that extends into the posterior fossa. Note the associated hydrocephalus.

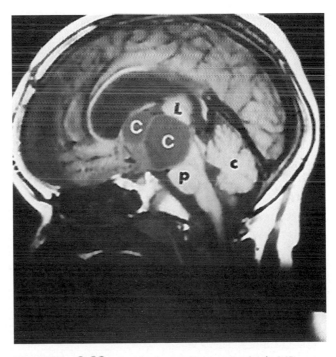

FIGURE **8-22** Craniopharyngioma. Sagittal MR scan demonstrates large multiloculated suprasellar mass with cystic (*C*) and lipid (*L*) components. c, Cerebellum; p, pons.

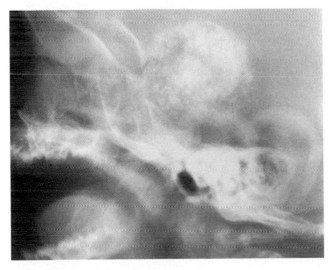

FIGURE **8-20** Craniopharyngioma. Plain skull radiograph shows large suprasellar calcified mass in a child.

New MR sequences—gradient-echo, fluid-attenuated inversion recovery, spectroscopy, and diffusion imaging—assist in differentiating tumor consistency.

Treatment

A new treatment is MR-guided stereotactic resection via microsurgery. Some tumors are completely resectable; for others, surgical debulking and radiation therapy are performed. Surgery and radiation, either alone or in combination, may provide long-term control in many patients.

Pineal Tumors

The most common tumors of the pineal gland are germinomas and teratomas, rapidly growing germ cell tumors, both of which occur predominantly in males less than 25 years of age and may be associated with precocious puberty.

Radiographic Appearance

Sagittal MR scans are ideal for showing pineal tumors, which typically compress the midbrain from above and lift up the splenium of the corpus callosum (Figure 8-23). Although most germinomas are isointense to brain on both T1- and T2-weighted images, teratomas may have mixed signal intensity because they contain cystic components and fat.

On CT, germinomas appear as hyperdense or isodense masses that tend to deform or displace the posterior aspect of the third ventricle and often obliterate the quadrigeminal cistern. Punctate calcification can often be detected within the mass. Intense enhancement of the tumor occurs after the injection of contrast material. Teratomas in the pineal region typically appear as hypodense masses with internal calcification (Figure 8-24). Occasionally, other formed elements (e.g., teeth) can occur. Contrast enhancement is usually much less pronounced than with germinomas. Large pineal tumors may cause obstructive hydrocephalus with ventricular dilatation.

A small number of tumors with the histologic appearance of pinealomas appear elsewhere in the brain at some distance from the normal pineal gland. These "ectopic pinealomas" generally occur in the anterior aspect of the third ventricle or within the suprasellar cistern. They may produce the clinical triad of bitemporal hemianopsia, hypopituitarism, and diabetes insipidus that simulates a craniopharyngioma.

Treatment

Surgery is the initial therapy of choice for pineal tumors. Radiation therapy following surgery may be helpful. Chemotherapy is used with radiation therapy if surgery is not a viable option.

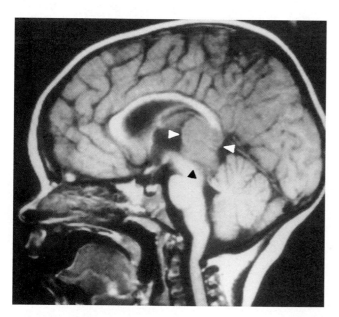

FIGURE 8-23 Pineal germinoma. Sagittal T1-weighted MR scan shows a large isointense mass *(white arrowheads)* that compresses the midbrain *(black arrowhead)* and elevates the splenium of the corpus callosum.

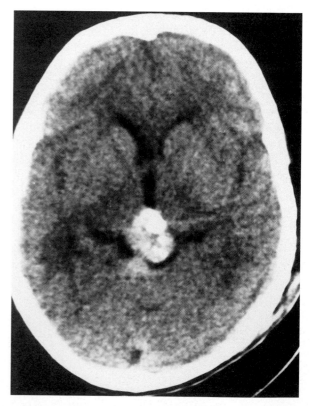

FIGURE 8-24 Pineal teratoma. Nonenhanced CT scan shows inhomogeneous mass containing a large amount of calcification.

Chordoma

Chordomas are tumors that arise from remnants of the notochord (the embryonic neural tube). Although any part of the vertebral column and base of the skull can be involved, the most common sites are the clivus and the lower lumbosacral region. The tumors are locally invasive, but do not metastasize. Chordomas arising at the base of the skull produce the striking clinical picture of multiple cranial nerve palsies on one or both sides combined with a retropharyngeal mass and erosion of the clivus.

Radiographic Appearance

On plain radiographs, a chordoma tends to be a bulky mass causing ill-defined bone destruction or cortical expansion. Flocculent (fluffy or cloudlike) calcification may develop within a large soft tissue mass (Figure 8-25, *A*). On CT scans, chordomas at the base of the skull tend to appear as lesions that are slightly denser than brain tissue and often demonstrate moderate contrast enhancement (Figure 8-25, *B*). Sagittal MR scans best demonstrate the clival origin of the mass and its effect on surrounding structures (Figure 8-26). Three-dimensional gradient-echo T1-weighted sequences are best for demonstrating the clival region. With gadolinium enhancement, chordomas have heterogeneous intensity and ring enhancement.

Treatment

Chordomas of the clivus region are difficult to completely remove surgically, and thus the patient usually is also treated with radiation. For chordomas of the lumbar region, complete surgical resection is usually possible.

Metastatic Carcinoma

Carcinomas usually reach the brain by hematogenous spread. Infrequently, epithelial malignancies of the nasopharynx can spread into the cranial cavity through neural foramina or by direct invasion through bone. The most common neoplasms that metastasize to the brain arise in the lung and breast. Melanomas, colon carcinomas, and testicular and kidney tumors also cause brain metastases.

Radiographic Appearance

On T2-weighted MR scans, metastases appear as single or multiple masses of high signal intensity that are most commonly situated at the junction between gray matter and white matter (Figure 8-27). Additional lesions can often be demonstrated after the injection of a paramagnetic contrast agent. On CT, brain metastases typically appear as multiple enhancing lesions of various sizes with surrounding amounts of low-density edema (Figures 8-28 and 8-29). On noncontrast scans, metastatic deposits may be hypodense, hyperdense, or similar in density to normal brain tissue, depending on such factors as cellular density, tumor neovascularity, and degree of necrosis. In general, metastases from lung, breast, kidney, and colon tend to be hypodense or isodense; hyperdense metastases often reflect hemorrhage or calcification within or adjacent to the tumor.

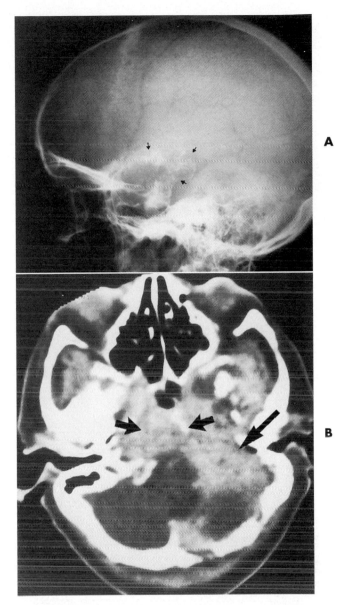

FIGURE 8-25 Chordoma. **A,** Plain skull radiograph shows dense calcification *(arrows)* within a large soft tissue mass that has an eroded dorsum sellae and upper portion of the clivus. **B,** In another patient, CT scan shows enlarging mass with destruction of the entire clivus *(short arrows)* and only small bone fragments remaining. Left petrous pyramid is also destroyed *(long arrow)*.

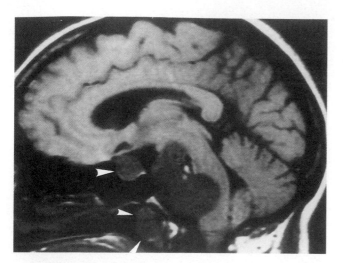

FIGURE 8-26 Clival chordoma. Sagittal MR scan shows a low-intensity multilobulated mass deforming and displacing the brainstem, destroying the clivus, and extending into the sella turcica *(upper arrowhead)* and nasopharynx *(two lower arrowheads)*.

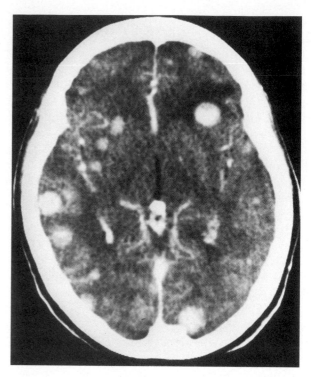

FIGURE 8-28 Metastases. CT scan shows multiple enhancing masses of various shapes and sizes representing hematogenous metastases from carcinoma of the breast.

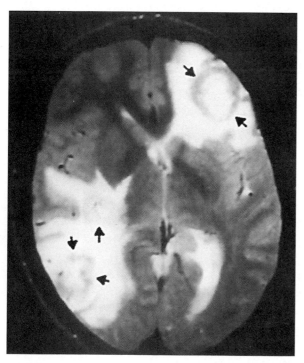

FIGURE 8-27 Metastases. Axial MR scan demonstrates three large masses *(arrows)* surrounded by extensive high signal intensity edema.

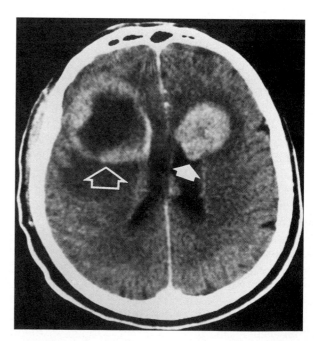

FIGURE 8-29 Metastases. CT shows enhancing metastases from squamous cell carcinoma of lung that are both ring enhancing *(open arrow)* and solid *(solid arrow)*.

disorder	location	radiographic appearance	treatment
Glioma	Glial cells in CNS	MRI—masses of high signal intensity on T2-weighted images, low signal intensity or isodense on T1-weighted images CT (nonenhanced)—a single heterogeneous mass (isodense to hypodense) CT (contrast enhanced)—a homogeneous lesion with an irregular ring of enhancement	Depends on location and histology Astrocytomas—good 5-year survival rate with surgery and radiation therapy Ependymomas of the filum terminale—surgical removal provides the most favorable prognosis
Meningioma	Arises from arachnoid lining and is attached to the dura Spinal	MRI—isodense lesion on T1- and T2-weighted images CT—rounded, sharply delineated, hyperdense (75%) tumor MRI—T1- and T2-weighted images that have been contrast-enhanced appear as homogenous intense lesions CT myelography—location of mass as a filling defect	Surgical resection is very successful because of the superficial position of the tumor and the lack of tumor infiltration
Acoustic neuroma	Schwann's cells of cranial nerve VIII	MRI—T1-weighted images show focal or generalized enlargement of cranial nerve VIII CT—best demonstrates bone involvement	Surgical excision of the lesion, or gamma knife radiosurgery, to improve symptoms
Pituitary adenoma	Most commonly from anterior lobe of the pituitary gland	CT—large tumor typically homogeneous and hyperdense in comparison with normal brain tissue, bone erosion, and tumor extension MRI—T1-weighted images show hypointense mass associated with contralateral deviation MRI (contrast enhanced)—the microadenoma becomes hypointense initially; delayed scans demonstrate hyperintensity of the tumor	Surgical resection by transsphenoidal approach Radiation therapy if tumor extends beyond pituitary gland Gamma knife radiosurgery—a new alternative
Craniopharyngioma	Usually superior to sella turcica	CT—(cystic and solid mass) with possible calcification mass with cystic and solid components MRI—cystic regions produce low signal intensity on T1-weighted images, high signal intensity on T2-weighted images; fatty regions produce hyperintense signals on T1-weighted images	MR-guided stereotactic microsurgery for resection For unresectable tumors, surgical debulking followed by radiation therapy
Pineal tumor	Germ cell tumors of the pineal gland	MRI—sagittal scans demonstrate compression of midbrain; germinomas are isointense on T1- and T2-weighted images; teratomas produce a mixed signal intensity because of their cystic components and fat CT—germinomas hyperdense or isodense, displacing third ventricle, and show intense contrast enhancement; teratomas are hypodense masses with internal calcifications	Surgery (first choice) followed by radiation therapy Chemotherapy with radiation therapy when surgery is not an option
Chordoma	Arises from the embryonic neural tube	Radiograph—ill-defined bone destruction or cortical expansion CT—base-of-skull mass is slightly denser than brain tissue and only moderately enhanced MRI—3D gradient-echo T1-weighted sequences in the sagittal plane best demonstrate the clival area and surrounding structures; gadolinium enhancement produces heterogeneous intensities with border-ring enhancement	Clival region—surgical resection followed by radiation therapy Lumbar region—complete surgical resection

Continued

SUMMARY of FINDINGS for Tumors of the Central Nervous System—cont'd

disorder	location	radiographic appearance	treatment
Metastatic carcinoma	Carcinoma reaching the brain by hematogenous spread	MRI—single or multiple masses of high signal intensity; additional lesions often seen with paramagnetic contrast agent CT—multiple enhancing lesions of various sizes with areas of low density surrounding edema	Single lesion—surgical resection Multiple lesions—whole brain radiation; chemotherapy if metastasis occurs after radiation therapy

Single metastatic deposits in the brain may be indistinguishable from primary tumors. However, because primary brain neoplasms are unusual in older patients, single lesions in this population should suggest metastatic disease.

Treatment

The number of lesions determines the choice of therapy. Single metastatic lesions or second-year postprimary (residual or regrowth) lesions require surgical intervention, which may provide relief from symptoms. Multiple metastases require radiation or chemotherapy. Radiation therapy can be to the whole brain or by the gamma knife. Systemic chemotherapy is used if metastasis occurs after radiation treatment. Surgery combined with whole-brain radiation therapy is the most successful treatment.

Traumatic Processes of the Brain and Skull

In the patient with head trauma, the purpose of radiographic imaging is to detect a surgically correctable hematoma. Emergency CT has virtually replaced all other radiographic investigations in patients with suspected neurologic dysfunction resulting from head injury. Because the presence or absence of a skull fracture does not correlate with intracranial abnormalities, plain radiographs of the skull are no longer indicated in the patient with head trauma.

Because of medicolegal reasons and the fear of missing a skull fracture, CT scans (and plain skull radiographs) are often overused. The following indications have been established for the use of radiographic procedures in the patient with head trauma:
1. Unexplained focal neurologic signs
2. Unconsciousness (including the unarousable alcoholic)
3. Documented decreasing level of consciousness or progressive mental deterioration
4. History of previous craniotomy with shunt tube in place

5. Skull depression or subcutaneous foreign body palpable or identified by a probe through a laceration or puncture wound
6. Hemotympanum or fluid discharge from the ear
7. Discharge of CSF from the nose
8. Ecchymosis over the mastoid process (Battle's sign)
9. Bilateral orbital ecchymoses (raccoon eyes)

Skull Fracture

Radiographic Appearance

A **linear skull fracture** appears on a plain radiograph as a sharp lucent line that is often irregular or jagged and occasionally branches (Figure 8-30). The fracture must be distinguished from suture lines, which generally have serrated edges and tend to be bilateral and symmetric, and vascular grooves, which usually have a smooth curving course and are not as sharp or distinct as a fracture line. The location of a linear skull fracture can indicate possible complications. A fracture that crosses a dural vascular groove may cause vessel laceration leading to an epidural hematoma. A fracture involving the sinuses or mastoid air cells may result in posttraumatic pneumocephalus, with air seen in the ventricles on plain radiographs. A **diastatic fracture** refers to a linear fracture that intersects a suture and courses along it, causing sutural separation.

More severe trauma, especially if localized to a small area of the skull, may force a fragment of bone to be separated and depressed into the cranial cavity (Figure 8-31). The underlying dura is frequently torn, and there is a relatively high incidence of cerebral parenchymal injury. **Depressed fractures** are often stellate (star shaped), with multiple fracture lines radiating outward from a central point. When the fracture is viewed en face, the overlap of fragments makes the fracture line appear denser than the normal bone. Tangential views are required to determine the amount of depression.

Fractures limited to the base of the skull are often hidden by the complex basal anatomy and may be very difficult to visualize on plain radiographs.

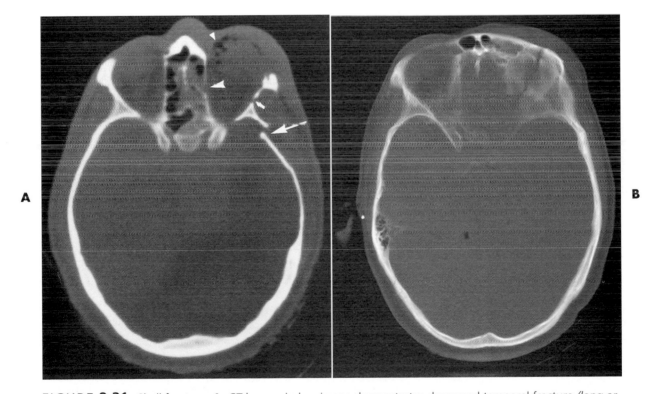

FIGURE 8-30 Skull fracture. **A,** Lateral projection of skull shows widely separated fracture *(arrow)* extending to star-shaped array of linear fractures. **B,** In another patient, lateral projection shows severely depressed skull fracture *(arrows).*

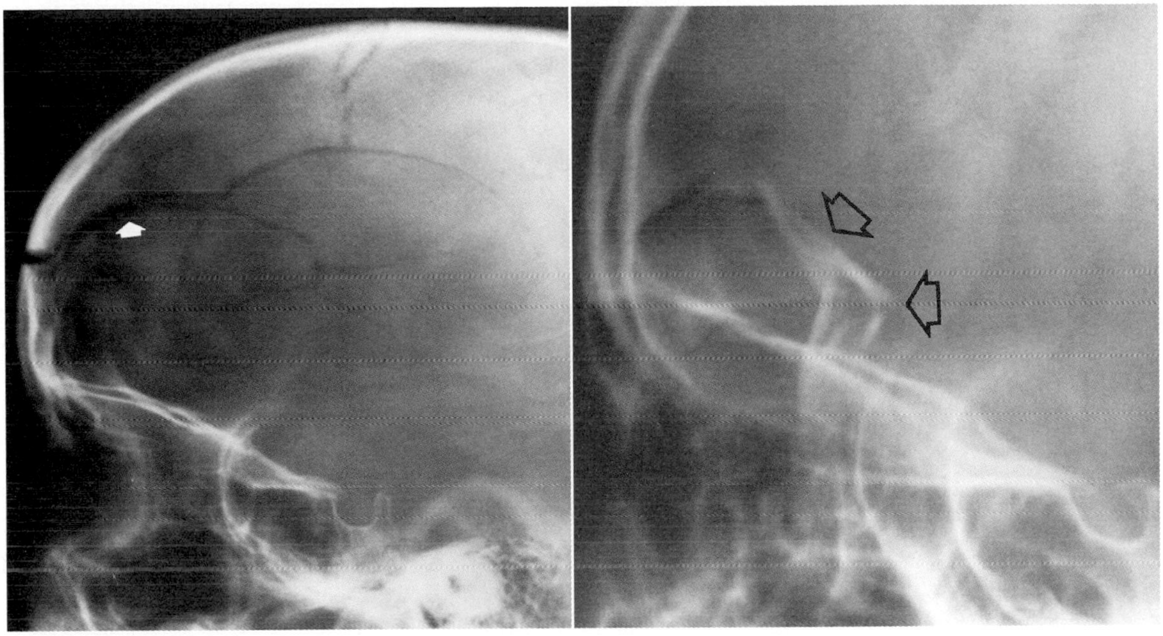

FIGURE 8-31 Skull fracture. **A,** CT bone-window image demonstrates depressed temporal fracture *(long arrow).* Note the lateral orbital wall fracture *(short arrow),* the medial orbital wall fracture *(large arrowhead),* and the ethmoid opacification caused by hemorrhage. Also, air can be seen in the orbital soft tissues *(small arrowhead),* resulting from medial fracture into the ethmoids. **B,** Trauma resulted in a nondisplaced fracture in the supraorbital plate in this 24-year-old woman.

A finding suggestive of a basilar skull fracture is an air-fluid level in the sphenoid sinus seen on an erect or cross-table lateral projection of the skull obtained with a horizontal x-ray beam. CT can demonstrate the presence of blood or fluid in the basilar cisterns and show some basilar skull fractures (using bone windows) that are not visible on routine skull radiographs. Potential complications of basal skull fractures include leakage of CSF, meningitis, and damage to the facial nerve or auditory apparatus within the petrous bone.

It must be emphasized that the presence or absence of a skull fracture does not correlate with intracranial abnormalities. Indeed, serious treatable intracranial hematomas can be present without skull fractures.

Treatment
The severity and location of the fracture and the complications resulting from the trauma determine the treatment.

Epidural Hematoma
Epidural hematomas are caused by acute arterial bleeding and most commonly form over the parieto-temporal convexity. Acute arterial bleeding is usually caused by laceration of the medial meningeal artery. Because of a high arterial pressure, epidural hematomas rapidly cause significant mass effect and acute neurologic symptoms.

Radiographic Appearance
Because the dura is very adherent to the inner table of the skull, an epidural hematoma typically appears as a biconvex (lens-shaped), peripheral, high-density lesion (Figure 8-32). There is usually a shift of the midline structures toward the opposite side unless a contralateral balancing hematoma is present. If not promptly recognized, an epidural hematoma can lead to rapid progressive loss of consciousness, dilatation of the ipsilateral pupil, compression of the upper midbrain, and eventually compression of the entire brainstem and death.

Treatment
To prevent death, emergency surgical decompression is required to relieve intracranial pressure.

Subdural Hematoma
Subdural hematomas reflect venous bleeding, most commonly from ruptured veins between the dura and meninges. Symptoms may occur within the first few minutes; however, because of the low pressure of venous bleeding, patients with subdural hematomas

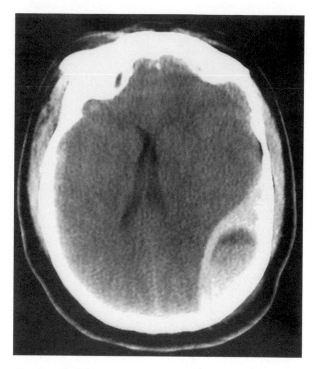

FIGURE 8-32 Acute epidural hematoma in a trauma patient. CT scan illustrates the characteristic lens-shaped epidural hematoma. Mass effect associated with the hematoma causes midline shift.

tend to have a chronic course with symptoms of headache, agitation, confusion, drowsiness, and gradual neurologic deficits.

Radiographic Appearance
An acute subdural hematoma typically appears on CT scans as a peripheral zone of increased density that follows the surface of the brain and has a crescentic shape adjacent to the inner table of the skull (Figure 8-33). On CT, the finding of isodense to hypodense areas within a hyperdense hematoma indicates rapid bleeding with an accumulation of unclotted blood. There is usually an associated mass effect with displacement of midline structures and obliteration of sulci over the affected hemisphere. The absence of displacement away from the side of a lesion may indicate the not infrequent presence of bilateral subdural hematomas. On MR scans, a subdural hematoma is detectable within a few days as an extraaxial mass of high signal intensity representing the accumulation of methemoglobin (Figure 8-34).

Serial CT scans demonstrate a gradual decrease in the attenuation value of a subdural hematoma over a period of weeks. With absorption and lysis of the blood clot, the hematoma becomes isodense with normal brain tissue, and the lesion may be identified

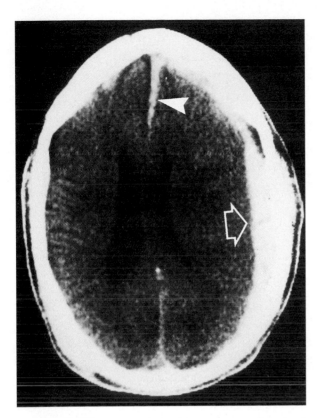

FIGURE 8-33 Acute subdural hematoma. High-density, crescent-shaped lesion *(arrow)* adjacent to the inner table of the skull. Hematoma extends into interhemispheric fissure *(arrowhead)*.

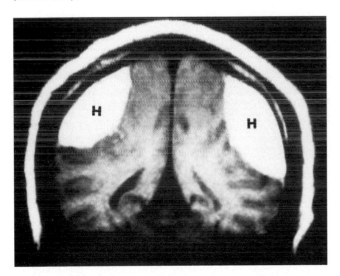

FIGURE 8-34 Bilateral subdural hematoma. Coronal MR image shows high signal intensity of bilateral subdural collections *(H)*.

only because of its mass effect. At this stage, scanning after the administration of contrast material may be of value because of enhancement of the membrane around the subdural hematoma and identification of the cortical veins. MR scanning of a lesion that is

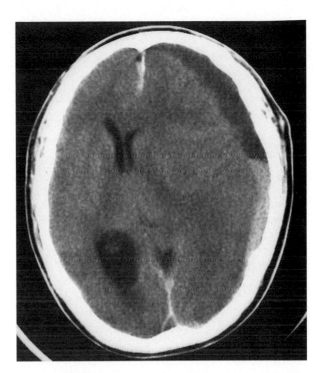

FIGURE 8-35 Chronic left subdural hematoma. Crescent-shaped high- and low-density regions in the left parietal area. The anterior is isodense (chronic hygroma); posteriorly, a hyperdense crescent shape resulting from acute bleeding can be seen. Midline shift and dilated right lateral ventricle are evident.

isodense by CT may show medial displacement of the superficial cerebral veins, an indication of an extracerebral mass and the entire extent of the hematoma over the cerebral convexity. A chronic subdural hematoma has a density similar to that of spinal fluid (Figure 8-35). At times, the small bridging veins associated with a chronic subdural hematoma may bleed and produce the difficult problem of an acute subdural hematoma superimposed on a chronic one.

Treatment

In small subdural hematomas without any inclination to rebleed, the hemorrhage resorbs naturally, and no treatment is necessary. Severe subdural hematomas require surgical ligation and evacuation of the hematoma to prevent transtentorial herniation. Less-invasive methods of decreasing intracranial pressure include drug therapy or placement of an intraventricular catheter to remove CSF, which may prevent herniation.

Cerebral Contusion

Cerebral contusion is an injury to brain tissue caused by movement of the brain within the calvaria after blunt trauma to the skull. Contusions occur when the brain contacts rough skull surfaces, such as the superior

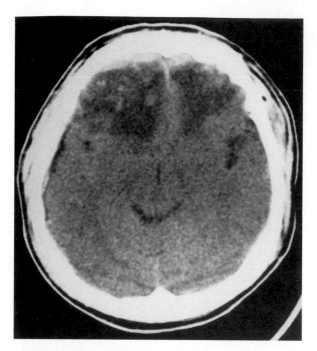

FIGURE 8-36 Cerebral contusion. CT scan shows small punctate hemorrhages (high density) within extensive areas of edema (low density).

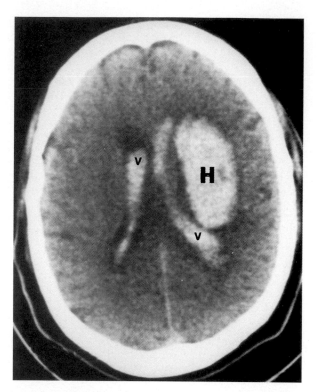

FIGURE 8-37 Intracerebral hematoma. Note the large, homogeneous, high-density area *(H)* with acute bleeding into lateral ventricles *(v)*.

orbital roof and petrous ridges. The patient loses consciousness and cannot remember the traumatic event.

Radiographic Appearance

Cerebral contusions typically appear on CT scans as low-density areas of edema and tissue necrosis, with or without nonhomogeneous density zones, reflecting multiple small areas of hemorrhage (Figure 8-36). The frontal and anterior temporal regions are the most common sites of injury. After the administration of intravenous contrast material, contusions generally enhance for several weeks after the injury because of a breakdown of the blood-brain barrier. On MR scans, the cerebral edema causes high signal intensity on T2-weighted images; associated areas of hemorrhage may produce high signal intensity regions on T1-weighted scans.

Treatment

The patient is hospitalized to allow observation of any changes in neurologic function. If the contusion causes swelling, medications to decrease intracranial pressure are prescribed. Surgery is usually not necessary.

Intracerebral Hematoma

Traumatic hemorrhage into the brain parenchyma can result from shearing forces to intraparenchymal arteries, which tend to occur at the junction of the gray and white matter. Injury to the intima of intracranial

vessels can cause the development of traumatic aneurysms, which can rupture.

Radiographic Appearance

On CT scans, an intracerebral hematoma appears as a well-circumscribed, homogeneous, high-density region that is usually surrounded by areas of low-density edema (Figure 8-37). As the blood components within the hematoma disintegrate, the lesion eventually becomes isodense with normal brain (usually 2 to 4 weeks after injury). On MR scans, the hematoma shows high signal intensity. A chronic hematoma filled with hemosiderin appears black on T2-weighted images.

Treatment

Although most intracerebral hematomas develop immediately after head injury, delayed hemorrhage is common. This is especially frequent after the evacuation of acute subdural hematomas that are compressing (tamponing) potential bleeding sites. Therefore a repeat CT (or MRI) scan is often performed within 48 hours in patients who have undergone decompressive surgery.

Subarachnoid Hemorrhage

Injury to surface veins, cerebral parenchyma, or cortical arteries can produce bleeding into the ventricular system.

Radiographic Appearance

On a CT scan, a subarachnoid hemorrhage appears as increased density within the basilar cisterns, cerebral fissures, and sulci. Identification of the falx cerebri, straight sinus, or superior sagittal sinus on noncontrast CT scans is often considered an indication of subarachnoid blood in the interhemispheric fissure. However, with high-resolution scanners this appearance may be seen in patients with a normal or calcified falx. MRI does not demonstrate the acute subarachnoid hemorrhage well unless a fluid-attenuated inversion recovery (FLAIR) sequence is used to demonstrate the increased signal intensity. However, T1-weighted scans can show subacute hemorrhage as a high signal intensity because of the conversion of fresh blood to methemoglobin.

Treatment

Subarachnoid hemorrhage may require surgical evacuation and vessel repair if bleeding continues. Less invasive methods of decreasing intracranial pressure include drug therapy and the placement of an intraventricular catheter to remove CSF.

Carotid Artery Injury

The extracerebral carotid arteries can be injured by penetrating trauma to the neck, as from gunshot wounds or stabbing. The internal carotid artery is associated in 50% of traumatic fistulas.

Radiographic Appearance

Angiography can demonstrate laceration of the artery or intimal damage, which may result in either dissection or thrombotic occlusion (Figure 8-38). Hyperextension injuries from motor vehicle collisions can cause intimal damage to the carotid or vertebral arteries, which may result in pseudoaneurysm formation. Traumatic arteriovenous fistulas usually arise between the internal carotid artery and the cavernous sinus. In this condition carotid arteriography demonstrates opacification of the cavernous sinus during the arterial phase. Reverse flow from the cavernous sinus may rapidly opacify a greatly dilated ophthalmic vein. The cavernous sinus and superior ophthalmic vein appear enlarged on a CT scan. MRI normally demonstrates strong enhancement of normal venous spaces (cavernous sinus). A fistula produces a signal void as a result of high flow.

Treatment

The placement of a detachable balloon catheter within the fistula using angiographic guidance may eliminate the need for surgical intervention.

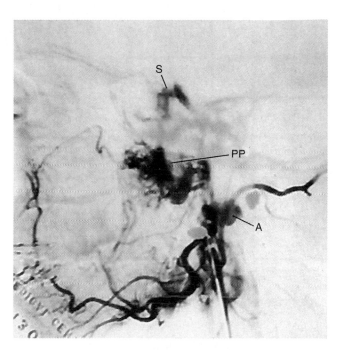

FIGURE 8-38 Posttraumatic caroticocavernous fistula. A lateral projection of an external carotid artery angiogram shows a pseudoaneurysm (A) and rapid filling of the cavernous sinus (S) and pterygoid plexus (PP). There is total interruption of the external carotid artery trunk beyond the takeoff of the facial artery.

Facial Fractures

Although it is padded by overlying skin, fat, and the muscles of expression, the face consists of thin and poorly supported bone, which can easily break in response to a traumatic force. The purpose of radiographic imaging in the patient with a facial injury is to demonstrate major disruptions of the facial skeleton and displacement of fracture fragments that will affect the surgical reduction and stabilization of the fracture.

Radiographic Appearance

Plain radiographs of the face are usually performed as an initial screening procedure, especially in a severely traumatized patient with substantial injuries to multiple organ systems. Whenever possible, films should be obtained with the patient in the erect position to demonstrate any air-fluid levels within the sinuses that could indicate recent hemorrhage and raise the suspicion of an underlying fracture. When erect films cannot be obtained, a cross-table lateral using a horizontal x-ray beam will demonstrate air-fluid levels. Complex-motion (pluridirectional) tomography can blur unrelated overlying structures and thus display details of injury that are obscure or only suspected on plain radiographs. CT can demonstrate soft tissue abnormalities, such as intraorbital or

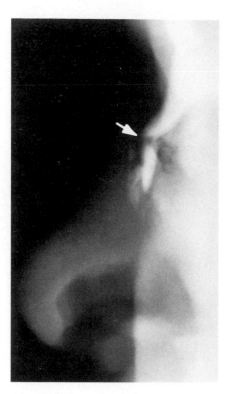

FIGURE 8-39 Depressed nasal fracture *(arrow)*.

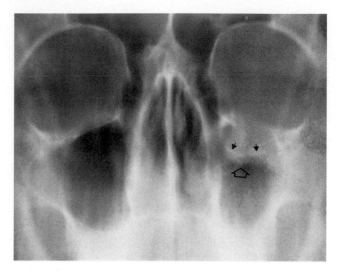

FIGURE 8-40 Blowout fracture. Conventional tomogram shows comminuted fracture of floor of left orbit with inferior displacement of fracture fragments *(solid arrows)*. Note characteristic soft tissue shadow *(open arrow)* protruding through floor into superior portion of maxillary sinus.

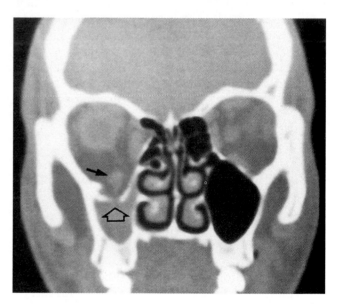

FIGURE 8-41 CT of orbital floor fracture. Coronal CT scan using bone window shows fractured orbital floor as double-hinged trap door with separation in center *(open arrow)*. There is opacification of the right maxillary sinus. Note displacement of inferior rectus muscle *(solid arrow)* in this patient who had limited upward gaze.

retrobulbar hematomas, that are impossible to detect by conventional means. In addition, bone detail and displacement can be exquisitely demonstrated when CT window and level settings are adjusted to optimize bony structures.

Nasal bone fractures are the most common facial fractures. Isolated nasal fractures vary from simple, nondisplaced linear fractures to comminuted lesions with depression of the septum and lateral splaying of the fracture fragments (Figure 8-39). These fractures are best demonstrated on right and left (underexposed) soft tissue lateral projections, which also can define interruption of the anterior nasal spine—the anterior projection of the maxilla at the base of the cartilaginous nasal septum. Most fractures are transverse and tend to depress the distal portion of the nasal bones.

A **blowout fracture** is caused by a direct blow to the front of the orbit that causes a rapid increase in intraorbital pressure. The fracture occurs in the thinnest, weakest portion of the orbit, which is the orbital floor just above the maxillary sinus. Plain radiographs (modified Waters' method), the preferred screening study, and thin-section tomography can demonstrate most blowout fractures (Figure 8-40), although CT may be necessary for better visualization and for detecting entrapment of the extraocular muscles in the upper portion of the adjacent maxillary sinus (Figure 8-41). The fracture segment can be comminuted, with a sagging, hammocklike appearance or can be of the trapdoor variety, with a displaced segment hanging into the antrum by a periosteal hinge. Herniation of orbital fat and extraocular muscles into the fractured orbital floor produces a characteristic soft tissue shadow protruding through the floor into the superior portion of the maxillary sinus. Opacification of the sinus caused by hemorrhage and mucosal edema is an indirect sign of orbital floor fracture.

SUMMARY
FINDINGS for Traumatic Processes of the Brain and Skull

disorder	location	radiographic appearance	treatment
Skull fracture	Any cranial bone	Linear—irregular or jagged sharp lucent line Depressed—stellate (star-shaped) fracture lines radiating outward CT—demonstrates fracture and associated intracranial complications	Treat associated complications
Epidural hematoma	Most commonly over parietotemporal convexity	CT—biconvex peripheral high-density lesion, showing midline shift	Emergency surgery to relieve increased intracranial pressure and to stop bleeding
Subdural hematoma	Most commonly from ruptured veins between dura and meninges	CT—acute: crescent-shaped peripheral high-density lesion; chronic: isodense lesion MRI—chronic; extracerebral mass with high signal intensity	Resorption in small hematomas Surgical ligation and evacuation of hematoma Control intracranial pressure with drugs or intraventricular drainage catheter
Cranial contusion	Injury to brain tissue Frontal and anterior temporal most common	CT—low-density areas that usually enhance for several weeks MRI—increased signal intensity on both T2-weighted (cerebral edema) and T1-weighted images (if hemorrhage)	Observation for neurologic change Surgery not usually required
Intracerebral hematoma	Hemorrhage into brain parenchyma	CT—well-circumscribed, homogeneous, high-density region surrounded by low-density regions of edema MRI high signal intensity region; chronic hematoma is black on T2-weighted image	Surgical evacuation of hematoma
Subarachnoid hemorrhage	Injury to surface veins or cortical arteries bleeding into the ventricles	CT—increased density within the basilar cisterns, cerebral fissures, and sulci MRI—acute hemorrhage on fluid-attenuated inversion recovery (FLAIR) shows as an increased signal intensity; subacute hemorrhage shows high intensity on T1-weighted images	Surgical evacuation of the hemorrhage and vessel repair Drug therapy or an intraventricular catheter to decrease intracranial pressure
Carotid artery injury	Extracerebral carotid arteries	Angiography—demonstrates laceration of artery or intimal damage CT—large cavernous sinus and superior ophthalmic vein MRI—signal void caused by large cavernous vein resulting from high flow	Placement of detachable balloon within fistula Surgical intervention to eliminate fistula
Facial fracture	Nasal bone (most common) Blowout (orbit) Tripod (zygoma separation from other facial and cranial bones) Mandible Le Fort (bilateral and horizontal fracture of maxillae)	Plain films—cranial and facial bones (upright or horizontal beam image shows fluid levels in the sinuses) CT—soft tissue abnormality and bone detail	Reduction of fracture Some require surgery to place internal or external fixation device

The presence of air within the orbit (orbital emphysema) indicates that there is a communication with a paranasal sinus, usually the ethmoid, as a result of an associated fracture of the medial wall of the orbit through the lamina papyracea.

The zygomatic arch is vulnerable to a blow from the side of the face, which can produce a fracture with inward displacement of the fragments centrally and outward displacement of the fragments at the zygomatic and temporal ends of the arch (Figure 8-42). **Zygomatic arch fractures** are best demonstrated on underexposed films taken in the basal (submentovertex) projection ("jug handle" view).

A **tripod fracture** consists of fractures of the zygomatic arch and the orbital floor or rim combined with separation of the zygomaticofrontal suture (Figure 8-43).

It is so named because it reflects separation of the zygoma from its three principal attachments. The resulting free-floating zygoma may cause facial disfigurement if not diagnosed and properly treated.

The mandible is a prominent, exposed segment of the facial skeleton and is thus a common site for both intentional and accidental trauma. Plain radiographs with oblique views, combined with panoramic tomography, can demonstrate most **mandibular fractures** (Figure 8-44). The angle of the mandible is the most common site of fracture, although fractures can involve any portion of the body and the condylar and coronoid processes. Because the mandible functions essentially as a bony ring, bilateral fractures are common.

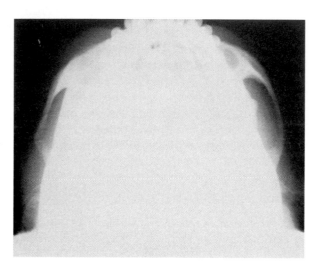

FIGURE 8-42 Zygomatic arch fracture. Submentovertex projection demonstrates two fractures on the right with depression of the zygomatic arch.

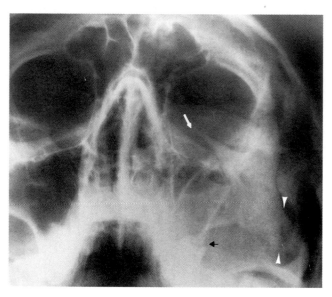

FIGURE 8-43 Tripod fracture. Interruption of the orbital rim *(white arrow)*, lateral maxillary fracture *(black arrow)*, and nondisplaced zygomatic arch fracture *(arrowheads)* are present.

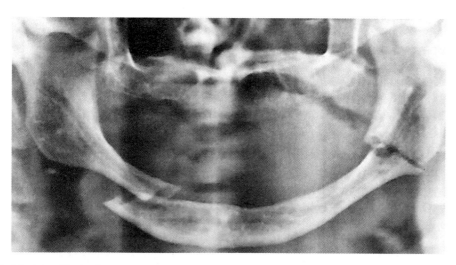

FIGURE 8-44 Mandibular fracture. Panoramic examination in edentulous (without teeth) patient shows fractures of left angle and right body of mandible.

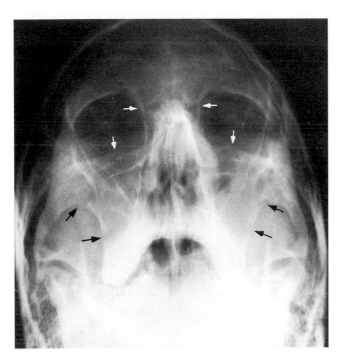

FIGURE 8-45 Le Fort II fracture. Waters' projection shows large separated fragment produced by multiple fractures *(arrows)*.

Le Fort fractures are severe injuries in which separation at the fracture site results in the formation of a large, complex, detached fragment that is unstable and may have its position altered relative to its site of origin. Le Fort fractures involve bilateral and horizontal fractures of the maxillae and are classified as type I, II, or III, depending on the extent of injury (Figure 8-45).

Treatment

Treatment for nasal bone fractures varies depending on the amount of bony displacement. Reduction is required for fractures causing deviation of the nasal septum. More severe facial fractures require surgical reconstruction, possibly using internal or external fixation devices to prevent disfigurement.

Vascular Disease of the Central Nervous System

The term **cerebrovascular disease** refers to any process that is caused by an abnormality of the blood vessels or blood supply to the brain. Pathologic processes causing cerebrovascular disease include abnormalities of the vessel wall, occlusion by thrombus or emboli, rupture of blood vessels with subsequent hemorrhage, and decreased cerebral blood flow caused by lowered blood pressure or narrowed lumen caliber. Cerebrovascular diseases include arteriosclerosis, hypertensive hemorrhage, arteritis, aneurysms, and arteriovenous malformations.

Radiographic Appearance

The radiographic evaluation of cerebrovascular disease depends on the symptoms and the most likely diagnosis. For ease of classification, cerebrovascular disease can be divided into three categories: completed stroke, transient ischemic attacks (TIAs), and intracranial hemorrhage. Imaging modalities used today include duplex color-flow Doppler ultrasound, MRA, CTA, conventional angiography, and digital subtraction angiography (DSA).

Stroke Syndrome

The term **stroke** denotes the sudden and dramatic development of a focal neurologic deficit, which may vary from dense **hemiplegia** (paralysis on one side of the body) and coma to only a trivial neurologic disorder. The specific neurologic defect depends on the arteries involved. A stroke, also known as an acute brain infarction, most commonly involves the circulation of the internal carotid arteries and is seen with symptoms that include acute **hemiparesis** (weakness of one side of the body) and **dysarthria** (difficulty speaking).

The purpose of radiographic evaluation in the acute stroke patient is not to confirm the diagnosis of a stroke but to exclude other processes that can simulate the clinical findings (e.g., parenchymal hemorrhage and subdural hematoma). Although the abrupt onset of a stroke may permit differentiation from other conditions that have a more gradual onset of symptoms, patients with focal neurologic deficits of various causes may initially be found comatose, so that the history of gradual onset is not elicited. Clearly it is essential to exclude an intracranial hemorrhage before considering the possibility of treating the stroke patient with anticoagulant therapy.

Radiographic Appearance

Noncontrast CT (or MRI, if available) is the examination of choice for the evaluation of the stroke patient. Intravenous contrast material is contraindicated because it is a toxic substance that can cross the disrupted blood-brain barrier in the region of a cerebral infarct and lead to increased edema and a slower recovery for the patient. CT and MR scans are normal in patients with small infarctions and in the early hours of large infarctions. The initial

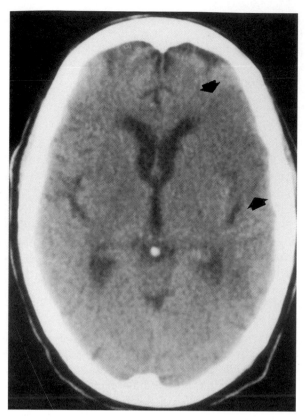

FIGURE 8-46 Acute left middle cerebral artery infarct. CT scan obtained 20 hours after onset of acute hemiparesis and aphasia shows obliteration of normal sulci *(arrows)* in involved hemisphere. The gray and white matter in the distribution of the left middle cerebral artery demonstrate low density.

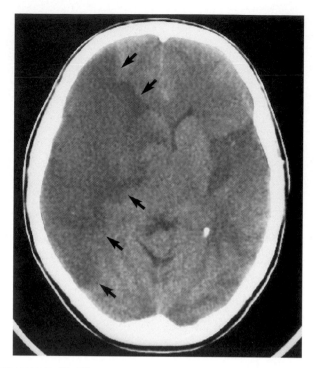

FIGURE 8-47 Chronic right middle cerebral artery infarct. Low-attenuation region *(arrows)* shows sharply defined borders and some midline shift.

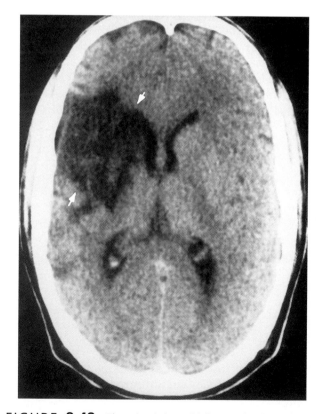

FIGURE 8-48 Chronic right middle cerebral artery infarct. Low-attenuation region shows sharply defined borders *(arrows)* and some dilatation of the adjacent ventricle.

appearance (within 8 to 24 hours) of a cerebral infarction is a triangular or wedge-shaped area of hypodensity on CT (Figure 8-46) and high signal intensity on T2-weighted MRI sequences involving both the cortex and the underlying white matter down to the ventricular surface. The abnormality is confined to the vascular territory of the involved artery. Although little or no mass effect is evident during the first day, progressive edema produces a mass effect that is maximal 7 to 10 days after the acute event (Figure 8-47). As an infarct ages, brain tissue atrophies, and the adjacent sulci and ventricular system enlarge (Figure 8-48). A combination of nonenhanced MRI and MRA is more sensitive than CT in detecting an infarct or ischemic edema, especially involving the brainstem. Occlusion or stenosis of an artery or vein can be demonstrated along with the associated hemorrhage as a result of ischemic infarction. A diffusion-weighted MR scan usually demonstrates a positive hyperintense signal within 2 hours of the incident and plays a critical role in diagnosing and determining the age of the stroke.

There is only a small window of 2 to 3 hours after the onset of a stroke in which fibrinolytic agents are effective in decreasing the amount of permanent neurologic deficits. A T2-weighted image detects edema sooner than CT and thus is considered more sensitive. In patients with classic stroke symptoms, follow-up CT or MR scans are not indicated.

Treatment

All stroke patients are placed on bed rest with reduced external stimuli to lower cerebral oxygen demands. Medications may be used to decrease intracranial pressure and intracranial edema. Patients with thrombotic strokes receive anticoagulants and possibly thrombolytic agents.

Transient Ischemic Attacks

TIAs present as focal neurologic deficits that completely resolve within 24 hours. They may result from emboli originating from the surface of an arteriosclerotic ulcerated plaque (embolic stroke), which causes temporary occlusion of cerebral vessels, or from stenosis of an extracerebral artery, which leads to a reduction in critical blood perfusion. Because almost two thirds of arteriosclerotic strokes are preceded by TIAs and the 5-year cumulative risk of stroke in patients with TIAs may be as high as 50%, accurate diagnosis and appropriate treatment are essential.

Radiographic Appearance

The most common location of surgically treatable arteriosclerotic disease causing TIAs is the region of the carotid bifurcation in the neck. In patients with an asymptomatic bruit (a rumbling noise heard by a stethoscope) or an unclear history of a TIA, carotid duplex color-flow Doppler scanning is often the initial screening study (Figure 8-49). This technique combines high-resolution ultrasound imaging and Doppler ultrasound with spectral analysis into a "duplex" unit that avoids many of the problems associated with each of these modalities when used alone. In most cases, carotid duplex scanning when combined with MRA can reliably determine whether the extent of the disease is sufficient to warrant more invasive procedures (angiography). Patients with a normal or near-normal carotid duplex scan do not need to undergo more invasive diagnostic procedures for assessment of the carotid bifurcation. Limitations of the usefulness of carotid duplex scanning include its extreme operator dependence and the fact that 10% of patients cannot be successfully imaged with carotid duplex scanning because of anatomic factors (patients with extremely high carotid bifurcations and those with short, thick necks). High-resolution,

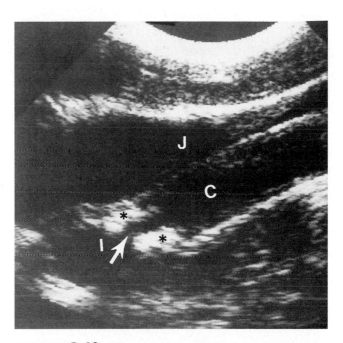

FIGURE 8-49 Ultrasound of carotid arteriosclerotic occlusive disease. There is severe narrowing *(arrow)* of the origin of the internal carotid artery *(I)* by densely echogenic arteriosclerotic plaque *(asterisks)*. *C,* Common carotid artery; *J,* jugular vein.

real-time ultrasound techniques provide hemodynamic information about blood flow velocity. Using ultrasound techniques, it may be impossible to differentiate patients with a total occlusion of the internal carotid artery from those with a tiny residual lumen. This is an important clinical distinction because patients with even a small remaining lumen can undergo a successful carotid endarterectomy (surgical removal of atherosclerotic plaque).

Noninvasive MRA provides accurate imaging of the carotid bifurcation and it demonstrates narrowing of the vertebral arteries (Figure 8-50). The reconstitution sign (flow gap) confirms a stenosis greater than 60%, indicating advanced disease requiring surgical intervention. Contrast-enhanced MRA also facilitates visualization of the aortic arch and the origins of the carotid and vertebral arteries.

Patients with a clear-cut episode of a TIA or a neurologic deficit usually are subjected to an angiographic study for evaluating the carotid arteries. Either intravenous or intraarterial DSA or selective intraarterial carotid arteriography can be used to demonstrate TIA-producing stenotic or ulcerative lesions that may be amenable to surgical therapy (Figures 8-51 to 8-53). Angiographic evaluation of the aortic arch and vertebral arteries is infrequently indicated in the evaluation of patients with TIAs because surgery on the origins of the great vessels and

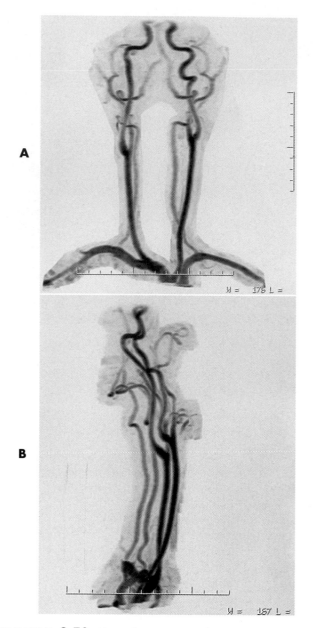

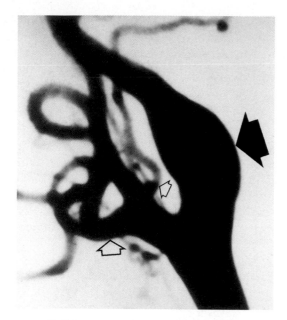

FIGURE **8-51** Normal carotid artery bifurcation. Common carotid arteriogram shows bulbous origin of the internal carotid artery *(solid arrow)* and multiple branches of the external carotid artery *(open arrows)*.

FIGURE **8-50** Normal MRA carotid study. **A,** The anteroposterior perspective of the neck demonstrates from the subclavian arteries to the origin of the basilar artery, and the bifurcation of the common carotid arteries. **B,** The off-lateral perspective offers a second view of the vessels.

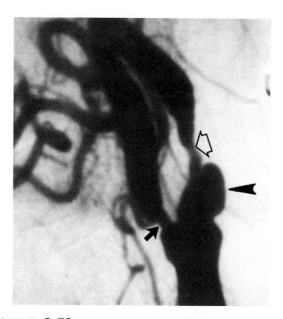

FIGURE **8-52** Ulceration of the internal carotid artery. Common carotid arteriogram shows ulcerated lesion *(arrowhead)* at the origin of the internal carotid artery, with severe stenosis of the internal carotid *(open arrow)* and external carotid *(black arrow)* arteries.

posterior circulation is both difficult and not commonly performed, and also because of the higher morbidity from arch and vertebral angiograms reported in some studies.

Treatment

Accurate diagnosis and appropriate treatment (antiplatelet therapy, anticoagulation therapy, or carotid endarterectomy) are essential to prevent permanent deficits. Thrombolytic agents may also be used.

Intraparenchymal Hemorrhage

Aside from head trauma, the principal cause of intraparenchymal hemorrhage (hemorrhagic stroke) is hypertensive vascular disease. Less frequent causes are rupture of a congenital berry aneurysm or an

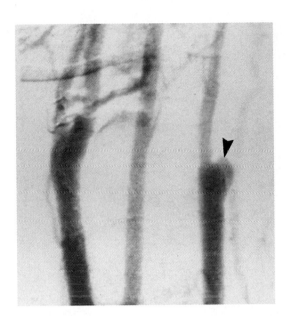

FIGURE 8-53 Occluded internal carotid artery. Intravenous DSA shows occlusion of the left internal carotid artery at its origin *(arrowhead)*.

arteriovenous malformation. Hypertensive hemorrhages result in oval or circular collections that displace the surrounding brain and can cause a significant mass effect. Although they can occur at any location within the brain, hypertensive hemorrhages are most frequent in the basal ganglia, white matter, thalamus, cerebellar hemispheres, and pons. A frequent complication is rupture of the hemorrhage into the ventricular system or subarachnoid space. Intraparenchymal hemorrhages resulting from congenital berry (saccular) aneurysms usually are associated with subarachnoid hemorrhage and tend to develop in regions where these congenital vascular anomalies most commonly occur. These include the sylvian fissure (middle cerebral artery) and the midline subfrontal area (anterior communicating artery). Arteriovenous malformations occur throughout the brain and tend to bleed into the white matter.

Radiographic Appearance

Patients with a suspected intraparenchymal hemorrhage should be evaluated with MRI or a noncontrast CT scan. A fresh hematoma appears on CT as a homogeneously dense, well-defined lesion with a round to oval configuration (Figure 8-54). Hematomas produce ventricular compression and, when large, considerable midline shift and brain herniation. A hematoma that is not homogeneously dense is suggestive of hemorrhage occurring within a tumor, an inflammatory process, or an infarction. As the hematoma ages, its density changes. On CT, after passing through an isodense stage, the hematoma becomes hypodense;

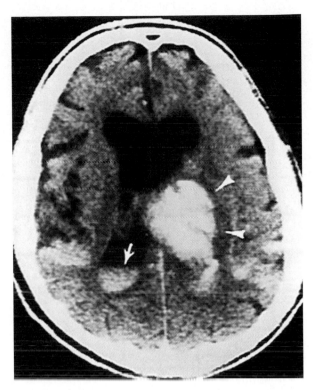

FIGURE 8-54 Intracerebral hematoma. Noncontrast CT scan shows homogeneous, high-density area in left thalamus. The low-density area *(arrowheads)* adjacent to the hematoma represents associated ischemia and edema. Hematoma has entered the ventricular system, and a prominent cerebrospinal fluid-blood level is seen in the dependent lateral ventricle *(arrow)*. Such extension of blood into the ventricular system is an extremely poor prognostic sign. Mass effect caused by hematoma has compressed the third ventricle and the foramen of Monro and has resulted in obstructive enlargement of the lateral ventricles.

by 6 months it appears as a well-defined, low-density region that is often considerably smaller than the original lesion. Contrast enhancement usually develops about the periphery of a hematoma after 7 to 10 days. On MRI, the preferred study, the high signal intensity within a hematoma (caused by the conversion of normal hemoglobin to methemoglobin) arises after a few days and continues for several months (Figure 8-55). Once the methemoglobin is completely converted to paramagnetic hemosiderin, the hematoma demonstrates very low signal intensity on T2-weighted sequences.

Arteriography is not indicated in patients with classic hypertensive hematomas. However, arteriography remains the gold standard for those patients in whom an aneurysm or arteriovenous malformation is suspected as the underlying cause of the hematoma. In patients with a suspected aneurysm, it is important to determine the number of aneurysms,

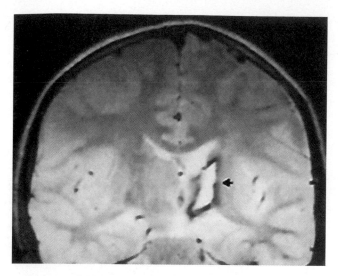

FIGURE 8-55 Intracerebral hematoma. Coronal T2-weighted MR scan shows a large hematoma in the left thalamic region *(arrow)*. Hematoma consists of two portions: central area of increased signal intensity representing methemoglobin and surrounding area of low signal intensity representing hemosiderin.

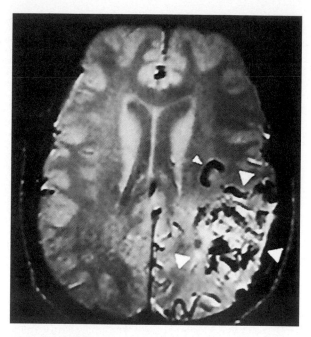

FIGURE 8-56 Arteriovenous malformation. Axial MR scan shows large left parietal mass *(large arrowheads)* consisting of vascular structures of varying intensity, depending on whether there is rapid flow *(black)* or slow flow *(white)*. Note greatly dilated vessel *(small arrowhead)* that feeds the malformation.

which aneurysm has ruptured, the location of the neck of the aneurysm, and the patency of the circle of Willis. Statistically the largest of multiple aneurysms is the one that has ruptured; it is rare for an aneurysm less than 5 mm in diameter to rupture. Because an aneurysm generally ruptures at its apex, an irregular, multiloculated dome is suggestive of a prior rupture. Spasm in adjacent vessels and adjacent hematomas also assist in identifying which of several aneurysms has bled. Noncontrast CT demonstrates an aneurysm as a slightly hyperdense region. The intravenous injection of contrast material produces a strong uniform enhancement. On MRI, an aneurysm produces a flow void on both T1- and T2-weighted images. Imaging has improved the ability to detect an aneurysm. CTA and MRA can visualize large and medium aneurysms, along with feeding and draining vessels associated with an arteriovenous malformation. Angiography remains, however, the gold standard for demonstrating abnormalities involving small vessels.

In patients less than 20 years of age, arteriovenous malformation is the most common cause of nontraumatic intraparenchymal hemorrhage. On MRI (Figure 8-56), a cerebrovascular malformation appears as a mass of vascular structures of varying intensity, depending on whether there is rapid flow (black) or slow flow (white). On CT, the malformation consists of an irregular tangle of vessels (best seen after the intravenous injection of contrast material) and greatly dilated veins draining from the central tangle (Figure 8-57, *A*). Arteriography demonstrates an irregular, racemose tangle of abnormal vessels that are fed by dilated cerebral or cerebellar arteries (Figure 8-57, *B*). There is rapid shunting of blood into dilated, tortuous draining veins. Because of the often multiple sources of blood flow to an arteriovenous malformation, the arteriographic evaluation should include selective injections of contrast material into both internal and external carotid arteries.

Treatment

Steroid therapy, especially in nontraumatic hematomas, usually controls the edema that produces much of the mass effect. In cases of hemorrhagic strokes, the first line of treatment consists of stopping the bleeding (i.e., correct any coagulopathy), and the second is to try to prevent a recurrence of bleeding (control blood pressure), and finally surgery is performed to correct pathology (aneurysm or arteriovenous malformation). For aneurysms, surgical placement of a clip at the neck of the lesion is required to close the pouch. Arteriovenous malformations (AVMs) require surgery or neurointerventional procedures.

Subarachnoid Hemorrhage

A major cause of subarachnoid hemorrhage (hemorrhagic stroke) is rupture of a berry aneurysm (Figure 8-58). Patients with this condition usually

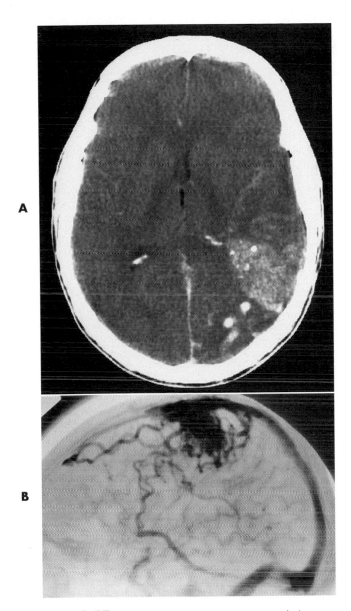

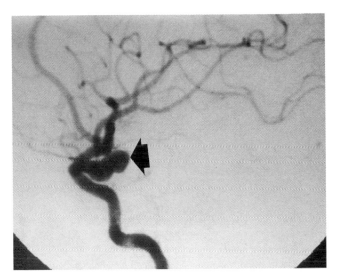

FIGURE 8-58 Ruptured berry aneurysm. Left carotid arteriogram demonstrates left supraclinoid aneurysm of the internal carotid artery. Posterior bulge of the aneurysm *(arrow)* represents the site of rupture.

FIGURE 8-57 Arteriovenous malformation with hemorrhage. **A,** CT scan shows an irregular tangle of vessels in the parietal lobe, seen without a contrast injection. **B,** In another patient, carotid arteriogram shows dilated blood vessels constituting an arteriovenous malformation.

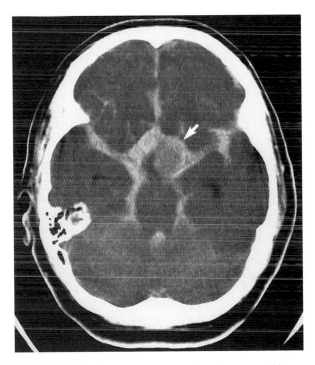

FIGURE 8-59 Berry aneurysm with subarachnoid hemorrhage. CT scan demonstrates subarachnoid bleed into the cisterns and ventricles (hyperdense) from a ruptured left middle cerebral aneurysm *(arrow)*.

have a generalized excruciating headache followed by unconsciousness. The most common locations for berry aneurysms are the origins of the posterior cerebral and anterior communicating arteries and the trifurcation of the middle cerebral artery. Because of the 20% incidence of multiple aneurysms, the angiographic procedure should include evaluation of the internal carotid and vertebral arteries bilaterally.

Radiographic Appearance
The radiographic procedure of choice is a noncontrast CT scan, which can demonstrate high-density blood in the subarachnoid spaces of the basal cisterns

in more than 95% of cases (Figure 8-59). Bleeding may extend into the brain parenchyma adjacent to the aneurysm. Contrast-enhanced CT scans are not indicated in subarachnoid hemorrhage because the surgeon will not operate for a suspected aneurysm without an angiogram, and the patient would thus

SUMMARY of FINDINGS for Vascular Disease of the Central Nervous System

disorder	location	radiographic appearance	treatment
Stroke syndrome	Neurologic deficit due to lack of circulation; internal carotid artery most common site	CT (initial exam)—a triangular or wedge-shaped hypodensity on noncontrast scan MRI—T2-weighted image produces high signal intensity of vascular territory involved Diffusion-weighted MRI—hyperintense signals within 2 hours of onset CT/MRI—mass effect seen 7-10 days after onset	Bed rest and reduced external stimuli for all stroke victims Medications to treat increased intracranial pressure if symptoms arise
Transient ischemic attack	Embolic stroke originating from arteriosclerotic ulcerated plaque	Duplex color-flow Doppler US—provides hemodynamic information including flow velocity (total occlusion vs. tiny residual flow) MRA—size and shape of diseased carotid and vertebral arteries; contrast-enhanced scan shows aortic arch and origins of vessels DSA—invasive study provides the highest resolution of intraluminal vascular pathology	Anticoagulants and/or thrombolytic agents to treat cause Surgical endarterectomy
Intraparenchymal hemorrhage	Hemorrhage into brain tissue	CT—new hematoma appears as homogeneously dense, well-defined, round or oval lesion, becoming isodense over time; 6-month-old hematoma appears as a well-defined, low-density lesion MRI—high signal intensity after a few days on T1- and T2-weighted images; with time, a low signal intensity is seen on T2-weighted images CTA/MRA—shows arteriovenous malformations in large and medium vessels and can detect an aneurysm Arteriography—used for small vessels	Steroid therapy Surgical clipping of aneurysm Surgery or neurointerventional procedures to correct arteriovenous malformation
Subarachnoid hemorrhage	Bleed beneath arachnoid layer of meninges	CT—noncontrast scan initially shows high attenuation of blood in the subarachnoid space MRI—best demonstrates chronic hemorrhages as hypointense areas on T2-weighted image CTA—high resolution demonstrates aneurysms greater than 3 mm MRA—shows large and medium vessels for detecting an aneurysm Arteriography—to localize and characterize small-vessel anatomy	Stop bleeding Prevent recurrence Surgical intervention to correct pathology

US, Ultrasound.

be exposed to the risk of an excessive load of contrast material. MRI is relatively insensitive for identifying acute subarachnoid bleeds, but it does demonstrate chronic blood staining of the meninges by a marked hypointensity on T2-weighted images. High-resolution CTA can demonstrate aneurysms greater than 3 mm and is becoming more accepted for presurgical planning.

The timing of angiography in subarachnoid hemorrhage depends on the philosophy of the surgeon. Blood in the subarachnoid space is an irritant that causes vasospasm of the vessels of the circle of Willis and the middle cerebral artery. This vasospasm, which can lead to cerebral ischemia and frank infarction, is greatest 3 to 14 days after the acute episode.

Treatment
If emergency surgery within the first 72 hours after the hemorrhage is planned, emergency selective angiography is indicated. If surgical intervention is to be delayed, angiography should be postponed until just before surgery.

SUMMARY of FINDINGS for Multiple Sclerosis

disorder	location	radiographic appearance	treatment
Multiple sclerosis	Most common demyelinating disorder of the CNS	MRI—plaques appear as a hyperintense signal on T2-weighted images and isointense to hypointense, possibly with beveled edges, on T1-weighted images MRI with contrast enhancement and fat suppression best demonstrates plaques involving the optic nerve and chiasm MRI—FLAIR, fast-spin echo, and spectroscopy—aid in determining extent of the disease	Immunosuppressive agents Antiviral drugs Subcutaneous injections of beta-interferon

Multiple Sclerosis

Multiple sclerosis is the most common demyelinating disorder; it presents as recurrent attacks of focal neurologic deficits that primarily involve the spinal cord, optic nerves, and central white matter of the brain. The disease has a peak incidence between 20 and 40 years of age, a strong predominance in women, and a clinical course characterized by multiple relapses and remissions. Impairment of nerve conduction caused by the degeneration of myelin sheaths leads to such symptoms as double vision, nystagmus (involuntary, rapid movement of the eyeball in all directions), loss of balance and poor coordination, shaking tremor and muscular weakness, difficulty in speaking clearly, and bladder dysfunction.

Radiographic Appearance

MRI is the modality of choice for demonstrating the scattered plaques of demyelination that are characteristic of multiple sclerosis. The plaques appear as multiple areas of increased signal intensity on T2-weighted images; these areas involve primarily the periventricular white matter, cerebellum, brainstem, and spinal cord (Figure 8-60). Lesions involving the optic nerve or chiasm require contrast enhancement and fat-suppression imaging (which increases the contrast difference between fat and water) to improve their detectability. On T1-weighted images, the plaques appear as isointense or hypointense lesions that may have a beveled edge. The use of MR fluid-attenuated inversion recovery, fast-spin echo, and spectroscopy aid in determining the extent of the disease. CT shows old inactive disease as well-defined areas of decreased attenuation in the deep white matter and periventricular regions. In the acute phase, CT performed after intravenous administration of contrast material demonstrates a mixture of nonenhancing focal areas of decreased density (representing old areas of demyelination) and enhancing regions that represent active foci.

Treatment

As the disease progresses and the symptoms increase in severity, immunosuppressive agents may help limit the autoimmune attack. Antiviral drugs may slow the progress of the disease. To reduce the number and severity of attacks, some patients receive subcutaneous injections of disease-modifying immunomodulatory agents (beta interferon). The treatments can only aid in slowing the progress of multiple sclerosis; there is no cure.

Epilepsy and Convulsive Disorders

Epilepsy is a condition in which brain impulses are temporarily disturbed, resulting in a spectrum of symptoms ranging from loss of consciousness for a few seconds to violent seizures (shaking and thrashing movements of all extremities). Although most cases of epilepsy are idiopathic, the disorder can be a result of injury (penetrating or nonpenetrating trauma, depressed skull fracture), birth trauma, or infection.

The mildest type of epilepsy, which occurs primarily in children, is called **petit mal**. This results in brief episodes of loss of consciousness, which may be associated with mild muscular twitching. Petit mal epilepsy usually disappears in young adulthood.

Grand mal epilepsy refers to generalized convulsions associated with the patient falling to the floor, hypersalivating (foaming at the mouth), and losing control of urine and sometimes feces. In many cases an approaching seizure is heralded by an aura, such

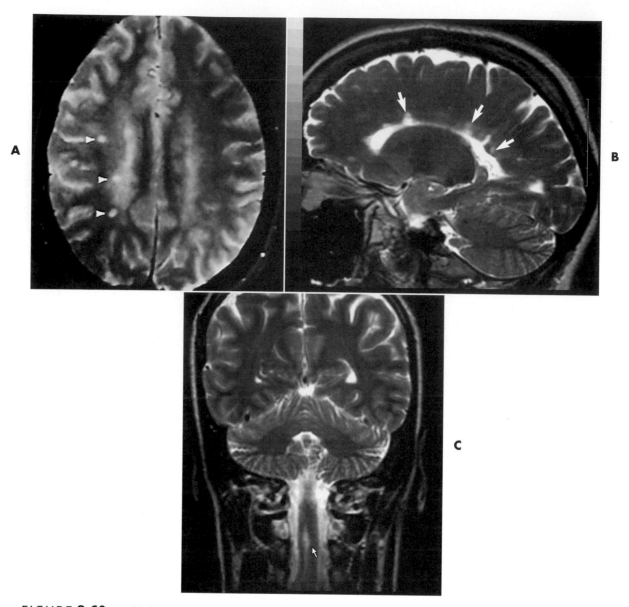

FIGURE 8-60 Multiple sclerosis. **A,** Axial T2-weighted MR image in a 35-year-old woman shows characteristic areas of increased signal intensity *(arrowheads)* in deep white matter. **B,** Sagittal image demonstrates periventricular plaques *(arrows)*. **C,** Coronal plane image shows increased intensity of cervical cord plaque *(arrow)*.

as a ringing in the ears, a tingling sensation in the fingers, or spots before the eyes. After a seizure, the patient tends to be groggy and unaware of what has happened (i.e., in a postictal state).

Radiographic Appearance

Whenever possible, the radiographic evaluation of a patient with a seizure disorder should be performed when the patient is clinically stable. The appropriate procedure is an MRI scan to search for an unsuspected brain tumor, arteriovenous malformation, or hippocampal sclerosis (Figure 8-61).

Hippocampal sclerosis (mesial temporal sclerosis) refers to neuronal loss and gliosis that occurs in the temporal region. High-resolution, thin-section, coronal T2-weighted images are the most specific. It is the most common cause of seizures that do not respond to medical therapy.

Since most seizure disorders are attributable to small areas of cortical brain injury resulting from trauma or infarction, CT or MR scans are usually normal. If the MR scan is normal, PET using ^{18}F-fluorodeoxyglucose (FDG) may localize the seizure focus in a patient with hippocampal sclerosis. PET

SUMMARY of FINDINGS for Epilepsy and Convulsive Disorders

disorder	location	radiographic appearance	treatment
Epilepsy and convulsive disorders	Brain impulses temporarily disrupted	MRI—high-resolution, thin-section T2-weighted image is most specific PET—localizes seizure foci	Stabilize patient for safety Reverse chemical causes Medications to decrease number of seizures Surgical resection

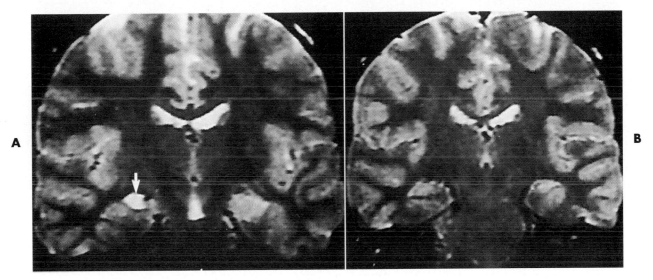

FIGURE 8-61 Seizure disorder caused by hippocampal sclerosis. **A,** Coronal T2-weighted MR scan shows high-intensity signal in the left hippocampal region *(arrow).* **B,** Normal scan for comparison.

has a 70% to 80% sensitivity and a very low rate of false-positive results (Figure 8-62).

Treatment

For the patient who has an acute seizure, initial efforts are directed toward stabilization (securing adequate ventilation and perfusion) and stopping the seizure. Subsequently, a careful history, physical examination, and appropriate laboratory studies should be performed to exclude reversible chemical causes of seizures, such as hypoglycemia, hyponatremia (decreased concentration of sodium in the blood) or hypernatremia, and hypocalcemia or hypercalcemia. If the patient does not respond to routine anticonvulsive treatment, CT may be indicated to search for causes of an acute seizure disorder (e.g., subdural hematoma, intracerebral hematoma), which may be amenable to surgical intervention. These conditions can be adequately assessed with a noncontrast CT scan; plain skull radiographs are not required. Medications may help decrease the number of seizures a patient

experiences. Surgical resection of the lesion is associated with a very good outcome.

Degenerative Diseases

Normal Aging

During normal aging, a gradual loss of neurons results in enlargement of the ventricular system and sulci (Figure 8-63).

Radiographic Appearance

Demyelination, which is also a part of normal aging, leads to the development of low density in the periventricular regions on CT and high signal intensity on T2-weighted MR images (Figure 8-64).

Alzheimer's Disease

Alzheimer's disease (presenile dementia) is a diffuse form of progressive cerebral atrophy that develops at an earlier age than the senile period.

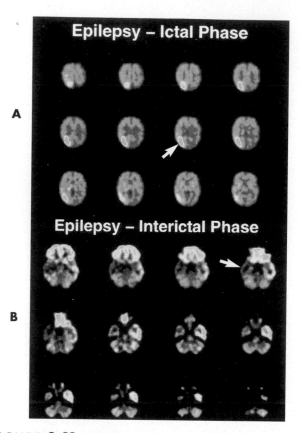

FIGURE 8-62 Epilepsy. In a patient with a history of epileptic seizures (ictal phase) **(A),** FDG-PET brain images demonstrate an area of increased activity: the highlighted region in the posterior portion of the cerebrum *(arrow).* **B,** The interictal phase (postseizure activity phase on the same patient) illustrates decreased activity in the temporal lobe *(arrow)* resulting from decreased blood flow during the seizure.

Radiographic Appearance

CT and MRI demonstrate nonspecific findings of cerebral atrophy, including symmetrically enlarged ventricles with prominence of the cortical sulci (Figure 8-65). T2-weighted MR images demonstrate periventricular hyperintensities. FDG-PET metabolic brain imaging used in conjunction with automated brain mapping can help distinguish changes associated with progressive neurodegenerative processes, such as Alzheimer's dementia. When superimposed into an Alzheimer's data base, areas of significantly reduced glucose metabolism correspond with Alzheimer's regions (Figure 8-66).

Treatment

Diet, education, memory aids, and safety issues may slow the progression of dementia, but there is no cure at this time. Medications available today help to slow the progression of the disease and may reverse early symptoms to some degree.

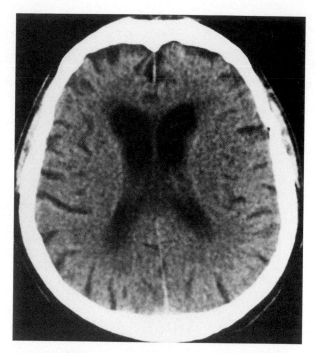

FIGURE 8-63 Normal aging. CT scan of 70-year-old man shows generalized ventricular dilatation with prominence of sulci over the surfaces of the cerebral hemisphere.

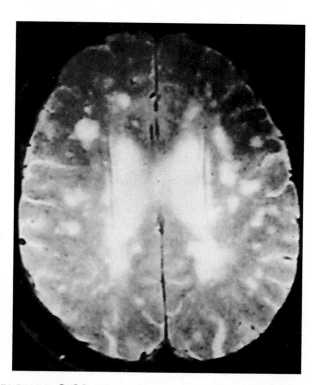

FIGURE 8-64 Degenerative changes of aging. Axial MR scan demonstrates multiple areas of increased signal intensity around ventricles and in deep white matter, consistent with cerebral ischemia or infarction.

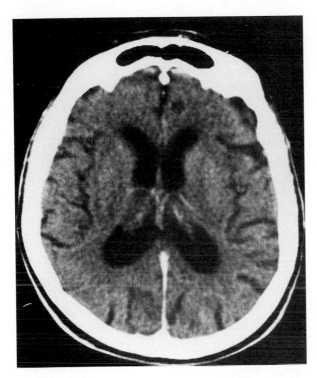

FIGURE 8-65 Alzheimer's disease. Noncontrast CT scan of a 56-year-old woman with progressive dementia shows generalized enlargement of ventricular system and sulci.

Huntington's Disease

Huntington's disease is an inherited (autosomal dominant) condition that predominantly involves men and appears in the early to middle adult years with dementia and typical choreiform movements (involuntary movements that are rapid, jerky, and continuous).

Radiographic Appearance

The pathologic hallmark of Huntington's disease is atrophy of the caudate nucleus and putamen, which produces the typical CT appearance of focal dilatation of the frontal horns and a loss of their normal concave shape (Figure 8-67) as a result of caudate nucleus atrophy. Generalized enlargement of the ventricles and dilatation of the cortical sulci can also occur.

Single-photon emission computed tomography (SPECT) images demonstrate a decrease in glucose metabolism, specifically in the caudate when compared with the putamen. On PET scans, a decrease in the dopamine receptor sites provides an opportunity to track the condition before its clinical onset.

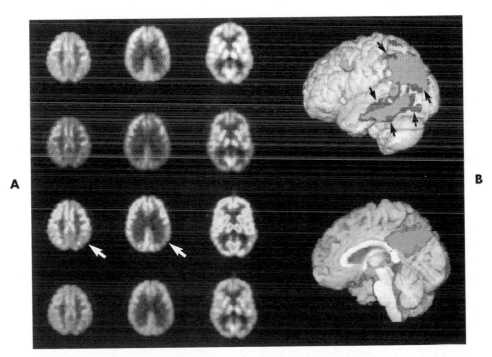

FIGURE 8-66 Alzheimer's dementia. **A,** FDG-PET metabolic brain imaging demonstrates significantly reduced glucose metabolism in the left cerebrum on transverse images *(arrows).* **B,** When the brain map was superimposed, the area of reduced uptake (represented by the *medium gray area*) superimposed the Alzheimer's control data (represented by the *dark gray area [black arrows]*). Significantly reduced glucose metabolism can be seen on the patient's left, which is consistent with a diagnosis of Alzheimer's dementia.

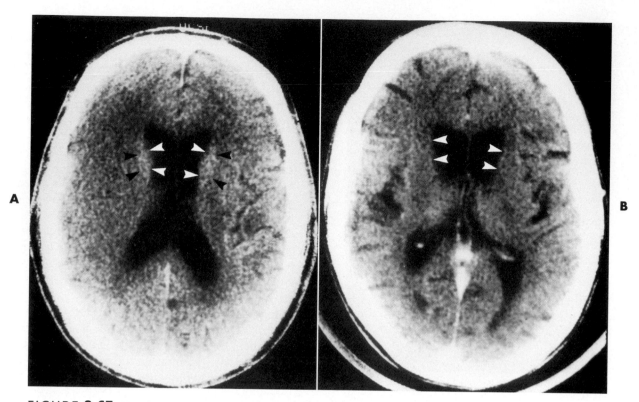

FIGURE 8-67 Huntington's disease. **A,** CT scan in a normal patient shows the heads of the caudate nucleus *(black arrowheads)* producing a normal concavity of the frontal horns *(white arrowheads)*. **B,** In a patient with Huntington's disease, atrophy of the caudate nucleus causes a characteristic loss of the normal concavity *(white arrowheads)* of the frontal horns.

Treatment

At present there is no cure. Treatment with acetylcholinesterase inhibitors increases cognition, but does not halt progression of the disease. Counseling is essential because of the hereditary genetic relationship.

Parkinson's Disease

Parkinson's disease (shaking palsy) is a progressive degenerative disease characterized by stooped posture, stiffness and slowness of movement, fixed facial expression, and involuntary rhythmic tremor of the limbs that disappears with voluntary movement. A disorder of middle or later life, Parkinson's disease is very gradually progressive and exhibits a prolonged course.

The major degenerative changes in nerve cells in Parkinson's disease occur in the basal ganglia, especially the globus pallidus, the substantia nigra, and the fibers of the corpus striatum. The essence of the condition seems to be an enzyme defect that results in an inadequate production of the neuronal transmitter substance dopamine. The most recent method of treatment is the administration of L-dopa,

a substance that is converted to dopamine in the brain. Although this drug therapy does not stop the neuronal degeneration, it dramatically improves both the appearance and behavior of the patient.

Radiographic Appearance

CT scans in patients with Parkinson's disease often demonstrate cortical atrophy. However, because this condition is usually seen in older individuals, the ventricular enlargement and prominent cortical sulci found on CT scans may be indistinguishable from those caused by the normal aging process. SPECT and PET are the most useful imaging modalities to demonstrate degenerative changes. The basal ganglia have decreased uptake and retention of 18F-DOPA in cases of Parkinson's disease.

Treatment

Drug treatment is the first choice for controlling symptoms because no cure currently exists. Stereotactic pallidotomy is a surgical option for some cases and may aid in long-term reduction of symptoms by creating lesions that destroy the globus pallidus.

SUMMARY of FINDINGS for Degenerative Diseases of the Central Nervous System

disorder	location	radiographic appearance	treatment
Normal aging	Cerebral atrophy, enlarged ventricular system, demyelination	CT—low-density periventricular regions MRI—high signal intensity of periventricular regions on T2-weighted images	None in normal aging process
Alzheimer's disease	Cerebral atrophy before senile period	CT—cerebral atrophy with enlarged ventricles and prominent cortical sulci MRI—similar to CT; periventricular intensity on T2-weighted images PET—reduced glucose metabolism consistent with Alzheimer's regions	No cure Diet, education, and safety factors to slow progression Medications to slow progression
Huntington's disease	Atrophy of caudate nucleus and putamen	CT—focal ventricular dilatation; loss of normal shape of frontal horns SPECT—demonstrate a decrease in glucose metabolism, specifically in the caudate when compared to the putamen PET—dopamine receptor sites decrease, providing early onset tracking prior to clinical onset	No treatment at present Acetylcholinesterase inhibitors increase cognition; however do not halt the disease progression Genetic counseling of families
Parkinson's disease	Degeneration of basal ganglia	CT—appearance similar to that of normal aging process SPECT/PET—demonstrate degenerative changes in the basal ganglia as decreased uptake and retention of 18F-DOPA	Drug treatment No cure known Stereotactic pallidotomy
Cerebellar atrophy	Degeneration of cerebellum	MRI—size changes in cerebellum	Discontinue prolonged use of drugs (alcohol and phenytoin)
Amyotrophic lateral sclerosis	Upper and lower motor neurons	CT/MRI/myelography—inconclusive for diagnostic purposes; can demonstrate other causes of similar symptoms	Incurable Psychological support Education

Cerebellar Atrophy

Isolated atrophy of the cerebellum may represent an inherited disorder, a degenerative disease, or the toxic effect of prolonged use of such drugs as alcohol and phenytoin (Dilantin) (Figure 8-68).

Amyotrophic Lateral Sclerosis (Lou Gehrig's Disease)

In this relentlessly progressive condition of unknown cause, there is widespread selective atrophy and loss of motor nerve cells leading to extensive paralysis and death from respiratory weakness or aspiration pneumonia.

Radiographic Appearance

Although this disease cannot be diagnosed radiographically, CT, MRI, or myelography is often performed to exclude a spinal malignancy, which could produce a similar clinical appearance.

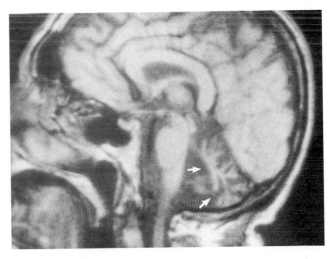

FIGURE 8-68 Cerebellar atrophy. Sagittal MR scan shows dramatic loss of substance of the vermis of the cerebellum *(arrows)* in a patient with severe alcoholism.

Treatment

Amyotrophic lateral sclerosis is uniformly fatal because there currently is no cure. Psychological support and education can be provided.

Hydrocephalus

Hydrocephalus refers to dilatation of the ventricular system that is usually associated with increased intracranial pressure. In **noncommunicating (obstructive) hydrocephalus**, there is an obstruction to the flow of CSF somewhere along the ventricular pathways from the lateral ventricles to the outlets of the fourth ventricle. Enlargement of the lateral ventricles with normal-sized third and fourth ventricles indicates an obstruction at the level of the foramen of Monro. This is most commonly attributable to a colloid cyst (Figure 8-69) or a suprasellar tumor, especially craniopharyngioma. Enlargement of the lateral and third ventricles with a normal-sized fourth ventricle indicates an obstruction at the level of the aqueduct of Sylvius (Figures 8-70 and 8-71). The most common causes of this appearance are congenital aqueduct stenosis or occlusion and neoplasm (pinealoma, teratoma). Enlargement of the entire ventricular system (with the fourth ventricle often dilated out of proportion

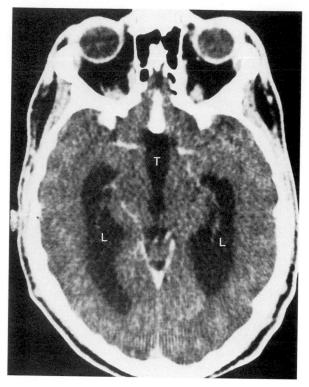

FIGURE 8-70 Hydrocephalus caused by obstruction at the level of the aqueduct. Dilatation of the lateral *(L)* and third *(T)* ventricles can be seen in this patient with congenital hydrocephalus. Symptoms of headache and papilledema resolved after ventricular shunting.

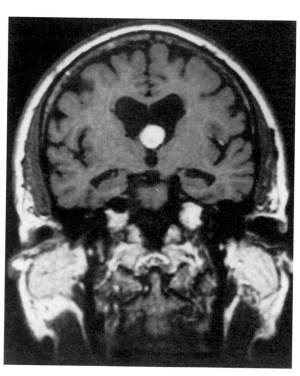

FIGURE 8-69 Hydrocephalus with obstruction at the level of the foramen of Monro. T1-weighted MR scan shows a hyperintense colloid cyst causing bilateral enlargement of the frontal horns.

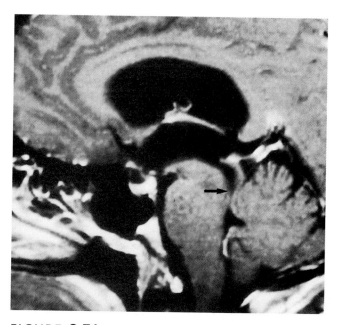

FIGURE 8-71 Aqueductal stenosis. T1-weighted sagittal MR scan shows pronounced narrowing of the inferior portion of the aqueduct *(arrow)*. There is flaring of the upper portion of the aqueduct and considerable enlargement of the third and lateral ventricles. Note that the fourth ventricle is of normal size.

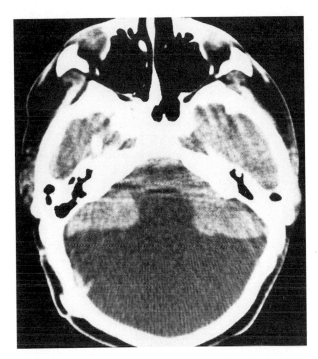

FIGURE 8-72 Hydrocephalus caused by obstruction at the level of the outlet of the fourth ventricle. Huge low-density cyst (a Dandy-Walker cyst) occupies most of the enlarged posterior fossa and represents an extension of the dilated fourth ventricle.

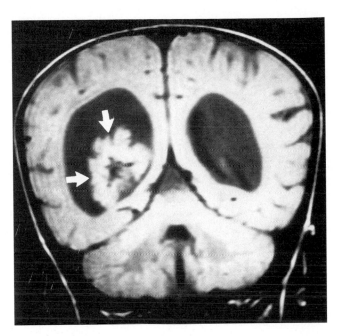

FIGURE 8-73 Choroid plexus papilloma. T1-weighted MR scan shows a lobulated isointense mass *(arrows)* in a greatly dilated right lateral ventricle.

[Dandy-Walker cyst]) indicates an obstruction at the level of the outlet of the fourth ventricle (Figure 8-72), a condition that may reflect congenital atresia, infection, neoplasm, or downward herniation of the cerebellar tonsils through the foramen magnum.

In the much more common **communicating hydrocephalus,** the ventricular fluid passes freely into the extraventricular subarachnoid space. There is generalized ventricular enlargement with normal or absent sulci. Obstruction of the normal CSF pathway distal to the fourth ventricle usually involves the subarachnoid space at the basal cisterns, cerebral convexity, or foramen magnum. Causes include infection (meningitis, empyema), subarachnoid or subdural hemorrhage, congenital anomalies, neoplasm, and dural venous thrombosis. A similar radiographic pattern is seen in **normal-pressure hydrocephalus**, a syndrome of gait ataxia, urinary incontinence, and dementia associated with ventricular dilatation and relatively normal CSF pressure.

Radiographic Appearance

CT clearly shows ventricular dilatation. MRI is more specific than CT in demonstrating the underlying cause of obstruction or in excluding obstruction (communicating hydrocephalus). Contrast-enhanced MRI may assist in distinguishing a congenital posterior fossa cyst from an enhancing cystic neoplasm. Ultrasound can demonstrate the ventricular dilatation either in utero or after birth as long as the sound waves can traverse the open fontanels.

Generalized enlargement of the ventricular system can also be attributable to the overproduction of CSF by a papilloma (Figure 8-73) or by carcinoma arising in the choroid plexus (CSF-secreting vascular tissue in the ventricles). These rare tumors usually occur in the fourth ventricle in adults and the lateral ventricles in children.

Treatment

Hydrocephalus can often be treated by the placement of a shunt between the dilated ventricles and the heart or the peritoneal cavity. Successful shunting causes a decrease in the intracranial pressure and ventricular size; the latter can be monitored by CT or MRI. If radiation exposure is of concern (patient age or pregnancy), MRI is the modality of choice.

Sinusitis

The paranasal sinuses (maxillary, ethmoid, frontal, and sphenoid) are paired, air-filled cavities that are lined with a mucous membrane that is directly continuous with the nasal mucosa. The size and shape of the sinuses vary in different age periods, in different individuals, and on the two sides of the

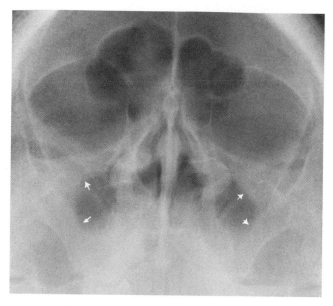

FIGURE 8-74 Chronic sinusitis. Mucosal thickening appears as soft tissue density *(arrows)* lining the walls of the maxillary antra.

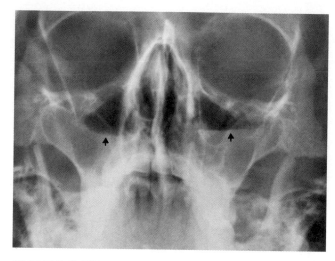

FIGURE 8-75 Acute sinusitis. There is mucosal thickening involving most of the paranasal sinuses and air-fluid levels *(arrows)* in both maxillary antra.

same individual. At birth, the maxillary sinus is only a slitlike space that later expands to fill the maxilla and is thus responsible for the growth of the face. The ethmoid sinuses can be seen radiographically by 6 years of age, whereas the frontal sinuses usually are not well demonstrated until about 10 years of age. The sphenoid sinuses begin to develop around 2 or 3 years of age and are fully developed by late adolescence.

Viral infection of the upper respiratory tract may lead to obstruction of drainage of the paranasal sinuses and the development of localized pain, tenderness, and fever.

Radiographic Appearance

Radiographically, acute or chronic sinusitis causes mucosal thickening, which appears as a soft tissue density lining the walls of the involved sinuses (Figure 8-74). The maxillary antra are most commonly affected and are best visualized on the Waters' projection. An air-fluid level in a sinus is usually considered a manifestation of acute inflammatory disease (Figure 8-75). To demonstrate this finding, it is essential that all sinus films be obtained with the patient erect and with the use of a horizontal beam. The destruction of the bony wall of a sinus is an ominous sign indicating secondary osteomyelitis (Figure 8-76). CT, the procedure of choice, demonstrates bony sinonasal anatomy; coronal images can show air-fluid levels (Figure 8-77). Coronal MRI provides the best method to detect suspected complications, such as mucocele, osteomyelitis, or underlying intracranial disease.

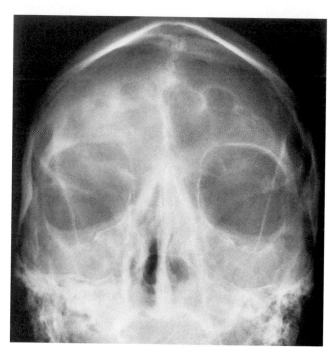

FIGURE 8-76 Mucormycosis causing pansinusitis with osteomyelitis. Destruction of the roof of the right orbit and outer margins of the right frontal sinus can be seen.

Treatment

Sinusitis caused by bacteria is treated with antibiotics to eradicate the infection. Decongestants may be taken to relieve symptoms and aid in sinus drainage. Steroid nasal sprays help reduce mucosal inflammation. Chronic sinusitis may require surgery to clean and drain the sinus, and to repair a deviated septum or nasal obstruction that may be the cause of recurrent inflammation.

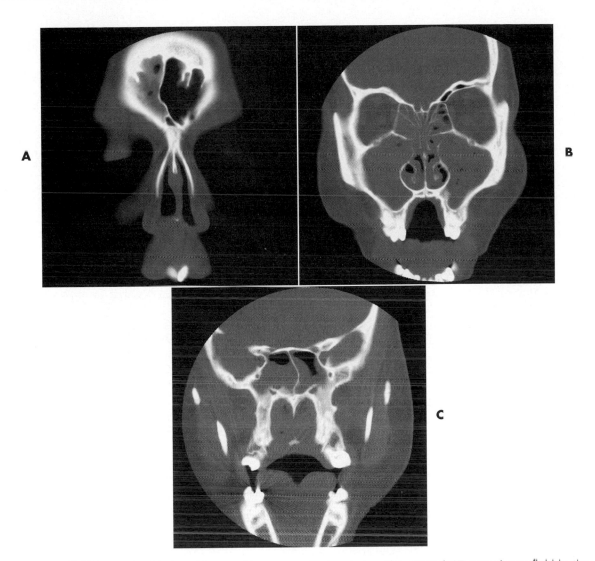

FIGURE 8-77 Pansinusitis in a 29-year-old woman with headache. The coronal CT scan shows fluid in the frontal sinus **(A),** in the maxillary and ethmoid sinuses **(B),** and in the sphenoid sinus **(C).**

SUMMARY of FINDINGS for Other Diseases of the Central Nervous System

disorder	location	radiographic appearance	treatment
Hydrocephalus	Cerebral ventricular system	CT—demonstrates ventricular dilatation MRI—may also show underlying cause	Shunt placement
Sinusitis	Paranasal sinuses; maxillary most common	Sinus radiograph—mucosal thickening and fluid levels CT—demonstrates sinonasal anatomy and fluid levels on coronal imaging MRI—suspected complications	Antibiotics for bacterial infection Decongestants Surgery

REVIEW QUESTIONS

1. The imaging modality of choice to evaluate patients with suspected neurologic dysfunction caused by head trauma is _____.
   A. ultrasound
   B. MRI
   C. CT
   D. skull radiographs

2. Arterial bleeding sometimes associated with head trauma can cause _____ hematomas.
   A. intracranial
   B. subdural
   C. epidural
   D. acute

3. Venous bleeding sometimes associated with head trauma can cause _____ hematomas.
   A. intracranial
   B. subdural
   C. epidural
   D. acute

4. Movement of the brain within the calvaria following blunt trauma to the skull sometimes results in a cerebral _____.
   A. subdural hematoma
   B. epidural hematoma
   C. acute hematoma
   D. contusion

5. Bleeding into the ventricular system caused by injury to surface veins, cerebral parenchyma, or cortical arteries can cause _____ hemorrhage.
   A. epidural
   B. subdural
   C. epiarachnoid
   D. subarachnoid

6. Plain radiographs of the facial bones should always be made with the patient in the _____ position if possible.
   A. supine
   B. erect
   C. lateral decubitus
   D. anterior

7. The most common primary brain tumor is a _____.
   A. glioma
   B. glioblastoma
   C. meningioma
   D. neurinoma

8. A benign tumor that arises from arachnoid lining cells and is attached to the dura is named _____.
   A. glioma
   B. glioblastoma
   C. meningioma
   D. neurinoma

9. The most common neoplasms that metastasize to the brain arise in the _____ and _____.
   A. lung, stomach
   B. lung, breast
   C. stomach, breast
   D. breast, prostate

10. A viral inflammation of the brain and meninges is called _____.
    A. meningitis
    B. hydrocephalus
    C. encephalitis
    D. encephalomalacia

11. The best imaging modality to evaluate brain abscesses is _____.

12. The two imaging procedures of choice to evaluate the extent of a stroke in the brain are _____ and _____.

13. The initials *TIA* stand for _____.

14. The imaging modality of choice to demonstrate the plaques of demyelination that are characteristic of multiple sclerosis is _____.

15. A condition in which brain impulses are temporarily disturbed, the results of which range from loss of consciousness to violent seizures, is termed _____.

16. A diffuse form of progressive cerebral atrophy that develops at an earlier age than the senile period is called _____.

17. A progressive degenerative disease characterized by involuntary tremors of the extremities that disappear with voluntary movement is named _____.

18. Sinus radiographs should be taken using a _____ beam and with the patient in the _____ position.

19. The pathologic condition that refers to dilatation of the ventricular system and is usually associated with increased intracranial pressure is _____.

20. If a patient needing facial or sinus radiographs is unable to stand or sit erect, a(n) _____ using a(n) _____ beam may be performed to demonstrate any air-fluid levels that may be present.

BIBLIOGRAPHY

Brant-Zawadzki M, Norman D: *Magnetic resonance imaging of the central nervous system*, New York, 1987, Raven Press.

Burgener FA, Kormano M: *Differential diagnosis in computed tomography*, New York, 1996, Thieme.

Callen PW: *Ultrasound in obstetrics and gynecology*, Philadelphia, 2000, Saunders.

eMedicine>Specialties>Neurology>: www.emedicine.com

eMedicine>Specialties>Radiology>: www.emedicine.com

Lee SH, Rao KCVG: *Cranial computed tomography and MRI*, New York, 1992, McGraw-Hill.

Osborn AG: *Handbook of neuroradiology*, St Louis, 1991, Mosby.

Ramsey RG: *Neuroradiology with computed tomography*, Philadelphia, 1987, Saunders.

Woodruff WW: *Fundamentals of neuroimaging*, Philadelphia, 1993, Saunders.

CHAPTER 9

HEMATOPOIETIC *System*

Chapter Outline

Physiology of the Blood
Diseases of Red Blood Cells
    Anemia
    Polycythemia
Diseases of White Blood Cells
    Leukemia
    Lymphoma
    Infectious Mononucleosis
Diseases of Platelets (Bleeding Disorders)
    Hemophilia
    Purpura (Thrombocytopenia)

Key Terms

anemia
basophil
coagulation factors
eosinophils
erythrocytes
hemoglobin
leukocytes
lymphatic leukemia
monocytes
myelocytic leukemia
neutrophils (polymorphonuclear leukocytes)
pernicious anemia
platelets
sickle cell anemia
spherocytosis
thalassemia

Prerequisite Knowledge

The student should have a basic knowledge of the physiology of the hematopoietic system.

Goals

To acquaint the student radiographer with the pathophysiology and radiographic manifestations of all the common and some of the unusual disorders of the hematopoietic system.

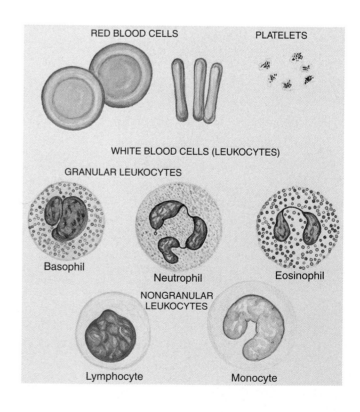

RED BLOOD CELLS   PLATELETS

WHITE BLOOD CELLS (LEUKOCYTES)

GRANULAR LEUKOCYTES

Basophil   Neutrophil   Eosinophil

NONGRANULAR LEUKOCYTES

Lymphocyte   Monocyte

RADIOGRAPHER *Notes*

Although the hematopoietic system cannot be directly imaged, many blood disorders result in abnormalities that can be demonstrated radiographically. It may be necessary to increase or decrease exposure factors when imaging patients who manifest advanced stages of these diseases (see the Box in Chapter 1 labeled Relative Attenuation of X-Rays in Advanced Stages of Diseases). The radiographer must be aware of the severe pain experienced by patients undergoing a sickle cell crisis. Patients with advanced leukemia or lymphoma who have an altered immune status may require protective isolation. Because many hematopoietic system diseases cause significant demineralization of bone, the radiographer must be alert to the possibility of pathologic fracture and thus exercise caution when moving and positioning these patients.

Radiographers need to be aware of the importance of using proper radiation safety shielding, pelvic shielding for patients, and aprons for technologists to prevent possible lack of blood cell formation in the pelvis, which could ultimately result in anemia.

Objectives

After reading this chapter, the reader will be able to:
1. Define all key terms in this chapter
2. Describe the physiology of the hematopoietic system
3. Identify the basic blood structures on diagrams
4. Differentiate the various pathologic conditions affecting the hematopoietic system as well as their radiographic manifestations

Physiology of the Blood

Blood and the cells within it are vital to life. An adequate blood supply to all body tissues is necessary to bring oxygen, nutrients, salts, and hormones to the cells and to carry away the waste products of cellular metabolism. The components of blood are also a major defense against infection, toxic substances, and foreign antigens.

Red bone marrow (found in vertebrae, proximal femurs, and flat bones such as the sternum, ribs, skull, and pelvis) and lymph nodes are the blood-forming tissues of the body. Red blood cells (**erythrocytes**) and platelets (thrombocytes) are made in red bone marrow, whereas white blood cells (**leukocytes**) are produced in both red marrow and lymphoid tissue. If a bone marrow puncture is necessary for diagnostic testing, the iliac rim and sternum are good sites.

Erythrocytes are biconcave disks without a nucleus that contain **hemoglobin,** an iron-based protein that carries oxygen from the respiratory tract to the body's tissues. In a normal person, there are 4.5 million to 6 million red blood cells in each cubic millimeter of blood. The amount of hemoglobin per deciliter is approximately 14 g in women and 15 g in men.

Leukocytes, or white blood cells, normally number from 5000 to 10,000/mm^3 of blood. Unlike erythrocytes, there are several types of white blood cells. **Neutrophils (polymorphonuclear leukocytes),** which make up 55% to 75% of white blood cells, defend the body against bacteria by ingesting these foreign organisms and destroying them (phagocytosis). The number of polymorphonuclear leukocytes in the blood enormously increases in acute infections because the bone marrow rapidly releases into the bloodstream the large numbers of these cells kept in reserve. **Eosinophils** (1% to 4%) are red-staining cells whose number greatly increases in allergic and parasitic conditions. The third type of leukocyte is the **basophil** (0% to 1%), which contains granules that stain blue. These three types of cells are formed in the sinusoids of bone marrow, and they, like red blood cells, go through immature stages before reaching the adult form.

Lymphocytes represent about 25% to 40% of white blood cells. They play a major role in the immune system and aid in the synthesis of antibodies and the production of immunoglobulins.

The final type of white blood cell is the monocyte, which is actively phagocytic and plays an important part in the inflammatory process. Monocytes are formed in the bone marrow and represent about 2% to 8% of white blood cells.

Platelets, the smallest blood cells, are essential for blood clotting. Normally there are about 150,000 to 400,000 platelets in every cubic millimeter of blood.

Diseases of Red Blood Cells

Anemia

Anemia refers to a decrease in the amount of oxygen-carrying hemoglobin in the peripheral blood. This reduction can be attributable to improper formation of new red blood cells, an increased rate of red blood cell destruction, or a loss of red blood cells as a result of prolonged bleeding. Regardless of the cause, a hemoglobin deficiency causes the anemic person to appear pale. This is best appreciated in the mucous membranes of the mouth and conjunctiva, and in the nail beds. A decrease in the oxygen-carrying hemoglobin impairs the delivery of an adequate oxygen supply to the cells and tissues, leading to fatigue and muscular weakness, and often to shortness of breath on exertion (dyspnea). To meet the body's need for more oxygen, the respiratory rate increases and the heart beats more rapidly.

Iron Deficiency Anemia

Iron deficiency is the most common cause of anemia. It most frequently results from chronic blood loss, as from an ulcer, a malignant tumor, or excessive bleeding during menstruation (menorrhagia). Other causes of iron deficiency anemia include inadequate dietary intake of iron and increased iron loss caused by intestinal parasites. Iron deficiency anemia also may develop during pregnancy because the mother's iron supply is depleted by red blood cell development in the fetus.

Treatment

If chronic blood loss causes the iron deficiency, the cause must be determined and treated. The first choice of treatment is for the patient to change dietary habits to include more foods rich in iron. The second option is on oral iron supplement: ferrous sulfate. When taking an iron supplement, it is important to remember that other products influence iron absorption. For example, increasing vitamin C intake enhances iron absorption. Iron deficiency can be treated successfully in most cases.

Hemolytic Anemia

The underlying abnormality in hemolytic anemia is a shortened life span of the red blood cells with resulting hemolysis and the release of hemoglobin into the plasma. Most hemolytic anemias are caused by a hereditary defect that may produce abnormal red cells or abnormal hemoglobin. Less commonly, hemolytic anemia is acquired and related to circulating antibodies from autoimmune or allergic reactions (e.g., drugs such as sulfonamide) or the malarial parasite.

Spherocytosis, sickle cell anemia, and **thalassemia** are the major hereditary hemolytic anemias. In spherocytosis the erythrocytes have a circular rather than a biconcave shape, making them fragile and susceptible to rupture. In sickle cell anemia, which is generally confined to blacks, the hemoglobin molecule is abnormal and the red cells are crescentic or sickle

shaped and tend to rupture. A defect in hemoglobin formation is also responsible for thalassemia, which predominantly occurs in persons living near the Mediterranean Sea, especially those of Italian, Greek, or Sicilian descent.

The breakdown of hemoglobin produces bilirubin, a pigmented substance that is normally detoxified by the liver and converted into bile. The accumulation of large amounts of this orange pigment in plasma causes the tissues to have a yellow appearance (jaundice).

Hemolytic anemia of the newborn (erythroblastosis fetalis) can result when the mother is Rh negative and the fetus has Rh-positive blood inherited from the father. Although the fetal and maternal circulations are separate, fetal blood can enter the mother's blood through ruptures in the placenta that occur at delivery. The mother thus becomes sensitized to the Rh factor of the fetus and makes antibodies against it. Any antibodies reaching the fetal blood through the placenta in future pregnancies cause hemolysis of the fetal red blood cells. The severity of the disease ranges from mild anemia with jaundice to fetal death.

Radiographic Appearance

The hemolytic anemias produce a variety of radiographic abnormalities. Although the radiographic findings are similar in the various types of hemolytic anemia, they tend to be most severe in thalassemia and least prominent in spherocytosis. Extensive marrow hyperplasia, the result of ineffective erythropoiesis and rapid destruction of newly formed red blood cells, causes generalized osteoporosis with pronounced widening of the medullary spaces and thinning of the cortices in long and tubular bones (Figure 9-1). As the fine secondary trabeculae are resorbed, new bone is laid down on the surviving trabeculae, thickening them and producing a coarsened pattern. Normal modeling of long bones does not occur because the expanding marrow flattens or even bulges the normally concave surfaces of the shafts.

In the skull, there is widening of the diploic space and thinning or complete obliteration of the outer table. When the hyperplastic marrow perforates or destroys the outer table, it proliferates under the invisible periosteum, and new bone spicules are laid down perpendicularly to the inner table. This produces the characteristic hair-on-end appearance of vertical striations in a radial pattern (Figure 9-2).

Extramedullary hematopoiesis is a compensatory mechanism of the reticuloendothelial system (liver, spleen, lymph nodes) in patients with prolonged erythrocyte deficiency resulting from the destruction of red blood cells or the inability of normal blood-forming organs to produce them. Paravertebral

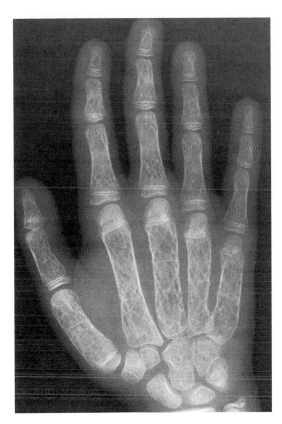

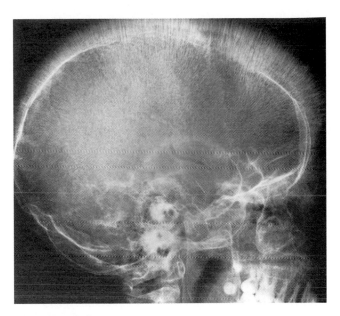

FIGURE 9-2 Thalassemia. Lateral projection of the skull demonstrates hair-on-end appearance. Note normal appearance of calvaria inferior to the internal occipital protuberance, an area in which there is no red marrow, and poor pneumatization of the visualized paranasal sinuses.

FIGURE 9-1 Thalassemia. Pronounced widening of medullary spaces with thinning of cortical margins. Note the absence of normal modeling caused by the pressure of expanding marrow space. Localized radiolucencies simulating multiple osteolytic lesions represent tumorous collections of hypoplastic marrow.

collections of hematopoietic tissue may appear on chest radiographs as single or multiple, smooth or lobulated, posterior mediastinal masses that are usually located at the lower thoracic levels (Figure 9-3).

In sickle cell anemia, expansile pressure of the adjacent intervertebral disks produces characteristic biconcave indentations on both the superior and inferior margins of the softened vertebral bodies, giving the appearance of fish vertebrae (Figure 9-4, *A*). Another typical appearance is the result of the development of localized steplike central depressions of multiple vertebral end plates (Figure 9-4, *B*). This is most often caused by circulatory stasis and ischemia, which retard growth in the central portion of the vertebral cartilaginous growth plate. The periphery of the growth plate, which has a different blood supply, continues to grow at a more normal rate.

Bulging of the abnormally shaped red blood cells in sickle cell anemia typically causes focal ischemia and infarction in multiple tissues. Bone infarcts commonly occur in infants and children. These most frequently involve the small bones of the hands and feet, producing an irregular area of bone destruction with overlying periosteal calcification, which may be indistinguishable from osteomyelitis. In older children and adults, bone infarction may initially appear as an ill-defined lucent area that becomes irregularly calcified.

Acute osteomyelitis, often caused by *Salmonella* infection, is a common complication in sickle cell disease. The resulting lytic destruction and periosteal reaction may be extensive, often involving the entire shaft and multiple bones (Figure 9-5). Radiographically, it may be impossible to distinguish between osteomyelitis and bone infarction without infection (Figure 9-6).

Throughout their lives, patients with sickle cell anemia are plagued by recurrent painful crises. These episodes are attributable to recurrent vaso-occlusive phenomena and may appear with explosive suddenness and attack various parts of the body, especially the abdomen, chest, and joints. It is often difficult to distinguish between a painful sickle cell crisis and some other type of acute process, such as biliary colic, appendicitis, or a perforated viscus. In the extremities, a sickle cell crisis may mimic osteomyelitis or an acute arthritis, such as gout or rheumatoid arthritis.

The most common extraskeletal abnormality in the hemolytic anemias is cardiomegaly caused by severe anemia and increased cardiac output. The heart has a globular configuration reflecting enlargement of

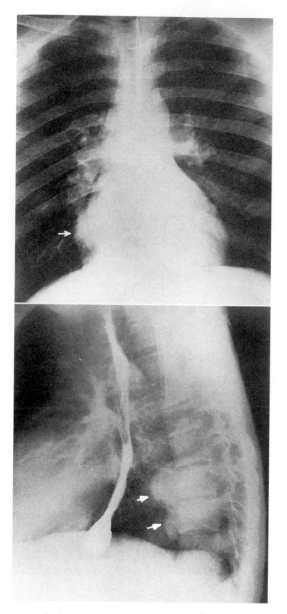

FIGURE 9-3 Extramedullary hematopoiesis in thalassemia. A lateral projection of the chest demonstrates lobulated posterior mediastinal masses of hematopoietic tissue *(arrows)* in the lower thoracic region.

all chambers. Increased pulmonary blood flow produces engorgement of the pulmonary vessels, giving a hypervascular appearance to the lungs. Pulmonary infarction, pulmonary edema and congestive failure, and pneumonia are frequent complications.

Renal abnormalities can be demonstrated by excretory urography in about two thirds of patients with sickle cell disease. A serious complication is renal papillary necrosis (see Figure 6-16), which is probably related to vessel obstruction within the papillae and may produce sinuses or cavity formation within one or more papillae.

Treatment

The cause and type of hemolytic anemia must be determined to successfully begin treatment. For spherocytosis, a splenectomy is curative.

For sickle cell anemia, no cure currently exists. Therefore treatment consists of management and control of symptoms. The most invasive treatment, a bone marrow transplant, offers a possible cure. During a crisis, bed rest, maintenance of oxygen levels to prevent sickling, folic acid to aid in red blood cell production, maintenance of fluids to keep electrolyte balance stable, and possible blood transfusion (of packed red cells) are appropriate. In some cases, prophylactic antibiotics are given. Gene therapy requires removal of a defective cell, fixing the gene, and replanting the new cell into the bone marrow. This may help manage and control symptoms, and in some cases even provide a cure.

If an Rh-negative mother delivers or aborts an Rh-positive infant, she is given a vaccine of Rh immunoglobulin within 24 hours to prevent the production of antibodies against the Rh factor. Blood testing to determine whether Rh incompatibility exists is now an essential part of prenatal care. An Rh-positive baby born to an Rh-negative mother receives a blood transfusion within 24 hours after birth.

Megaloblastic Anemia

A deficiency of vitamin B_{12} or of folic acid leads to defective deoxyribonucleic acid (DNA) synthesis and an anemia in which there is a decreased number of red blood cells, although each cell contains the normal amount of hemoglobin. The most common cause of vitamin B_{12} deficiency is **pernicious anemia,** in which there is inadequate intrinsic factor secretion related to atrophy of the gastric mucosa. Intrinsic factor acts as a carrier in the small bowel absorption of vitamin B_{12}, which is essential for erythrocyte development.

A deficiency of folic acid (and vitamin B_{12}) may also be related to intestinal malabsorption. This in turn may be related to intestinal parasites or bacterial overproduction, especially in patients with stasis of bowel contents, as in blind loop syndrome and multiple jejunal diverticula. Other causes of megaloblastic anemia include a poor diet, such as strict vegetarianism, in which there are no sources of vitamin B_{12}, or long-term alcoholism, in which no folic acid is available.

Radiographic Appearance

Gastric atrophy is seen radiographically as a tubular stomach with a bald appearance that reflects a decrease or absence of the usually prominent rugal

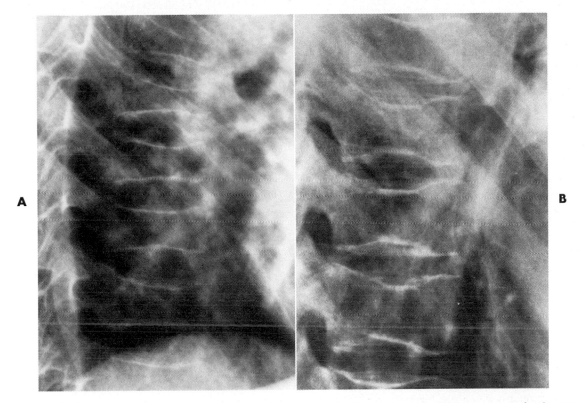

FIGURE 9-4 Sickle cell anemia. **A,** Biconcave indentations on both superior and inferior margins of soft vertebral bodies produce characteristic fish vertebrae appearance. **B,** Localized step-like central depressions of multiple vertebral end plates.

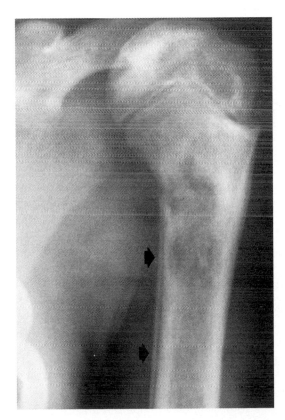

FIGURE 9-5 Acute osteomyelitis in sickle cell anemia. Diffuse lytic destruction of the proximal humerus can be seen along with extensive periosteal reaction *(arrows)*.

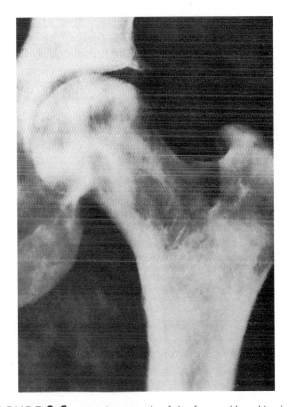

FIGURE 9-6 Aseptic necrosis of the femoral head in sickle cell anemia. Mottled areas of increased and decreased density reflect osteonecrosis without collapse. Trabeculae in neck and intertrochanteric region are thickened by apposition of new bone. Solid layer of new bone along the inner aspect of the cortex of the femoral shaft causes narrowing of the medullary canal.

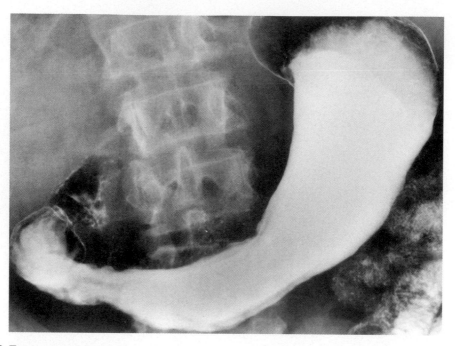

FIGURE 9-7 Megaloblastic anemia in a patient with chronic atrophic gastritis, which is recognized by the tubular stomach with a striking decrease in the usually prominent rugal folds.

folds (Figure 9-7). It must be emphasized, however, that radiographic findings of atrophic gastritis are often seen in older persons with no evidence of pernicious anemia.

Treatment

The treatment of megaloblastic anemia consists of correcting the deficiency of vitamin B_{12} or folic acid. Vitamin B_{12} deficiency requires an injection because taking vitamin B_{12} orally does not reverse the process. Folic acid deficiency can be treated with an oral supplement. If needed, a blood transfusion is given.

Aplastic Anemia

A generalized failure of the bone marrow to function (aplastic anemia) results in decreased levels of erythrocytes, leukocytes, and platelets. In addition to anemia, the patient cannot fight infection (a white blood cell function) and has a bleeding tendency (platelet depletion). Causes of aplastic anemia include exposure to chemical agents or drugs, infections, and invasion of the bone marrow by cancer.

Treatment

Patient prognosis depends on the severity and duration of the bone marrow aplasia. Regular blood transfusions are generally necessary for survival and to reduce symptoms. Because the patient has a suppressed immune response, preventive antibiotics are sometimes prescribed. Situations exposing the patient to an infection or a viral illness should be avoided. Some clinicians recommend medications to stimulate the bone marrow to produce more blood cells. Bone marrow transplantation is a new technique for treating these patients.

Myelophthisic Anemia

Infiltration of bone marrow with nonhematopoietic cells, such as tumor cells, or encroachment on marrow cavities caused by cortical thickening can result in severe myelophthisic anemia and pancytopenia (decreased red and white blood cells and platelets). Tumors may arise from cells that are normally found in the bone marrow (leukemia, lymphoma, myeloma), or the marrow may be invaded by extensive metastases to bone (from carcinomas of the breast, prostate, lung, thyroid). Less common causes of marrow replacement include lipid storage disorders (Gaucher's disease), osteopetrosis (marble bones), and myelofibrosis.

Radiographic Appearance

Skeletal films may demonstrate lytic or blastic lesions, depending on the progression of metastases. A radionuclide bone scan detects bone marrow abnormalities and skeletal metastases. Magnetic resonance imaging (MRI) can demonstrate the extent of bone marrow infiltration.

Treatment

Treatment is focused on the underlying cause of the myelophthisic anemia. A packed red blood cell transfusion is used to treat the anemia and help stabilize the patient.

SUMMARY of FINDINGS for Diseases of Red Blood Cells

disorder	location	radiographic appearance	treatment
Hemolytic anemias	Shortened life span of red blood cells	Long bones—osteoporosis, widened medullary spaces with thinning of cortices; later stages: thickened, coarsened trabecular patterns Skull—thinning of outer table; vertical striation results from new bone formation	Spherocytosis—splenectomy curative Rh-negative mother and Rh-positive fetus—blood transfusion for baby and Rh immunoglobulin vaccine for mother
	Sickle cell anemia—hemoglobin molecule abnormal; red cells crescentic or sickle shaped	Spine—characteristic biconcave indentations superiorly and inferiorly on vertebral body Chest—cardiomegaly IVU/US—renal papillary necrosis	Sickle cell anemia—no cure exists Most invasive treatment—bone marrow transplant, offers possible cure Crisis—bed rest, maintenance of oxygen, folic acid, maintenance of fluids, possible blood transfusion
Megaloblastic anemia	Lack of small bowel absorption of vitamin B_{12} or folic acid	GI series—tubular stomach with bald appearance (decreased or absence of rugal folds)	Vitamin B_{12} deficiency requires an injection Folic acid deficiency can be treated with an oral supplement Possible blood transfusion
Polycythemia	Primary (neoplastic)—increased production of erythrocytes, granulocytes, and platelets	Chest film—prominent vascular markings without cardiomegaly	Bloodletting Chemotherapy Splenectomy
	Secondary (nonneoplastic)—elevated hemoglobin concentration	Chest film—normal Skull (of child)—thickened tables, hair-on-end appearance; similar to congenital hemolytic anemia	

GI, Gastrointestinal; IVU, intravenous urography.

Polycythemia

Primary Polycythemia (Polycythemia Vera)

Polycythemia vera is a hematologic disorder characterized by hyperplasia of the bone marrow (neoplastic) that results in increased production of erythrocytes, granulocytes, and platelets. The disease is slowly progressive and produces symptoms associated with increased blood volume and viscosity. Cerebrovascular and peripheral vascular insufficiencies are common, and many patients give a history of some thrombotic or hemorrhagic event during the course of their disease. There is an increased incidence of peptic ulcer disease, and the excessive cellular proliferation often results in increased levels of uric acid with secondary gout and the formation of urate stones. The spleen is often massively enlarged and may be seen as a left upper quadrant mass.

Radiographic Appearance

Increased blood volume in polycythemia vera can lead to prominence of the pulmonary vascular shadows, usually without the cardiomegaly associated with the increased pulmonary vascularity that occurs in patients with congenital heart disease (Figure 9-8). Intravascular thrombosis may cause pulmonary infarctions that appear as focal areas of consolidation or as bands of fibrosis.

Secondary Polycythemia

Secondary polycythemia may be the result of long-term inadequate oxygen supply in patients with severe chronic pulmonary disease or congenital cyanotic heart disease, or it may develop in persons living at high altitudes. An elevated hemoglobin concentration may also be caused by certain

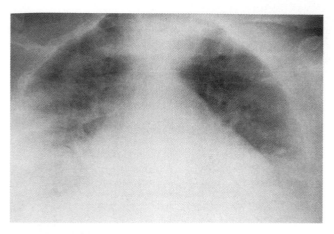

FIGURE 9-8 Primary polycythemia. Severe hypoventilation caused by profound obesity causes engorgement of pulmonary vessels. Although cardiomegaly is uncommon in polycythemia, in this case it reflects pronounced elevation of the diaphragm as a result of a huge abdominal girth and some underlying cardiac decompensation.

neoplasms (renal cell carcinoma, hepatoma, cerebellar hemangioblastoma) that result in an increased production of erythropoietin, which stimulates red blood cell formation.

Radiographic Appearance

Because secondary polycythemia is a compensatory phenomenon, the pulmonary vasculature is normal in appearance and there is no evidence of the disease on chest radiographs. In children with severe secondary polycythemia caused by cyanotic heart disease, the skull may show thickened tables and a hair-on-end appearance similar to the findings in congenital hemolytic anemias. Computed tomography (CT) may be used to investigate the kidneys and their function if a suspicion of tumor exists.

Treatment of Polycythemias

Treatment for both primary and secondary polycythemias starts with bloodletting to remove excessive cellular elements. This improves circulation by lowering blood viscosity and is continued until the hemoglobin and hematocrit levels become normal. Chemotherapy helps to lower the platelet count, and it suppresses production of blood elements by the marrow. For primary polycythemia, clinicians may consider a splenectomy to alleviate painful enlargement of the organ and for patients with repeated episodes of thrombosis causing splenic infarction. Patients who receive these treatments can expect to live about 15 to 20 years after their condition is diagnosed.

Diseases of White Blood Cells

Leukemia

Leukemia is a neoplastic proliferation of white blood cells. The two major types of leukemia are named for the site of malignancy. **Myelocytic leukemia** is a cancer of the bone marrow (myelocytes are the primitive white blood cells in bone marrow). In this condition, a huge increase in the number of circulating granulocytes occurs, and there is decreased production of red blood cells and platelets. **Lymphatic leukemia** is a malignancy of the lymph nodes; in lymphocytic leukemia, the only white blood cells that dramatically increase are lymphocytes.

Leukemia may be chronic or acute. Acute lymphocytic leukemia, which has an abrupt onset and progresses rapidly, is the most common form in children. Acute myelocytic leukemia is more common in adults. Chronic leukemias run a more prolonged course and may involve either cell type.

Because of the exuberant white cell production, there is generally a decrease in the number of circulating red blood cells and platelets. This results in a typical clinical appearance of weakness, shortness of breath, and cardiac palpitations. A decrease in the number of platelets interferes with the blood-clotting mechanism and results in a bleeding tendency. Even though there are more circulating white blood cells than normal, most are immature and thus the patient becomes highly susceptible to infection. Diffuse infiltration of white cells into the spleen and liver may cause massive enlargement of these organs (hepatosplenomegaly).

Radiographic Appearance

In childhood leukemia, radiographically detectable skeletal involvement is extremely common as a result of the infiltration of leukemic cells into the marrow. The earliest radiographic sign of disease is usually a transverse radiolucent band at the metaphyseal ends of the long bones, most commonly about the knees, ankles, and wrists (Figure 9-9). In infancy this appearance is nonspecific because it also occurs with malnutrition or systemic disease. The presence of these transverse lucent metaphyseal bands after 2 years of age is strongly suggestive of acute leukemia.

As the proliferation of neoplastic cells in the marrow becomes more extensive, actual destruction of bone may occur. This may cause patchy lytic lesions, a permeative moth-eaten appearance, or diffuse destruction with cortical erosion (Figure 9-10). A reactive response to proliferating leukemic cells can cause patchy or uniform osteosclerosis; subperiosteal proliferation incites the formation of periosteal new

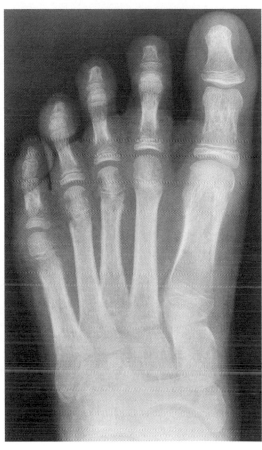

FIGURE 9-9 Acute leukemia. In addition to radiolucent metaphyseal bands, there is frank bone destruction with cortical erosion involving many metatarsals and proximal phalanges.

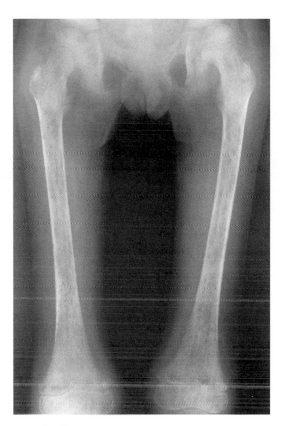

FIGURE 9-10 Acute leukemia. Proliferation of neoplastic cells in the marrow has caused extensive destruction of bone in both femurs.

bone. Diffuse skeletal demineralization may result in vertebral compression fractures.

Enlargement of mediastinal and hilar lymph nodes is the most common abnormality on chest radiographs. Diffuse bilateral reticular changes may simulate lymphangitic spread of carcinoma. The nonspecific pulmonary infiltrates seen in patients with acute leukemia are usually attributable to hemorrhage or secondary infection.

The radiographic abnormalities in chronic leukemia are often similar to those in the acute disease, although their frequency and degree may vary. Skeletal changes are much less common and are usually limited to generalized demineralization in the flat bones, where active marrow persists in adulthood. The demonstration of focal areas of destruction, or periosteal new bone formation, indicates probable transformation into an acute phase of the disease.

Hilar and mediastinal adenopathy are common, especially in chronic lymphocytic leukemia. Congestive heart failure commonly results from the associated severe anemia.

Splenomegaly is an almost constant finding in patients with chronic leukemia (Figure 9-11). Leukemic infiltration of the gastrointestinal tract can produce single or multiple intraluminal filling defects, and the infiltrative process may be indistinguishable from carcinoma. Renal infiltration can cause bilateral enlargement of the kidneys. In chronic lymphocytic leukemia, enlargement of retroperitoneal or mesenteric lymph nodes can cause displacement or obstruction of structures in the genitourinary or gastrointestinal tracts.

Treatment

Leukemia treatment may require multidrug chemotherapy, bone marrow transplant, antibiotics to aid in preventing infections, or a transfusion to reverse the blood cell imbalance. Interferon therapy is a drug regimen to aid the body in producing antiviral proteins that decrease the production of leukemia cells, resulting in an increase in the effectiveness of the immune system. Stem cell transplantation (SCT), although controversial and very expensive, helps by increasing the production of normal cells to replace cells damaged or destroyed by radiotherapy and chemotherapy.

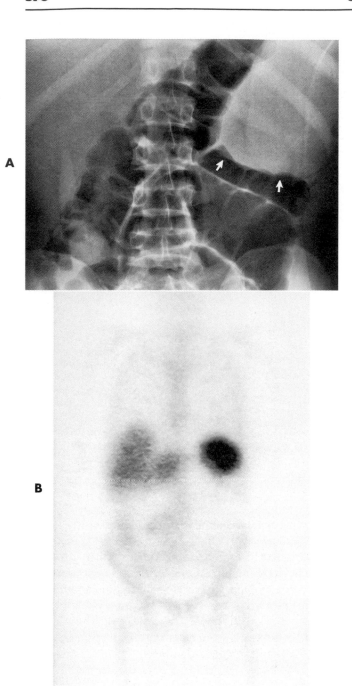

FIGURE **9-11** Chronic leukemia. **A,** Massive splenomegaly causes downward displacement of splenic flexure of colon. Arrows point to inferior margin of spleen. **B,** Indium-111 whole-body scan. Indium-111 tagged to white blood cells illustrates a grossly enlarged spleen on images taken 27 hours after injection.

Lymphoma

Lymphomas are neoplasms of the lymphoreticular system, which includes the lymph nodes, the spleen, and the lymphoid tissues of parenchymal organs, such as the gastrointestinal tract, lung, and skin. They are usually divided into two major types: Hodgkin's

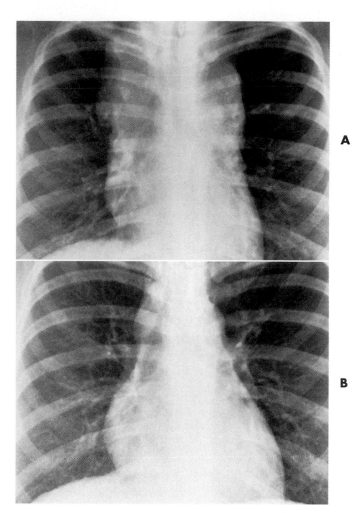

FIGURE **9-12** Lymphoma. **A,** Initial chest film demonstrates considerable widening of upper half of the mediastinum caused by pronounced lymphadenopathy. **B,** After chemotherapy, there is dramatic decrease in the width of the upper mediastinum.

and non-Hodgkin's lymphomas. Ninety percent of cases of Hodgkin's disease originate in the lymph nodes; 10% are of extranodal origin. In contrast, parenchymal organs are more often involved in non-Hodgkin's lymphomas, about 40% of which are of extranodal origin.

Radiographic Appearance

Mediastinal lymph node enlargement is the most common radiographic finding in lymphoma (Figure 9-12). It is seen on initial chest radiographs of about half the patients with Hodgkin's disease and about one third of those with non-Hodgkin's lymphoma. Mediastinal lymph node enlargement is usually bilateral but asymmetric.

Involvement of anterior mediastinal and retrosternal nodes is common, a major factor in differentiating lymphoma from sarcoidosis, which rarely produces radiographically visible enlargement of nodes in the anterior compartment. Calcification may develop in intrathoracic lymph nodes after mediastinal irradiation.

Involvement of the pulmonary parenchyma and pleura usually occurs by direct extension from mediastinal nodes along the lymphatic vessels of the bronchovascular sheaths. Radiographically, this may appear as a coarse interstitial pattern (Figure 9-13), as solitary or multiple ill-defined nodules, or as patchy areas of parenchymal infiltrate that may coalesce to form a large homogeneous mass. At times, it may be difficult to distinguish a superimposed infection after radiation therapy or chemotherapy from the continued spread of lymphomatous tissue. Pleural effusion occurs in up to one third of patients with thoracic

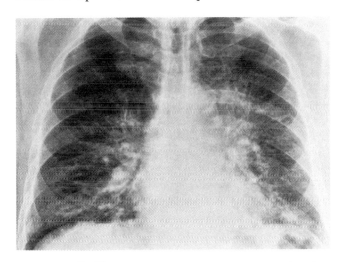

FIGURE 9-13 Lymphoma. Diffuse reticular and reticulonodular changes causing prominence of interstitial lung markings. Note enlargement of left hilar region.

lymphoma. Extension of the tumor to the pericardium can cause pericardial effusion.

About 5% to 10% of patients with lymphoma have involvement of the gastrointestinal tract, primarily of the stomach and small bowel. Gastric lymphoma often is seen as a large, bulky polypoid mass, usually irregular and ulcerated, that may be indistinguishable from a carcinoma (Figure 9-14). A multiplicity of malignant ulcers or an aneurysmal appearance of a single huge ulcer (the diameter of which exceeds that of the adjacent gastric lumen) is characteristic of lymphoma. Additional findings suggestive of lymphoma include relative flexibility of the gastric wall, enlargement of the spleen, and associated prominence of retrogastric and other regional lymph nodes that cause extrinsic impressions on the barium-filled stomach. Other manifestations of gastric lymphoma include thickening, distortion, and nodularity of rugal folds (Figure 9-15) and generalized gastric narrowing caused by a severe fibrotic reaction.

Lymphoma can produce virtually any pattern of abnormality in the small bowel. The disease may be localized to a single intestinal segment, it may be multifocal, or it may cause diffuse involvement. The major radiographic appearances include irregular thickening of mucosal folds, large ulcerating masses, and multiple intraluminal or intramural filling defects simulating metastatic disease.

Skeletal involvement can be demonstrated in about 15% of patients with lymphoma. Direct extension from adjacent lymph nodes causes bone erosion, especially of the anterior surface of the upper lumbar and lower thoracic spine. Paravertebral soft tissue masses may occur. The hematogenous spread of lymphoma produces a mottled pattern of destruction

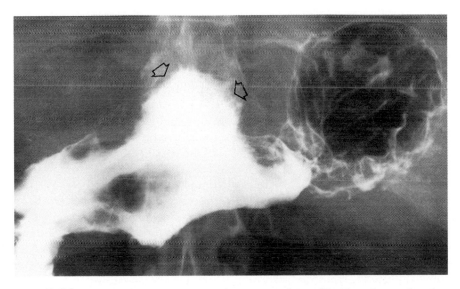

FIGURE 9-14 Lymphoma presenting as a large mass almost filled by a huge ulcer *(arrows)*.

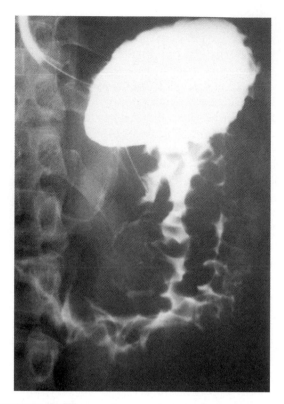

FIGURE 9-15 Lymphoma of the stomach. Note the diffuse thickening, distortion, and nodularity of the gastric folds.

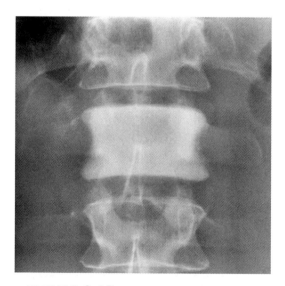

FIGURE 9-16 Lymphoma. Ivory vertebra.

and sclerosis, which may simulate metastatic disease. Dense vertebral sclerosis (ivory vertebra) may develop in Hodgkin's disease (Figure 9-16).

Diffuse lymphomatous infiltration may cause renal enlargement, with distortion, elongation, and compression of the calyces (Figure 9-17). Single or multiple renal nodules or perirenal masses may displace or distort the kidney. Diffuse retroperitoneal

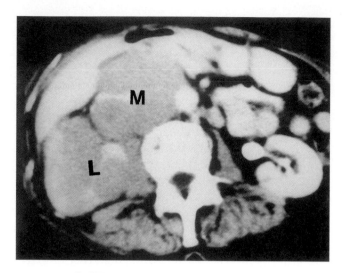

FIGURE 9-17 Lymphoma. Right kidney is completely replaced by a lymphomatous mass *(L)*. Note the extensive involvement of lymph nodes *(M)*.

lymphoma can displace the kidneys or ureters and obliterate one or both psoas margins.

Staging

Once the diagnosis of lymphoma is made, it is essential to determine the status of the abdominal and pelvic lymph nodes. This is necessary both for the initial staging and treatment planning and for assessing the efficacy of treatment and detecting tumor recurrence.

Although lymphography was the procedure of choice in the past, MRI and positron emission tomography (PET) are now the noninvasive techniques employed to demonstrate lymphomatous involvement of the abdominal and pelvic nodes. In practice, CT of the chest, abdomen, and pelvis is generally the first imaging procedure used in staging lymphoma patients. This is especially true for those with non-Hodgkin's lymphoma, which tends to produce bulky masses in the mesenteric and high retrocrural areas. An abnormal CT scan may eliminate the need for more invasive procedures (Figure 9-18); a normal CT scan obtained at 2-cm intervals can exclude retroperitoneal adenopathy with a high degree of confidence. CT is usually used because of standardization and repeatability for patients. Malignant nodes appear round or oval and their transverse-to-longitudinal ratio is greater than 2. A narrow or absent hilus of the node also suggests malignancy.

Ultrasound can detect enlarged retroperitoneal nodes, characterize them, and measure them accurately. For retroperitoneal adenopathy, ultrasound is 80% to 90% accurate, and it has the ability to detect extranodal disease, which typically produces discrete hyperechoic masses. MRI is considered the superior technique because it can detect subtle detail using multiple sequences.

Gallium scans may illustrate increased nodal uptake (indicating swelling or inflammation), and it can assess the response to treatment and detect early recurrence of tumor tissue. PET imaging using fluorodeoxyglucose (FDG) uptake is considered superior to the gallium scan and CT because it can detect microscopic tumor foci and alterations in function within normal-size nodes. PET also has the ability to distinguish large nodes that contain tumor from those that have only benign reactive changes. PET can also be used to monitor the effectiveness of the therapy and identify tumor recurrence (Figure 9-19).

To ensure proper diagnosis and staging of both Hodgkin's and non-Hodgkin's lymphoma, biopsies are performed to extract cell and tissue samples.

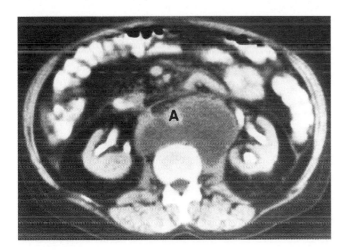

FIGURE 9-18 Lymphoma. CT scan demonstrates anterior displacement of abdominal aorta *(A)* away from the spine, caused by lymphomatous involvement of retroaortic and paraaortic nodes.

Free-hand fine needle aspiration biopsy works best for superficial nodes, whereas CT-guided or ultrasound-guided biopsy is required for deep node evaluation. Patients unable to tolerate surgical procedures may undergo a large-needle core biopsy to determine the extent of the disease before beginning treatment.

Treatment

The best treatment available for Hodgkin's lymphoma is multidrug chemotherapy and high-dose radiation therapy. For non-Hodgkin's lymphoma, more aggressive chemotherapy is required if the disease process is diffuse (Figure 9-20), whereas conservative chemotherapy is used for low-level disease. Bone marrow transplant may be necessary.

Infectious Mononucleosis

Mononucleosis is a self-limited viral disease of the lymphoreticular system characterized by vague symptoms of mild fever, fatigue, sore throat, and swollen lymph nodes caused by an intense increase of lymphoid cells. The Epstein-Barr virus may cause this disease process. It primarily infects young adults and, although often termed the "kissing disease," is not particularly contagious. Blood tests show an elevated white cell count with an abnormally high percentage of atypical lymphocytes, which resemble monocytes. The diagnosis is based on the presence of antibodies to the virus in the blood.

Radiographic Appearance

Generalized lymphadenopathy and splenomegaly are characteristic clinical and radiographic findings in infectious mononucleosis. Hilar lymph node enlargement, usually bilateral, can be demonstrated in about 15% of cases (Figure 9-21). Pneumonia is a rare complication that can appear as a diffuse reticular pattern indicating interstitial disease, or as a patchy, nonspecific air-space consolidation.

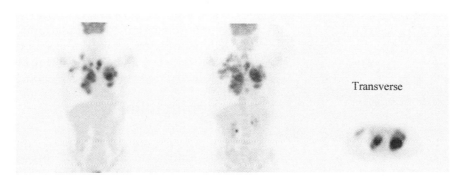

FIGURE 9-19 Lymphoma in a 16-year-old girl with a 3-week history of supraclavicular adenopathy. The PET body scan demonstrates FDG uptake in the supraclavicular fossae, the mediastinum, and the lungs; this indicates a metabolically active neoplasm, which is consistent with the clinically suspected lymphoma.

SUMMARY of FINDINGS for Diseases of White Blood Cells

disorder	location	radiographic appearance	treatment
Leukemia	Neoplastic proliferation of white blood cells	Skeletal radiograph in child—radiolucent bands at metaphyses on long bones after 2 years of age, bone destruction (moth-eaten appearance with resulting osteosclerosis), possible pathologic fractures Chest film—enlarged mediastinal and hilar lymph nodes, bilateral reticular changes; congestive heart failure KUB/US—splenomegaly Organ infiltration—displacement or obstruction of GI or GU system	Multidrug chemotherapy Bone marrow transplant Antibiotics Blood transfusion
Lymphoma	Neoplasm of lymphoreticular system	Chest film—asymmetric, bilaterally enlarged mediastinal lymph nodes GI series—irregular and ulcerated polypoid mass (multiple ulcers or a huge single ulcer); thickening of rugal folds Skeletal radiograph—bone erosion of thoracolumbar spine with mottled pattern and sclerosis (ivory vertebra) CT—detects increased node size PET—metabolically active neoplasm	Hodgkin's lymphoma— multidrug chemotherapy and radiation therapy Non-Hodgkin's lymphoma—aggressive chemotherapy for diffuse disease; conservative chemotherapy for low-level disease Bone marrow transplant
Infectious mononucleosis	Viral disease of lymphoreticular system	Generalized lymphadenopathy and splenomegaly	Self-limited—supportive treatment, bed rest, and hydration

GI, Gastrointestinal; *GU,* genitourinary; *KUB,* kidney–ureter–bladder radiograph; *US,* ultrasound.

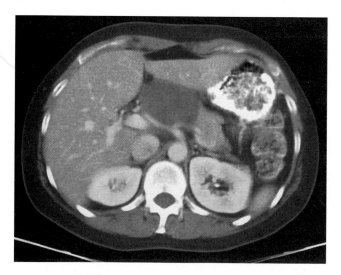

FIGURE 9-20 CT scan of patient with non-Hodgkin's lymphoma. The patient was diagnosed 8 months earlier with a pancreatic tumor measuring 4 × 6 × 4 cm. After chemotherapy, this scan shows a smaller tumor (3 × 5 × 3 cm) and no mass in the tail.

Treatment

Because infectious mononucleosis is a self-limited disease, the usual treatment includes supportive therapy, adequate bed rest, and hydration.

Diseases of Platelets (Bleeding Disorders)

Blood coagulation (clotting) is a complicated mechanism requiring platelets, calcium, and 12 coenzymes and proteins called **coagulation factors**. A deficiency in quantity or activity of any of these elements may lead to an inability to control hemorrhage or may even lead to spontaneous bleeding.

Hemophilia

Hemophilia is an inherited (by a sex-linked recessive gene) anomaly of blood coagulation that appears clinically only in males. Patients with this disease have a decreased or absent serum concentration of antihemophilic globulin (factor VIII) and suffer a lifelong tendency to spontaneous hemorrhage or severe bleeding from even minor cuts or injuries.

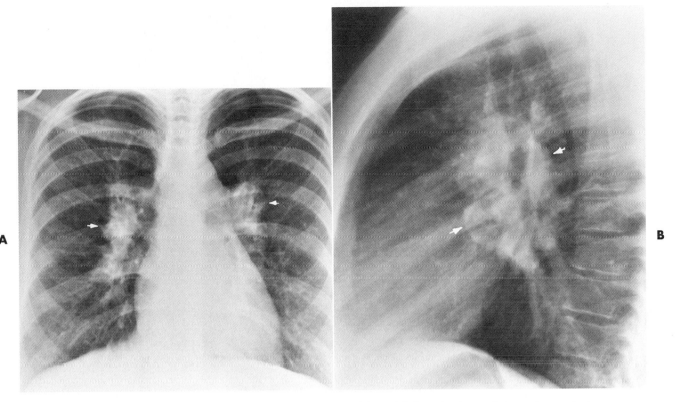

FIGURE **9-21** Infectious mononucleosis. Frontal **(A)** and lateral **(B)** projections of chest demonstrate pronounced enlargement of hilar lymph nodes bilaterally *(arrows).*

Radiographic Appearance

The major radiographic changes in hemophilia are complications of recurrent bleeding into the joints, most commonly involving the knees, elbows, and ankles. Initially the hemorrhage produces a generalized nonspecific soft tissue prominence of the distended joint. Deposition of iron pigment may produce areas of cloudy, increased density in the periarticular soft tissues. Although complete resorption of intraarticular blood may leave no residual change, subsequent episodes of bleeding result in synovial hypertrophy. In chronic disease, the hyperplastic synovium causes cartilage destruction and joint space narrowing and often leads to the development of multiple subchondral cysts of varying sizes in the immediate juxtaarticular bone (Figure 9-22, *A*). Destruction of articular cartilage and continued use of the damaged joint lead to subchondral sclerosis and collapse, extensive and bizarre spur formation, and often pronounced soft tissue calcification. Hemorrhage extending into the adjacent bony structures may cause extensive destruction (pseudotumor of hemophilia), which can mimic a malignant tumor (Figure 9-22, *B*).

Repeated joint hemorrhages lead to increased blood flow in the region of the epiphysis and growth plate. These structures may ossify prematurely, become abnormally large, or fuse prematurely with the metaphysis. The increased blood flow and atrophy of bone and muscle that may follow an episode of joint bleeding result in severe osteoporosis. Common signs suggestive of, though not pathognomonic for, hemophilia include widening and deepening of the intercondylar notch of the femur (Figure 9-23) and "squaring" of the inferior border of the patella. Asymmetric growth of the distal tibial epiphysis may result in "slanting" of the talotibial joint. Hemarthrosis can cause occlusion of epiphyseal vessels and result in avascular necrosis. This most commonly involves the femoral and radial heads, both of which have a totally intracapsular epiphysis and are therefore especially vulnerable to deprivation of their vascular supply from compression by a tense joint effusion.

As in the other bleeding disorders, submucosal bleeding into the wall of the gastrointestinal tract may develop in patients with hemophilia. This most commonly involves the small bowel and produces a short or long segment with regular thickening of folds. In the colon, bleeding may produce the thumbprint pattern of sharply defined, fingerlike, marginal indentations along the contours of the colon wall.

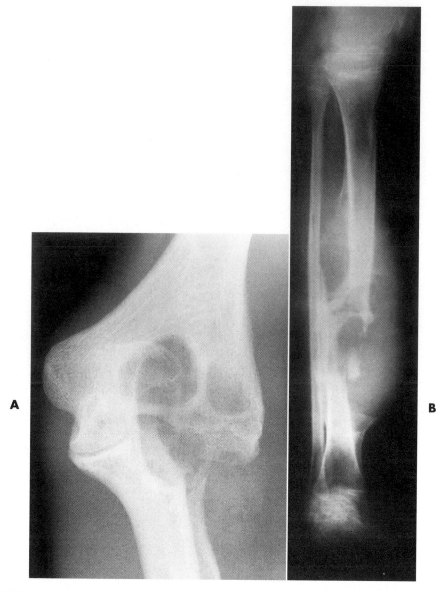

FIGURE 9-22 Hemophilia. **A,** Large subchondral cysts about the elbow. **B,** Destructive, expansile lesion of the lower tibial shaft.

Treatment
Hemophilia is usually treated with transfusions and factor VIII replacement.

Purpura (Thrombocytopenia)
Purpura refers to a deficiency in the number of platelets, and it results in spontaneous hemorrhages in the skin, mucous membranes of the mouth, and internal organs. The decreased number of platelets results from decreased production, increased destruction, or splenic sequestration of platelets. In the skin, purpura leads to the development of small, flat, red spots (petechiae) or larger hemorrhagic areas (ecchymoses).

Acute idiopathic thrombocytopenic purpura typically has the sudden onset of severe purpura 1 to 2 weeks after a sore throat or upper respiratory infection in an otherwise healthy child. In most patients, the disorder is self-limited and clears spontaneously within a few weeks. Unlike the acute form, chronic idiopathic thrombocytopenic purpura occurs primarily in young women and has an insidious onset with a relatively long history of easy bruising and menorrhagia. This condition is generally considered to be an autoimmune disorder because most patients have a circulating platelet autoantibody that develops without underlying disease or significant exposure to drugs.

Purpura can also be a complication of conditions that suppress the bone marrow (aplastic anemia) or infiltrate the bone marrow with tumor cells (leukemia, lymphoma, myeloma, metastases).

Radiographic Appearance

The radiographic changes caused by either acute or chronic idiopathic thrombocytopenic purpura primarily involve the gastrointestinal tract. Hemorrhage into the small bowel produces characteristic uniform, regular thickening of mucosal folds in the affected intestinal segment (Figure 9-24). Splenomegaly is commonly present; splenectomy is often required to remove this important site of platelet destruction and major source of synthesis of platelet antibodies.

Treatment

Blood platelet transfusions are being used to increase low platelet counts. Anti–human immunodeficiency virus (anti-HIV) drugs are effective in slowing or stopping the production of auto-antibodies that attack the platelets. Drug-induced thrombocytopenia responds well to discontinuing the offending drug. Virus-induced thrombocytopenia shows improvement following a cure of the infection.

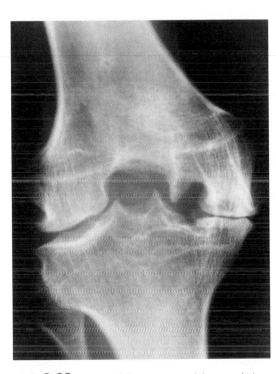

FIGURE 9-23 Hemophilia. Intercondylar notch is greatly widened, and coarse trabeculae, narrowing of joint space, and hypertrophic spurring can be seen.

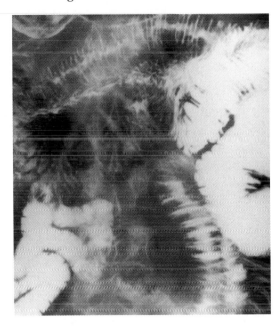

FIGURE 9-24 Chronic idiopathic thrombocytopenic purpura. Hemorrhage into the wall of the small bowel causes regular thickening of the mucosal folds.

SUMMARY of FINDINGS for Bleeding Disorders

disorder	location	radiographic appearance	treatment
Hemophilia	Anomaly of blood coagulation	Joint films—cloudy increased density in periarticular soft tissues Chronic—cartilage destruction with joint narrowing, multiple subchondral cysts; widening and deepening of intracondylar notch	Blood transfusion Factor VIII replacement
Purpura	Deficiency in number of platelets	Small bowel—uniform regular thickening of mucosal folds Splenomegaly	Self-limited—spontaneous recovery Drug-induced—discontinuation of drug Virus-induced—improves with cure of infection Splenectomy

REVIEW QUESTIONS

1. When diseases of the hematopoietic system result in demineralization of bone, the radiographer must be alert to the possibility of _____.
   A. patient infection　　C. pathologic fracture
   B. self-infection　　　D. syncope

2. Red blood cells are called _____.
   A. erythrocytes　　　C. thrombocytes
   B. leukocytes　　　　D. hemoglobin

3. Platelets are called _____.
   A. erythrocytes　　　C. thrombocytes
   B. leukocytes　　　　D. lymphocytes

4. White blood cells are called _____.
   A. erythrocytes　　　C. thrombocytes
   B. leukocytes　　　　D. paracytes

5. The smallest blood cells, platelets, are essential for what process?
   A. immunity　　　　C. carrying oxygen
   B. clotting　　　　D. fighting infection

6. Lymphocytes play a major role in the _____ system.
   A. endocrine　　　　C. immune
   B. hematopoietic　　D. metabolic

7. Which term refers to a decrease in the amount of oxygen-carrying hemoglobin in the blood?
   A. spherocytosis　　C. anemia
   B. thalassemia　　　D. hematopoiesis

8. What type of anemia can cause painful bone infarcts and is generally confined to the black race?
   A. spherocytosis　　C. sickle cell
   B. thalassemia　　　D. *Salmonella*

9. A hematologic disorder characterized by an increase in the production of erythrocytes, granulocytes, and platelets is _____.
   A. polycythemia vera　　C. sickle cell anemia
   B. erythrocytosis　　　D. hemolytic anemia

10. A cancerous disease of the hematopoietic system characterized by an increase in white blood cells is _____.
    A. anemia　　　　　C. leukemia
    B. thrombocytopenia　D. hemophilia

11. What is the name of an inherited anomaly of blood coagulation?
    A. sickle cell anemia　C. leukemia
    B. hemophilia　　　　D. leukocytosis

12. What pathologic condition refers to a deficiency in the number of platelets resulting in spontaneous hemorrhages in the skin, internal organs, and mucous membranes of the mouth?
    A. hemophilia　　　C. leukemia
    B. purpura　　　　D. sickle cell anemia

BIBLIOGRAPHY

Estrada DA: Lymphoma, non-Hodgkin's, *eMedicine Journal* 2:9, 2001. http://www.emedicine.com/med/tomic1363.htm.

Korsten J et al: Extramedullary hematopoiesis in patients with thalassemia anemia, *Radiology* 95:257-264, 1970.

Pear BL: Skeletal manifestations of the lymphomas and leukemias, *Semin Roentgenol* 9:229-240, 1974.

Reynolds J: Radiologic manifestations of sickle cell hemoglobulinopathy, *JAMA* 238:247-250, 1977.

Stoker DJ, Murray RO: Skeletal changes in hemophilia and other bleeding disorders, *Semin Roentgenol* 9:185-193, 1974.

ENDOCRINE *System*

Chapter Outline

Key Terms

acromegaly
androgens
follicular carcinoma
gigantism
glucocorticoids
hyperactive
hyperglycemia
hypoactive
medullary carcinoma
mineralocorticoids
papillary carcinoma
parathormone
primary hyperparathyroidism
primary hypoparathyroidism
secondary hyperparathyroidism
tertiary hyperparathyroidism
thyroxine

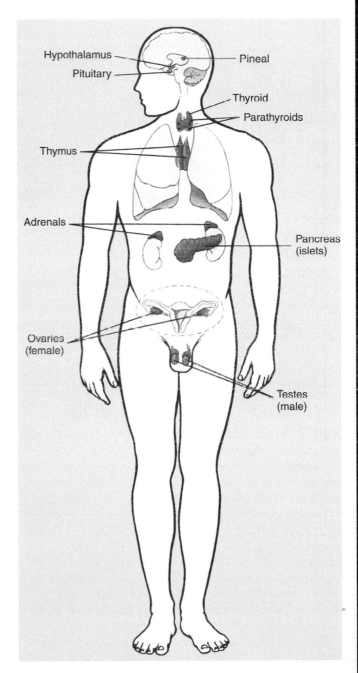

Prerequisite Knowledge

The student should have a basic knowledge of the anatomy and physiology of the endocrine system. In addition, proper learning and understanding of the material will be facilitated if the student has some clinical experience in general radiography and image evaluation, including a

RADIOGRAPHER *Notes*

Imaging modalities are used to diagnose both the underlying endocrine disorder and the secondary changes that may occur in various areas of the body. Disorders of the endocrine glands themselves are usually evaluated by ultrasound, computed tomography (CT), magnetic resonance imaging (MRI), and radionuclide scanning. Secondary pathologic manifestations elsewhere in the body are generally evaluated on plain radiographs, for which the routine exposure techniques may have to be altered (see the Box in Chapter 1 labeled Relative Attenuation of X-Rays in Advanced Stages of Diseases). For example, Cushing's syndrome causes extensive osteoporosis, which requires a decrease in kilovolts-peak for adequate visualization of the demineralized bones. It should also be noted that patients with this condition can easily sustain pathologic fractures and thus should always be handled with caution.

concept of the newer imaging modalities used to study the various body systems affected by endocrine abnormalities. These modalities include ultrasound, CT, MRI, and positron emission tomography (PET).

Goals

To acquaint the student radiographer with the pathophysiology and imaging manifestations of all of the common and some of the unusual disorders of the endocrine system.

Objectives

After reading this chapter, the reader will be able to:
1. Define all key terms in this chapter
2. Describe the physiology of the endocrine system
3. Identify anatomic structures on both diagrams and images of the endocrine system
4. Differentiate the various pathologic conditions affecting the endocrine system and their radiographic manifestations

Physiology of the Endocrine System

The endocrine system is a biochemical communication network through which several small glands control a broad range of vital body activities. The endocrine glands secrete chemical messengers called hormones, which circulate in the blood and may affect a single target organ or the entire body. Hormones may be proteins (growth hormone), steroids (cortisone), peptides (antidiuretic hormone [ADH]), amino acids (thyroxine), or amines (epinephrine). They range from small to large molecules and have chemical structures of various complexities.

The major endocrine glands are the pituitary, adrenal, thyroid, and parathyroid glands. Inadequate (hypoactive) or excess (hyperactive) production of hormones from these endocrine glands can give rise to a wide variety of clinical symptoms and radiographic abnormalities.

Because hormones are powerful chemicals, it is essential that their circulating levels be carefully controlled. One type of control is called the negative feedback mechanism. In this system, an adequate level of a hormone in the blood automatically stops the release of additional hormone (somewhat like a thermostat). As the blood level of the hormone decreases, the gland is stimulated to secrete more of it. Another control mechanism is the production of two different hormones whose actions are opposite to each other. For example, insulin is secreted by the pancreas when the blood glucose level rises. When the blood glucose level falls below normal, a second hormone, glucagon, is secreted by the pancreas to raise the blood glucose level. Thus these two hormones are balanced so that a proper blood glucose level is continually maintained.

Adrenal Glands

Physiology of the Adrenal Glands

The adrenal glands, which are situated at the top of each kidney, consist of an outer cortex and an inner medulla. The adrenal cortex secretes several different types of steroid hormones, which can be divided into three general groups. The **mineralocorticoids** (primarily aldosterone) regulate salt and water balance by controlling sodium retention and potassium excretion by the kidneys. The production of aldosterone is primarily regulated by the secretion of renin from specialized cells (the juxtaglomerular apparatus) in the kidney. Reduced blood volume (as in hemorrhage) causes low blood pressure, which is detected by the juxtaglomerular apparatus and eventually results in increased aldosterone secretion from the adrenal cortex.

Glucocorticoids (especially cortisone) regulate carbohydrate metabolism and are under the regulation of adrenocorticotropic hormone (ACTH) from the anterior pituitary gland. Cortisone also depresses the inflammatory response to almost all forms of injury, thus leading to its use in the treatment of trauma, rheumatoid arthritis, bursitis, and asthma, and as an immunosuppressive agent to help limit rejection after organ transplantation.

Androgens are sex hormones that tend to masculinize the body, to retain amino acids, and to enhance protein synthesis. It is these hormones that are used both illegally and unwisely by athletes in an attempt to increase body strength.

The adrenal medulla secretes epinephrine (adrenaline) and norepinephrine. These fight-or-flight hormones are secreted in stress situations when additional energy and strength are needed. Epinephrine stimulates heart activity, raises blood pressure, and increases the level of blood glucose. By constricting some blood vessels and dilating others, epinephrine shunts blood to active muscles where oxygen and nutrients are urgently needed.

Diseases of the Adrenal Cortex

Cushing's Syndrome

The excess production of glucocorticoid hormones in Cushing's syndrome may be attributable to generalized bilateral hyperplasia of the adrenal cortex, or it may be a result of a functioning adrenal or even nonadrenal tumor. It can also be the result of the exogenous administration of cortisone. Excess secretion of glucocorticoid hormones mobilizes lipids and increases their level in the blood. This produces a characteristic obesity that is confined to the trunk of the body and is associated with a round, moon-shaped face and a pathognomonic fat pad that forms behind the shoulders (buffalo hump). Retention of salt and water results in hypertension.

Radiographic Appearance

Generalized enlargement of the adrenal glands is best demonstrated by CT, which shows thickening of the wings of the adrenal gland, which appear to have a stellate or Y-shaped configuration in cross section. Ultrasound can also show diffuse adrenal gland enlargement.

Benign and malignant tumors of the adrenal cortex are less common causes of Cushing's syndrome than is nontumorous adrenal hyperfunction. As a general rule, the larger the adrenocortical tumor and the more abrupt the onset of clinical symptoms and signs, the more likely the tumor is to be malignant (Figure 10-1). However, the differentiation between

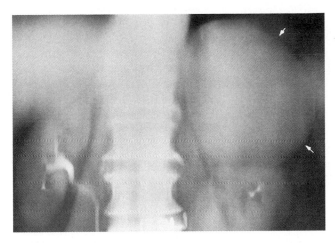

FIGURE **10-1** Cushing's syndrome caused by large adrenal adenoma. Nephrotomogram demonstrates huge suprarenal mass *(arrows)* causing indentation and downward displacement of left kidney.

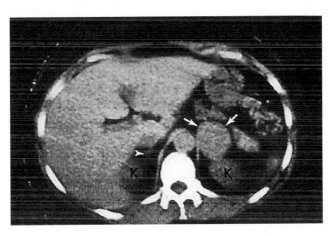

FIGURE **10-2** Cushing's syndrome caused by functioning cortical adenoma. A 4-cm mass in the left adrenal gland *(arrows)* is seen posterior to the tail of the pancreas and anterior to the kidney *(K)*. Arrowhead points to the normal right adrenal gland.

adenoma and carcinoma may be impossible at the time of histologic examination, and the nature of the tumor may have to be defined by the clinical course alone. Both CT and ultrasound can demonstrate an adrenal tumor (Figure 10-2), but CT is often more valuable because the abundance of retroperitoneal fat may prevent an optimal ultrasound examination. Adrenal venography has been widely used to demonstrate adrenal masses, and it also permits the aspiration of blood samples for assessment of the level of adrenal hormones.

Cushing's syndrome produces radiographic changes in multiple systems. Diffuse osteoporosis causes generalized skeletal demineralization, which may lead to the collapse of vertebral bodies, spontaneous fractures, and aseptic necrosis of the head of the femur or humerus. Widening of the mediastinum as a result of excessive fat deposition sometimes develops in Cushing's syndrome and can be confirmed by CT. Hypercalciuria caused by elevated steroid levels can lead to renal calculi and nephrocalcinosis.

Imaging of the sella turcica by conventional tomography or CT is important in the routine assessment of the patient with Cushing's syndrome. Most patients with nontumorous adrenal hyperfunction are found at surgery to have an intrasellar lesion. It is important to emphasize, however, that small pituitary microadenomas may be present in asymptomatic patients. The modality of choice to detect a functioning microadenoma causing adrenal hyperplasia is contrast-enhanced MRI. After adrenal surgery, a pituitary adenoma develops in up to one third of the patients and produces progressive sellar enlargement. For this reason, yearly follow-up sellar tomograms may be indicated after adrenalectomy.

Nonpituitary tumors producing ACTH may cause adrenal hyperfunction and Cushing's syndrome. The most common sites of origin are the lung, thymus, and pancreas; about half of these tumors can be demonstrated on chest radiographs. Octreotide scintigraphy (a nuclear medicine exam) detects ectopic ACTH tumors based on increased uptake of tumor cell surface receptors for somatostatin.

Treatment

Treatment for Cushing's syndrome depends on the cause of the excess production of glucocorticoid hormones. Surgical resection is the treatment of choice to eliminate the excessive hormone production. Medical suppression of abnormal endocrine stimulation and radiation therapy directed to the hyperfunctioning tumor are alternatives if the tumor is inoperable.

Aldosteronism

An overproduction of mineralocorticoid hormones produced by the most superficial layer of the adrenal cortex causes retention of sodium and water and abnormal loss of potassium in the urine. This results in hypertension, muscular weakness or paralysis, and excessive thirst (polydipsia). Aldosteronism may be attributable to an adrenocortical adenoma (Conn's syndrome) or to bilateral hyperplasia of the superficial cortical layer. Aldosteronism may also be the result of renin-secreting tumors, renal artery stenosis, malignant hypertension, and bilateral chronic renal disease. The biochemical assay is the basis for diagnosing aldosteronism, and CT or MR images are used for adrenal identification.

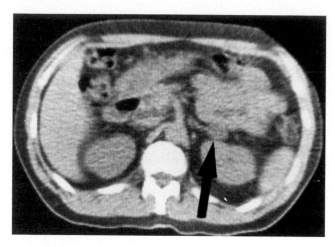

FIGURE 10-3 Aldosteronoma. Note the small mass *(arrow)* anterior to the left kidney.

Radiographic Appearance

The role of diagnostic imaging is to demonstrate the location of adenomas that may otherwise be difficult to detect during exploratory surgery.

Noncontrast CT, the most widely used imaging modality, demonstrates the small adrenocortical adenoma as a contour abnormality of the gland (Figure 10-3). Using CT or MRI, the adrenal gland can be measured quite accurately; the normal adrenal measures 3 to 6 mm thick, 4 to 6 mm long, and 2 to 3 cm wide. However, the scan may not demonstrate any abnormal findings. With newer scanners, specificity has increased to 75%, and tumors larger than 1 cm can be consistently identified. Adenomas may be isointense or hypointense relative to the liver on T1-weighted MR images. On T2-weighted images, they have slight hyperintensity. Chemical-shift imaging can aid in identifying and characterizing the adrenal mass. In adenomas smaller than 1 cm, nuclear medicine studies using iodine-131 attached with a cholesterol binder can differentiate a normal gland from hyperplasia based on the time course of radionuclide uptake. Early uptake (less than 5 days) in both adrenal glands indicates hyperplasia, whereas unilateral early uptake implies an adrenal adenoma. Adrenal venography with biochemical assay of a sample of adrenal blood is another important technique for localizing aldosteronomas and determining primary versus secondary hyperaldosteronism.

Treatment

Hypertension and other clinical manifestations of aldosteronism can be cured by the resection of an adenoma, but are little affected by the removal of both adrenal glands in the patient with bilateral hyperplasia. Medical antihypertensive agents, especially long-acting calcium channel blockers, are available if the adenoma is inoperable.

Adrenogenital Syndrome

The adrenogenital syndrome (adrenal virilism) is caused by the excessive secretion of androgenically active substances by the adrenal gland. In the congenital form, a specific enzyme deficiency that prevents the formation of androgenic hormones causes continuous ACTH stimulation and bilateral hyperplasia. The elevated levels of androgens result in accelerated skeletal maturation along with premature epiphyseal fusion, which may lead to dwarfism.

In women the tumor causes masculinization, with the development of hair on the face (hirsutism). The breasts diminish, the clitoris enlarges, and ovulation and menstruation cease.

Radiographic Appearance

Most cases of acquired adrenogenital syndrome are caused by adrenocortical tumors, which can be detected by CT (Figure 10-4), ultrasound, or adrenal venography. CT is currently the imaging modality of choice.

Treatment

Surgical resection of a hyperfunctioning tumor with replacement therapy allows normal development. Medical suppression of abnormal stimuli prevents the excessive release of ACTH, allowing female features to develop normally. If not treated, a masculinized woman may require reconstructive surgery.

Hypoadrenalism

The clinical manifestations of adrenal insufficiency vary from those of a chronic insidious disorder (easy fatigability, anorexia, weakness, weight loss, and increased melanin pigmentation) to those of an acute collapse with hypotension, rapid pulse, vomiting, and diarrhea.

The most common cause of adrenal insufficiency is the excessive administration of steroids. Primary adrenocortical insufficiency (Addison's disease) results from progressive cortical destruction, which must involve more than 90% of the glands before clinical signs of adrenal insufficiency appear. In the past, Addison's disease was usually attributed to tuberculosis; at present most cases reflect idiopathic atrophy, probably on an autoimmune basis. In areas where the disease is endemic, histoplasmosis is an occasional cause of adrenal insufficiency.

Radiographic Appearance

Acute inflammatory disease causes generalized enlargement of the adrenal glands, which can be demonstrated by a variety of imaging techniques (Figure 10-5). MRI can differentiate adrenal masses better than CT, but MRI cannot distinguish a tumor from an inflammatory process. Other radiographic findings occasionally seen in patients with adrenal insufficiency include a small heart and calcification of the cartilage of the ear.

Treatment

Corticosteroids produce a fast recovery and must be administered regularly for the patient's survival. Morbidity and mortality are high without treatment.

Adrenal Carcinoma

About half of adrenal carcinomas are functioning tumors that cause Cushing's syndrome, virilization, feminization, or aldosteronism. The tumors grow rapidly and are usually large necrotic masses at the time of clinical presentation.

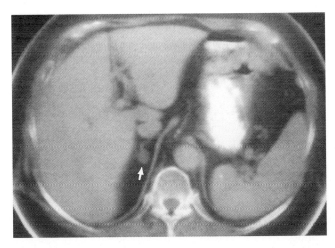

FIGURE 10-4 Adrenogenital syndrome caused by a functioning adrenocortical tumor *(arrow)*.

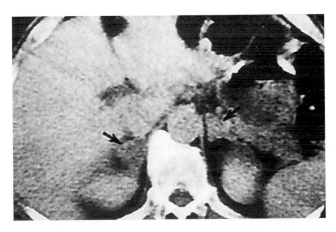

FIGURE 10-5 Adrenocortical insufficiency caused by disseminated histoplasmosis. CT scan demonstrates bilateral adrenal enlargement *(arrows)*.

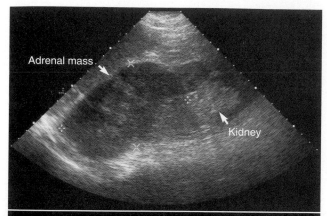

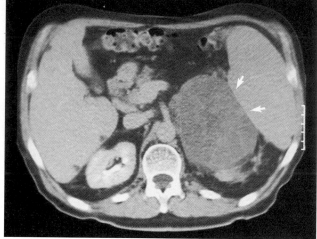

FIGURE 10-6 Adrenal carcinoma. **A,** Ultrasound identifies a heterogeneous lobulated mass (12 × 7 × 11 cm) involving the upper pole of the left kidney. **B,** CT scan 1 month later shows diffuse inhomogeneous enhancement with the appearance of some low-density areas suggesting necrosis.

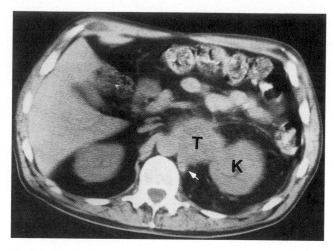

FIGURE 10-7 Adrenal carcinoma. Large soft tissue tumor *(T)* invades the anteromedial aspect of the left kidney *(K)* and the left crus of the diaphragm *(arrow)*.

Radiographic Appearance

Ultrasound demonstrates the tumor as a complex mass that may be difficult to separate from an upper pole renal tumor (Figure 10-6). CT demonstrates an adrenal carcinoma as a large unilateral mass with an irregular edge that often contains low-density areas resulting from central necrosis or prior hemorrhage (Figure 10-7) and high-density calcifications. On contrast-enhanced CT, the tumor enhancement is irregular and greatest on the periphery. For adrenal exams, spiral CT with 3- to 5-cm section reconstructions offers the best resolution and may identify tumors 1 cm or smaller.

Because lymphatic and hepatic metastases are common at the time of clinical presentation, CT scans at multiple abdominal levels are necessary to define the extent of the primary tumor and to detect metastases before surgical resection is attempted. Extension of the tumor into the renal vein and inferior vena cava can also be detected by CT, especially after the injection of intravenous contrast material, or by MRI (Figure 10-8). On MR scans, the higher signal intensity of the tumor in comparison with the liver on T2-weighted images (lower signal on T1-weighted images) may distinguish adrenal carcinoma from nonfunctioning adenomas and pheochromocytomas.

Treatment

The treatment of choice is surgical resection by open laparotomy or laparoscopy. Chemotherapy using mitotane, an adrenocortical cytotoxin and adrenal inhibitor, may improve symptoms if resection is not an option.

Metastases to the Adrenal Gland

The adrenal gland is one of the most common sites of metastatic disease. The primary tumors that most frequently metastasize to the adrenal gland are carcinomas of the lung, breast, kidney, ovary, and gastrointestinal tract, and melanomas.

Radiographic Appearance

Metastatic enlargement of an adrenal gland can cause downward displacement of the kidney with flattening of the upper pole. Ultrasound and CT demonstrate adrenal metastases as solid, soft tissue masses that vary considerably in size and are frequently bilateral (Figure 10-9). However, the ultrasound (hypoechoic lesions) and CT patterns are indistinguishable from those of primary malignancies of the gland. Therefore when a known primary tumor exists elsewhere, it is usually assumed that an adrenal mass is metastatic.

On MR imaging, metastases typically have higher signal intensity on T2-weighted images than do benign

SUMMARY
FINDINGS *for* Diseases of the Adrenal Cortex

disorder	location	radiographic appearance	treatment
Cushing's syndrome	Bilateral adrenal hyperplasia, cortical	CT (noncontrast)—thickening of adrenal wings, which appear stellate or in a Y-shape US—diffuse adrenal gland enlargement	Surgical resection for erosive hormone production Medical suppression of endocrine stimulation if tumor is inoperable Radiation therapy if tumor is inoperable
	Adrenal tumor	CT—to evaluate sella turcica MRI—detects functioning pituitary microadenoma causing adrenal hyperplasia	
Aldosteronism	Overproduction of mineralocorticoid hormones	CT—locates small adrenocortical adenoma as a contour abnormality of the gland MRI—hypointense or isointense to liver on T1-weighted images; T2-weighted images demonstrate a hyperintense lesion NM—unilateral early uptake of the affected gland Venography (adrenal)—to acquire material for biochemical assay	Resection of altered adrenal gland Therapeutic option: antihypertensive drugs
Adrenogenital syndrome	Excessive secretion of androgenically active substances	CT/US—demonstrates underlying adrenal neoplasm or hyperplasia Venography (adrenal)—to acquire material for biochemical assay	Surgical resection Medical suppression Reconstructive surgery if necessary
Hypoadrenalism	Adrenal insufficiency	CT—enlarged adrenal glands or atrophic adrenals	Corticosteroids Morbidity and mortality high without treatment
Adrenal carcinoma	Tumor of adrenal cortex	US—complex tabulated mass above upper pole of kidney; homogeneous when small; heterogeneous when large, with central necrosis or hemorrhage CT—irregular mass containing low-density areas often with calcifications; contrast enhancing periphery; metastasis also detected MRI—higher signal intensity than liver on T2-weighted images	Surgical resection Chemotherapy
Adrenal metastases	Adrenal gland	US/CT—demonstrates type of mass and whether bilateral MRI—high signal intensity on T2-weighted images; greater contrast enhancement with metastases than benign adenoma Chemical-shift imaging—lipid-laden adenoma produces low signal intensity on an out-of-phase image US/CT—guided biopsy	Adrenalectomy with replacement therapy

US, Ultrasound.

adenomas, and they also demonstrate increased contrast enhancement on T1-weighted, fat-suppressed images. In-phase and out-of-phase pulse sequences (also known as chemical shift imaging) are highly accurate for distinguishing between adrenal adenomas and metastases. Lipid-laden adenomas show low signal intensity on out-of-phase images and intermediate to high signal intensity on in-phase images.

If necessary, a needle biopsy using ultrasound or CT guidance may be of value to determine whether the adrenal lesion is primary or metastatic.

Treatment
The most common form of treatment is an adrenalectomy followed by replacement therapy; however, as metastasis has occurred, the prognosis is unfavorable.

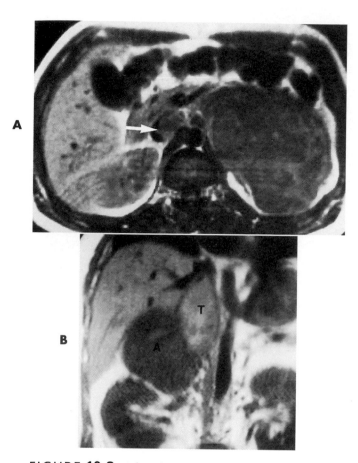

FIGURE 10-8 Adrenal carcinoma. **A,** Axial MR scan demonstrates a large left adrenal tumor invading the left renal vein and inferior vena cava *(arrow).* **B,** In another patient, a coronal MR scan shows an adrenal mass *(A)* above the kidney with a tumor thrombus of slightly higher signal intensity filling the inferior vena cava *(T).*

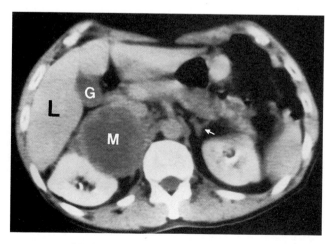

FIGURE 10-9 Adrenal metastases. Note huge irregular low-attenuation mass *(M)* representing adrenal metastasis from oat cell carcinoma of the lung. The left adrenal gland *(arrow)* is normal. *G,* Gallbladder; *L,* liver.

Diseases of the Adrenal Medulla

Pheochromocytoma

A pheochromocytoma is a tumor that most commonly arises in the adrenal medulla and produces an excess of vasopressor substances (epinephrine and norepinephrine), which can cause an uncommon but curable form of hypertension. About 10% of pheochromocytomas are extraadrenal in origin. About 10% of patients have bilateral tumors, and a similar percentage of pheochromocytomas are malignant.

Because in almost all patients the diagnosis of a pheochromocytoma can be made with biochemical tests, radiographic imaging serves as a confirmatory study and as a means of localizing the tumor. Excretory urography, even with nephrotomography, may be of limited value because the kidney is often not displaced even when the adrenal pheochromocytoma is large.

Radiographic Appearance

CT and ultrasound (Figure 10-10) are very useful in the localization of pheochromocytomas. The cross-sectional images not only detail the extent of the adrenal lesion, but also define the status of adjacent structures and can demonstrate bilateral or multiple pheochromocytomas, extraadrenal tumors, and metastases. Pheochromocytomas generally appear as round, oval, or pear-shaped masses, often greater than 3 cm, that are slightly less echogenic than liver and kidney parenchyma on ultrasound and have an attenuation value less than these organs on CT (Figure 10-11). Necrosis, hemorrhage, and fluid levels are common findings in larger lesions. Most extraadrenal pheochromocytomas arise in the abdomen (Figure 10-12); a few are found in the chest or neck. The tumor may be located anywhere along the sympathetic nervous system, in the organ of Zuckerkandl, and in chemoreceptor tissues such as the carotid body or the glomus jugulare, in the wall of the urinary bladder, or even in the kidney or ureter. Masses may displace the ureter or kidney or may appear as filling defects in the bladder.

MRI can demonstrate the relationship of the tumor to surrounding structures in the coronal plane (Figure 10-13) and has a higher sensitivity than CT. On T2-weighted spin-echo images, the extreme hyperintensity of the tumor (because of its water content) makes it stand out from the surrounding structures. When CT and MRI are inconclusive, a radionuclide scan using metaiodobenzylguanidine is highly sensitive for localizing ectopic pheochromocytomas, but this agent is not readily available.

In patients with pheochromocytomas, the arterial injection of contrast material causes a sharp elevation

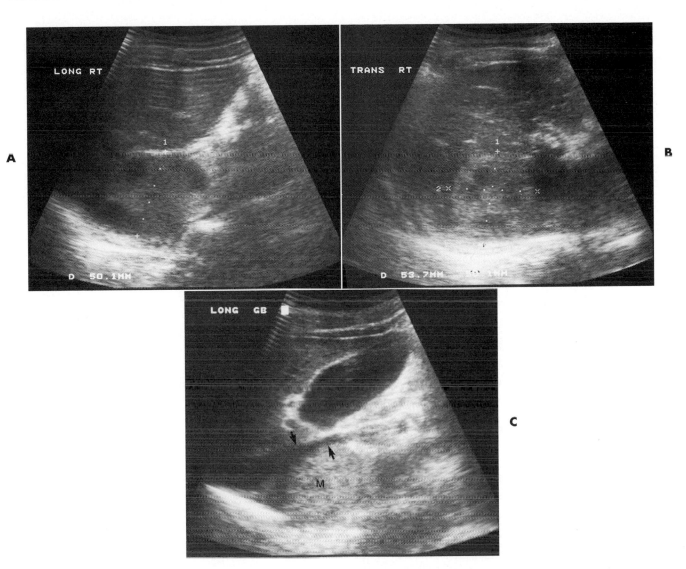

FIGURE 10-10 Pheochromocytoma. Longitudinal **(A)** and transverse **(B)** ultrasound images show a cystic and necrotic mass superior to the right kidney (note measuring markers). **C,** The mass *(M)* elevates the inferior vena cava *(arrows)*. The patient's history of increased heart rate (up to 200 beats per minute) and elevated blood pressure are consistent with a diagnosis of pheochromocytoma.

in blood pressure, which must be controlled by α-adrenergic blocking agents. Therefore arteriography is hazardous in these patients.

Treatment

Surgical removal of the tumor results in stabilizing the blood pressure and curing the hypertension. Most tumors are benign and well encapsulated, which makes removal successful.

Neuroblastoma

Neuroblastoma, a tumor of adrenal medullary origin, is the second most common malignancy in children. About 10% of these tumors arise outside the adrenal gland, primarily in sympathetic ganglia in the neck,

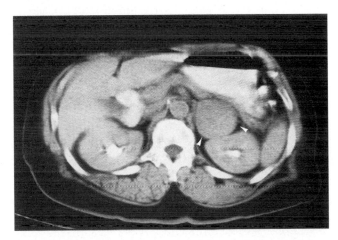

FIGURE 10-11 Pheochromocytoma. Large pear-shaped mass *(arrows)* is seen anterior to left kidney.

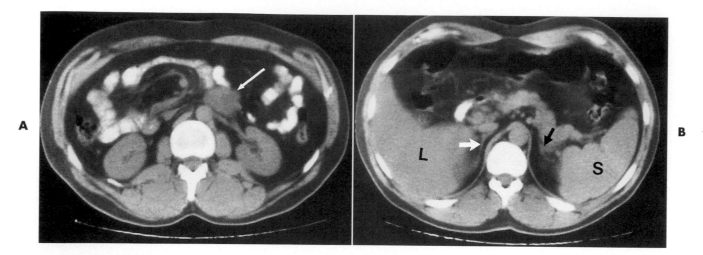

FIGURE 10-12 Ectopic pheochromocytoma. **A,** Soft tissue mass *(arrow)* is seen adjacent to the aorta and in front of the left renal vein. **B,** CT scan taken at a higher level demonstrates that both right and left adrenal glands are normal *(arrows)*. *L,* Liver; *S,* spleen.

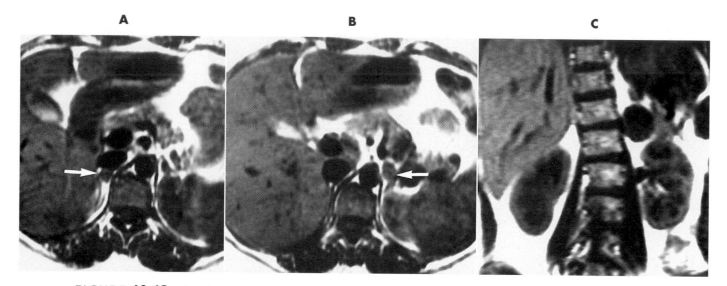

FIGURE 10-13 Pheochromocytoma. Axial MR scans (**A** and **B**) at two levels demonstrate bilateral low-intensity lesions *(arrows)*. Coronal MR scan (**C**) in a different patient shows a left suprarenal mass.

chest, abdomen, or pelvis. The tumor is highly malignant and tends to attain great size before detection.

Radiographic Appearance

Calcification is common in neuroblastoma (occurring in about 50% of cases) in contrast to the relatively infrequent calcification in Wilms' tumor, from which neuroblastoma must be differentiated. Calcification in a neuroblastoma has a fine granular or stippled appearance (Figure 10-14, *A*). Occasionally, there may be a single mass of amorphous calcification. Calcification can also develop in metastases of neuroblastoma in paravertebral lymph nodes and liver.

Excretory urography usually demonstrates downward and lateral renal displacement by the tumor mass (Figure 10-15). Neuroblastoma tends to cause the entire kidney and its collecting system to be displaced as a unit, unlike Wilms' tumor, which has an intrarenal origin and thus tends to distort and widen the pelvicalyceal system.

Because of its nonionizing character, ultrasound is a superb modality for evaluating abdominal masses in children. A neuroblastoma appears as a solid or semisolid mass that is separate from the kidney. It appears as a poorly defined heterogenic mass, unlike the well-defined and relatively homogeneous Wilms'

SUMMARY *of* FINDINGS *for* Diseases of the Adrenal Medulla

disorder	location	radiographic appearance	treatment
Pheochromocytoma	Adrenal medulla—excessive epinephrine and norepinephrine	CT—round, oval, or pear-shaped mass with lower attenuation than liver or kidney parenchyma; larger lesions may present with necrosis; hemorrhage and fluid levels may be apparent US—mass shows lower echogenicity than normal liver and kidney parenchyma MRI—T2-weighted spin-echo hyperintense signal NM metaiodobenzylguanidine scan—supersensitive for localizing lesions ectopic	Surgical resection
Neuroblastoma	Adrenal medullary origin	Radiograph—calcification of tumor; destructive metastatic bone lesions IVU—inferior and lateral kidney displacement US—solid to semisolid mass separate from kidney; poorly defined, heterogeneous mass with irregular hyperechoic areas CT—heterogeneous and lobulated appearance MRI—T1-weighted lesions are hypointense; with enhancement the T1 signal becomes hyperintense	Combination treatment: surgical resection, chemotherapy, and radiation therapy

IVU, Intravenous urography; *NM*, nuclear medicine; *US*, ultrasound.

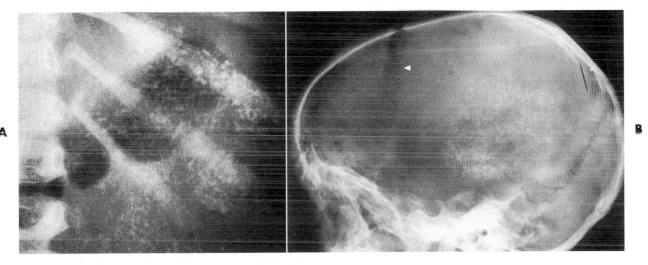

FIGURE 10-14 Neuroblastoma metastatic to bone. **A,** Plain film of the upper abdomen shows diffuse granular calcification within a large primary tumor. **B,** Lateral projection of the skull shows similar calcified deposits within a metastatic lesion in the calvaria. Note sutural widening *(arrowhead)* consistent with increased intracranial pressure.

tumor. The tumor is often diffusely hyperechogenic, probably because of necrosis, calcification, and hemorrhage. On contrast-enhanced CT, necrosis and hemorrhage cause the tumor to appear heterogeneous and often lobulated. Because CT can demonstrate evidence of tumor spread to lymph nodes and the sympathetic chain, widening of the paravertebral stripe (also seen on plain films) (Figure 10-16), and metastases to the liver and chest, it has become the most commonly used imaging study to diagnose neuroblastomas. This modality is also used to assess the response to treatment. MRI, which like ultrasound does not use ionizing radiation, may offer a safer approach to demonstrating characteristics typical

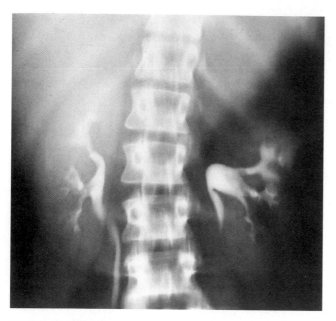

FIGURE **10-15** Neuroblastoma. Nephrotomogram demonstrates downward and lateral displacement of the upper pole of the left kidney.

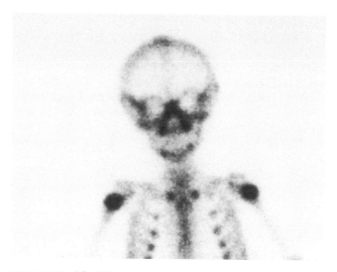

FIGURE **10-17** Neuroblastoma. Bone scan performed in a 1-year-old baby boy with left adrenal neuroblastoma to evaluate for osseous involvement. Temporal bones and orbital zygomatic region demonstrate increased uptake appearing as "raccoon eyes."

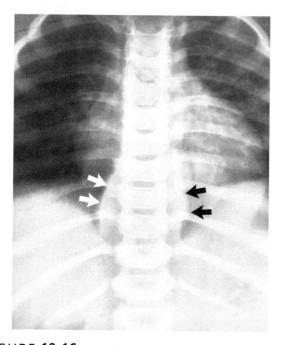

FIGURE **10-16** Neuroblastoma. Bilateral widening of the paravertebral stripes *(arrows)* represents metastatic deposits.

of tumor tissue. Neuroblastomas usually produce a hypointense signal on T1-weighted images and are hyperintense on T2-weighted images. On contrast-enhanced T1-weighted images, hemorrhage appears as a hyperintense signal.

Metastases to bone, liver, and lungs are common in neuroblastoma. Metastases to the skull typically cause spreading of cranial sutures because of plaques

of tumor tissue growing along the surface of the brain (Figure 10-17). Bone destruction leads to a granular pattern of osteoporosis that is often associated with thin, whiskerlike calcifications coursing outward and inward from the tables of the skull (see Figure 10-14, *B*). Metastases in long tubular bones are often multiple and relatively symmetric and present a permeative destructive pattern. On T2-weighted MR images, bone metastases appear as hyperintense (bright) and heterogeneous signals.

Neuroblastomas arising in the chest appear as posterior mediastinal masses. Metastases to the chest most commonly cause asymmetric enlargement of mediastinal nodes; metastases to the pulmonary parenchyma are infrequent.

Treatment

Combining surgery, multiple-agent chemotherapy, and radiation therapy has dramatically improved the prognosis to about a 90% cure rate. Infants tend to have a more favorable outcome when chemotherapy and surgery are the combined treatment.

Pituitary Gland

Physiology of the Pituitary Gland

The pituitary gland is often called the master gland because the many hormones it secretes control the level of most glandular activity throughout the body. The hormone secretion of the pituitary gland itself is controlled by the hypothalamus.

The pituitary is a tiny gland, about the size of a pea, that is suspended from the base of the brain by a slender stalk (infundibulum) and sits in the bony depression of the sella turcica. It is divided into anterior and posterior portions, each of which secretes different hormones.

The anterior lobe of the pituitary gland secretes growth hormone, thyroid-stimulating hormone (TSH), ACTH, and a group of hormones that affect the sex organs, or gonads. These gonadotropins include follicle-stimulating hormone (FSH) and luteinizing hormone (LH), which regulate the menstrual cycle and secretion of male and female sex hormones, and prolactin, which stimulates the production of milk during pregnancy and after delivery.

Growth hormone affects all parts of the body by promoting the growth and development of the tissues. Before puberty, it stimulates the growth of long bones (increasing the child's height) and the size of such organs as the liver, heart, and kidneys. After adolescence, growth hormone is secreted in lesser amounts, but continues to function in promoting tissue replacement and repair. TSH controls the secretion of thyroid hormone, which regulates the body's metabolism (production and use of energy). ACTH controls the level of activity of the adrenal cortex.

The posterior lobe of the pituitary gland (neurohypophysis) produces two hormones: vasopressin (antidiuretic hormone) and oxytocin. ADH increases the rate of reabsorption of water and electrolytes by the renal tubules, thus decreasing the output of urine and protecting the individual from excessive water loss. Oxytocin causes contraction of smooth muscle, especially in the uterus, and thus strengthens contractions during labor and helps to prevent hemorrhage after delivery.

Diseases of the Pituitary Gland

Hyperpituitarism

Hyperpituitarism results from an excess of growth hormone produced by a tumor (see Figures 8-18 and 8-19) or generalized hyperplasia of the anterior lobe of the pituitary gland. The development of this condition before enchondral bone growth has ceased results in **gigantism;** hyperpituitarism beginning after bone growth has stopped produces **acromegaly.**

Generalized overgrowth of all the body tissues is the underlying abnormality in acromegaly. Although the long bones can no longer grow because the epiphyses are closed, the bones of the hands, feet, and face enlarge, and there is excessive growth of soft tissues. Proliferation of cartilage may cause joint space widening, especially of the metacarpophalangeal and hip joints. The slight increase in length of each of the

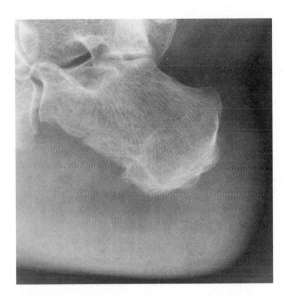

FIGURE 10-18 Acromegaly. Prominent thickening of the heel pad measuring 32 mm, which is highly suggestive of acromegaly.

seven articular cartilages for each digit leads to perceptible lengthening of the fingers. Overgrowth of the tips of the distal phalanges produces thick bony tufts with pointed lateral margins. The associated hypertrophy of the soft tissues produces the characteristic square, spade-shaped hand of acromegaly. Degenerative changes develop early and are associated with prominent hypertrophic spurring. Unlike typical osteoarthritis, acromegaly results in joint spaces that remain normal or are even widened.

Radiographic Appearance

Thickening of the heel pads (the soft tissue inferior to the plantar aspect of the calcaneus) to greater than 23 mm is highly suggestive of acromegaly (Figure 10-18). However, a similar appearance may also be seen in patients with obesity, myxedema, or generalized edema.

The bones of the skull become thickened and have increased density, often with obliteration of the diploic space. This bone thickening is especially prominent in the frontal and occipital regions, leading to characteristic frontal bossing and enlargement of the occipital protuberance (Figure 10-19). The paranasal sinuses (especially the frontal) become enlarged, and the mastoid processes are usually overpneumatized. Lengthening of the mandible and an increased mandibular angle produce prognathism, one of the typical clinical features of acromegaly. Thickening of the tongue may lead to slurred speech. Pituitary enlargement causes expansion and erosion of the sella turcica (Figure 10-20).

In the spine, hypertrophy of cartilage causes an increased width of the intervertebral disk spaces. An increase in the size of the vertebral bodies is best seen on lateral projections. Hypertrophy of soft tissues may produce an increased concavity of the posterior aspect of the vertebral bodies (scalloping) that is most prominent in the lumbar spine (Figure 10-21).

Extraskeletal manifestations of acromegaly include visceral enlargement, especially of the heart and kidney, enlargement of the tongue, and calcification of cartilage in the pinna of the ear.

Gigantism is manifested as an excessively large skeleton. If hypersecretion of growth hormone con-

tinues after epiphyseal closure, the soft tissue and bony changes of acromegaly are superimposed.

To diagnose the pituitary tumor causing the excessive growth, MRI provides the most exact definition of the sella turcica and tissue contained within. Its superior sensitivity and multiplanar capabilities make MRI the modality of choice. Thin-section coronal and sagittal T1-weighted spin-echo images permit clear distinction of the sphenoid sinus and carotid artery for surgical planning. After gadolinium injection, normal pituitary tissue enhances more than an adenoma, which appears as a hypoenhancing lesion.

Treatment

Surgical resection of the tumor remains the treatment of choice. Even with treatment, any changes or damage in the skeleton will remain unchanged. Radiation therapy or medications to decrease growth hormone levels may provide some relief if resection is not a viable option for the patient.

Hypopituitarism

Because the pituitary gland controls the level of secretion of gonadal and thyroid hormones and the production of growth hormone, decreased function of the pituitary gland causes profound generalized disturbances in bone growth and maturation. In children, hypopituitarism typically leads to a type of dwarfism

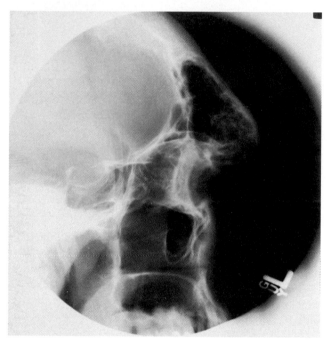

FIGURE 10-19 Acromegaly. Lateral skull demonstrating a thickened frontal bone with characteristic frontal bossing.

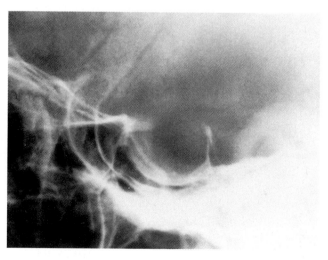

FIGURE 10-20 Pituitary adenoma causing acromegaly. Ballooning of the sella turcica with downward displacement of the floor is demonstrated.

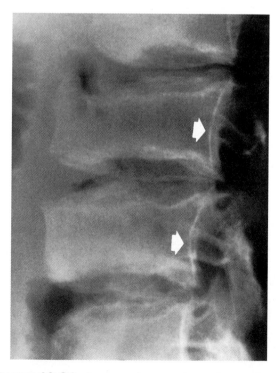

FIGURE 10-21 Acromegaly. Posterior scalloping *(arrows)* associated with enlargement of vertebral bodies (especially in anteroposterior dimension).

in which the delayed appearance of epiphyseal centers causes the failure of bones to grow normally in length or width. This results in a person who is small in stature and sexually immature, although well proportioned and of normal mentality. In many patients, there is a delay in the eruption of the teeth, which tend to become impacted because their size is not affected. The arrest in the growth of the skeleton occurs during childhood, when the cranial vault is proportionally greater in relation to the facial bones than in the adult. Because this discrepancy remains into adulthood in hypopituitary dwarfism, the relatively large skull may be mistakenly believed to result from hydrocephaly.

Hypopituitarism occurring after adolescence results in hypofunction of the thyroid gland, adrenal glands, and gonads, but usually causes few radiologic findings. The heart and kidneys are often small, and calcification or ossification may develop in the articular cartilages.

Radiographic Appearance

MRI is the preferred imaging modality because it has superb sensitivity and can directly image the sellar and parasellar regions in multiple planes. The use of contrast enhancement may help define a microadenoma or detect sarcoidosis in an older patient with Addison's disease.

Treatment

For children a subcutaneous injection of recombinant growth hormone several times per week during puberty and earlier is recommended to prevent the arrest in growth. Tumor location and type will determine whether surgery is needed. In adults usually no treatment is required.

Diabetes Insipidus

The impaired ability of the kidneys to conserve water in diabetes insipidus results from low blood levels of ADH, reflecting deficient vasopressin release by the posterior lobe of the pituitary gland in response to normal physiologic stimuli. In response to excessive water loss in the urine (polyuria), the body compensates by developing an insatiable thirst (polydipsia). Another type of diabetes insipidus occurs when the kidneys fail to respond to circulating ADH; this is known as nephrogenic diabetes insipidus. It must be stressed that diabetes insipidus is completely unrelated to diabetes mellitus.

Radiographic Appearance

On T1-weighted MR images, an absence of signal in the posterior pituitary indicates diabetes insipidus. Severe polyuria can lead to massive dilatation of the renal pelves, calyces, and ureters. This probably represents a compensatory alteration to accommodate the huge volume of excreted urine.

Treatment

Treatment for diabetes insipidus consists of taking drugs that mimic ADH, delivered most commonly in a nasal spray. For the nephrogenic type, treatment with thiazide diuretics allows the kidney to resorb an increased amount of fluid.

SUMMARY FINDINGS *for* Diseases of the Pituitary Gland

disorder	location	radiographic appearance	treatment
Hyperpituitarism	Excessive growth hormone—anterior pituitary	Radiograph—widened joints, thickened heel pad, thickened skull tables with frontal bossing, paranasal sinus enlargement, mandibular changes, vertebral enlargement with scalloping, hypertrophy of cartilage MRI—superior sensitivity and multiplanar imaging to evaluate the pituitary gland; post enhancement—T1-weighted spin-echo appears as a hypoenhancing lesion	Surgical resection of pituitary tumor
Hypopituitarism	Loss of secretion of any anterior pituitary hormone	Radiograph—skeletal changes in size; dwarfism MRI—detects pituitary tumor by multiplanar imaging; loss of signal of posterior pituitary on T1-weighted images	Children—subcutaneous injection of growth hormone Adults—usually no treatment required
Diabetes insipidus	Deficient release of hormones from the posterior lobe of the pituitary	MRI—detection of pituitary tumor by multiplanar imaging as an absence of signal in the posterior pituitary gland	Drugs to mimic antidiuretic hormone

Thyroid Gland

Physiology of the Thyroid Gland

The thyroid is a butterfly-shaped gland located in the neck at the level of the larynx. It consists of two lobes, one on each side of the trachea, and a connecting strip (the isthmus) that runs anterior to the trachea and connects the lower portions of the two lobes. The thyroid lies just below the Adam's apple, the protrusion formed by the cricoid cartilage of the larynx. Microscopically the thyroid gland consists of innumerable follicles surrounding a central core of colloid, the storage form of the active material known as thyroxine, which is the only natural iodine-containing substance in the body.

The thyroid gland picks up iodine from the bloodstream and combines it with the amino acid tyrosine to synthesize thyroid hormones, which are stored in the gland until released into the bloodstream when stimulated by TSH from the anterior lobe of the pituitary gland. The active hormone, **thyroxine,** is a small molecule that may contain either three iodine molecules (T_3) or four iodine molecules (T_4). These substances stimulate cellular metabolism in response to the body's need for increased energy production. The increased cellular metabolism requires that additional oxygen be circulated to the cells and that more waste materials be removed, which in turn requires increased blood flow and greater cardiac output. The increased demand for oxygen stimulates the respiratory center and results in a faster rate and greater depth of breathing. Increased cellular metabolism produces heat, which is dissipated by perspiration and by increased blood flow through dilated vessels in the skin, giving the person a flushed appearance. Thyroid hormone also increases the secretion of digestive juices and the movement of ingested material through the intestinal tract.

The release of thyroid hormone is controlled by TSH, which is secreted by the anterior lobe of the pituitary gland. This process is a negative feedback mechanism, in which a high blood level of thyroxine inhibits the anterior pituitary and TSH release, whereas a low level of thyroxine forces the anterior pituitary to release TSH again.

Diseases of the Thyroid Gland

Radioactive Iodine Scanning

Scanning after the administration of radioactive iodine is the superior imaging modality for demonstrating both functioning and nonfunctioning thyroid tissue. This technique is used to localize palpable nodules, to determine the function of nodules, to detect nonpalpable lesions (especially in patients with a history of neck irradiation), and to evaluate the extent of residual tissue after surgical or radioisotopic thyroid ablation. Radionuclide scanning may be combined with uptake, stimulation, or suppression techniques to better characterize the thyroid lesions.

Radiographic Appearance

The distribution of radioactivity is uniform throughout the normal thyroid gland (Figure 10-22). Diffuse thyroid enlargement without hyperthyroidism most frequently represents a multinodular goiter of Hashimoto's thyroiditis. In a patient with hyperthyroidism, diffuse thyroid enlargement is suggestive of Graves' disease.

Masses within the thyroid gland appear as hyperfunctioning ("hot") or poorly functioning ("cold") nodules. A hot nodule demonstrates increased radionuclide uptake compared with surrounding thyroid tissue (Figure 10-23). These hot nodules usually represent autonomously functioning thyroid tissue and are rarely malignant, although malignancy is sometimes reported elsewhere in the same gland. Large hyperfunctioning nodules may completely suppress the remaining thyroid tissue so that only the nodule itself is visualized. An autonomous nodule may eventually develop central hemorrhage or cystic change and evolve into a nonfunctioning (cold) nodule.

Cold thyroid nodules contain less radionuclide per unit tissue mass than adjacent normal thyroid tissue (Figure 10-24). Most cold nodules represent poorly functioning adenomas. Thyroid cysts, carcinoma, and thyroiditis can also produce this appearance. In a young patient, the absence of uptake in the region of a solitary cold thyroid nodule is associated with a 10% to 25% probability that the nodule is malignant. Ultrasound can establish the precise location of the

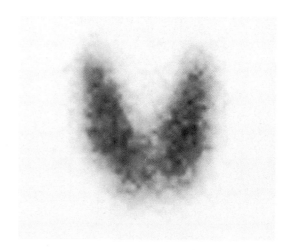

FIGURE 10-22 Normal radioactive iodine scan. There is uniform distribution of nuclide activity throughout the thyroid gland.

palpable mass and determine whether it is within the thyroid or in adjacent tissue. In patients who are at risk because of irradiation of the neck during their youth or because of a family history, but who have no palpable lesion, ultrasound may detect an occult thyroid nodule. Although ultrasound can distinguish a thyroid cyst from the other causes of cold nodules, this modality is of little value in further characterizing noncystic thyroid masses.

Hyperthyroidism

Hyperthyroidism results from the excessive production of thyroid hormone, either from the entire gland (Graves' disease) or from one or more functioning adenomas. Graves' disease is a relatively common disorder that most often develops in the third and fourth decades and has a strong female predominance. The major clinical symptoms include nervousness, emotional lability, an inability to sleep, tremors, rapid pulse rate (tachycardia), palpitations, excessive sweating, and heat intolerance. Weight loss is common, usually despite an increased appetite. A characteristic physical finding is exophthalmos, outward protrusion of the eyeball caused by edema in the tissue behind the eyes.

Radiographic Appearance

Radioactive iodine scans in patients with Graves' disease typically demonstrate diffuse enlargement of the thyroid gland with increased radioiodine uptake (Figure 10-25), which rules out a single toxic adenoma. The degree of increased uptake on the scan helps to determine the dose of radioactive iodine for treatment.

In severe cases, high-output cardiac failure may develop along with generalized cardiomegaly and pulmonary congestion. Unilateral or bilateral exophthalmos as a result of Graves' disease can be demonstrated by CT as thickening of the extraocular muscles. Ultrasound imaging helps determine the size and location of the thyroid (Figure 10-26), and the image can be correlated with the radioactive scans.

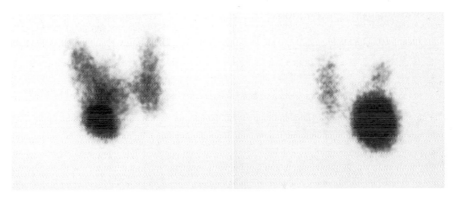

FIGURE 10-23 Hyperfunctioning (hot) nodules in two patients. Notice the variable amount of suppression in the remainder of the thyroid gland.

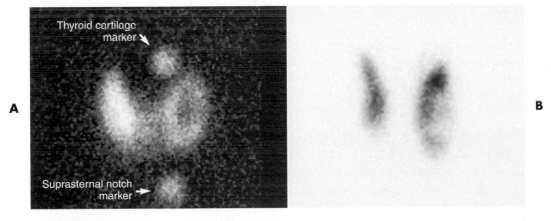

FIGURE 10-24 Nonfunctioning (cold) nodules in two patients. **A,** Uptake within the gland is normal. A cold nodule in the left lobe of the thyroid corresponds to the nodule seen on the ultrasound. The upper marker is at the thyroid cartilage; the inferior marker is at the suprasternal notch. **B,** Inhomogeneous right and left lobes demonstrate multiple cold nodules. There is a dominant cold nodule in the inferior left pole.

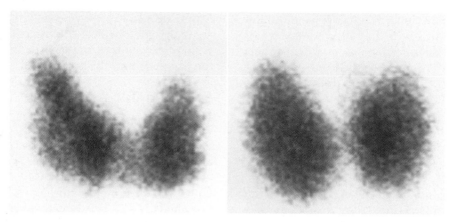

FIGURE 10-25 Hyperthyroidism. Radionuclide scans in two patients with Graves' disease show symmetrically enlarged thyroid glands with homogeneous increased iodine uptake.

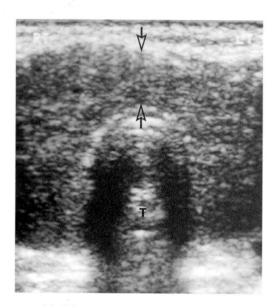

FIGURE 10-26 Thyroid goiter. Ultrasound image shows thickened isthmus *(arrows)* and enlarged bilateral lobes. *T,* Trachea.

Treatment

Antithyroid drugs are used to decrease thyroid response. Destruction of thyroid cells by radioactive iodine (^{131}I) or total thyroidectomy results in hypothyroidism.

Hypothyroidism

Hypothyroidism can result from any structural or functional abnormality that leads to an insufficient synthesis of thyroid hormone. Hypothyroidism dating from birth (cretinism) results in multiple developmental abnormalities. Children with cretinism typically have a short stature; coarse features with a protruding tongue, a broad, flattened nose, and widely set eyes; sparse hair; dry skin; and a protuberant abdomen with an umbilical hernia.

Adult hypothyroidism has an insidious onset with nonspecific symptoms including lethargy, somnolence (sleeping up to 16 hours a day), constipation, cold intolerance, slowing of intellectual and motor activity, and weight gain despite a decreased appetite. Dry skin; stiff, aching muscles; and a deepening voice with hoarseness often occur. The facial features are thickened, and there is a doughy thickening of the skin (myxedema).

Radiographic Appearance

The major radiographic abnormalities in children include a delay in the appearance and subsequent growth of ossification centers and retarded bone age. Skull changes are common and include an increase in the thickness of the cranial vault, underpneumatization of the sinuses and mastoid air cells, widened sutures with delayed closure, and a delay in the development and eruption of the teeth (Figure 10-27).

Radiographically the heart in adults is typically enlarged because of pericardial effusion. Soft tissue thickening is often seen on films of the extremities, and adynamic ileus is a common finding on abdominal radiographs.

Treatment

If a tumor is the cause of hypothyroidism, a combination of surgery, chemotherapy, and radiation therapy is the treatment of choice. For functional hypothyroidism, the thyroid hormone is replaced with a synthetic product (thyroxine).

Goiter

A goiter is an enlargement of the thyroid gland that does not result from an inflammatory or neoplastic process and is not initially associated with hyperthyroidism or myxedema. A simple (nontoxic) goiter results when one or more factors impair the capacity

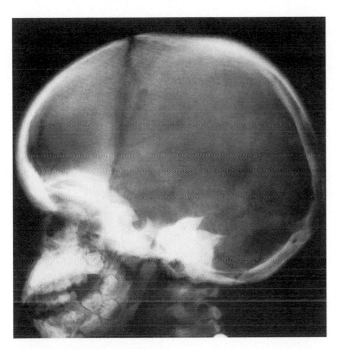

FIGURE 10-27 Cretinism. Lateral projection of skull shows increased density at the base, small underdeveloped sinuses, and hypoplasia of teeth with delayed eruption. Retardation of facial maturation makes face appear small relative to size of calvaria.

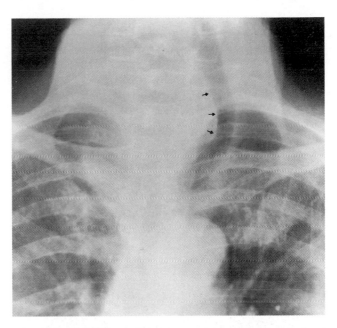

FIGURE 10-28 Goiter. Greatly enlarged thyroid gland appears as a soft tissue mass impressing the trachea *(arrows)* and displacing it to the left.

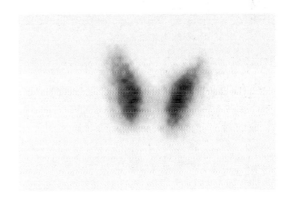

FIGURE 10-29 Multinodular goiter. Radioactive iodine scan shows patchy uptake of the nuclide caused by increased and decreased uptake by the thyroid.

of the thyroid gland in the basal state to secrete the quantities of active hormones necessary to meet the needs of the body. Because the blood level of thyroid hormone is low, there is nothing to inhibit the anterior pituitary, which continues to secrete TSH, causing the thyroid gland to enlarge. In most cases, there is a sufficient increase in both the functioning thyroid mass and the cellular activity to overcome the mild or moderate impairment of hormone synthesis, permitting the patient to remain metabolically normal although goitrous.

Although goiters were once endemic in areas where there was insufficient iodine in the diet, this situation is now rare because iodine is added commercially to salt and bread.

Radiographic Appearance

On a radioactive iodine scan, a nontoxic goiter usually appears as a symmetric or an asymmetric enlargement of the thyroid gland. Plain radiographs and esophagrams often show the enlarged thyroid gland impressing or displacing the trachea and esophagus (Figure 10-28).

A toxic multinodular goiter may be a consequence of a long-standing nontoxic goiter. In this condition, one or more areas of the gland become independent of TSH stimulation. Radioactive iodine scans most commonly show accumulation of iodine in diffuse but

patchy foci throughout the gland (Figure 10-29). Another pattern consists of iodine accumulation in one or more discrete nodules within the gland, with the remainder of the gland being essentially nonfunctional.

Ultrasound is indicated to determine if a nonfunctioning mass detected on a radioactive iodine scan is cystic or solid (Figure 10-30). Ultrasound may be used to monitor growth of thyroid nodules. CT or MRI is employed only when there is a substernal thyroid that cannot be seen with ultrasound.

Treatment

The first-line treatment of small goiters is to control the nodule size with oral thyroxine. If the goiter continues to enlarge, the thyroid is surgically resected to relieve

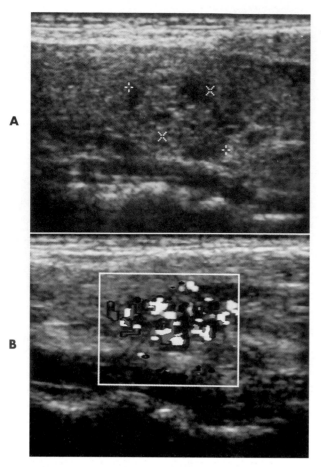

FIGURE **10-30** Multinodular goiter. **A,** Ultrasound image demonstrates solid nodular lesions (8 ×15 mm) in both lobes of the thyroid (left lobe shown here). **B,** The Doppler image demonstrates increased vascularity.

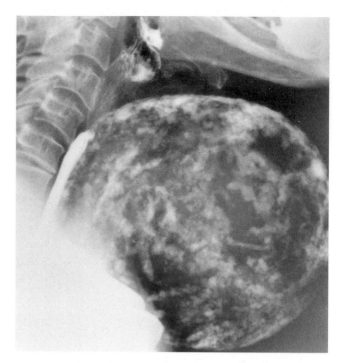

FIGURE **10-31** Thyroid adenoma. Lateral projection of the neck shows a huge calcified thyroid mass.

the compression of anatomic structures in the neck (trachea, esophagus).

Benign Thyroid Adenomas

Benign thyroid adenomas are encapsulated tumors that vary greatly in size and usually compress adjacent tissue. They may be located within the neck, where they tend to cause deviation or compression of the trachea, or they may extend substernally and appear as masses in the superior portion of the anterior mediastinum.

Radiographic Appearance of Thyroid Adenomas

Calcification may develop within the mass (Figure 10-31). Thyroid adenomas can appear as hot or cold nodules on radionuclide imaging, depending on their functional capacity. Ultrasound usually demonstrates an adenoma as a solid mass with a consistent echogenicity. There is often a thick and smooth peripheral hypoechoic halo caused by the fibrous capsule and blood vessels. Cystic lesions as small as 2 mm and solid lesions of 3 mm can be visualized.

Thyroid Carcinomas

The three major types of thyroid carcinomas are papillary, follicular, and medullary. **Papillary carcinoma,** the most common type, has peaks of incidence occurring in adolescence and young adulthood and again in later life during the third to fifth decades. The tumor is usually slow growing and cystic, and it typically spreads to regional lymph nodes, where it may remain silent for many years. Distant metastases to the lungs are rare and often cause only mild, nonspecific thickening of bronchovesicular markings, although the metastases may also appear as miliary and nodular densities that predominantly involve the lower lobes.

Follicular carcinoma has a histologic appearance that closely mimics normal thyroid tissue. Typically (in about 75% of cases), this tumor occurs in women more than 40 years of age. The tumor usually undergoes early hematogenous spread, especially to the lung and bone. Skeletal metastases, which may be the initial presentation, tend to produce entirely lytic, expansile destruction that extends into the soft tissues and is associated with little or no periosteal reaction.

Medullary carcinoma is the least common type of thyroid malignancy. At least 10% of the cases are familial, most often appearing as a component of a syndrome in which there are multiple endocrine tumors. Dense, amorphous calcifications can often be seen within the tumor. Medullary carcinomas readily metastasize via the lymphatic channels.

There is a substantially increased risk of thyroid cancer in persons with a history of therapeutic neck irradiation in childhood. In the past, such radiation was used for benign disease, such as enlargement of the tonsils, adenoids, and thymus; middle ear disease; and a variety of skin disorders, including acne.

Radiographic Appearance of Thyroid Carcinomas

On radioactive iodine scans, thyroid carcinoma usually appears as a solitary cold nodule that corresponds to a palpable mass (Figure 10-32). A nodule

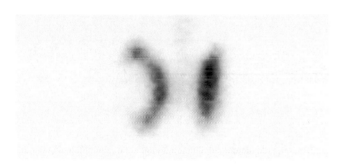

FIGURE 10-32 Thyroid carcinoma. Radioactive iodine scan shows a solitary cold nodule that corresponds to the patient's palpable mass.

that is functioning (hot) can essentially be excluded from a diagnosis of thyroid carcinoma.

On ultrasound, 90% of papillary carcinomas appear as solid hypoechoic masses that may contain microcalcifications, which appear as tiny hyperechoic foci (Figure 10-33). Follicular carcinomas, which have similar tissue consistency, cannot be distinguished from adenomas unless they demonstrate irregular tumor margins and a thick irregular halo (Figure 10-34). On color Doppler, tortuous or disordered blood vessel arrangement is common. Medullary carcinomas appear similar to papillary carcinomas, with bright echogenic foci caused by calcifications.

MRI and CT demonstrate substernal thyroids that ultrasound cannot detect because of bone interference. MRI may aid in defining the extent of the neoplasm.

Treatment of Thyroid Tumors

Thyroid adenoma treatment may be as simple as observation or as complex as a surgical lobectomy. Drug therapy options include TSH suppression or radioactive iodine. Appropriate treatment will depend on the size and location of the thyroid adenoma.

Thyroidectomy is the first choice of treatment, especially for papillary carcinomas. About 80% of patients survive longer than 10 years. If the patient cannot undergo surgery, alternative choices are suppressive drugs and chemotherapy with radioactive iodine, which may result in hypothyroidism. For patients with follicular carcinoma and widespread metastases, radioactive iodine treatment is the best treatment.

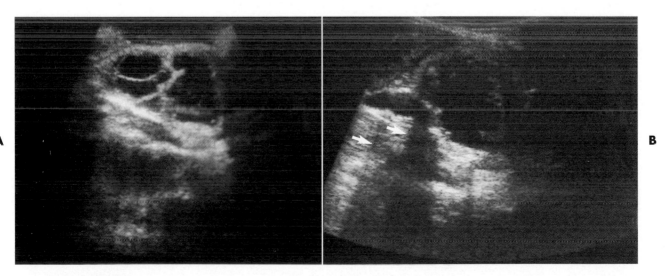

A   **B**

FIGURE 10-33 Ultrasound images of a complex thyroid mass. **A,** The mass has solid components and intercystic septations of various thicknesses. **B,** Echogenic foci with shadowing are evident *(arrows)*. Together with the radioactive iodine scan, which showed a cold nodule, this suggests a malignant lesion.

SUMMARY *of* FINDINGS *for* Diseases of the Thyroid Gland

disorder	location	radiographic appearance	treatment
Hyperthyroidism	Excessive hormone production	NM radionuclides—diffuse enlarged thyroid with increased uptake	Antithyroidal drugs Radioactive iodine Partial or total resection of thyroid
Hypothyroidism	Insufficient synthesis of thyroid hormone	Imaging not used for diagnosis Radiograph—retarded bone age; increased skull thickness with widened sutures and delayed suture closure Chest film (in adult)—enlarged heart with pericardial effusion	Replacement therapy If caused by tumor—surgery, radiation, and chemotherapy
Goiter	Enlarged thyroid gland	NM radionuclides—enlargement of thyroid gland Esophagram—thyroid gland impresses or displaces trachea and esophagus	Thyroxine to manage goiter size Resection of enlarged portion of thyroid
Benign thyroid adenomas	Encapsulated tumor	X-ray calcification NM radionuclides—hot or cold nodule US—solid homogeneous mass with peripheral hypoechoic halo	Observation Lobectomy Drug therapy
Thyroid carcinomas	Papillary, follicular, or medullary	NM radionuclides—solitary cold nodule US—papillary carcinoma appears as a solid hypoechoic mass with hyperechoic foci, follicular carcinoma has irregular tumor margins and a thick irregular halo Color Doppler—tortuous or disordered blood vessel arrangement; medullary carcinomas appear similar to papillary carcinomas with bright echogenic foci MRI/CT—demonstrates substernal thyroid and may aid in defining the extent of the neoplasm	Thyroidectomy Suppressive drugs Chemotherapy with radioactive iodine Radiation therapy

NM, Nuclear medicine; *US*, ultrasound.

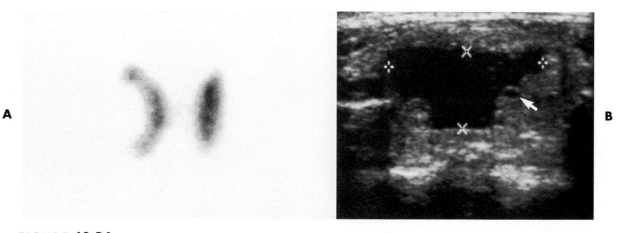

A   **B**

FIGURE 10-34 Degenerative follicular adenoma. **A,** Radioactive iodine scan shows a prominent cold nodule. **B,** Ultrasound illustrates a lesion that is not smooth (note papillary projections, *arrow*) and that lacks back wall enhancement. These features most often indicate a degenerative follicular adenoma.

Parathyroid Glands

Physiology of the Parathyroid Glands

The parathyroids are four tiny glands, two on each side, that lie behind the upper and lower poles of the thyroid gland. They secrete **parathormone** (parathyroid hormone—PTH), which is responsible for regulating the blood levels of calcium and phosphate. Parathormone raises a low serum calcium level by three mechanisms. First, it increases the amount of calcium absorbed from the intestinal tract by interaction with ingested vitamin D. Second, the hormone prevents a loss of calcium through the kidneys and releases calcium from bones by stimulating osteoclastic activity. Third, serum phosphate levels are reduced.

Diseases of the Parathyroid Glands

Hyperparathyroidism

Excessive secretion of parathormone leads to a generalized disorder of calcium, phosphate, and bone metabolism that results in elevated serum levels of calcium and phosphate. **Primary hyperparathyroidism** may be caused by a discrete adenoma (80%) or carcinoma (2%) or by generalized hyperplasia (18%) of all glands. Other causes include nonparathyroid tumors that secrete a parathormone-like substance and the familial syndrome of multiple endocrine neoplasia. **Secondary hyperparathyroidism** occurs more frequently than the primary form and is most often attributable to chronic renal failure. **Tertiary hyperparathyroidism** refers to the development of autonomous functioning parathyroid glands in patients who demonstrate progressive bone disease in the presence of biochemical and clinically controlled renal disease.

Radiographic Appearance

The radiographic findings of primary and secondary hyperparathyroidism are similar, except that in the secondary form brown tumors (focal areas of bone destruction) are rare and osteosclerosis is more common. As a result of the predominant skeletal changes, conventional radiography is the primary image modality used for diagnosis. The earliest change is subperiosteal bone resorption, which particularly involves the radial margins of the middle phalanges (Figure 10-35), the distal clavicles (Figure 10-36), and the medial aspect of the upper third of the tibias. Loss of normal cortical definition is followed by an irregularly lacy resorption, with the endosteal margin initially remaining intact. Erosions of the terminal tufts of the fingers and loss of the lamina dura of the teeth often occur, although these are nonspecific findings that also are seen in other conditions.

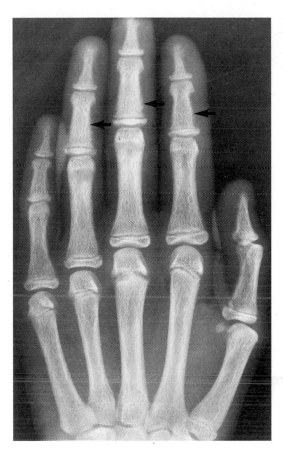

FIGURE 10-35 Hyperparathyroidism. Subperiosteal bone resorption can be seen that predominantly involves the radial margins of the middle phalanges of the second, third, and fourth digits *(arrows)*. Notice also resorption of terminal tufts.

Generalized loss of bone density may produce a ground-glass appearance. So-called brown tumors may become large and expansile and even simulate a malignant process (Figure 10-37). Pathologic fractures may lead to bizarre deformities. Irregular demineralization of the calvaria produces the characteristic salt-and-pepper skull (Figure 10-38).

A generalized increase in bone density (osteosclerosis) may develop in patients with hyperparathyroidism, especially when it is a result of renal failure. Thick bands of increased density adjacent to the superior and inferior margins of vertebral bodies produce the characteristic "rugger-jersey" spine (Figure 10-39).

Soft tissue calcification is common, especially in secondary hyperparathyroidism. Calcific deposits may develop in vessels, articular cartilages, menisci, joint capsules, and periarticular tissues (Figure 10-40). Elevated serum calcium and decreased excretion of calcium in the urine may result in nephrocalcinosis and urinary tract stones. Increased incidences

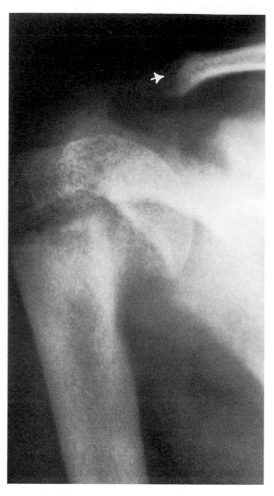

FIGURE 10-36 Hyperparathyroidism. Characteristic erosion of the distal clavicle *(arrow)* is shown. Metaphyseal subperiosteal resorption beneath the proximal humeral head has led to a pathologic fracture with slippage of the humeral head.

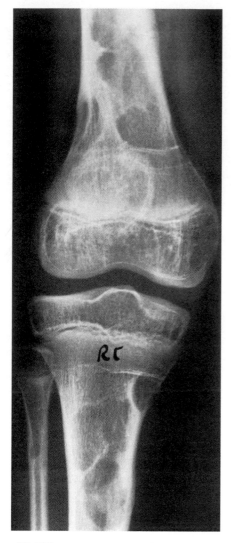

FIGURE 10-37 Hyperparathyroidism. Brown tumors have produced multiple lytic lesions about the knee.

of pancreatic calculi and pancreatitis, peptic ulcer, and gallstones have also been reported in patients with hyperparathyroidism.

The preoperative localization of a functioning parathyroid adenoma has long been a difficult imaging problem. Ultrasound can detect 80% to 85% of the parathyroid abnormalities. Parathyroid carcinomas usually have a more heterogeneous internal structure than adenomas. Preoperative parathyroid localization is not required unless the patient has had previous neck surgery. Plain radiographs and barium studies are of virtually no value unless the tumor is very large.

The major role of sophisticated imaging modalities in the localization of functioning parathyroid adenomas is in patients who remain hypercalcemic, or in whom hypercalcemia recurs (Figure 10-41), after neck surgery for hyperparathyroidism. In these patients,

normal anatomic relationships are disturbed, landmarks may be absent, and scarring and adhesions distort the field and complicate the surgical technique. Also, the elusive parathyroid tumor is more likely to be situated in an ectopic position (Figure 10-42). Indeed, the success rate for parathyroid reexploration without help from imaging is less than 65%.

Thus CT and MRI are required to detect ectopic parathyroid tissue location (such as in the thymus). Radionuclide subtraction imaging using technetium-99m (Figure 10-43, *A*) and thallium can detect parathyroid adenomas with a fairly high sensitivity and specificity. An adenoma takes up only the thallium (Figure 10-43, *B*) and a residual focus of activity appears when the technetium is subtracted from the initial image (Figure 10-43, *C*). The normal thyroid can be distinguished from the tumor because it concentrates both radionuclides.

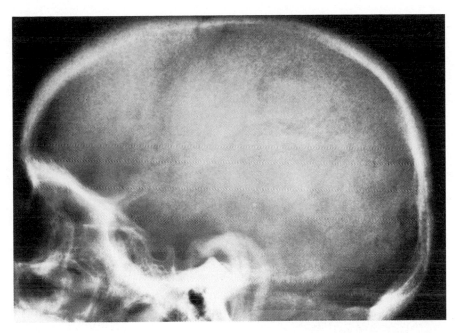

FIGURE **10-38** Hyperparathyroidism. Characteristic salt-and-pepper skull.

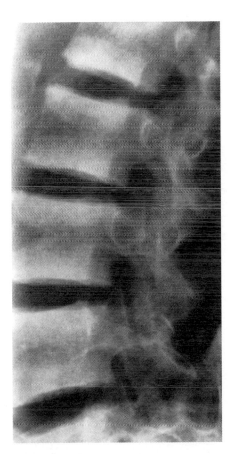

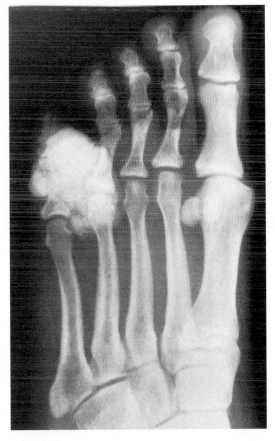

FIGURE **10-39** Hyperparathyroidism. Lateral projection of the lumbar spine demonstrates osteosclerosis of the superior and inferior margins of the vertebral bodies ("rugger-jersey" spine).

FIGURE **10-40** Hyperparathyroidism. Dense mass of tumoral calcification is seen in the joint capsules and periarticular soft tissues on the lateral aspect of the foot in a patient with chronic renal disease.

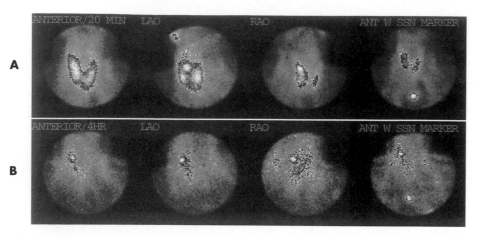

FIGURE 10-41 Parathyroid adenoma. **A,** Technetium-99m sestamibi was injected, and the patient was scanned 20 minutes later; normal distribution was noted. **B,** After 4 hours, washout of the activity in the thyroid tissue and a focal area of increased activity verify that the cause of hypercalcemia is a parathyroid adenoma.

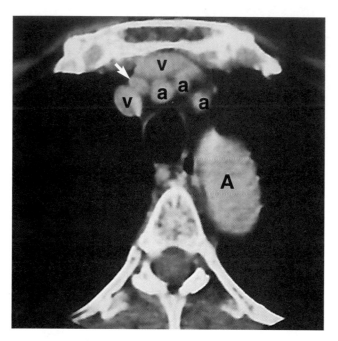

FIGURE 10-42 Ectopic parathyroid adenoma. CT scan shows small soft tissue mass *(arrow)* in anterior mediastinum. *A,* Aorta; *a,* three major branches of the aorta (from the patient's right to left, brachiocephalic, left carotid, and left subclavian arteries); *v,* right and left brachiocephalic veins.

Using ultrasound or CT guidance for preoperative fine-needle aspiration biopsy can increase the specificity of localizing and confirming the exact site of a parathyroid adenoma, especially in patients who have undergone previous neck dissection. When a successful aspiration biopsy of the neck shows the presence of parathyroid cells, there is no doubt that abnormal parathyroid tissue is situated at this site, and this eliminates the need for extensive surgical dissection.

Ultrasound, radionuclide scanning, CT, and MRI are complementary modalities for investigating the patient with hypercalcemia after parathyroid surgery. If these techniques fail to demonstrate a lesion, arteriography and venography with venous sampling may be performed for localization.

Treatment
A standard bilateral neck dissection by an experienced parathyroid surgeon can be expected to have a 95% success rate in controlling hyperparathyroidism. For hypercalcemia, specific drugs such as steroids and calcium-losing diuretics may be used.

Hypoparathyroidism
Clinically, hypoparathyroidism causes sustained muscular contraction (tetany), muscle cramps in hands and feet, and numbness and tingling of the extremities. Spasm of laryngeal muscles can cause fatal obstruction of the respiratory tract.

Radiographic Appearance
Hypoparathyroidism usually results from injury or accidental removal of the glands during thyroidectomy, and this type of hypoparathyroidism is not associated with any significant radiographic abnormalities.

In **primary hypoparathyroidism,** which is less common, the most common radiographic finding on plain skull radiographs or CT of the skull is cerebral calcification, especially involving the basal ganglia (Figure 10-44), the dentate (tooth-shaped) nuclei of the cerebellum, and the choroid plexus. A pattern of increased density may develop in the long bones, usually localized to the metaphyseal area.

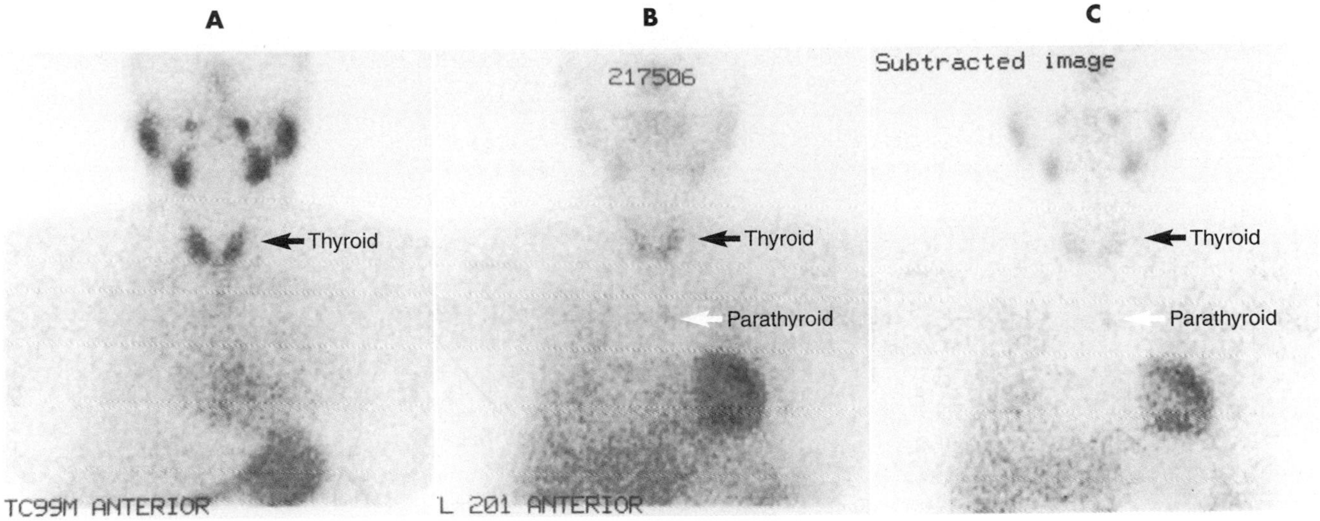

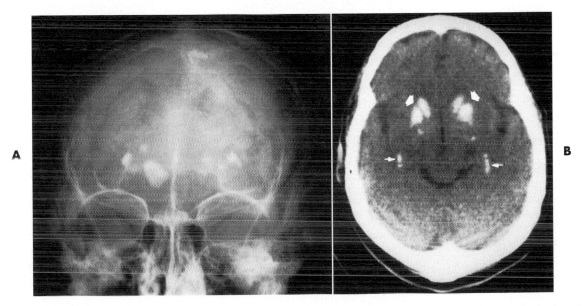

FIGURE 10-43 Radionuclide subtraction imaging. **A,** Technetium uptake. **B,** Thallium uptake. **C,** The residual focus of thallium activity after the technetium activity is subtracted. In this case a substernal parathyroid is demonstrated. *Black arrow,* Thyroid; *white arrow,* parathyroid.

FIGURE 10-44 Hypoparathyroidism. **A,** Frontal projection of the skull demonstrates calcification in the basal ganglia bilaterally. **B,** CT scan shows characteristic bilateral calcification in the basal ganglia *(broad arrows).* Note also the small calcific deposits in the tail of the caudate nuclei *(thin arrows).*

Treatment

Synthetic parathormone decreases symptoms to a tolerable level.

Pseudohypoparathyroidism and Pseudopseudohypoparathyroidism

Pseudohypoparathyroidism is a hereditary disorder in which there is failure of normal end-organ response to normal levels of circulating parathyroid hormone. Most patients are obese and have short stature, with round faces, opacities in the cornea or lens of the eye, short fingers, and mental retardation.

Radiographic Appearance

The most common radiographic abnormality is shortening of the tubular bones of the hands and feet (especially the fourth and fifth metacarpals) (see Figure 12-16) and calcific or bony deposits in the skin or subcutaneous tissues. An appearance similar to rickets may develop. As in idiopathic hypoparathyroidism,

SUMMARY of FINDINGS for Diseases of the Parathyroid Glands

disorder	location	radiographic appearance	treatment
Hyperparathyroidism	Excessive secretion of parathormone	Skeletal radiograph—subperiosteal bone resorption, erosion of distal clavicles, sclerotic stripes in vertebral bodies, salt-and-pepper skull US—carcinomas produce a more heterogeneous echo than adenomas CT/MRI—detect ectopic parathyroid tissue NM subtraction imaging—thallium appears as residual focal activity on technetium subtraction scan	Surgical resection by standard bilateral neck resection For hypercalcemia, steroids and calcium-losing diuretics
Hypoparathyroidism	Decreased secretion of parathormone	Radiograph/CT—cerebral calcification and increased density of metaphysis	Replacement therapy— synthetic parathormone
Pseudohypoparathyroidism	Failure of response by target organ	Radiograph—shortening of metacarpals and metatarsals	Some form of calcium supplement
Pseudopseudohypoparathyroidism	Similar skeletal anomalies in family members	Radiograph—shortening of metacarpals and metatarsals	Some form of calcium supplement

NM, Nuclear medicine; *US,* ultrasound.

calcification is often found in the brain, especially the basal ganglia (best demonstrated on CT or MRI).

Pseudopseudohypoparathyroidism refers to the presence of similar skeletal anomalies in other members of the patient's family in the absence of biochemical disturbances.

Treatment

Therapy consists of some form of calcium supplement, either calcium carbonate or calcitriol combined with vitamin D.

Diabetes Mellitus

Diabetes mellitus is a common endocrine disorder in which beta cells in the islets of Langerhans of the pancreas fail to secrete insulin, or target cells throughout the body fail to respond to this hormone. A lack of insulin prevents glucose from entering the cells, thus depriving them of the major nutrient needed for energy production. The blood glucose level increases **(hyperglycemia)**.

The severity and age of onset of diabetes vary. Juvenile-onset diabetes, which develops in childhood, and insulin-dependent diabetes require the patient to undergo daily insulin injections. Non–insulin-dependent diabetes, which tends to develop later in life, is less severe and can often be controlled by diet alone. The precise cause of diabetes is unknown, although it is generally considered that heredity is an important factor.

Polyuria (excessive urination) and polydipsia (drinking large quantities of liquid) are common manifestations of diabetes. The large amount of sugar filtered through the kidneys exceeds the amount that the renal tubules can absorb. This leads to the excretion of glucose in the urine (glycosuria), which is a major sign of diabetes.

Glucose is the major fuel of the body. However, as glucose cannot enter the cells without the action of insulin, diabetic patients are forced to metabolize a large amount of fat. This produces a large number of fatty acids and ketones, which can be detected in the urine. Production of fatty acids lowers the body's pH (acidosis). Severe acidosis and dehydration in a diabetic patient who fails to take enough insulin or eats a high-sugar diet can lead to diabetic coma, which may be fatal if not treated rapidly with fluids and a large dose of insulin.

A major complication of diabetes is the deposition of lipids within the walls of blood vessels (atherosclerosis). This causes arterial narrowing and even occlusion, resulting in myocardial infarction (coronary artery), stroke (carotid artery), or gangrene (peripheral artery). Excess glucose in tissues provides an excellent bacterial culture medium and leads to the frequent development of infections, which tend to heal poorly because of the generally poor circulation in diabetic patients. The kidneys are always affected by long-standing diabetes, and kidney failure is frequently the cause of death. Another complication is narrowing and rupture of minute retinal blood vessels, which may lead to blindness. Poor circulation to the nervous system may produce intractable pain, tingling sensations, loss of feeling, and paralysis.

A patient with diabetes must also be wary of developing insulin shock (hypoglycemic shock), which results from too much insulin, not enough food, or excessive exercise. The patient feels lightheaded and faint, trembles, and begins to perspire. In the radiology department, this may occur in diabetic patients who have not eaten or drunk before gastrointestinal examination or other special procedures. It is essential that this condition be rapidly recognized and sugar given, usually in the form of orange juice or candy.

Radiographic Appearance

Diabetes mellitus produces a variety of radiographic findings that involve multiple organ systems. Atherosclerotic disease and subsequent ischemia involving the coronary, extracerebral, and peripheral circulations occur earlier and are more extensive in diabetics, especially those who smoke. Calcifications in peripheral vessels, especially those of the hands and feet, are virtually pathognomonic of the disease (Figure 10-45). Men with diabetes may demonstrate characteristic calcification of the vas deferens, which appears as bilaterally symmetric parallel tubular densities that run medially and caudally to enter the medial aspect of the seminal vesicles at the base of the prostate gland (Figure 10-46).

Diabetic persons have an increased susceptibility to infection; this especially affects the feet and may lead to severe osteomyelitis, which produces bone destruction without periosteal reaction. Diabetic neuropathy with gait abnormalities and the loss of deep pain sensation may lead to repeated trauma on an unstable joint. Degeneration of cartilage, recurrent fracture and fragmentation of subchondral bone, soft tissue debris, and considerable proliferation of

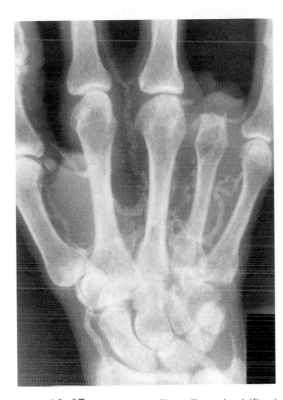

FIGURE 10-45 Diabetes mellitus. Typical calcification in moderate-size vessels of the hand and wrist. Evidence of a prior surgical resection of the phalanges of the fourth digit can be seen

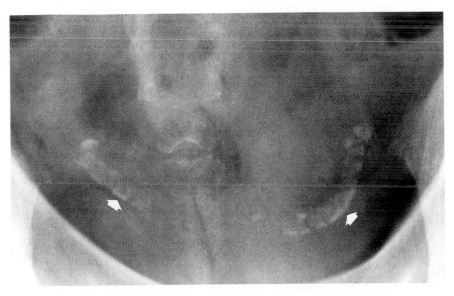

FIGURE 10-46 Diabetes mellitus. Bilateral calcification of the vas deferens.

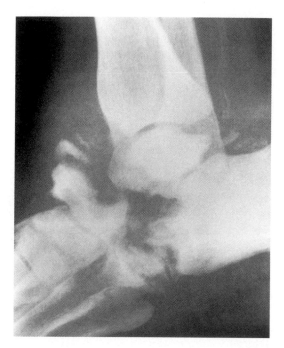

FIGURE **10-47** Neuropathic joint in diabetes mellitus. Severe destructive changes with calcific debris can be observed about the intertarsal joints. Notice the characteristic vascular calcification posterior to the ankle joint.

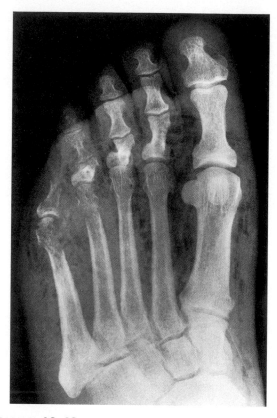

FIGURE **10-48** Diabetic gangrene. There is diffuse destruction of the phalanges and the metatarsal head of the fifth digit. Notice the large amount of gas in the soft tissues of the foot.

adjacent bone can lead to total disorganization of the joint (Charcot's, or neuropathic, joint) (Figure 10-47). Vascular disease with diminished blood supply can lead to gas gangrene, in which bubbles or streaks of gas develop in the subcutaneous or deeper tissues (Figure 10-48).

Diabetic neuropathy often causes radiographically evident abnormalities in the gastrointestinal tract. Findings include decreased primary peristalsis and tertiary contractions in the esophagus, delayed gastric emptying, and dilatation of the small bowel. Emphysematous cholecystitis with gas in the lumen and wall of the gallbladder (see Figure 5-86) is a severe complication that occurs almost exclusively in diabetic patients.

Renal disease is a common complication and a leading cause of death in persons with diabetes. Acute and chronic pyelonephritis, renal papillary necrosis, and cystitis often occur. Diabetic neuropathy can cause dilatation and atony (lack of normal tone) of the bladder with incomplete emptying.

Mucormycosis infection is a devastating fungal disease that occurs virtually only in uncontrolled diabetics. It usually originates in the nose and paranasal sinuses, from which it can extend to destroy the walls of the sinus and invade the substance of the brain. Pulmonary mucormycosis is a progressive severe pneumonia that is widespread and confluent and often cavitates (Figure 10-49).

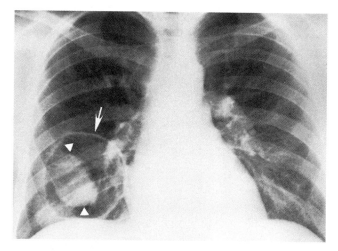

FIGURE **10-49** Mucormycosis in a diabetic patient. Large, thin-walled cavity (arrow) contains a smooth, elliptic, homogeneous mass (arrowheads) representing the fungus ball.

Treatment

The purpose of therapy is to keep the blood glucose levels constant with a minimal variation. Insulin is used when proper diet and exercise cannot maintain normal levels. Recent advances in therapy include islet cell transplantation and insulin gene therapy.

CHAPTER 11

REPRODUCTIVE *System*

Chapter Outline

Infectious Diseases of Both Genders
    Syphilis
    Gonorrhea
Male Reproductive System
Physiology of the Male Reproductive System
Benign Prostatic Hyperplasia
Carcinoma of the Prostate Gland
Undescended Testis (Cryptorchidism)
Testicular Torsion and Epididymitis
Testicular Tumors
Female Reproductive System
Physiology of the Female Reproductive System
Pelvic Inflammatory Disease
Cysts and Tumors
    Ovarian Cysts and Tumors
    Dermoid Cyst (Teratoma)
    Uterine Fibroids
    Endometrial Carcinoma
    Endometriosis
    Carcinoma of the Cervix
Breast Lesions
    Breast Cancer
    Benign Breast Disease
Imaging in Pregnancy
    Ectopic Pregnancy
    Trophoblastic Disease
    Female Infertility

Key Terms

chorion
congenital syphilis
corpus luteum
cystadenoma
ectopic pregnancy
epididymis
estrogen
hydrosalpinx
menarche
menopause
menstrual phase
oligohydramnios
ovulation
polyhydramnios
primary cystadenocarcinoma

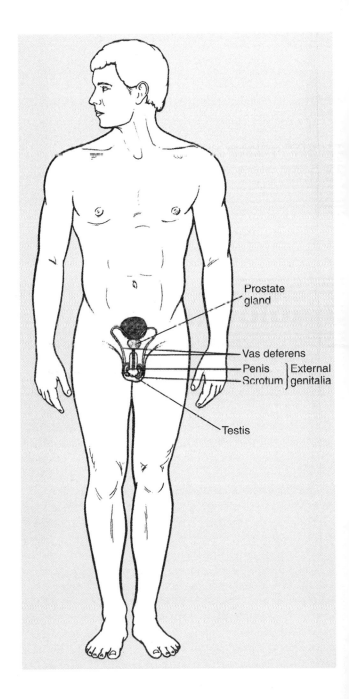

Prostate gland

Vas deferens

Penis] External
Scrotum } genitalia

Testis

primary stage
progesterone
proliferative, or postmenstrual, phase
prostate gland

pyosalpinx
secondary stage
secretory, or postovulatory, phase
seminal vesicle
spermatogenesis

tertiary stage
testosterone
vas deferens
vasectomy

Prerequisite Knowledge

The student should have a basic knowledge of the anatomy and physiology of the reproductive system. In addition, proper learning and understanding of the material will be facilitated if the student has some clinical experience in reproductive system imaging and image evaluation.

Goals

To acquaint the student radiographer with the pathophysiology and radiographic manifestations of all the common and some of the unusual disorders of the reproductive system.

Objectives

After reading this chapter, the reader will be able to:
1. Define all key terms in this chapter
2. Describe the physiology of the reproductive system
3. Identify anatomic structures on both diagrams and radiographs of the reproductive system

4. Differentiate various pathologic conditions affecting the reproductive system and their radiographic manifestations
5. Initiate alterations that must be made in routine exposure techniques to obtain optimal-quality radiographs

Infectious Diseases of Both Genders

Syphilis

Syphilis is a chronic, sexually transmitted systemic infection caused by the spirochete *Treponema pallidum*. The baby of an infected mother may be born with **congenital syphilis**. In the **primary stage** of infection, a chancre, or ulceration, develops on the genitals (usually the vulva of the female and the penis of the male). If untreated, the **secondary stage** of the disease appears as a nonitching rash that affects any part of the body. At this stage, the patient is still

RADIOGRAPHER *Notes*

Because of its nonionizing character, ultrasound has become the major modality for imaging both the male and female reproductive systems. Computed tomography (CT) and magnetic resonance imaging (MRI) are used for staging malignant tumors when ultrasound is inconclusive, and radionuclide studies are used to differentiate testicular torsion from epididymitis.

Conventional plain film radiography is virtually never indicated for disorders of the pregnant patient. The once common pelvimetry and gravid uterus examinations have been almost completely replaced by nonionizing ultrasound imaging. The two radiographic studies of the female reproductive system that are in current use are hysterosalpingography and mammography. Hysterosalpingography, which is performed by use of fluoroscopic guidance, evaluates the patency (openness) of the fallopian tubes. Plain radiographs are obtained only to provide a

permanent record. Mammography requires dedicated equipment and a specially trained radiographer. Properly performed mammograms can detect early stage breast cancer before it is symptomatic, thus decreasing the incidence of metastases and greatly improving patient survival rates. However, mammograms performed by poorly trained radiographers or with inadequate equipment may fail to demonstrate early lesions and condemn a woman with an otherwise curable disease to unnecessary suffering and even death.

It is essential that the radiographer attempt to put the patient at ease when performing an examination of the reproductive system. Although these procedures are not actually painful, they may at times be uncomfortable and are frequently embarrassing for the patient. A good professional attitude goes a long way in reassuring the patient and making these examinations as comfortable as possible.

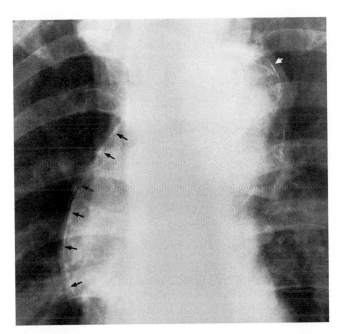

FIGURE 11-1 Syphilitic aortitis. Aneurysmal dilatation of the ascending aorta with extensive linear calcification of the wall (*black arrows*). Some calcification is also seen in the distal aortic arch (*white arrow*).

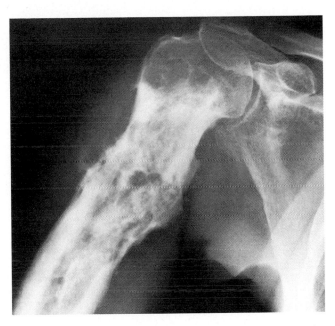

FIGURE 11-2 Syphilitic osteomyelitis. Diffuse lytic destruction of the proximal humerus with reactive sclerosis and periosteal new bone formation.

infectious. If still untreated, the disease may become dormant for many years before the development of the most serious or **tertiary stage** of the disease in which radiographic abnormalities become apparent. The young black male population is most often affected, though the incidence of the disease has decreased recently.

Radiographic Appearance

Cardiovascular syphilis involves primarily the ascending aorta, which may become aneurysmally dilated and often demonstrates linear calcification of the wall (Figure 11-1). Syphilitic aortitis often involves the aortic valvular ring and produces aortic regurgitation with enlargement of the left ventricle.

Syphilitic involvement of the skeletal system most commonly produces radiographic findings of chronic osteomyelitis, which usually affects the long bones and the skull. The destruction of bone incites a prominent periosteal reaction, with dense sclerosis as the most outstanding feature (Figure 11-2). Syphilis is a major cause of neuropathic joint disease (Charcot's joint), in which bone resorption and total disorganization of the joint are associated with calcific and bony debris (Figure 11-3).

Syphilitic lesions developing in the cerebral cortex can cause mental disorders, deafness, and blindness. The cerebral lesions (intracerebral gummata) containing syphilis bacteria are hypodense on nonenhanced CT. On T1-weighted MR images, the lesions

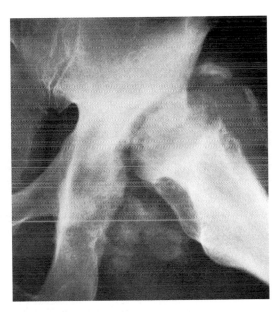

FIGURE 11-3 Neuropathic joint disease in syphilis. Joint fragmentation, sclerosis, and calcific debris about the hip.

appear hypointense or isointense, and they become hyperintense on T2-weighted images. The intracerebral gummata densely enhance with the administration of gadolinium. Single-photon emission computed tomography (SPECT) demonstrates the significant decrease of blood flow in the frontal and temporal cortices bilaterally. Scans following therapy

SUMMARY *of* FINDINGS *for* Infectious Diseases of the Reproductive System

disorder	location	radiographic appearance	treatment
Syphilis	Male and female reproductive organs	Cardiovascular—aortic dilatation with possible calcification Skeletal radiograph—chronic osteomyelitis of long bones and skull; periosteal reaction with dense sclerosis CT—intracerebral gummata are hypodense on nonenhanced scans MRI—On T1-weighted images, the lesions appear hypo- or isointense; they are hyperintense on T2-weighted images; intracerebral gummata densely enhance with contrast SPECT—decreased cortical flow in frontal and temporal cortices bilaterally; post-therapeutic scans demonstrate a marked improvement in flow	Primary and secondary—antibiotics Tertiary—incurable
Gonorrhea	Male and female reproductive organs	Skeletal—septic arthritis with articular erosion and joint space narrowing PID—US or CT demonstrates thick, dilated fallopian tubes or abscess formation	Penicillin; if penicillin-resistant, ceftriaxone

GI, Gastrointestinal; *PID,* pelvic inflammatory disease; *US,* ultrasound.

demonstrate a marked improvement in flow. Diffuse thickening of the gastric wall can cause narrowing of the lumen indistinguishable from carcinoma.

Multiple bone abnormalities can occur in infants with congenital syphilis who are born to infected mothers (Figure 11-4). Mental retardation, deafness, and blindness are common complications.

Treatment

In the primary and secondary stages of syphilis, antibiotic therapy cures the disease. The ulcerations in primary syphilis and the skin lesions and rash in secondary syphilis heal in a few days with penicillin, doxycycline, or tetracycline. The tertiary stage is incurable.

Gonorrhea

Gonorrhea is a bacterial infection that is one of the most common and widespread of the venereal diseases and occurs more commonly in men (1.5:1). Persons of Asian and Pacific Island descent are least likely affected, whereas the African-American population is experiencing the greatest increase. Symptoms usually occur a few days after infection. An acute urethritis with copious discharge of pus develops in men. Women may be asymptomatic or have minimal symptoms of urethral or cervical inflammation. If untreated, the inflammation may become chronic, spread upward, and produce fibrosis, leading to urethral stricture in men (Figure 11-5) and pelvic inflammatory disease (PID) or sterility in women. A serious complication is fibrous scarring of the fallopian tubes that may result in sterility or an ectopic pregnancy.

Radiographic Appearance

Gonorrheal infection can cause septic arthritis leading to articular erosion and joint space narrowing.

For patients suspected of PID, ultrasound or CT is the modality of choice for demonstrating thick, dilated fallopian tubes or abscess formation. Ultrasound is superior for showing ectopic pregnancy.

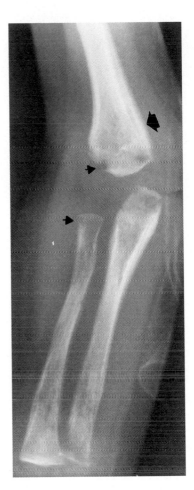

FIGURE 11-4 Congenital syphilis. Transverse bands of decreased density across the metaphyses *(small arrows)* associated with patchy areas of bone destruction in the diaphyses. Solid periosteal new bone formation *(large arrow)* is best seen about the distal humerus.

Treatment

Gonorrhea usually responds rapidly to antibiotic therapy (penicillin). Recently, penicillin-resistant gonorrhea has been reported that requires a single intramuscular dose of ceftriaxone.

MALE REPRODUCTIVE SYSTEM

Physiology of the Male Reproductive System

The major function of the male reproductive system is the formation of sperm **(spermatogenesis)**, which begins at about 13 years of age and continues throughout life. Under the influence of follicle-stimulating hormone (FSH) secreted by the anterior lobe of the pituitary gland, the seminiferous tubules of the testes are stimulated to produce the male germ cells called spermatozoa. In addition to producing sperm cells, the testes secrete the male hormone **testosterone**. This substance stimulates the development and activity of the accessory sex organs (prostate, seminal vesicles) and is responsible for adult male sexual behavior. Testosterone causes the typical male changes that occur at puberty, including the development of facial and body hair and alterations in the larynx that result in a deepened voice. Testosterone also helps regulate metabolism by promoting growth of skeletal muscles and is thus responsible for the greater male muscular development and strength.

The final maturation of sperm occurs in the **epididymis**, a tightly coiled tube enclosed in a fibrous

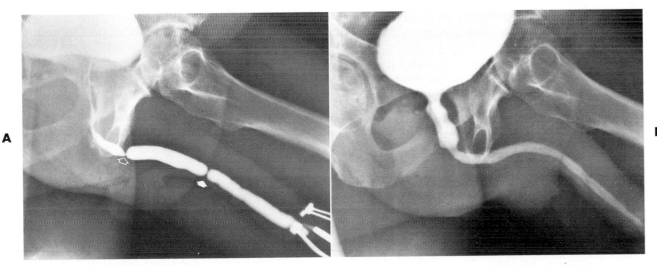

FIGURE 11-5 Gonococcal urethral stricture. **A,** Initial retrograde urethrogram shows diffuse stricture of the bulbar urethra and high-grade stenoses in proximal *(solid arrow)* and distal *(open arrow)* portions of the urethra. **B,** After balloon dilation, a voiding urethrogram shows considerable improvement in the appearance of the urethra.

casing. The sperm spend about 1 to 3 weeks in this segment of the duct system, where they become motile and capable of fertilizing an ovum. The tail of the epididymis leads into the **vas deferens,** a muscular tube that passes through the inguinal canal as part of the spermatic cord and joins the duct from the **seminal vesicle** to form the ejaculatory duct. Depending on the degree of sexual activity and frequency of ejaculation, sperm may remain in the vas deferens up to 1 month with no loss of fertility. Severing of the vas deferens **(vasectomy)** is an operation performed to make a man sterile. Vasectomy interrupts the route from the epididymis to the remainder of the genital tract.

The seminal vesicles lie on the posterior aspect of the base of the bladder and secrete a thick liquid that is rich in fructose, a simple sugar that serves as an energy source for sperm motility after ejaculation. The seminal vesicles also secrete prostaglandin, which increases uterine contractions in the woman and helps propel the sperm toward the fallopian tubes.

The **prostate gland** lies just below the bladder and surrounds the urethra. It secretes a thin alkaline substance that constitutes the major portion of the seminal fluid volume. The alkalinity of this material is essential to sperm motility, which would otherwise be inhibited by the highly acidic vaginal secretions.

Intense sexual stimulation causes peristaltic contractions in the walls of the epididymis and vas deferens, propelling sperm into the urethra. At the same time, the seminal vesicles and prostate gland release their secretions, which mix with the mucous secretion of the bulbourethral glands to form semen. The ejaculation of semen occurs when intense muscular contractions of erectile tissue cause the semen to be expressed through the urethral opening.

Male fertility is related not only to the number of sperm ejaculated but also to their size, shape, and motility. Although only one sperm fertilizes an ovum, millions of sperm seem to be necessary for fertilization to occur. Indeed, it is estimated that sterility may result when the sperm count falls below about 50 million/ml of semen.

Benign Prostatic Hyperplasia

Enlargement of the prostate gland is common in men more than 60 years of age and may be detected on a digital rectal examination. The enlargement is probably related to a disturbance of hormone secretions from the sex glands that occurs as the period of reproductive activity declines. The major effect of prostatic enlargement is an inability to empty the bladder completely, leading to partial urinary tract obstruction, bilateral ureteral dilatation, and hydronephrosis.

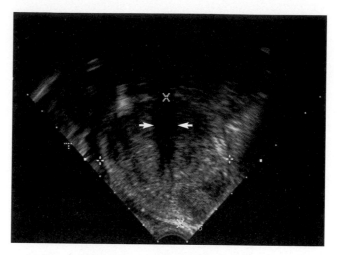

FIGURE 11-6 Benign prostatic hyperplasia. Transrectal ultrasound in the sagittal plane demonstrates enlargement of the central periurethral soft tissue consistent with benign prostatic hyperplasia *(measurement markers)*. The Eiffel Tower sign is caused by an enlarged urethra *(arrows)*.

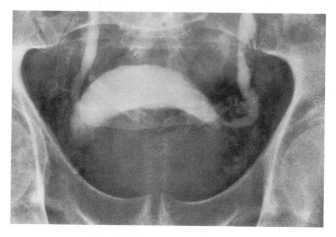

FIGURE 11-7 Benign prostatic hyperplasia. Large, smooth filling defect at the base of the bladder. Notice the fish-hook as appearance of the distal ureters and calcification in the vas deferens.

Radiographic Appearance

Transrectal ultrasound, performed by means of a probe inserted into the rectum, demonstrates gland enlargement and heterogeneous signal intensity of the central portion (Figure 11-6). A circumferential surgical pseudocapsule, discrete nodules, and a thickened bladder wall may also be visualized. Moreover, an abdominal-pelvic scan can demonstrate residual urine volume and aids in the evaluation of the kidneys for the presence of hydronephrosis.

On excretory urography, the enlarged prostate typically produces elevation and a smooth impression on the floor of the contrast material–filled bladder (Figure 11-7). Elevation of the insertion of the ureters on the trigone of the bladder produces a characteristic J-shaped, or fish-hook, appearance of the distal ureters. Residual urine in the bladder provides a growth medium for bacterial infection, which produces cystitis; the infection may ascend from the bladder to the kidney, resulting in pyelonephritis.

On MR images, benign prostatic hyperplasia causes a diffuse or nodular area of homogeneous low signal intensity on T1-weighted images and an inhomogeneous, mixed (intermediate to high) signal intensity on T2-weighted images (Figure 11-8). A pseudocapsule, representing compression of adjacent tissue visualized as a low signal intensity rim, often accentuates focal enlargement. Diffuse enlargement shows similar intensity changes, though the pseudocapsule is not present. Unfortunately, the intensity of benign prostatic hyperplasia may often be similar to that of the normal prostate or a region of prostatitis.

Treatment

Surgical resection of the prostate (transurethral resection, or TUR) can relieve the obstructive symptoms.

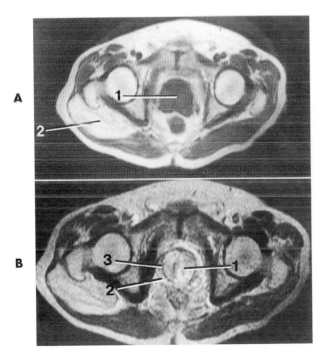

FIGURE **11-8** Benign prostatic hyperplasia. **A,** T1-weighted MR image shows prostatic enlargement of homogeneous low signal intensity (1). Notice high signal intensity of the large lipoma (2) in the right gluteal region. **B,** On T2-weighted image, intermediate signal intensity of the enlarged transitional zone (1) shows increased inhomogeneity and is separated from the high signal intensity peripheral zone (2) by a low signal intensity rim of pseudocapsule.

Carcinoma of the Prostate Gland

Carcinoma of the prostate gland is the second most common malignancy in men, with a slightly higher incidence in black men. The disease rarely occurs before 50 years of age, and the incidence increases by about 40% with advancing age. The tumor can be slow growing and asymptomatic for long periods or can behave aggressively with extensive metastases. Prostate carcinoma occurs most often in the peripheral zone (70%). Carcinoma of the prostate is best detected by palpation of a hard, nodular, and irregular mass on a routine rectal examination. The presence of an elevated serum PSA (prostate specific antigen) indicates an abnomality, though this blood test is not specific for malignancy.

Radiographic Appearance

Radiographically, carcinoma of the prostate often elevates and impresses the floor of the contrast-filled bladder. Unlike the smooth contour seen in benign prostatic hyperplasia, in carcinoma the impression on the bladder floor is usually more irregular (Figure 11-9). Bladder neck obstruction, infiltration of the trigone, or invasive obstruction of the ureters above the bladder may produce obstruction of the upper urinary tract.

Transrectal ultrasound is the preferred technique for detecting carcinoma of the prostate (Figure 11-10). The normal prostate has a generally homogeneous

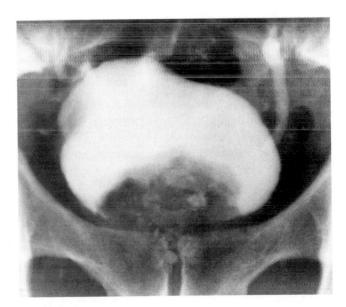

FIGURE **11-9** Carcinoma of the prostate. A large, irregular mass elevates and impresses the floor of the contrast agent–filled bladder.

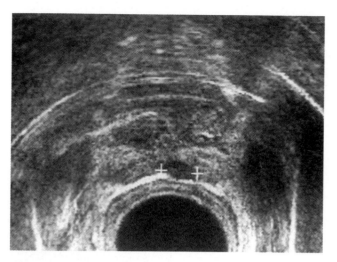

FIGURE 11-10 Cancer of the prostate. Transrectal ultrasound demonstrates hypoechoic mass (between cursors) with the capsule still intact.

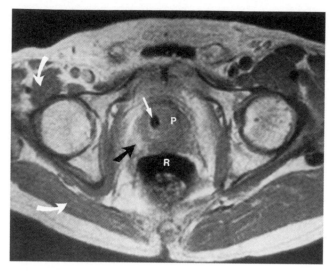

FIGURE 11-11 Carcinoma of the prostate. Axial MR image through the pelvis demonstrates an abnormal area of increased signal intensity *(black arrow)* within the prostate gland *(P)*. A Foley catheter is in place *(straight white arrow)*, and the rectum *(R)* contains air and feces. Note the decreased size of the pelvic musculature on the right *(curved white arrows)* in this patient with an above-knee amputation.

appearance with a moderate echo pattern. Early studies indicated that prostatic carcinoma appeared as hyperechoic areas. However, with the development of newer and higher frequency transducers, many carcinomas appear as areas of low echogenicity within the prostate. Up to 40% of carcinomas are isoechoic with normal prostate tissue and thus cannot be visualized on ultrasound. The most recent studies have concluded that the wide range of sonographic patterns in carcinoma indicates that ultrasound cannot reliably differentiate prostatic malignancy from benign disease.

Staging

MRI can superbly delineate the prostate, seminal vesicles, and surrounding organs to provide accurate staging of pelvic neoplasms. When the spin-echo technique is used, the central and peripheral zones of the prostate are well demonstrated and distinctly separate from the surrounding levator ani muscles. In the sagittal plane, the relation of the prostate to the bladder, rectum, and seminal vesicles is clearly shown. Prostatic carcinoma is best demonstrated on long TR images, where it appears as disruption of the normally uniform high signal intensity of the peripheral zone of the prostate (Figure 11-11). T2-weighted images demonstrate low intensity that is surrounded by the hyperintense signal of the normal tissue. The new technique of MR lymphography aids in visualizing nonenlarged pelvic lymph nodes. However, there is much controversy over whether MRI is reliable for detection and diagnosis of prostate cancer, and therefore a precise diagnosis requires a biopsy and histologic examination. It has been demonstrated that a normal-appearing

prostate gland on MRI does not exclude the presence of a neoplasm. In addition, inhomogeneity of the gland is a common nonspecific finding that can also be seen in patients with adenoma or prostatitis.

Carcinoma of the prostate may spread by direct extension or by way of the lymphatics or the bloodstream. Spread of carcinoma of the prostate to the rectum can produce a large, smooth, concave pressure defect; a fungating ulcerated mass simulating primary rectal carcinoma; or a long, asymmetric annular stricture. Both ultrasound and CT, especially the arterial phase of multislice CT, aid in defining extension of tumor into the bladder and seminal vesicles and in detecting metastases in enlarged lymph nodes (Figure 11-12).

The most common hematogenous metastases are to bone. They involve primarily the pelvis, thoracolumbar spine, femurs, and ribs. These lesions are most commonly osteoblastic and appear as multiple rounded foci of sclerotic density (Figure 11-13) or occasionally diffuse sclerosis involving an entire bone ("ivory vertebra"). Patients with bony metastases usually have strikingly elevated levels of serum acid phosphatase. Because significant bone destruction or bone reaction must occur before a lesion can be detected on plain radiographs, the radionuclide bone scan is the best screening technique for detection of asymptomatic skeletal metastases in patients with carcinoma of the prostate. However, since the radionuclide scan is very sensitive but not specific and may show increased

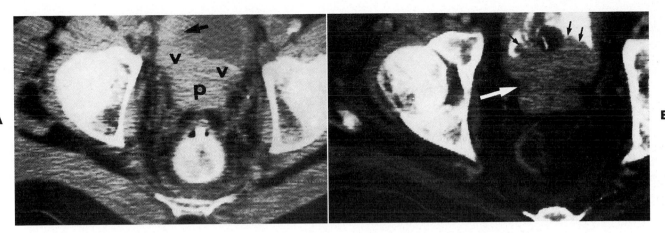

FIGURE 11-12 Metastatic carcinoma of the prostate gland. **A,** CT scan shows prostatic carcinoma *(p)* invading the wall of the bladder *(arrow)* and the seminal vesicles *(v)*. **B,** In another patient, CT scan shows prostatic carcinoma involving the bladder *(black arrows)* and seminal vesicles. The normally sharp angle between the seminal vesicles and the prostate is lost *(white arrow)*.

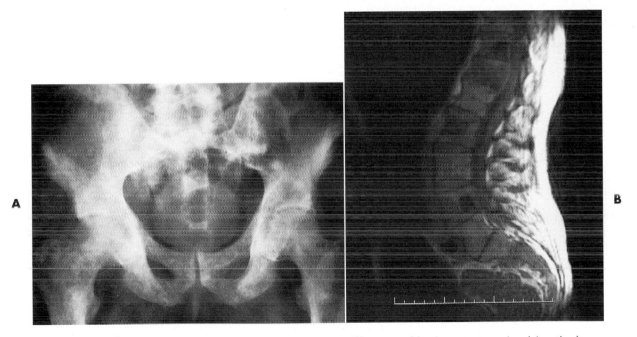

FIGURE 11-13 Metastatic carcinoma of the prostate. **A,** Diffuse osteoblastic metastases involving the bones about the pelvis. **B,** T1-weighted spin-echo MR image illustrates osteoblastic lesions throughout the spine.

uptake in multiple disorders of the bone, conventional radiography of the affected site should be performed when an abnormal scan is obtained.

Treatment

For a tumor confined to the prostate gland, a successful cure can be achieved by a radical prostatectomy or radiation therapy. Prostate tumors with local invasion require both a radical prostatectomy and radiation therapy. Radiation therapy may consist of iodine-125 seed implantation. Stage D prostate cancers, the most progressive, require hormonal therapy (antiandrogen drugs) to slow the spread of disease and palliative measures to reduce pain. In some cases orchiectomy (removal of the testes) is performed.

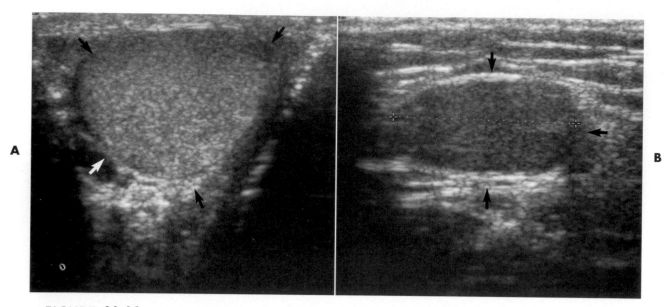

FIGURE 11-14 Undescended testes. Ultrasound in the transverse plane **(A)** illustrates a normal right testis and in the longitudinal plane **(B)** demonstrates the undescended left testis, smaller and less echogenic, located in the inguinal canal.

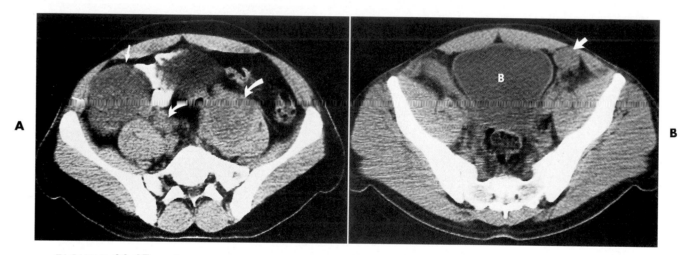

FIGURE 11-15 Malignant neoplasms developing in one of the bilateral undescended testes. **A,** Undescended right testis is enlarged by carcinoma *(straight arrows)*. The tumor has metastasized to the lymph nodes *(curved arrows)*, which are enlarged. **B,** Nontumorous intraabdominal left testis *(arrow)* appears as a smaller, rounded structure adjacent to the bladder *(B)*.

Undescended Testis (Cryptorchidism)

Near the end of gestation, the testis normally migrates from its intraabdominal position through the inguinal canal into the scrotal sac. This condition is more common in premature males and can cause infertility. If one of the testicles cannot be palpated within the scrotum, it is important to determine whether this represents an absent testis or an ectopic position of the testis. The rate of malignancy is up to 40 times higher in the undescended (intraabdominal) than in the descended testicle.

Radiographic Appearance

In the absence of a palpable testicle, ultrasound is usually used as a screening technique. This modality carries no radiation risk and has a high diagnostic accuracy in demonstrating undescended testicles that are located in the inguinal canal (Figure 11-14). However, sonography is not successful in detecting ectopic testicles in the pelvis or abdomen. If ultrasound fails to demonstrate an undescended testis, MRI or CT is indicated (Figures 11-15 and 11-16). MRI typically demonstrates a low signal mass on T1-weighted images that has high signal intensity on T2-weighted scans. The uniform oval soft tissue mass

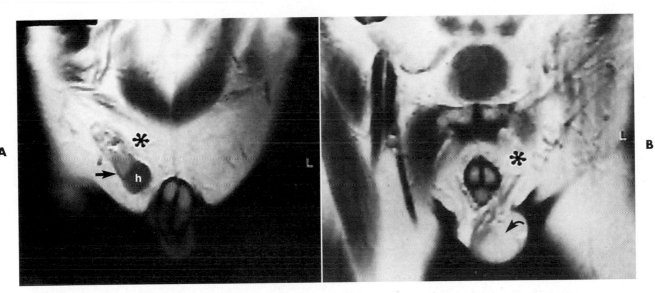

FIGURE 11-16 Atrophic undescended testis. **A,** Coronal MR scan shows a small, intermediate signal intensity testis *(arrow)* associated with low signal intensity hydrocele *(h)*. The signal intensity of the testis is low compared with that of fat *(*)*. **B,** Image slightly posterior to **A** shows the normally descended contralateral testis *(curved arrow)*, which demonstrates high signal intensity similar to that of fat *(*)*.

of an undescended testis demonstrates contrast enhancement on CT.

Treatment

Because of the extremely high rate of malignancy, the diagnosis of undescended testis usually leads to orchiopexy (surgical fixation of an undescended testis into the scrotum) in patients younger than 10 years of age. Spontaneous descent may occur in the first 6 months, and hormonal therapy may stimulate descent. Surgical placement of the testis through the inguinal canal into the scrotal sac, a procedure known as orchiopexy, may be an alternative to salvage fertility. Orchiectomy (surgical removal) is recommended in those seen after puberty.

Testicular Torsion and Epididymitis

Testicular torsion refers to the twisting of the gonad on its pedicle, which leads to the compromise of circulation and the sudden onset of severe scrotal pain. Although primarily a clinical diagnosis, the scrotal pain and swelling of testicular torsion may be difficult to distinguish from those caused by inflammation of the epididymis (epididymitis). In such cases, color Doppler ultrasound or radionuclide studies are of value.

Radiographic Appearance

The preferred imaging modality depends on the patient's age—generally color Doppler ultrasound in adults and radionuclide studies for children. As

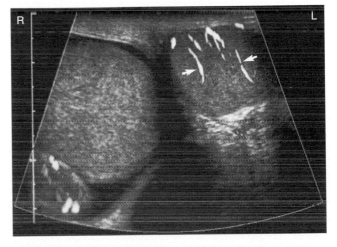

FIGURE 11-17 Testicular torsion. Doppler ultrasound on a 3-year-old boy demonstrates an abnormal to absent blood flow in the right testicle and a normal blood flow *(arrows)* in the left testicle. Surgical correction was performed, saving the testis.

new technology improves color and power, Doppler ultrasound is the modality of choice in most cases. Doppler ultrasound demonstrates the presence of intratesticular arterial pulsations. In testicular torsion, the arterial perfusion is diminished or absent (Figures 11-17 and 11-18), whereas in epididymitis there is increased blood flow (Figure 11-19). Similarly, the radionuclide angiogram shows isotope activity on the twisted side that is either slightly decreased or at the normal, barely

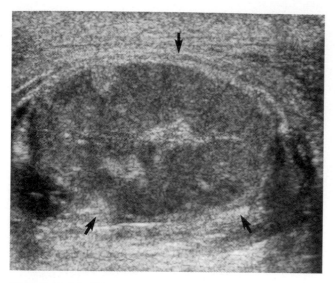

FIGURE 11-18 Testicular torsion. Scrotal ultrasound on a 16-year-old boy demonstrates the left testicle *(arrows)* without arterial blood flow, a complex heterogeneous echogenicity (indicates necrotic tissue), and a thickened scrotal wall. At surgery the testicle remained discolored and was removed.

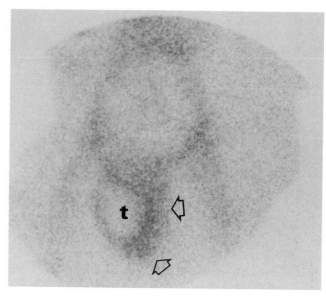

FIGURE 11-20 Testicular torsion. Severe diminished arterial perfusion causes the testicle to appear as a rounded, cold area *(t)* on a radionuclide scan. The surrounding rim of increased activity represents the blood supply to the scrotal sac *(arrows)*.

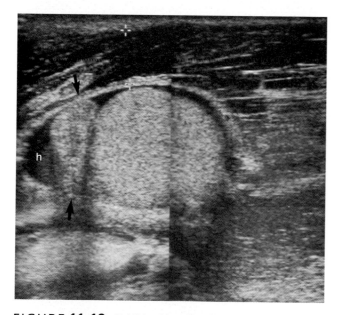

FIGURE 11-19 Epididymitis. A longitudinal ultrasound scan from an 80-year-old man demonstrates an enlarged hypoechoic epididymis *(arrows)* with a moderate-sized hydrocele *(h)*.

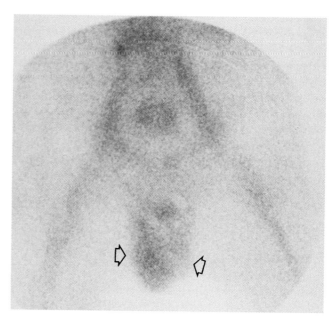

FIGURE 11-21 Epididymitis. Radionuclide scan shows high isotope uptake in the region of the testicle *(arrows)* caused by increased blood flow.

perceptible level. On the uninvolved side, the perfusion should be normal. When compared with the decreased activity on the involved side, the perfusion appears increased. Static nuclear scans demonstrate a rounded, cold area replacing the testicle in

patients with torsion (Figure 11-20), but a hot area in those with epididymitis (Figure 11-21). A nuclear testicular scan is superior to Doppler ultrasound for distinguishing between testicular torsion and epididymitis.

Treatment

Immediate surgery must be performed within 5 or 6 hours of the onset of pain to preserve the testis. For epididymitis, bed rest, scrotal support, and antibiotics are prescribed for all bacterial infections.

Testicular Tumors

Testicular tumors are the most common neoplasms in men between 20 and 35 years of age. Almost all testicular tumors are malignant, and they tend to metastasize to the lymphatics that follow the course of the testicular arteries and veins and drain into paraaortic lymph nodes at the level of the kidneys.

There are two major types of testicular tumors. Seminomas constitute about 45% of germ cell tumors; the remaining 55% are nonseminomas that consist of teratomas and other germ cell tumors. Seminomas arise from the seminiferous tubules, whereas teratomas arise from a primitive germ cell and consist of a variety of tissues.

Radiographic Appearance

Testicular tumors are best diagnosed on ultrasound examination (with 98% to 100% accuracy). The normal testis has a homogeneous, medium-level echogenicity. A localized testicular tumor appears as a circumscribed mass with either increased or decreased echogenicity in an otherwise uniform-echo testicular structure. Seminomas appear as uniform hypoechoic masses without calcification or cystic areas (Figure 11-22). A teratoma appears inhomogeneous with cystic and solid areas of calcification and cartilage (Figure 11-23). Testicular tumors can also be detected on MRI (Figure 11-24), which is required when ultrasound is equivocal or when there is discrepancy between the ultrasound and the physical examination.

Lymphatic metastases from testicular tumors typically occur at the level of the renal hilum (where the gonadal veins drain) and are best detected by CT (Figure 11-25). This modality also can detect spread of tumor to the lung or liver.

Treatment

All testicular cancers are removed (orchiectomy). Seminomas are radiosensitive, and early diagnosis and irradiation have resulted in many cures. Teratomas are surgically removed; if malignant, surgery is followed by radiation therapy and chemotherapy (consisting of several cytotoxic drugs in combination). Follow-up examinations are required to rule out metastasis.

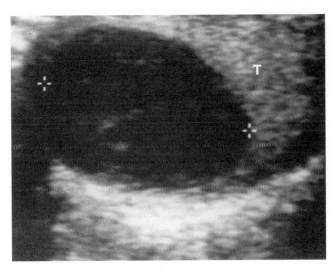

FIGURE 11-22 Seminoma. A well-circumscribed, predominantly hypoechoic, intratesticular mass *(cursors)* with echogenicity markedly less than that of the normal adjacent testis *(T)* is characteristic of a seminoma.

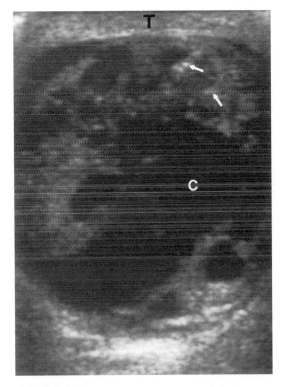

FIGURE 11-23 Malignant teratoma. A transverse testicular scan demonstrates a large malignant teratoma replacing most of the testis. Cystic *(C)* and solid elements with small echogenic foci *(arrows)* from small calcifications are present. *T,* Residual normal testis.

SUMMARY *of* FINDINGS *for* Diseases of the Male Reproductive System

disorder	location	radiographic appearance	treatment
Benign prostatic hyperplasia	Enlargement of prostate gland	US—transrectal inner gland enlargement (relatively hypoechoic compared with the peripheral zone) IVU—elevation and smooth impression of floor in a contrast agent–filled bladder; distal ureters produce a characteristic J-shaped appearance MRI—diffuse or nodular area of homogeneous low signal intensity on T1-weighted images and an inhomogeneous, mixed (intermediate-to-high) signal intensity on T2-weighted images	Surgical resection to relieve symptoms
Carcinoma of the prostate gland	Prostate gland	IVU—irregular elevation of floor of a contrast agent–filled bladder with possible obstruction US—transrectal wide range of sonographic patterns, depending on glandular area involved MRI—on long TR images, loss of uniform high signal intensity of the peripheral zone	Radical prostatectomy Local invasion—surgery and radiation therapy (seeds) Stage D—hormonal therapy, palliative measures
Undescended testis	Inguinal or ectopic testicle	US—demonstrates inguinal testicle MRI—demonstrates ectopic undescended testis; low signal mass on T1-weighted images that has high signal on T2-weighted images CT—uniformly enhanced, oval soft tissue mass	Spontaneous descent Hormonal therapy Orchiopexy—surgical attachment in the scrotum Orchiectomy
Testicular torsion	Testes	Color Doppler US—in torsion the arterial perfusion is diminished or absent; epididymitis causes increased blood flow	Immediate surgery to preserve testis
Epididymitis	Inflammation of the epididymis	Radionuclide angiogram—torsion has a slightly decreased normal intake, cold areas on static scan; epididymitis appears as a hot area on a static scan	Bed rest, scrotal support, and antibiotics
Testicular tumors	Seminomas (seminiferous tubules) Teratomas (primitive germ cell)	US—seminomas appear uniformly hypoechoic without calcifications; teratomas inhomogeneous mass with cystic and solid areas MRI—T2-weighted image demonstrates inhomogeneous signal intensity CT—demonstrates lymphatic involvement as low attenuation nodules	Orchiectomy Seminomas—radiosensitive Cancerous teratomas—surgery, radiation therapy, and chemotherapy

IVU, Intravenous urography; *US,* ultrasound.

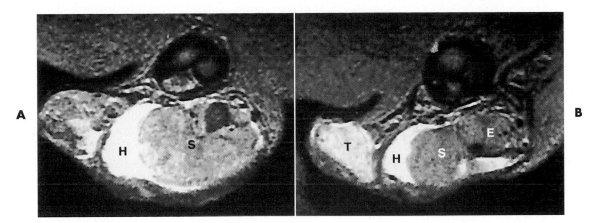

FIGURE 11-24 Testicular seminoma. **A,** T2-weighted MR scan shows that the signal intensity of the semi-noma *(S)* in the left testis is inhomogeneous, and its contrast is markedly different from that of the adjacent hydro-cele *(H)*. **B,** Inhomogeneous intermediate signal intensity of intratesticular tumor *(S)* extends into the epididymis *(E)*. Note that the normal contralateral testis *(T)* demonstrates a much higher signal intensity.

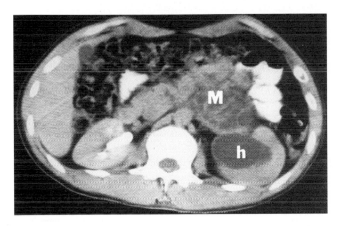

FIGURE 11-25 Metastatic testicular seminoma. CT scan through the level of the kidneys shows diffuse nodal metas-tases *(M)* containing characteristic low-attenuation areas. Extrinsic pressure on the lower left ureter has caused severe hydronephrosis with dilatation of the renal pelvis *(h)*.

FEMALE REPRODUCTIVE SYSTEM

Physiology of the Female Reproductive System

The ovaries are the equivalent of the testes in the male and are responsible for the production of ova and the secretion of female hormones. A woman's reproductive life begins with the onset of menstruation, **menarche,** which generally occurs between 11 and 15 years of age. Once each month, on about the first day of men-struation, several primitive graafian follicles and their enclosed ova begin to grow and develop, and the fol-licular cells start to secrete **estrogen**. In most cycles, only one follicle matures and migrates to the surface

of the ovary, where it ruptures and expels the mature ovum into the pelvic cavity **(ovulation)**.

After the release of the ovum, the remaining cells of the ruptured follicle enlarge and a golden colored pigment (lutein) is deposited in their cytoplasm. This **corpus luteum** continues to grow for 7 to 8 days and secretes **progesterone** in increasing amounts. If fer-tilization of the ovum has not occurred, the size and secretions of the corpus luteum gradually diminish until the nonfunctional structure is reduced to a white scar (corpus albicans) that moves into the cen-tral portion of the ovary and eventually disappears. If fertilization does occur, however, the corpus luteum remains intact throughout pregnancy.

The cyclic changes in the ovaries are controlled by a variety of substances secreted by the anterior pituitary gland. Growth of the primitive graaf-ian follicles and ova and the secretion of estrogen are controlled by FSH, whereas rupture of the fol-licle, expulsion of its ripe ovum, and the secretion of progesterone are under the control of luteinizing hormone (LH).

The fallopian tubes serve as ducts for the ovaries, even though they are not directly attached to them. The union of an ovum and a spermatozoon (fer-tilization) normally occurs in the fallopian tubes. About 1 day later, the resulting embryo reaches the uterus, where it begins to implant itself in the endo-metrium. Occasionally, implantation occurs in the fallopian tube or pelvic cavity instead of the uterus, resulting in an **ectopic pregnancy**. Within 10 days, there is the earliest development of the placenta, which is derived in part from both the develop-ing embryo and the maternal tissues and serves to nourish the fetus and anchor it to the uterus. Al-though they are closely related, maternal and fetal blood do not mix, and the exchange of nutrients occurs across the important fetal membrane termed the **chorion**.

The menstrual cycle refers to the changes in the endometrium of the uterus that occur in women throughout the childbearing years. Each cycle lasts about 28 days and is divided into three phases: proliferative, secretory, and menstrual. Although the first day of menstruation is normally considered as the first day of the cycle, for ease of description the menstrual phase will be described last.

The **proliferative, or postmenstrual, phase** occurs between the end of the menses and ovulation. Production of estrogen by ovarian follicular cells under the influence of FSH causes proliferation of the endometrium of the uterus. In a typical 28-day cycle, the proliferative phase usually includes cycle days 6 to 13 or 14. However, there is far more variability in the length of this phase than in the others.

The **secretory, or postovulatory, phase** occurs between ovulation and the onset of the menses. The high level of estrogen in the blood after ovulation inhibits the secretion of FSH, and the anterior lobe of the pituitary gland begins to secrete LH. This stimulates the corpus luteum to produce the hormone progesterone, which stimulates a further increase in the thickness of the endometrium and prepares the uterus for implantation of the ovum should fertilization occur. The length of the secretory phase is fairly constant and usually lasts 14 days.

If fertilization of the ovum does not occur, the high level of progesterone in the blood inhibits the secretion of LH so that the corpus luteum begins to degenerate and ceases to produce progesterone. As the superficial layers of the hypertrophied endometrium begin to break down, denuded bleeding areas are exposed. The flow of blood, mucus, and sloughed endometrium from the uterus is called the menstrual flow. This **menstrual phase** of the cycle lasts about 4 to 6 days, until the low level of progesterone causes the pituitary gland to again secrete FSH and a new menstrual cycle begins. Of course, if the ovum is fertilized, the corpus luteum does not degenerate, and the endometrium remains intact throughout pregnancy.

The reproductive years terminate with the cessation of menstrual periods **(menopause),** which usually begins when a woman is in her late 40s or early 50s.

Pelvic Inflammatory Disease

Inflammation of the pelvic reproductive organs is usually the result of venereal disease (especially gonorrhea) in women of childbearing age, with the peak incidence between the ages of 20 and 24. It can also develop from an unsterile abortion or delivery, multiple sexual partners, or it may be a complication of intrauterine devices. If PID is not promptly and adequately treated, spread of infection to the fallopian tubes may cause fibrous adhesions that obstruct the inner portion near the uterus. If the outer ends of the tubes remain open, the spill of purulent material can lead to peritonitis and the formation of a pelvic abscess. More commonly the outer ends close, and the fallopian tubes fill with pus **(pyosalpinx)**. After antibiotic therapy, the infection subsides, and the tubes may remain filled with a watery fluid **(hydrosalpinx)**. Obstruction of the fallopian tubes can result in infertility or ectopic pregnancy. Spread of infection to involve the ovaries can produce tubo-ovarian abscesses, which are usually bilateral.

Radiographic Appearance

Ultrasound is the imaging procedure of choice for detecting PID and pelvic abscesses. The transabdominal approach best demonstrates the extent of the disease process, whereas the endovaginal approach is most sensitive for detecting dilated tubes, inflammatory changes, and abscesses. The fluid-filled urinary bladder provides an excellent acoustic window and permits confusing loops of small bowel to be displaced out of the pelvis. Endometritis may occur after childbirth or in association with PID. Ultrasound demonstrates a thickened endometrium, possibly with irregularity that may contain fluid (Figure 11-26). Pyosalpinx and tubo-ovarian abscesses typically are seen as tubular adnexal masses that are sonolucent and compatible with fluid collections (Figure 11-27). However, abscesses may also have thick and irregular (or "shaggy") walls or may contain echoes or fluid levels representing the layering of purulent debris (Figure 11-28). In severe cases, CT may aid in assessing the full extent of the disease. MRI is unnecessary unless the patient has an iodine allergy.

The status of the fallopian tubes can be assessed radiographically by hysterosalpingography, in which the uterine cavity and fallopian tubes are opacified after the injection of contrast material into the uterus. In the woman with normal patent fallopian tubes, contrast material extravasating into the pelvic peritoneal cavity outlines the peritoneal surfaces and often loops of bowel within the pelvis (Figure 11-29). If the fallopian tubes are occluded by fibrosis from PID or developmental anomalies, there is no evidence of the contrast material reaching the peritoneal cavity (Figure 11-30).

Plain abdominal or pelvic radiographs are of little value in detecting PID and pelvic abscesses. Abnormal gas collections can be masked by fecal material in the rectum and in loops of small bowel.

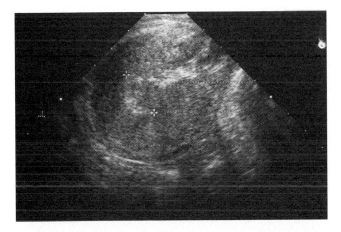

FIGURE 11-26 Endometritis. Ultrasound illustrates an enlarged endometrial cavity with a heterogeneous echogenicity (between *cursors*) associated with a therapeutic abortion.

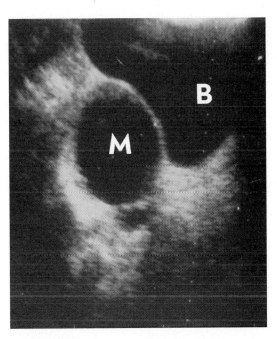

FIGURE 11-27 Tubo-ovarian abscess. Ultrasound scan demonstrates a large sonolucent mass *(M)* posterior to the bladder *(B)*.

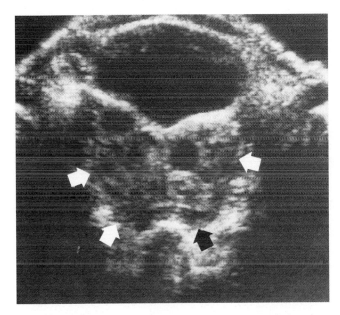

FIGURE 11-28 Chronic PID. Transverse sonogram demonstrates large, complex cystic and echogenic masses *(arrows)* posterior to the echo-free bladder.

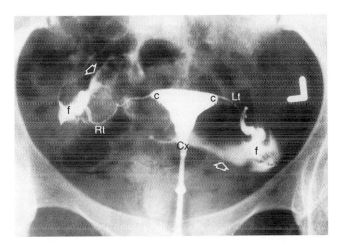

FIGURE 11-29 Normal hysterosalpingogram. Arrows point to a bilateral spill of contrast material into the peritoneal cavity. *Cx,* internal cervical os; *c,* cornua of the uterus; *f,* fimbriated portion of fallopian tube; *Rt* and *Lt,* right and left fallopian tubes.

Treatment

Antibiotic therapy and abstaining from sexual intercourse until the inflammation subsides are the usual treatments. In more complex instances, ultrasound-guided aspiration and drainage may be required. Thick purulent materials require catheter drainage; most nonpurulent abscesses need only aspiration. The healing phase may leave the fallopian tubes scarred and obstructed.

Cysts and Tumors

Ovarian Cysts and Tumors

Physiologic ovarian cysts are most common in the female infant and in women of childbearing age. They include follicular cysts (unruptured, enlarged follicles) and corpus luteum cysts, which occur after continued hemorrhage or lack of resolution of the corpus luteum. Polycystic ovarian syndrome (PCOS) is characterized by multiple ovarian cysts, which may interfere with the physiology of the ovary. This is considered the most common genital disorder found in young women.

The most common malignancies involving the ovaries are metastatic tumors, which primarily arise from carcinomas of the breast, colon, and stomach. They are frequently bilateral and often asymptomatic.

Radiographic Appearance

On ultrasound, cysts appear as rounded, anechoic adnexal masses (Figure 11-31). On ultrasound, PCOS demonstrates 10 or more cysts peripherally in the echodense stroma. **Primary cystadenocarcinoma** of

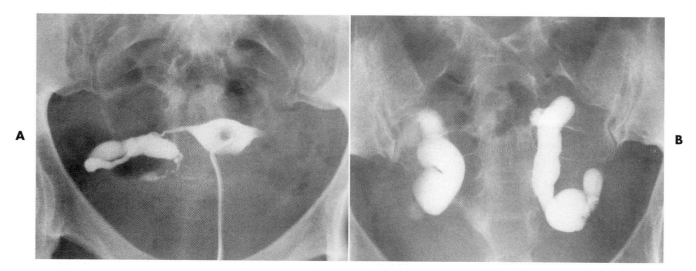

FIGURE 11-30 Hydrosalpinx. Unilateral **(A)** and bilateral **(B)** gross dilatation of fallopian tubes without evidence of free spill of contrast material into peritoneal cavity.

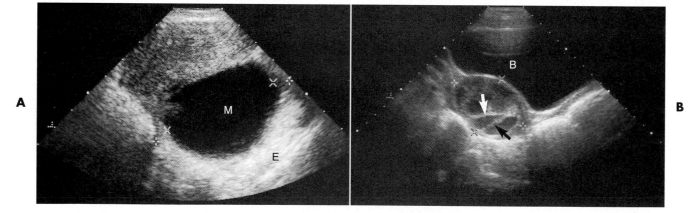

FIGURE 11-31 Ovarian cysts. **A,** Ultrasound scan demonstrates a large (5 × 6 cm) sonolucent mass *(M)* with back wall enhancement *(E)* involving the right ovary. **B,** In another patient, the longitudinal scan of the right ovary demonstrates a septated *(arrows)* mass (between *cursors*) with homogeneous sonolucent components measuring 5 × 6.7 cm located posterior to the bladder *(B)*.

the ovary often contains psammomatous bodies, depositions of calcium carbonate located in the fibrous stroma of the tumor that can be detected on plain abdominal radiographs. These psammomatous calcifications appear as scattered, fine, amorphous shadows that are barely denser than the normal soft tissues and can therefore be easily missed unless they are extensive (Figure 11-32). On ultrasound examination, cystadenocarcinoma typically appears as a large cystic mass with internal septa. It may be

difficult to distinguish cystadenocarcinoma (Figure 11-33) from **cystadenoma** (Figure 11-34), its benign counterpart. The more solid and irregular the areas within the mass on ultrasound images, the more likely it is that it represents a malignant tumor. In addition, the association of ascites with an ovarian mass is strongly suggestive of underlying malignancy. MRI is a more definitive study to determine whether the tumor has benign or malignant characteristics.

Ovarian carcinomas usually spread by implanting widely on the omental and peritoneal surfaces. This can produce the characteristic CT appearance of an "omental cake," an irregular sheet of soft tissue densities beneath the anterior abdominal wall (Figure 11-35). CT is also of value in detecting tumor adherence to bowel, ureteral involvement, and retroperitoneal adenopathy. This makes CT the modality of choice for staging and surgical planning. Positron emission tomography (PET) may be used in determining recurrence of ovarian carcinoma (Figure 11-36).

Treatment

Simple ovarian cysts are common, and many resolve without treatment. Cysts larger than 10 mm or complex may require drainage or surgery. With surgical treatment, ovarian carcinoma currently has a 25% to 30% survival rate.

Dermoid Cyst (Teratoma)

A dermoid cyst, the most common type of germ cell tumor, contains skin, hair, teeth, and fatty elements, all of which typically derive from ectodermal tissue.

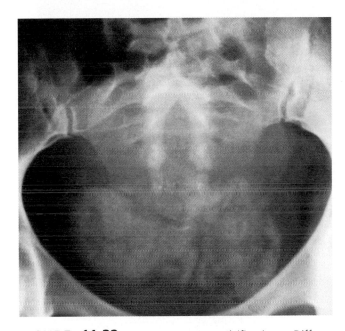

FIGURE 11-32 Psammomatous calcifications. Diffuse, ill-defined collections of granular amorphous calcification are visible within this cystadenocarcinoma of the ovary.

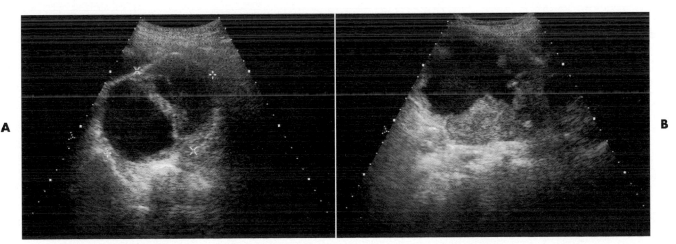

FIGURE 11-33 Endovaginal sonogram of a cystadenocarcinoma. **A,** The transverse image demonstrates a thickened wall and septations within the ovary, the left measuring 9 × 7 × 10 cm. **B,** The longitudinal image illustrates an enlarged uterus with a large, complex mass. The CT scan had demonstrated posterior wall thickening in the cyst and irregular densities within the liver—highly suggestive of cystadenocarcinoma.

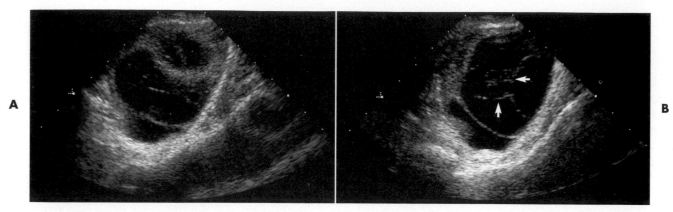

FIGURE 11-34 Cystadenoma. Longitudinal **(A)** and transverse **(B)** sonograms demonstrate a complex, predominantly cystic mass (sonolucent) containing several thin and well-defined septations *(arrows)*, which suggest a benign lesion—a mucinous cystadenoma.

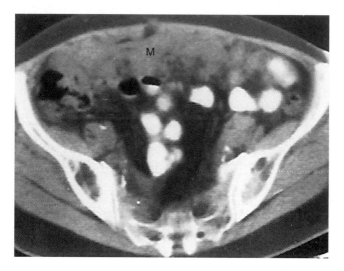

FIGURE 11-35 "Omental cake." Metastases *(M)* resulting from cystadenocarcinoma of the ovary cause an irregular sheet of soft tissue densities beneath the anterior abdominal wall that posteriorly displaces the adjacent contrast-filled bowel loops.

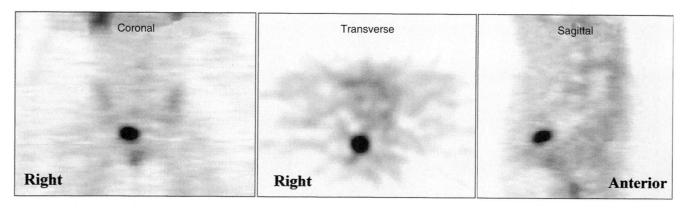

FIGURE 11-36 Recurrence of ovarian carcinoma. PET scan revealed a solitary focus of intense fluorodeoxyglucose (FDG) uptake in the right paramidline retrocystic location, suggestive of an active neoplasm and consistent with regional recurrence of the patient's ovarian carcinoma. The finding resulted in a change in treatment: the tumor focus, identified by PET-FDG to be in the right posterior pelvis, was successfully resected.

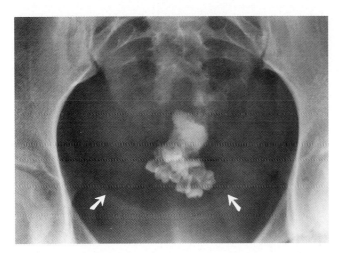

FIGURE 11-37 Dermoid cyst containing multiple well-formed teeth. Notice the relative lucency of the mass *(arrows)*, which is composed largely of fatty tissue.

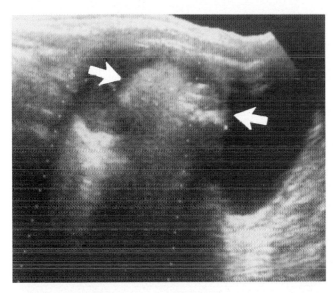

FIGURE 11-38 Dermoid cyst. Sagittal sonogram demonstrates only the near wall of the dermoid because of acoustic shadowing from a hairball *(arrows)*, producing the so-called tip of the iceberg sign.

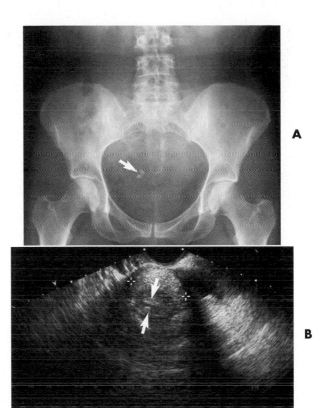

FIGURE 11-39 Dermoid cyst. **A,** Kidney-ureter-bladder study demonstrates two toothlike densities *(arrow)* beside the coccyx. **B,** A transverse sonogram has a heterogeneous mass (between *cursors*) with a high-amplitude echogenic focus *(arrows)* as a result of the toothlike densities.

These cysts are of no clinical significance unless they grow so large that they produce symptoms by compressing adjacent structures. About half of all ovarian dermoid cysts contain some calcification. This is usually in the form of a partially or completely formed tooth (Figure 11-37); less frequently the wall of the cyst is partially calcified.

Radiographic Appearance
The characteristic calcification combined with the relative radiolucency of the lipid material within the lesion is pathognomonic of an ovarian dermoid cyst.

The most common ultrasound appearance of a dermoid cyst is a complex, primarily solid mass containing high-level echoes arising from hair or calcification within the mass (Figures 11-38 and 11-39). The highly echogenic nature of these masses may make it difficult to delineate the lesion completely or to distinguish it from surrounding gas-containing loops of bowel.

Treatment
Surgical removal is recommended since the cyst may undergo transformation and become malignant.

Uterine Fibroids
Fibroids (leiomyomas) of the uterus are benign smooth-muscle tumors that are very common; they are often multiple and vary greatly in size. Growth of fibroid tumors is stimulated by estrogen. They develop only during the reproductive years and tend to shrink after menopause. Abnormal bleeding between periods or excessively heavy menstrual flow is the most common symptom. Large tumors may project

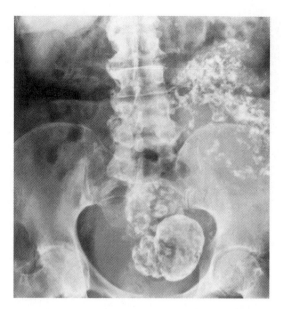

FIGURE 11-40 Calcified uterine fibroid. Calcified mass extends well beyond the confines of the pelvis.

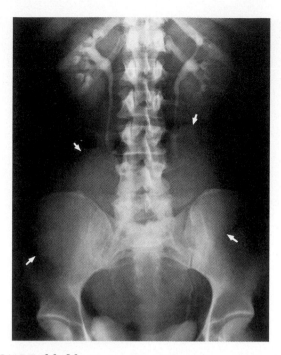

FIGURE 11-41 Uterine fibroid. Excretory urogram demonstrates persistent dense opacification of a huge uterine leiomyoma *(arrows)*.

from the uterus, causing pressure on surrounding organs, resulting in pelvic pain. They can also interfere with delivery or, if on a stalk (pedunculated), protrude into the vagina.

Radiographic Appearance

Uterine fibroids are by far the most common calcified lesions of the female genital tract. They have a characteristic mottled, mulberry, or popcorn type of calcification and appear on plain abdominal radiographs as smooth or lobulated nodules with a stippled or whorled appearance. A very large calcified fibroid occasionally occupies the entire pelvis or even extends out of the pelvis to lie in the lower abdomen (Figure 11-40).

During excretory urography, persistent uterine opacification is often seen in patients with an underlying uterine fibroid tumor (Figure 11-41). The tumor typically presses on the fundus of the bladder, causing a lobulated extrinsic impression that differs from the smooth impression usually seen with ovarian cysts. Extension of a fibroid into the adjacent tissues (parametrium) may cause medial displacement of the pelvic ureter or ureteral compression leading to hydronephrosis.

The classic ultrasound appearance of a uterine fibroid is a hypoechoic, solid, contour-deforming mass in an enlarged, inhomogeneous uterus (Figure 11-42). Fatty degeneration and calcification cause focal increased echogenicity; the calcification may result in acoustic shadowing. A subserosal fibroid projecting from the uterus, but attached to it by a large stalk,

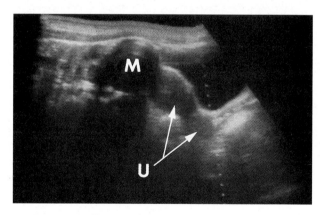

FIGURE 11-42 Uterine fibroid. Longitudinal sonogram demonstrates a pedunculated leiomyoma as a hypoechoic mass *(M)* projecting from the fundus of the uterus *(U)*. Decreased sound transmission through the mass indicates its solid nature.

may occasionally simulate an adnexal mass or an ovarian tumor.

Endovaginal (transvaginal) ultrasound is the best modality to demonstrate small and submucosal uterine fibroids (Figure 11-43). MRI is more sensitive than CT or ultrasound, but it is indicated only when ultrasound is inconclusive in differentiating between uterine and adnexal masses or between leiomyoma and adenomyosis, and when searching for submucosal fibroids in the patient with unexplained bleeding.

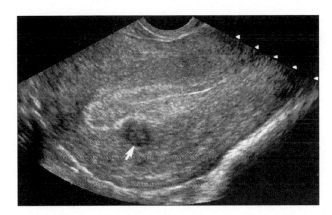

FIGURE 11-43 Submucosal uterine fibroid. Endovaginal ultrasound of the uterus in the sagittal plane demonstrates a fibroid filling the superior endometrial cavity *(arrow)*.

Treatment

In many cases no treatment is required. Medications can induce a temporary chemical menopause that causes a temporary shrinkage of the fibroid. If bleeding and fibroid size cannot be controlled with medications, surgery is performed. In younger women and for superficial fibroids, a myomectomy (removal of the leiomyoma) is performed to preserve the uterus. Large or multiple tumors usually require hysterectomy, especially if childbearing is complete. Many new therapeutic techniques are available—multilaser technique, myolysis (electrical coagulation of the myoma), uterine artery embolization—and various medications have proven to be effective.

Endometrial Carcinoma

Adenocarcinoma of the endometrium is the predominant neoplasm of the uterine body and is the most common invasive gynecologic neoplasm. It usually occurs in postmenopausal women, especially those who have never had children. About 75% of patients are 50 years or older and seen clinically for postmenopausal bleeding.

Radiographic Appearance

Excretory urography may demonstrate an enlarged uterus impressing or invading the posterior wall and fundus of the bladder. The typical ultrasound appearance of endometrial carcinoma is an enlarged uterus with irregular areas of low-level echoes and bizarre clusters of high-intensity echoes (Figure 11-44). Unless evidence of local invasion can be demonstrated, the ultrasound findings are indistinguishable from those of fibroid tumors, which often occur in patients with endometrial carcinoma. The endovaginal approach is generally preferred to measure endometrial thickness and to determine

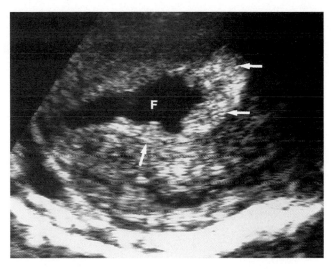

FIGURE 11-44 Endometrial carcinoma. Endovaginal scan localizing irregular endometrial thickening *(arrows)* with echogenic polypoid projections into the fluid-filled endometrial canal *(F)*.

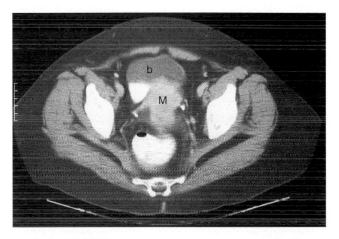

FIGURE 11-45 Bladder invasion by endometrial carcinoma. CT scan shows a mass *(M)* obliterating the fat planes between the bladder *(b)* and the uterus. Urine within the bladder outlines thickening of the posterior bladder wall. Nodular extension into the ischiorectal fossa indicates local extension of the tumor.

whether dilation and curettage (D & C—dilation of the cervix to allow scraping of the uterine wall) is required for histologic examination.

CT demonstrates focal or diffuse enlargement of the body of the uterus (Figure 11-45). This modality is especially useful for detecting clinically unsuspected omental and nodal metastases in patients with advanced disease, for evaluating patients with suspected neoplastic recurrence, and for checking the response to chemotherapy or radiation treatment.

MRI allows differentiation of the endometrium (the inner lining) from the myometrium (the muscle

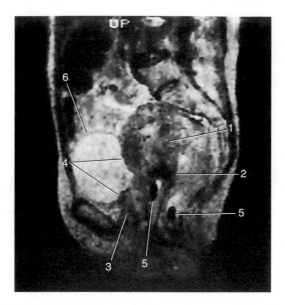

FIGURE **11-46** Endometrial carcinoma. Sagittal T2-weighted MR scan shows extensive tumor of mixed-signal intensity *(1)* that has invaded the endocervix and permits identification only of the ectocervix *(2)*. Tumor has extended inferiorly along the serosal surface of the uterus into the vesicovaginal septum *(3)* and bladder wall *(4)*. Low-intensity foci in the vagina represent radiotherapy implants *(5)*. Note the normal urinary bladder wall superiorly *(6)*.

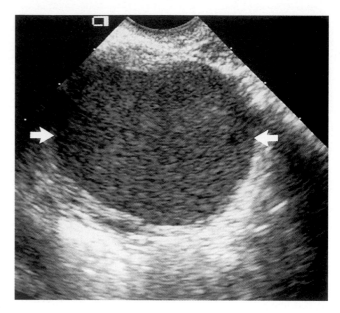

FIGURE **11-47** Endometrioma. Endovaginal scan demonstrating diffuse, homogeneous, low-level echoes throughout the cystic mass *(arrows)*.

layer) of the uterus and has been shown to be useful for demonstrating focal or diffuse endometrial tumors (Figure 11-46). The excellent contrast resolution of this technique may allow determination of the depth of myometrial invasion. For staging purposes, MRI is superior to CT for demonstrating extension of the tumor into the cervix, broad ligaments, and ovaries. Lymphatic involvement of the pelvis and retroperitoneal lymph nodes can also be visualized; the use of a contrast agent increases the contrast resolution.

Treatment
The first option for treatment is a hysterectomy with resection of the enlarged lymph nodes. Radiation therapy may follow surgery, especially in cases of advanced disease or an incomplete resection. For inoperable cancers, the preferred choice is chemotherapy.

Endometriosis
Endometriosis is the presence of normal-appearing endometrium in sites other than their normal location inside the uterus. Although tissues next to the uterus (ovaries, uterine ligaments, rectovaginal septum, and pelvic peritoneum) are most frequently involved in endometriosis, the gastrointestinal and urinary tracts can also be affected. Current theories of the cause of

endometriosis include (1) reflux of endometrial fragments backward through the fallopian tubes during menstruation, with implantation into the pelvis; (2) transformation of multipotential cells in the abdomen and pelvis; (3) implantation of endometrial fragments during surgery or delivery; and (4) spread of endometrial tissue by way of the bloodstream or lymphatic system.

Radiographic Appearance
Even though the endometrial tissue lies outside the uterus, it still responds to hormonal changes and undergoes a proliferative and secretory phase along with sloughing and subsequent bleeding. Thus an endometrial implant within a closed space can continue to grow with each menstrual cycle (Figure 11-47). Clinical symptoms include abnormal bleeding, painful menstruation (dysmenorrhea), and pain during sexual intercourse (dyspareunia). Because endometriosis is usually clinically apparent only when ovarian function is active, most women who are symptomatic for endometriosis are between 20 and 45 years of age. Ultrasound may demonstrate cystic masses filled with old blood. However, differentiation of endometriosis from other adnexal masses requires MRI.

Endometriosis involving the urinary tract most commonly produces ureteral obstruction below the level of the pelvic brim. The condition mimics a ureteral tumor and may appear as an intraluminal mass or stricture or as a smooth, rounded, or multilobular filling defect in the bladder. In the gastrointestinal

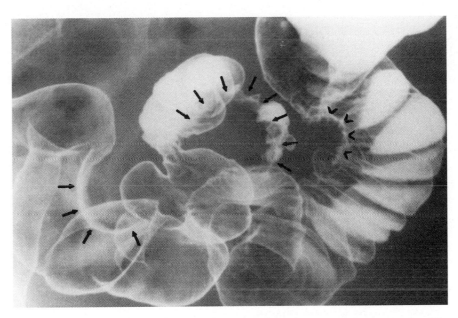

FIGURE 11-48 Endometriosis. Three separate endometrial implants (*arrows* and *arrowheads*) are seen in the sigmoid colon. The most distal lesion has a smooth interface with the bowel wall, indicating no intramural invasion. The two more proximal lesions have irregular borders, indicating intramural or submucosal invasion.

tract, endometriosis primarily affects those segments that are situated in the pelvis (especially the rectosigmoid colon). It typically causes abdominal cramps and diarrhea during the menstrual period and may appear as single or multiple masses in the colon (Figure 11-48). Repeated shedding of endometrial tissue and blood into the peritoneal cavity can lead to the development of dense adhesive bands causing small bowel obstruction.

A rare complication of endometriosis with intrathoracic implants of endometrial tissue is recurrent catamenial pneumothorax, which is usually right sided and occurs during menstrual flow.

Treatment

The main functions of treatment include pain management, reduction of disease progression, and prevention or reversal of infertility. To manage pain and reduce disease progression, drugs can be used to interrupt the menstrual cycle by stopping proliferation and secretion of extrauterine cells. A conservative surgical treatment, laser surgery, is used to remove visible endometrial implants that obstruct the fallopian tubes. When pain is unbearable, the radical surgical treatment is a complete hysterectomy.

Carcinoma of the Cervix

Carcinoma of the cervix is the third most common form of cancer in women. Development of the tumor appears to be related to chronic irritation, infection, and poor hygiene. A higher incidence occurs in women who have begun sexual activity at an early age and have had multiple sexual partners. The development of the Pap smear examination has permitted detection of cervical carcinoma at a very early stage (carcinoma in situ—confined to the site of origin), when it has not yet invaded the underlying tissues and is surgically curable. Widespread cervical cancer becomes inoperable, and radiation therapy is the usual treatment.

Radiographic Appearance

At the time of the initial staging, one third of patients have unilateral or bilateral hydronephrosis that can be demonstrated by excretory urography or ultrasound. Indeed, the most common cause of death in patients with carcinoma of the cervix is impairment of renal function caused by ureteral obstruction. Extension of the tumor to the bladder may cause an irregular filling defect; direct infiltration of the perirectal tissues may produce irregular narrowing of the rectosigmoid colon and widening of the retrorectal space. Distant metastases to the skeleton or lungs are uncommon, even in patients with advanced disease.

Ultrasound usually demonstrates a cervical carcinoma as a solid mass behind the bladder (Figure 11-49). CT is more accurate in detecting pelvic side wall invasion and therefore is usually the initial staging procedure in patients in whom there is a clinical suspicion of advanced disease (Figures 11-50

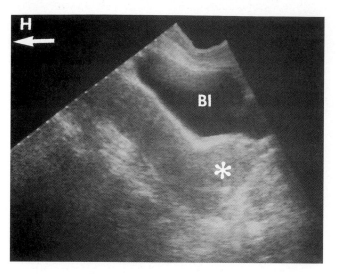

FIGURE **11-49** Carcinoma of cervix. Sonogram demonstrates a solid, echogenic mass *(asterisk)* lying behind the bladder *(Bl)* that is indistinguishable from a benign cervical myoma.

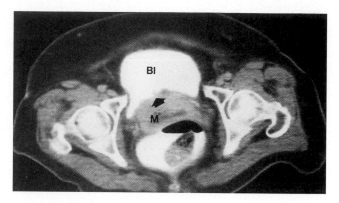

FIGURE **11-51** Bladder invasion by carcinoma of the cervix. CT scan shows irregularity *(arrow)* of the posterior margin of a contrast-filled urinary bladder *(Bl)* and the adjacent inhomogeneous cervical mass *(M)*.

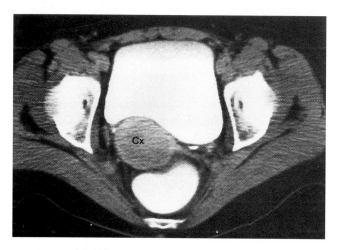

FIGURE **11-50** Carcinoma of cervix. CT scan demonstrates the inhomogeneity of an enlarged cervix *(Cx)* without evidence of bladder invasion.

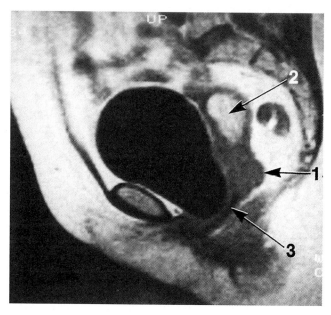

FIGURE **11-52** Cervical carcinoma. On this sagittal T1-weighted MR scan, posterior cervical lobulation *(1)* is the only primary sign of infiltrating cervical neoplasm. Note the considerable widening of the central uterine high-intensity zone *(2)* caused by an accumulation of menstrual products in the endometrial canal resulting from tumor occlusion of the endocervical canal. Urine *(3)* within the vagina produces low signal intensity on this imaging sequence.

and 11-51). This modality is also the procedure of choice for monitoring tumor response to treatment and for assessing suspected recurrence.

MRI is superior to CT and is the preferred study to distinguish the cervix from the uterus and vagina. Thus MRI is of value in detecting and staging cervical carcinoma (Figures 11-52 and 11-53). CT cannot always differentiate tumor from adjacent normal tissue.

After radiation therapy for carcinoma of the cervix (and other types of pelvic carcinoma), it may be difficult to distinguish chronic rectal narrowing and widening of the retrorectal space caused by radiation

effects from that caused by recurrence of tumor. Radiation therapy can also lead to the development of fibrous inflammatory adhesions between loops of bowel and the bladder, resulting in the development of fistulas between bowel loops (enteric-enteric) and between a bowel loop and the urinary bladder (enteric-vesicular).

SUMMARY *of* FINDINGS *for* Diseases of the Female Reproductive System

disorder	location	radiographic appearance	treatment
Pelvic inflammatory disease	Infection of uterus and fallopian tubes	US—fallopian tubes appear as adnexal masses that are sonolucent; multiloculated, irregular mass with scattered internal echoes CT—shows full extent of severe disease Hysterosalpingography—for nonvisualized fallopian tubes	Antibiotics Drainage or aspiration of abscesses
Ovarian cysts	Follicular or corpus luteum	US—round, anechoic adnexal masses	Self-resolve Aspiration and drainage Surgery
Polycystic ovarian syndrome	Mulitple cysts	US—10 or more cysts peripherally	Insert durgs to induce ovulation
Ovarian tumors		KUB—scattered tumor calcifications US—solid irregular mass with associated ascites	Surgery
	Ovarian metastasis	CT—irregular sheet of soft tissue densities beneath the anterior abdominal wall—omental cake PET—determines recurrence	
Dermoid cyst (teratoma)	Germ cell tumor of ovary	Radiograph—calcifications US—complex, primarily solid mass containing high-level echoes	Surgery
Uterine fibroids (leiomyomas)	Uterine smooth muscle	KUB—mottled mulberry, popcorn calcification IVU—lobulated extrinsic impressions of fundus of bladder US—hypoechoic, solid, contour-deforming mass in an enlarged inhomogeneous uterus (endovaginal demonstrates small and submucosal fibroids) MRI—to differentiate anatomy and distinguish fibroid from adenomyosis	Medications Myomectomy Myolysis Hysterectomy
Endometrial carcinoma	Uterine body	IVU—cancer invading posterior wall and fundus of bladder US—enlarged uterus with irregular hypoechoic areas and bizarre clusters of high signal intensity echoes CT—diffuse enlargement of the uterine body; omental and nodal metastases MRI—to determine depth of myometrial invasion	Hysterectomy Radiation therapy for incomplete resection Chemotherapy for inoperable tumors
Endometriosis	Endometrium outside normal location	US—sonolucent masses MRI—differentiates endometriosis from other adnexal masses	Medications to interrupt menstrual cycle Conservative surgery—laser technique Radical surgery—hysterectomy
Carcinoma of the cervix	Cervix	US—solid mass posterior to bladder CT—demonstrates pelvic side-wall invasion MRI—differentiates uterus from vagina; used for staging	Stage I and II—hysterectomy followed by radiation Advanced stages—surgery with radiation and chemotherapy

IVU, Intravenous urography; *KUB*, kidney–ureter–bladder radiograph; *US*, ultrasound.

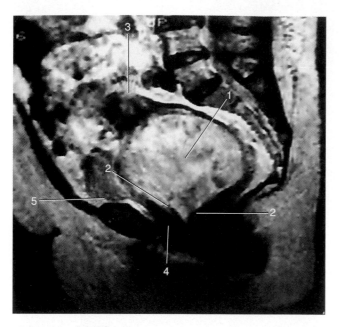

FIGURE 11-53 Carcinoma of the cervix. Sagittal T2-weighted MR image shows a bulky cervical neoplasm *(1)* with mottled high signal intensity. The lesion has invaded the upper third of the vaginal stroma *(2)* anteriorly and posteriorly, but has spared the uterus *(3)*. The urethra *(4)* and urinary bladder *(5)* are anteriorly displaced by the tumor.

Treatment

A hysterectomy with resection of the involved nodes and surrounding tissues and followed by radiation is recommended for stage I and II cervical cancers. Advanced lesions require surgery with a combination of radiation and chemotherapy. A pelvic exenteration (removal of all the pelvic organs to debulk the tumor) is used as a last resort.

Breast Lesions

Breast Cancer

Breast cancer is the most common malignancy among women between ages 44 and 50. Most tumors are classified as infiltrating duct carcinomas, which occur most frequently in the upper lateral quadrant. Current surgical and radiation therapy techniques provide highly effective treatment, but only if the cancers are detected when localized to the breast itself. Today many breast tumors are diagnosed before they are palpable because routine screening is available (especially in the United States). In these instances, the prognosis is considerably better because the mass has not extended into surrounding tissue or beyond the breast. Breast cancers diagnosed in Stage I have a survival rate of approximately 98%. Unfortunately, most breast tumors are discovered accidentally rather than in the course of regular survey examinations. By this time, the majority have spread either to regional lymph nodes or systemically, accounting for the current high mortality (about 50%) that makes breast cancer the leading cause of cancer death in women.

Periodic careful physical examination of the breast, done either by a trained health professional (clinical breast examination–CBE) or by the patient herself (breast self-examination–BSE), will discover cancers that are small and more likely to be localized. Even smaller, nonpalpable, and potentially more curable lesions can be detected by mammography, a radiographic examination that is by far the most effective diagnostic procedure for breast cancer. Indeed, routine mammography combined with physical examination is the only approach currently available that promises to significantly reduce breast cancer mortality. Following a general clinical history, the accepted assessment of a suspected breast mass is a three-pronged approach—physical examination, imaging (usually mammography), and needle biopsy.

From screening mammography, 7% to 10% of the patients are recalled for more extensive imaging. Of these, 15% to 20% will require a biopsy, and 5% to 7% will have cancer detected. On screening examinations, 40% of the cancers detected are in situ (at the origin) and approximately 75% have no nodal involvement.

Radiographic Appearance

The two major radiographic techniques for diagnosing breast cancer are screen-film mammography and the digital direct-capture system. Screen-film imaging uses a specially designed x-ray screen that permits the proper exposure of film by many fewer x-rays than would otherwise be necessary. This produces a conventional black-and-white image at a very low radiation dose. A direct-capture system relies on radiation captured by multiple cells that convert the radiation energy to electrical energy to produce a numerical value (i.e., a digitized image). The advantages of digital mammography are faster image acquisition with lower dose (shorter exposure), increased contrast with the ability to manipulate images to visualize specific areas of interest, decreased repeats, and the ease of sharing images with other professionals.

Almost all breast cancers are seen mammographically as a tumor mass, clustered calcifications, or both. Either feature, when clearly demonstrated, is so indicative of malignancy that prompt biopsy is required whether the lesion is palpable or not. Secondary changes of breast carcinoma include skin thickening and nipple retraction. Magnification imaging and compression techniques greatly improve the diagnostic value of the image.

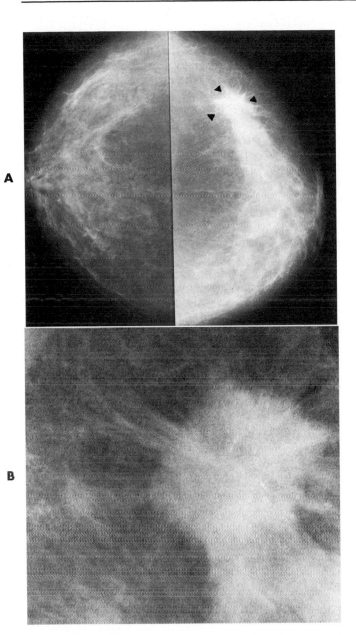

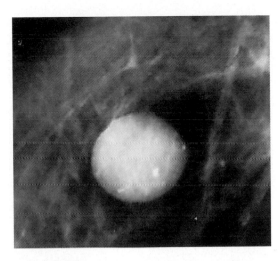

FIGURE **11-55** Benign breast mass. Screen-film mammogram demonstrates smooth, round fibroadenoma with clearly defined margins.

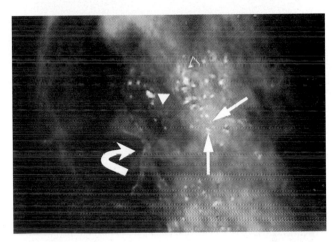

FIGURE **11-56** Malignant calcifications in breast cancer. Numerous tiny calcific particles with linear *(straight arrows)*, curvilinear *(solid arrowhead)*, and branching *(open arrowhead)* forms characteristic of malignancy. Note the benign calcification in the arterial wall, which is easily recognized by its large size and tubular distribution *(curved arrow)*.

FIGURE **11-54** Breast cancer. Full **(A)** and magnified coned **(B)** views of the breast demonstrate an ill-defined, irregular mass with radiating spicules *(arrowheads)*.

The typical malignant tumor mass is poorly defined with areas of distortion, has irregular margins, and demonstrates numerous fine linear strands or spicules radiating out from the mass (Figure 11-54). This appearance is characteristic but not diagnostic of malignancy and is in stark contrast to the typical mammographic picture of a benign mass, which has well-defined, smooth margins and a round, oval, or gently lobulated contour (Figure 11-55).

Clustered calcifications in breast cancer are typically numerous, very small, and localized to one segment of the breast. They demonstrate a wide variety of shapes, including fine linear, curvilinear, and branching forms (Figure 11-56). Although only about half of breast cancers are seen mammographically as clusters of calcifications, typical calcifications are seen in many of the nonpalpable intraductal cancers that often do not form mass lesions and may otherwise escape detection.

Ultrasound provides a secondary diagnostic tool that can differentiate a benign cyst from a solid mass, and thus it substantially reduces the number of biopsies performed for benign cysts (Figures 11-57 and 11-58) and normal fibroglandular tissue. Ultrasound is best in determining the size of a mass, and Doppler ultrasound permits visualization of blood flow patterns. However, ultrasound is of limited value in detecting nonpalpable cancers, particularly those that

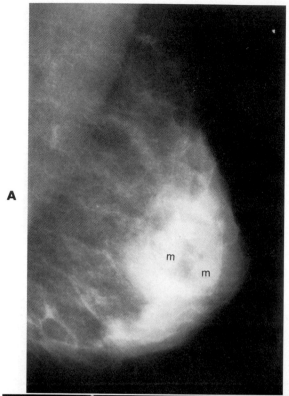

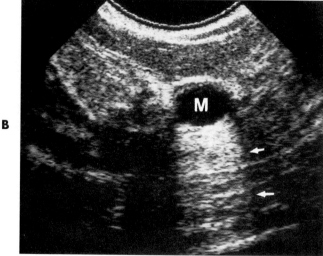

FIGURE 11-57 Sonography for breast disease. **A,** Mammogram shows several rounded masses *(m)* that could be solid or cystic in a breast that is very dense anteriorly. **B,** Sonogram clearly shows that the largest mass *(M)* is cystic because it contains no internal echoes and shows considerable posterior enhancement *(arrows)*.

have calcifications alone, and thus it cannot substitute for mammography as a screening examination. In cases of ruptured silicone implants, an inflammatory process causes the development of silicone granulomas. These produce a "snowstorm" appearance (Figure 11-59) causing shadowing posteriorly that obscures the posterior border.

MRI with multiple sequences and contrast enhancement now has the ability to help differentiate between benign adenomas and carcinomas. The use of image subtraction (noncontrast image subtracted from the enhanced image) assists in highlighting the contrast-enhanced regions. Benign masses tend to have smooth borders, whereas malignancies appear as high signal intensity lesions with spiculation. Using longer sequences, carcinomas produce high signal intensity, whereas adenomas assume a lower signal intensity (and are not apparent). Fat suppression using water excitation best demonstrates the functional parenchyma, and this technique helps differentiate among various lesions. MRI is used in questionable cases for surgical preplanning to determine whether lumpectomy or mastectomy is the best operative approach. For patients with breast implants, MRI may best demonstrate the surrounding breast tissue (Figure 11-60). This modality also demonstrates implant twisting or rupture, which may not be visible on other imaging techniques.

Although not used routinely, CT can assist in determining extension of the disease (Figure 11-61). SPECT fusion imaging aids in determining lymphatic involvement for breast malignancies (Figure 11-62). The most sensitive imaging modality is PET. Although PET is the least used modality because of its expense and limited availability, as a molecular imaging technique it can demonstrate the metabolic activity and vascularization of the tumor at its earliest stages. Currently, PET is used to detect recurrences in scarred breasts because postoperative scarring makes mammography less effective for visualizing new lesions.

Although relatively infrequent (1 in 100), breast cancer also can develop in men. Breast cancer in men usually has a poor prognosis because it is often diagnosed in a later stage. Breast enlargement in men results from a proliferation of the glandular component and is known as gynecomastia.

Treatment

Imaging also plays a role in surgical planning by providing guidance (by ultrasound or mammography) for needle localization (Figure 11-63). A conservative surgical approach is lumpectomy, which is used for isolated lesions. Mastectomy, a more aggressive surgical approach, includes the removal of all breast tissue and a dissection of the lymph nodes. If the lymph nodes contain cancerous cells, the axillary nodes are removed (radical mastectomy). Chemotherapy and radiation therapy are used in more advanced cases, depending on the type of cancer cells and whether the axillary nodes are involved. Hormonal chemotherapy with synthetic antiestrogens may be used if the tumor contains estrogen receptors.

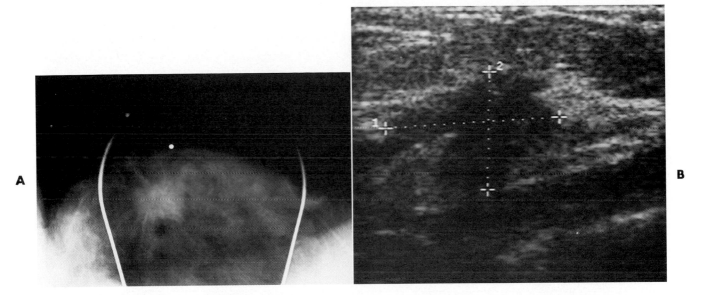

FIGURE 11-58 Spiculated lesion. **A,** Mammography using magnification-spot compression demonstrates microcalcifications and a spiculated lesion. **B,** Breast sonography demonstrates fingerlike projections emanating from the lesion measuring 1.8 × 1.25 cm.

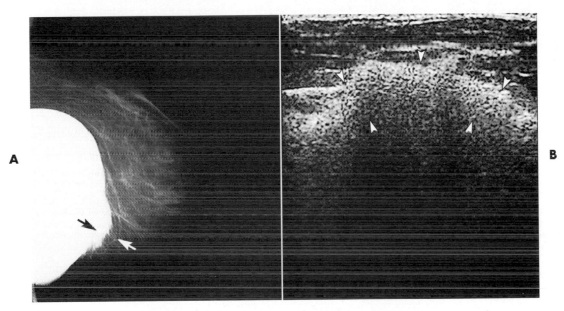

FIGURE 11-59 Ruptured silicone breast implants. **A,** Mammogram shows retroglandular implant with extra-capsular silicone *(arrows)*. **B,** Ultrasound image of the same patient shows typical "snowstorm" appearance of free extracapsular silicone *(arrowheads)*.

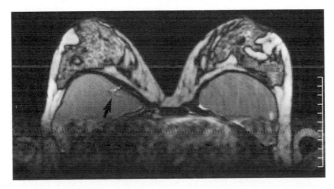

FIGURE 11-60 Breast implants. MRI distinguishes between breast tissue and the implant. A fold in the implant is also visualized *(arrow)*.

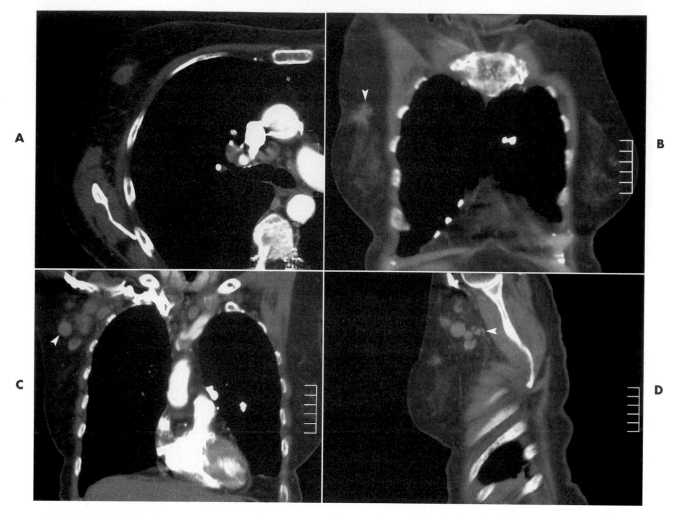

FIGURE 11-61 Breast cancer. CT images demonstrates an enhancing breast lesion *(arrows)* in the axial **(A)** and coronal projections **(B)**. The lymph nodes *(arrows)* are enlarged as seen on the coronal **(C)** and sagittal projections **(D)**. On lung window images, pulmonary metastatic nodules were demonstrated.

SUMMARY *of* FINDINGS *for* Breast Lesions

disorder	location	radiographic appearance	treatment
Breast carcinoma	Breast tissue	Mammography—poorly defined with areas of distortion, irregular margins with numerous fine linear strands or spicules radiating from the mass US—differentiates benign cysts from a solid mass and its size; blood flow patterns with Doppler; ruptured silicone implants produce "snowstorm" appearance MRI (subtraction imaging)—benign masses tend to have smooth borders, whereas malignancies demonstrate high signal intensity with spiculation; fat suppression best demonstrates the functional parenchyma and helps differentiate lesions; best demonstrates the surrounding breast tissue in patients with implants PET—demonstrates metabolic activity and vascularization of the tumor at the earliest stages; utilized to detect recurrences in scarred breast tissue	Lumpectomy Mastectomy Radical mastectomy Chemotherapy or hormonal therapy
Benign breast disease	Fibrocystic breast or single cysts	Mammography—smooth, well-circumscribed mass without invasion of surrounding tissue US—simple cyst appears as an anechoic center with a thin echogenic capsule	Pain management through diet Hormonal therapy Surgery for single cysts

US, Ultrasound.

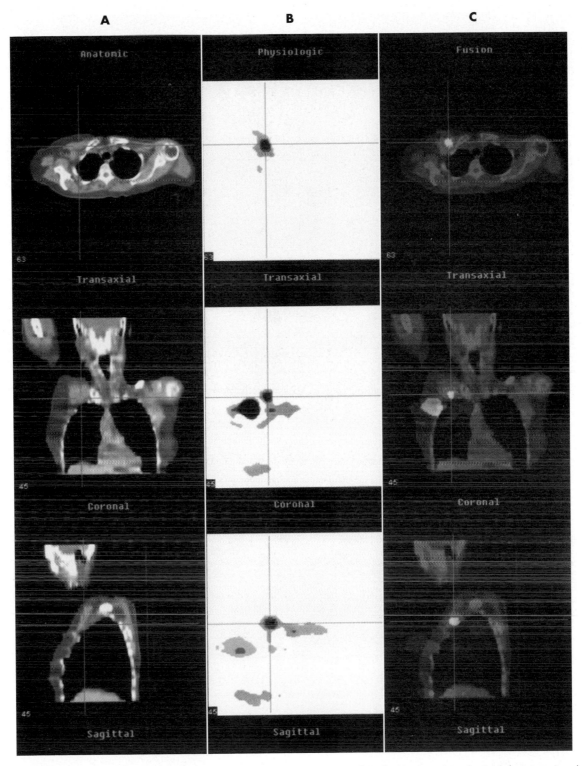

FIGURE 11-62 Right sentinel lymph node studied with SPECT and CT fusion imaging. **A,** A triplanar anatomic CT image. **B,** A triplanar SPECT physiologic image. **C,** A triplanar fusion image. One sentinel node is located and marked for intraoperative removal.

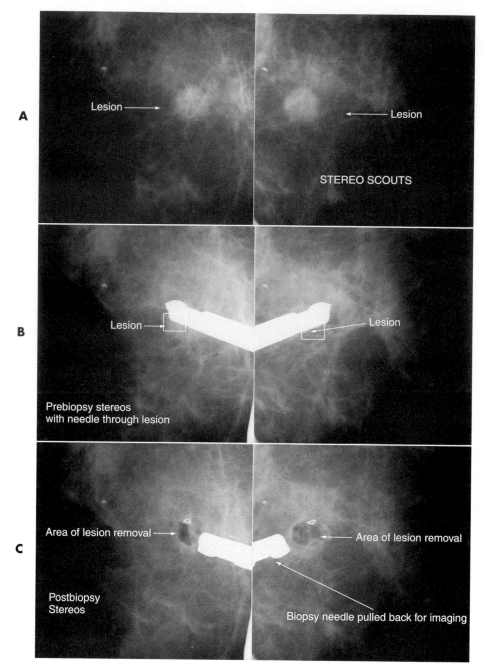

FIGURE 11-63 Stereotaxic needle biopsy. **A,** Stereotaxic scout images of breast lesion. **B,** Stereotaxic images showing needle localization. **C,** Postbiopsy images of lesion with needle pulled back to demonstrate lesion removal.

Benign Breast Disease

Fibrocystic disease of the breast is a common benign condition that occurs in about 20% of premenopausal women. It is usually bilateral, with cysts of various sizes distributed throughout the breasts that also contain an increased amount of fibrous tissue. The size of the cyst usually changes with the menstrual cycle, as does the amount or type of fluid in it.

Radiographic Appearance

A fibroadenoma is the most common benign breast tumor. It generally appears as a smooth, well-circumscribed mass with no invasion of surrounding tissue (see Figure 11-55). Ultrasound permits differentiation of a solid fibroadenoma from a fluid-filled breast cyst. Sonographically, a simple cyst has an anechoic center with a thin echogenic capsule (see Figure 11-57).

High-risk patients require monitoring of the cystic lesions for possible conversion to a cancerous process. Equivocal lesions may require imaging with other modalities.

Treatment

The most conservative treatment addresses pain management, usually by dietary modifications and reducing caffeine intake. If dietary changes do not reduce pain to a tolerable level, drainage of the cyst may be performed. Hormonal therapy with synthetic antiestrogens that block estrogen and progesterone is used in cases of cyclical pain. However, these drugs may produce intolerable side effects. Surgery is not the most effective treatment unless there is only a single cyst (and most patients have multiple cysts).

Imaging in Pregnancy

Because of its noninvasive and nonionizing character, ultrasound is the modality of choice in the evaluation of possible complications of pregnancy. A major role of ultrasound is to assess the gestational age, a measurement that is often highly inaccurate when based on the date of the last menstrual period. Knowledge of the true gestational age may be critically important for obstetric decisions because the length of pregnancy is a major factor in interpreting the graphs that indicate the status of the fetus.

Measurements of fetal age by ultrasound include the longest biparietal diameter (BPD), the crown-to-rump length, and the length of the fetal femur. The BPD is measured from the outer margin of the skull on one side to the inner margin on the other side at the level of the thalami (Figure 11-64). A single measurement of the BPD has its greatest accuracy between 12 and 26 weeks; after this time, the size of the head and thus the BPD may be affected by a growth disturbance. The crown-to-rump length refers to the distance between the tip of the head and the bottom of the fetal trunk (Figure 11-65). This measurement is highly accurate for assessing gestational age in early pregnancy (less than 11 weeks). Fetal femoral length (Figure 11-66) aids in determining fetal age in the second and third trimesters by identifying epiphyseal cartilage at the knee, which indicates a gestational age beyond 33 to 35 weeks.

An early diagnosis of multiple pregnancies can be made by ultrasound (Figure 11-67). This is essential so that therapeutic measures can be taken to reduce the high complication rate associated with twin (or more) fetuses.

Ultrasound can be used to detect an abnormal volume of amniotic fluid, which is often associated with

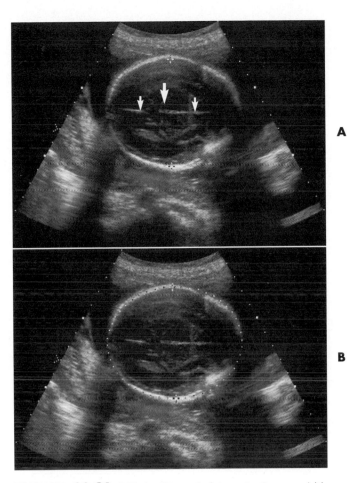

FIGURE 11-64 BPD in 27-week fetus. **A,** Cursor width indicates BPD, which is measured from outer margin of skull on one side to inner margin on other side. Arrows point to midline falx. **B,** Dotted line indicates head circumference.

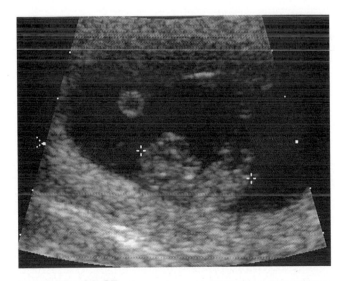

FIGURE 11-65 Crown-to-rump length measurement. Cursors delineate the length of the fetus from the top of the head to the bottom of the torso.

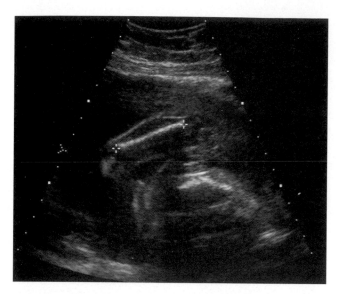

FIGURE 11-66 Fetal femur. Cursor measures a femur length of 3.96 cm, and cartilage is not demonstrated, indicating a fetal age earlier than 33 weeks.

underlying fetal anomalies. **Polyhydramnios** refers to an excessive accumulation of amniotic fluid that may be caused by maternal disorders, such as diabetes mellitus and Rh isoimmunization (Figure 11-68). Polyhydramnios is also caused by fetal abnormalities, especially those related to the central nervous system, the gastrointestinal tract, the circulatory system, and dwarfism. **Oligohydramnios** refers to a very small volume of amniotic fluid. This condition results primarily from fetal urinary tract disorders, such as renal aplasia, renal dysplasia, and urethral obstruction. Oligohydramnios is also associated with intrauterine growth retardation.

Clinically significant errors of morphologic development occur in up to 5% of all children. The in utero detection of these anomalies by ultrasound may permit in utero medical or surgical therapy, may provide an indication for termination of the pregnancy, or may influence the mode of delivery. Although a detailed description of the rapidly expanding field of prenatal sonography is beyond the scope of this book, some of the abnormalities that can be detected, and often treated, in utero are osseous (bony) and neural anomalies of the fetal cranium (Figures 11-69 and 11-70) and spine, gastrointestinal atresias and developmental cysts, cystic and obstructive lesions of the genitourinary tract, and congenital cardiac diseases and skeletal anomalies (Figure 11-71).

Because ultrasound examinations can demonstrate the fetus and placenta with no apparent risk to the mother or unborn child, ultrasonography is unquestionably the imaging study of choice for evaluating

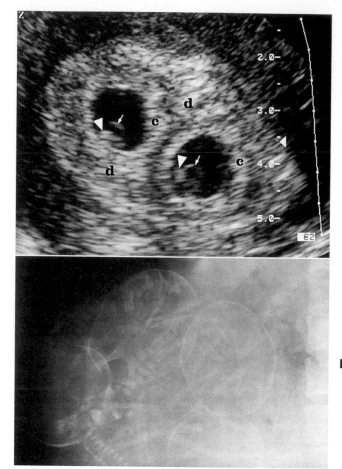

FIGURE 11-67 Multiple pregnancies. **A,** Endovaginal sonogram shows two gestational sacs surrounded by the echogenic chorionic ring *(c)* composed of the decidua capsularis and the chorion laeve within the decidua vera *(d)*. A yolk sac *(small arrow)* and live embryo *(arrowhead)* are present within each gestational sac. The crown-to-rump lengths measure 5.4 mm and 4.7 mm, corresponding to a gestational age of 6.5 weeks. **B,** Lateral abdominal radiograph of a woman with quadruplets clearly shows four separate fetal skulls and spines.

the gravid (pregnant) woman. In extremely rare instances, there may be justification for performing radiographic pelvimetry to demonstrate the architecture of the maternal pelvis and to compare the size of the fetal head with the size of the maternal bony pelvic outlet to determine whether the pelvic diameters are adequate for normal delivery or whether a cesarean section will be required. In almost all cases, however, the combination of careful clinical evaluation and ultrasonography is sufficient to make these decisions without the need to resort to radiographic pelvimetry with its high radiation dose. There is absolutely no indication ever to perform fetography, the radiographic demonstration of the fetus in utero. Ultrasound can provide far better diagnostic information and is not associated with the danger of producing radiation-induced fetal malformations.

Ectopic Pregnancy

Although ectopic pregnancy is a life-threatening condition, responsible for up to one fourth of maternal deaths, the diagnosis is missed by the initial examining physician in up to three fourths of cases. More than 95% of ectopic pregnancies occur within the fallopian tubes, and more than half the patients with this complication of pregnancy have a history or pathologic evidence of PID. Ectopic pregnancies

are often associated with urine or plasma levels of human chorionic gonadotropin (HCG) that are substantially lower for the expected date of gestation than those in patients with normal intrauterine pregnancies.

Radiographic Appearance

Ultrasound is the major imaging modality for diagnosing ectopic pregnancy. The classic appearance consists of an enlarged uterus that does not contain a gestational sac and is associated with an irregular adnexal mass, an "ectopic fetal head," or fluid in the cul-de-sac (Figure 11-72). The unequivocal demonstration of an intrauterine pregnancy virtually excludes an ectopic pregnancy because the incidence of coexisting ectopic and intrauterine pregnancies is only 1 in 30,000.

Treatment

Emergency surgical intervention before a fatal hemorrhage occurs is required.

Trophoblastic Disease

Trophoblastic disease refers to a spectrum of pregnancy-related disorders ranging from benign hydatidiform mole to the more malignant and frequently metastatic choriocarcinoma. A hydatidiform mole results from abnormal fertilization when there is an absence of the female chromosome. About half of choriocarcinomas follow pregnancies complicated by hydatidiform mole. The remainder occur after spontaneous abortion, ectopic pregnancy, or normal deliveries.

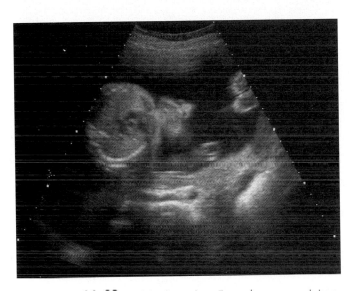

FIGURE 11-68 Polyhydramnios. Excessive accumulation of amniotic fluid (hypoechoic area) surrounds the fetus in the mother of advanced maternal age.

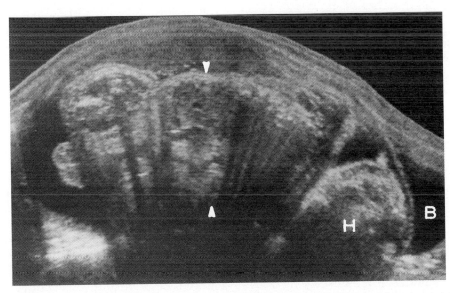

FIGURE 11-69 Anencephaly. Long-axis image of third-trimester fetus shows that the head *(H)* is irregularly shaped, echogenic, and much smaller than the body *(arrowheads)*. B, Maternal bladder.

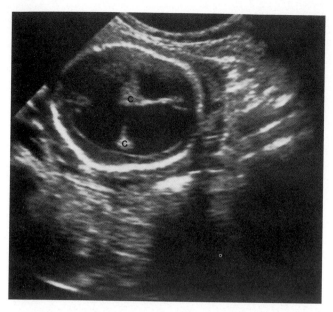

FIGURE 11-70 Ventriculomegaly. Cranial axial ultrasound image at 27 menstrual weeks shows obvious ventricular enlargement with convex surface of the lateral ventricle wall that parallels the bony calvaria. Note the dangling choroids *(c)*.

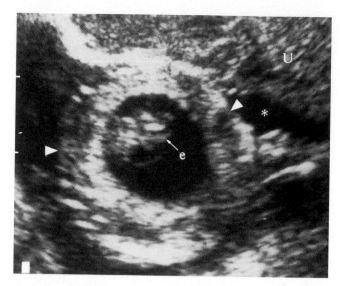

FIGURE 11-72 Ectopic pregnancy with live embryo in the adnexa. Endovaginal sonography shows tubal ring *(arrowheads)* and gestational sac, containing yolk sac and live embryo *(e)*. Asterisk indicates free fluid. *U,* Uterus.

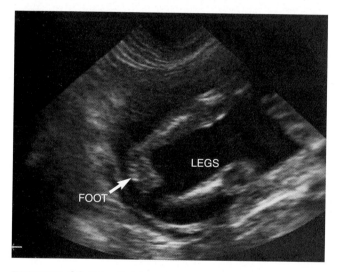

FIGURE 11-71 Clubfoot. Prenatal ultrasound scan shows the feet with the foot at a right angle to the leg.

Radiographic Appearance

A hydatidiform mole typically appears on an ultrasound image as a large, soft tissue mass of placental (trophoblastic) tissue filling the uterine cavity and containing echoes of low to moderate amplitude ("bunch of grapes") (Figure 11-73) without any signs of fetal movement. Endovaginal sonography confirms that there is no evidence of a developing fetus. On ultrasound images, choriocarcinoma resembles benign hydatidiform mole and usually appears as a large complex mass of central hemorrhage, with necrosis found in the expected position of the uterus. Choriocarcinoma tends to metastasize to the lungs, where it typically produces multiple large masses that rapidly regress once appropriate chemotherapy is instituted.

Treatment

Hydatidiform moles are treated by removal of all placental tissue by suction curettage of the uterus. If suction curettage does not lower the patient's HCG, the disease progresses, and the patient requires chemotherapy. For choriocarcinoma, folic acid antagonists have a cure rate of approximately 80% if treatment begins before brain metastasis occurs.

Female Infertility

The causes of infertility in young women include anomalies in the reproductive organs, such as an abnormal uterus that cannot hold a fetus (Figure 11-74), obstructed fallopian tubes, ovaries that are unable to produce mature ova, and disruption of the path the ova normally follow en route to the uterus.

Radiographic Appearance

The major radiographic procedure for evaluating infertile women is hysterosalpingography, in which the uterine cavity and fallopian tubes are opacified after the injection of contrast material into the uterus. In a woman with normal patent fallopian tubes, contrast material extravasating into the pelvic peritoneal

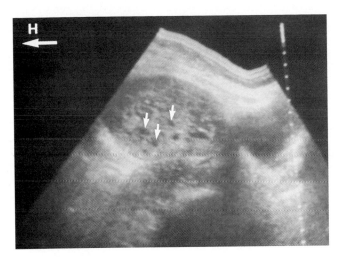

FIGURE 11-73 Hydatidiform mole. Longitudinal sonogram in a patient in her second trimester of pregnancy demonstrates large, moderately echogenic mass filling the central uterine cavity. Note the numerous small cystic spaces *(arrows)* that represent greatly hydropic chorionic villi.

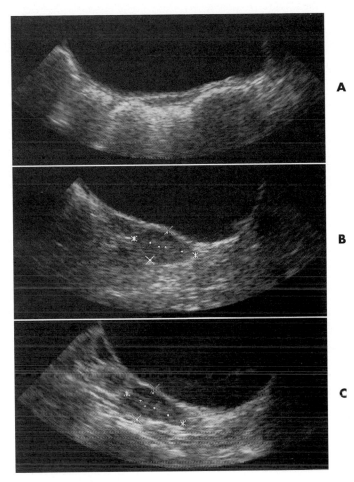

FIGURE 11-74 Uterine agenesis. Ultrasound on a 16-year-old girl who has never had a menstrual cycle. Midline sagittal view **(A)** demonstrates the bladder *(dark area)* with no uterus found posteriorly. Normal left **(B)** and right **(C)** ovaries are shown in the parasagittal plane.

cavity outlines the peritoneal surfaces and often loops of bowel within the pelvis (see Figure 11-29). Developmental anomalies or fibrosis from PID may cause occlusion of one or both of the fallopian tubes; in such cases, there is no evidence of the contrast material reaching the peritoneal cavity (see Figure 11-30). In addition to assessing tubal patency, hysterosalpingography can also demonstrate uterine abnormalities that contribute to infertility, such as intrauterine fibroids, severe uterine flexion or retroversion, and other congenital and acquired malformations.

Treatment

For women who receive ovulation-induction agents as treatment for infertility, ultrasound can be used to monitor the maturation of ovarian follicles. Low level internal echoes in mature ovarian follicles appear to be a prognostic indicator of fertility. They may represent a periovulatory state, which is an appropriate time for artificial insemination or in vitro fertilization.

Ultrasound can also demonstrate the characteristic bilateral multicystic ovarian enlargement in the ovarian hyperstimulation syndrome, which may develop in women receiving menotropins (Pergonal) therapy for infertility.

SUMMARY FINDINGS *for* Pregnancy

disorder	location	radiographic appearance	treatment
Uterine pregnancy	Fetus within the uterus	US—demonstrates the fetus and placenta	Normal birth
Ectopic pregnancy	Fertilization outside the uterus	US—enlarged uterus without gestational sac and an appearance of an irregular adnexal mass	Surgical intervention

Continued

SUMMARY of FINDINGS for Pregnancy—cont'd

disorder	location	radiographic appearance	treatment
Trophoblastic disease Hydatidiform mole	Abnormal fertilization	US—large soft tissue mass with "bunch of grapes" appearance	Suction curettage
Choriocarcinoma	Malignant transformation of hydatidiform mole	US—large complex mass with necrosis	Chemotherapy of folic acid antagonist
Female infertility	Lack of fertilization or implantation	Radiograph—hysterosalpingography to demonstrate the ovaries, fallopian tubes, and uterus US—screening for congenital anomalies, and to monitor treatment	Ovulation-induction agents

US, Ultrasound.

REVIEW QUESTIONS

1. Why has ultrasound become the major imaging modality for both the male and the female reproductive systems?

2. In addition to ultrasound, what are the main radiographic studies currently used for the female reproductive system?

3. The formation of sperm is known as _____.

4. What male hormone helps to regulate metabolism by promoting growth of skeletal muscles and is considered responsible for the greater degree of muscle development in men?

5. Severing of the vas deferens to create sterility is termed _____.

6. The second most common cause of malignancy in men is _____.

7. What imaging modality for demonstrating the prostate gland uses a probe inserted into the rectum?

8. Ultrasound studies of the prostate gland *cannot* always determine the malignant or benign status of prostatic disease. Is this true or false?

9. Prostatic carcinoma can often spread through the bloodstream to the bone and can sometimes cause sclerosis of an entire vertebra. This pathologic condition is termed _____.

10. What screening technique is usually employed to identify the location of an undescended testicle?

11. What is the term used to describe the twisting of the male gonad on its pedicle?

12. The most common neoplasms in men between 20 and 35 years of age are tumors that tend to metastasize through the _____ system.

13. The rupture and expulsion of the mature ovum into the pelvic cavity is termed _____.

14. A pregnancy that occurs in a fallopian tube or in the pelvic cavity is termed _____.

15. What is the name of the radiographic procedure used to demonstrate the patency or status of the fallopian tubes?

16. Untreated _____ can lead to cerebral cortical lesions causing mental disorders and involvement of the skeletal system and affects infants born to infected mothers.

17. The most common type of germ cell tumor, often containing teeth, hair, and fatty material, is called a(n) _____.

18. Leiomyomas, more commonly referred to as _____, are benign smooth-muscle tumors of the uterus.

19. The most common malignancy among women occurs in the _____.

20. The second most common form of cancer in women is _____.

BIBLIOGRAPHY

Callen PW: *Ultrasonography in obstetrics and gynecology*, Philadelphia, 2000, Saunders.

de Paredes ES: *Atlas of film-screen mammogram*, Baltimore, 1992, Williams & Wilkins.

Eisenberg RL, Margulis AR: *What to order when*, ed 2, Philadelphia, 2000, Lippincott Williams & Wilkins.

eMedicine Specialties > Neurology > Neurological Infections: emedicine.com.

eMedicine Specialties > Medicine, Ob/Gyn, Psychiatry, and Surgery > Obstetrics/gynecology: emedicine.com.

Rumack CM, Wilson SR, Charborneau JW: *Diagnostic ultrasound*, St Louis, 1998, Mosby.

Sanders RC, James AE: *Ultrasonography in obstetrics and gynecology*, Norwalk, Conn, 1992, Appleton-Century-Crofts.

Tabar L, Dean PB: *Teaching atlas of mammography*, ed 2, New York, 1985, Thieme.

MISCELLANEOUS
Diseases

Chapter Outline

Key Terms

arachnodactyly
ascorbic acid
aseptic necrosis
fat-soluble vitamins
gonadal dysgenesis
microcephaly
niacin
nutritional deficiency
osteomalacia
pectus excavatum
Pelken spur
syndrome
testicular dysgenesis
thiamine
vitamins
water-soluble vitamins
Wimberger's sign of scurvy

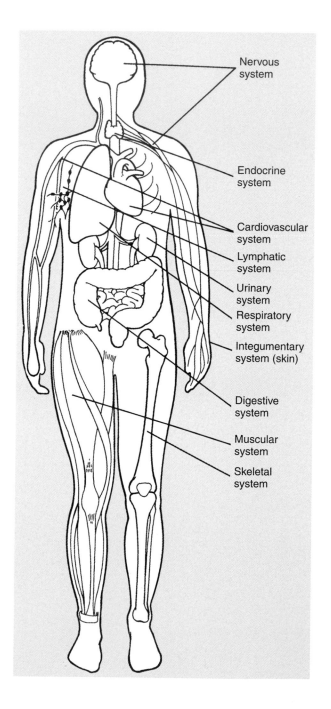

Nervous system

Endocrine system

Cardiovascular system

Lymphatic system

Urinary system

Respiratory system

Integumentary system (skin)

Digestive system

Muscular system

Skeletal system

Prerequisite Knowledge

The student should have a basic understanding of the physiology of the various body systems. In addition, proper learning and understanding of the material will be facilitated if the student has some clinical experience in general radiography.

Goals

To acquaint the student with the pathophysiology and radiographic manifestations of both common and unusual disorders caused by vitamin deficiencies, hereditary abnormalities, and some disease processes that do not fit neatly into a single body system, and to understand the use, positioning, and complications of various tubes, catheters, and wires in the chest.

Objectives

After reading this chapter, the reader will be able to:

1. Describe nutritional disorders and their possible relationship to disorders of other organs
2. Define terminology relating to nutritional disorders
3. Define all key terms in this chapter
4. Distinguish the pathologic conditions caused by various vitamin deficiencies
5. Describe the pathologic conditions associated with sarcoidosis, muscular dystrophy, melanoma, and systemic lupus erythematosus
6. Differentiate hereditary abnormalities including chromosomal aberrations and genetic amino acid disorders
7. Locate placement for an endotracheal tube, central venous catheter, Swan-Ganz catheter, and transvenous cardiac pacemaker
8. Recognize the most common complications involved with improper placement of the aforementioned catheters and how chest radiography plays an important role in the diagnosis of these complications

Nutritional Diseases

Disorders of nutrition range from malnutrition and vitamin deficiency to obesity and hypervitaminosis. In addition to inadequate intake, **nutritional deficiency** may be related to disorders of the liver, pancreas, and gastrointestinal tract that result in an inability of the body to digest and properly use proteins, carbohydrates, and lipids. In diabetes mellitus, the absence of insulin prevents entry of glucose into the cells and thus deprives the body of its major source of energy. Abnormalities of the pancreas, liver, and gastrointestinal tract causing nutritional diseases are discussed elsewhere; this section deals with diseases caused by vitamin deficiency, malnutrition, and obesity.

Vitamin Deficiencies

Vitamins are an essential part of the enzymatic systems that are vital to the body's cellular metabolism. Vitamins are formed (synthesized) only by plants, not by animals. Therefore man's supply of vitamins comes directly from eating fruits and vegetables or from animals (including fish) that have eaten plants and have stored the vitamins. Vitamins are generally divided into two categories: fat soluble and water soluble. The **fat-soluble vitamins** (A, D, E, and K) can be stored within body tissues. **Water-soluble vitamins** (B and C) cannot be stored and must be a regular part of the diet to prevent a deficiency. The major B vitamins include thiamine, riboflavin, niacin, pantothenic acid,

RADIOGRAPHER *Notes*

Radiography of patients with various nutritional diseases can be challenging because of the many effects these diseases have on all body systems. Some produce deformities; others can cause mental disorders. Obese patients can present unique problems in positioning and in selecting radiographic settings. The radiographer must be especially empathetic when dealing with these patients, who often are embarrassed because of their size and thus difficult to deal with. The manifestations of systemic lupus erythematosus cause considerable discomfort for patients. Patients with melanoma that has already metastasized or those who are facing extensive surgical intervention are usually very depressed and sometimes require special handling. Patients with muscular dystrophy can be easily agitated and are usually frustrated at their inability to control themselves. Hereditary diseases causing abnormalities require special understanding on the part of the technologist to attain optimal patient cooperation that will result in good diagnostic radiographs. In general, patients suffering from the various diseases in the miscellaneous category can be very demanding and require considerable patience on the part of the radiographer.

cobalamin (vitamin B$_{12}$), and folic acid. Vitamin deficiency diseases are rare in the United States, but are all too prevalent in underdeveloped countries.

Beriberi (Thiamine)

Beriberi results from a deficiency in thiamine (vitamin B$_1$), a coenzyme essential for carbohydrate metabolism that promotes growth and maintains muscle tone and heart function. Beriberi occurs primarily in rice-eating countries, such as China, where the main staple is polished rice that has had the vitamin-containing skin and germ removed. Infantile beriberi is common in breast-fed infants 2 to 4 months of age if the mother has a **thiamine** deficiency. Noninflammatory degeneration of the myelin sheath caused by thiamine deficiency produces a peripheral neuropathy characterized by weakness of the limbs and a "pins and needles" sensation in the extremities.

Radiographic Appearance

Initially, peripheral vasodilatation in beriberi causes increased cardiac output, which then produces a generalized enlargement of the cardiac silhouette and increased pulmonary vascular markings. With progression of disease, the myocardium becomes edematous and flabby and cannot function properly, leading to congestive heart failure and generalized edema (Figure 12-1).

Pellagra (Niacin)

Pellagra, caused by a deficiency of **niacin** (vitamin B$_3$), is characterized by reddening and scaling of the skin on exposed parts of the body, vomiting and severe diarrhea, and nervous and mental disorders (ranging from chronic depression to violent, irrational

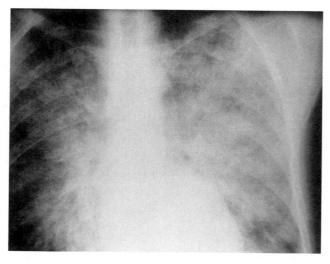

FIGURE 12-1 Beriberi. Diffuse pulmonary edema caused by severe high-output heart failure.

behavior). The body requires niacin to complete the cellular process called respiration, in which nutrients and oxygen reach the cells through a series of chemical reactions. As a result of dietary supplements, epidemics of pellagra no longer exist; however, sporadic incidences occur among chronic alcoholics and those suffering from malabsorption.

Scurvy (Vitamin C)

In patients with scurvy, the deficiency of **ascorbic acid** (vitamin C) leads to an inability of the supporting tissues to produce and maintain vascular endothelium and the cementing substances that hold epithelial cells together (collagen, osteoid, dentin). Scurvy was classically a disease of sailors and explorers deprived of fresh fruit and vegetables containing vitamin C.

Weakening of capillary walls in scurvy often results in bleeding into the skin, joints, and internal organs. The gums are especially affected and bleed easily. The open lesions provide an entry for bacteria, leading to necrosis of gum tissue and tooth loosening and loss. Impaired synthesis of collagen leads to poor and delayed wound healing.

Radiographic Appearance

In children, disordered chondroblastic and osteoblastic activity cause radiographic bone changes that are most prevalent where growth is normally most rapid (especially about the knee and wrist). The bones are generally osteoporotic with blurring or disappearance of trabecular markings and severe cortical thinning. Widening and increased density of the zone of provisional calcification produce the characteristic "white line" of scurvy (Figure 12-2). A relatively lucent osteoporotic zone forms on the diaphyseal side of the white line. This osteoporotic zone is easily fractured, permitting the dense bone to become impacted on the shaft and to jut laterally beyond it, thus giving rise to characteristic marginal spur formation (**Pelken spur**). The epiphyseal ossification centers are demineralized and surrounded by dense, sharply demarcated rings of calcification (**Wimberger's sign of scurvy**). If epiphyseal dislocations have not occurred, the appearance of the skeletal structures usually returns to normal after appropriate therapy.

Subperiosteal hemorrhage often occurs along the shafts of the long bones. Calcification of the elevated periosteum and underlying hematoma is a radiographic sign of healing.

Rickets (Vitamin D)

Rickets is a bone disease of young children in which a lack of vitamin D leads to decreased absorption of calcium from the gastrointestinal tract, resulting in weak, deformed bones. In adults, lack of vitamin D

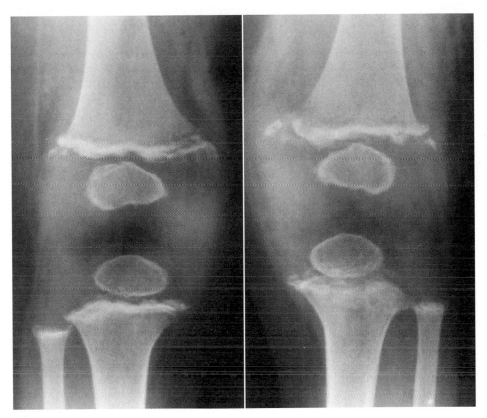

FIGURE 12-2 Scurvy. Frontal projections of both knees demonstrate widening and increased density of the zone of provisional calcification, producing the characteristic "white line" of scurvy. Notice also the submetaphyseal zone of lucency and characteristic marginal spur formation (Pelken spur). Epiphyseal ossification centers are surrounded by a dense, sharply demarcated ring of calcification (Wimberger's sign).

causes generalized softening of bones (**osteomalacia**). The radiographic findings of rickets and osteomalacia are found in Chapter 4.

Vitamin A Deficiency

Vitamin A, or retinol, is essential for vision because it is a vital component of the pigment that absorbs light in the rods of the retina. A lack of vitamin A results in night blindness, an inability to see in dim light. Vitamin A also is important for maintaining the integrity of the mucous membranes lining the respiratory, gastrointestinal, and urogenital tracts. A lack of vitamin A makes these membranes dry and susceptible to cracking, permitting infectious organisms to enter the underlying tissues.

Vitamin A is derived from β-carotene, a yellow plant pigment that is converted into vitamin A by the liver. Good sources of vitamin A include dairy products, egg yolks, fish, and vegetables such as carrots, spinach, and sweet potatoes.

Vitamin K Deficiency

Vitamin K, a fat-soluble vitamin, is necessary for the formation of prothrombin, an essential ingredient in the blood-clotting mechanism. It is primarily found in green leafy vegetables. A deficiency of vitamin K results in excessive bleeding.

Treatment of Vitamin Deficiencies

Three different approaches can be used to treat vitamin deficiencies: (1) the patient's diet is modified to include foods that contain the recommended daily requirements, (2) the patient is given synthetic oral supplements, or (3) vitamins are injected. Some deficiencies may be associated with absorption abnormalities resulting from a lack of the specific vitamins needed to absorb and process vitamins.

Dietary modifications for vitamin B deficiencies include increasing the intake of protein (meat), green leafy vegetables, and milk. For vitamin C deficiencies, an increase in consumption of fresh fruits and green leafy vegetables may help. Vitamin D deficiencies require adding cod liver oil, egg yolks, butter, and oily fish to the diet. Fortified milk and exposure to sunlight also provide vitamin D. To increase vitamin A, a diet including more liver, meat, eggs, milk, and dark green and yellow vegetables is of value. Eating more spinach, lettuce, broccoli, Brussels sprouts, and cabbage increases dietary vitamin K.

Hypervitaminosis

Chronic excessive intake of vitamin A produces a syndrome characterized by bone and joint pain, hair loss, itching, anorexia, dryness and fissuring of the lips, hepatosplenomegaly, and yellow tinting of the skin. This condition usually affects young children, who become irritable and fail to gain weight.

Radiographic Appearance

Excess vitamin D causes too much calcium to be absorbed from the gastrointestinal tract. The resulting hypercalcemia leads to the deposition of calcium in the kidney, heart, lungs, and wall of the stomach (Figure 12-3).

Treatment

Because there is an excess of vitamins, treatment requires a decrease in vitamin intake and monitoring of the patient to ensure that the levels are stable.

Protein-Calorie Malnutrition (Kwashiorkor)

Severe protein-calorie malnutrition (kwashiorkor) affects millions of young children (under age 5) in developing countries (approximately 182 million in 2000) and produces abnormalities involving the gastrointestinal tract and nervous system. In those affected, an imbalance between the body's supply of nutrients and its demand for energy causes a wasting away or emaciation. Fatty replacement of liver tissue and the resulting decreased levels of albumin lead to diffuse edema and ascites and the characteristic clinical appearance of a considerably protuberant abdomen. Damage to the pancreas and intestinal mucosa prevents proper digestion and absorption of nutrients.

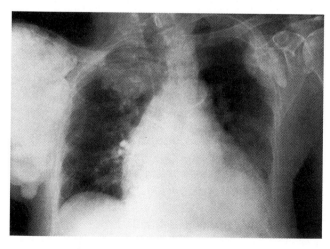

FIGURE 12-3 Hypervitaminosis D. Huge masses of calcification near the shoulder joints bilaterally.

Radiographic Appearance

Retarded bone growth with thinned cortices usually occurs. Atrophy of the thymus gland and lymphoid tissues diminishes the child's resistance to infection from organisms that enter the body through skin lesions and the damaged mucous membranes of the gastrointestinal tract. Mental development is also impaired, and brain atrophy can be demonstrated radiographically.

Treatment

The initial approach is to correct the child's fluid and electrolyte balance. Milk and supplementary vitamins are added to the diet. The mortality rate of 15% to 40% results from the dangerous fluid imbalance.

Obesity

Obesity refers to an excess of adipose (fatty) tissue that develops when the caloric intake (from food) consistently exceeds the amount of calories required by the body to perform its daily activities. It may be related simply to personal habits of excessive eating combined with a lack of activity, or it may be a result of such conditions as hypothyroidism, Cushing's disease, insulinoma, and hypothalamic disorders.

Radiographic Appearance

Excess adipose tissue can cause displacement of normal abdominal structures, producing such radiographic patterns as widening of the retrogastric (Figure 12-4) and retrorectal spaces. An extreme increase in the intraabdominal volume causes diffuse elevation of the diaphragm with a relatively transverse position of the heart (simulating cardiomegaly), prominence of pulmonary markings, and atelectatic changes at the lung bases. In the most severe form of obesity (pickwickian syndrome), the excursion of the diaphragm is limited, and the lungs can barely expand with breathing. This results in profound hypoventilation, hypoxia, retention of carbon dioxide, secondary polycythemia, and pulmonary hypertension with right heart failure. An excessive deposition of fatty tissue can also appear radiographically as widening of the mediastinum and prominence of the pericardial fat pads.

Treatment

The simplest treatments include weight management by dieting, using nutritional counseling and behavioral therapy, and dietary drugs. Patients with morbid obesity may undergo surgical procedures in an attempt to lose large amounts of weight. Gastric restrictive operations attempt to limit gastric capacity and restrict gastric outflow, thus making the patient feel full after a small meal. This causes the patient

SUMMARY of FINDINGS for Nutritional Diseases

disorder	cause	radiographic appearance	treatment
Beriberi	Deficiency in vitamin B_1 Decrease in carbohydrate metabolism	Enlarged cardiac silhouette with increased pulmonary markings	Increase intake by diet modification Increase intake with synthetic supplements Receive injections of the specific vitamin Increase absorption of vitamin by association with other dietary products
Pellagra	Deficiency in vitamin B_3	Not specific	
Scurvy	Deficiency in vitamin C	Osteoporosis with blurring of trabecular markings and severe cortical thinning Widening and increased density of the zone of provisional calcification, producing a white line	
Rickets	Deficiency of vitamin D Leads to decrease in absorption of calcium	See Osteomalacia in Chapter 4	
Vitamin A	Deficiency of vitamin A Visual deficiencies and decreased integrity of mucous membranes	Not specific	
Vitamin K	Deficiency of vitamin K Decreased prothrombin production	Not specific	
Hypervitaminosis	Usually excessive vitamin A or D	Vitamin A—not specific Vitamin D—hypercalcemia leads to deposition of calcium in the kidney, heart, lungs, and wall of the stomach	Decrease vitamin intake
Protein-caloric malnutrition	Severe protein-calorie deficiency	Retarded bone growth Thinned cortices Brain atrophy	Balance fluids and electrolytes Provide milk and supplemental vitamins
Obesity	Excessive adipose tissue—due to caloric intake consistently exceeding calories required	Displacement of anatomic structures Elevated diaphragm Widened mediastinum	Weight management by dieting Nutritional counseling and behavioral therapy Dietary drugs Surgical resection to limit gastric capacity

to limit his or her oral intake and results in weight control. The major procedure is a gastroplasty, in which a small upper gastric remnant is connected to a larger lower gastric pouch by a narrow channel. A new procedure, gastric banding, is the placement of an adjustable band (accessed by an external port) that can be inflated to control gastric emptying. Complications of gastric restrictive procedures can occur in the early and late postoperative periods and include leakage, perforation, widening of the channel, and obstruction.

Lead Poisoning

Lead poisoning results from the ingestion of lead-containing materials (especially paint) or from the occupational inhalation of lead fumes. Environmental exposure occurs when drinking water (leaded pipes) and eating food that is processed, preserved, or stored in containers made with lead. Currently, lead is the number one major environmental pollutant worldwide; however, the incidence in the United States has decreased as a result of public education and governmental restrictions of its use. The chronic form of lead poisoning may cause mental retardation, seizures, behavioral disorders, or delayed development. Ingested lead affects all systems of the body. Children are more susceptible to lower doses, and the effect on their central nervous system is more severe, causing interference in the cognitive thought process.

Radiographic Appearance

In children, because lead and calcium are used interchangeably by bone, high concentrations of lead are deposited in the most rapidly growing portions of the skeleton, especially the metaphyses at the distal ends of the femur. This results in classic lead lines, dense transverse bands extending across the metaphyses of the long bones (Figure 12-5) and along the margins of flat bones, such as the iliac crest. In young children who eat lead-containing paint (pica), plain abdominal radiographs may show extensive mottled opacities, which are suggestive of intestinal barium, even though no contrast material has been administered (Figure 12-6). Computed tomography (CT) is the modality of choice for demonstrating cerebral edema and structural changes.

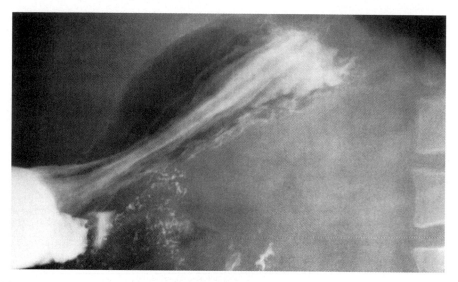

FIGURE 12-4 Obesity. Enlargement of the retrogastric space caused by a massive deposition of fatty tissue.

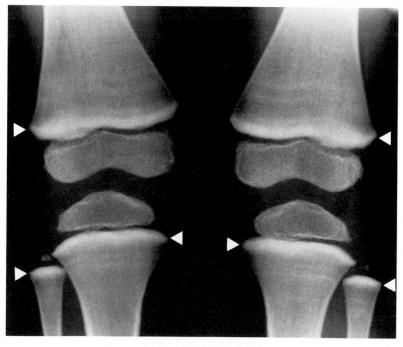

FIGURE 12-5 Lead lines. Dense transverse bands of sclerosis *(arrowheads)* extend across the metaphyses of the distal femurs and the proximal tibias and fibulas.

Treatment

First, the source must be eliminated. If the drop in lead is not quick enough, chelation therapy to aid in the urinary excretion of lead is prescribed for those who do not have kidney or liver disease. The objective is to keep the level of lead less than 60 µg/dl to prevent potential encephalopathy.

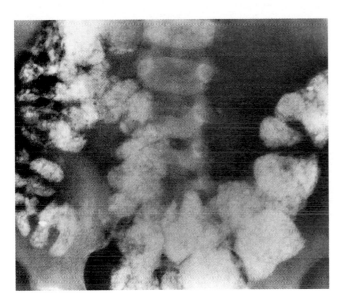

FIGURE 12-6 Pica. Large amounts of lead-containing material ingested by a young child who had received no contrast material.

Sarcoidosis

Sarcoidosis is a multisystem granulomatous disease of unknown cause that is most often detected in young adults. Women are affected slightly more often than men, and the disease is far more prevalent among African-Americans than among whites. Histopathologic findings include multiple epithelioid granulomas.

Radiographic Appearance

Ninety percent of patients with sarcoidosis have radiographic evidence of thoracic involvement. Indeed, in most cases the presence of the disease is first identified on a screening chest radiograph of an asymptomatic individual.

Bilateral, symmetric, hilar lymph node enlargement, with or without diffuse parenchymal disease, is the classic radiographic abnormality in sarcoidosis. Usually, enlargement of the right paratracheal nodes occurs, producing the typical 1-2-3 pattern (Figure 12-7). Conventional tomography frequently reveals additional enlargement of the left paratracheal nodes, which usually cannot be seen on routine frontal radiographs because they are obscured by the superimposed aorta and brachiocephalic vessels. Unilateral hilar enlargement, which is a common manifestation of primary tuberculosis or lymphoma, is rare in sarcoidosis. High-resolution CT (HRCT) is more sensitive than chest radiographs for detecting

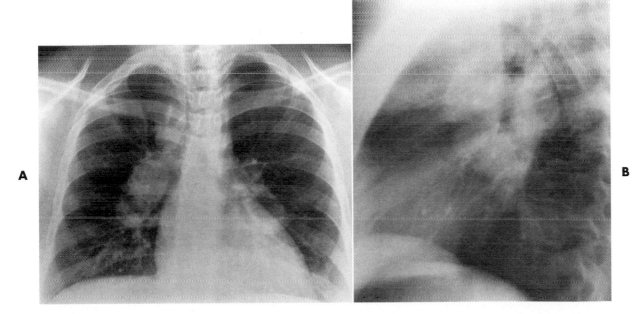

FIGURE 12-7 Sarcoidosis. Frontal **(A)** and lateral **(B)** projections of the chest demonstrate enlargement of the right hilar, left hilar, and right paratracheal lymph nodes, producing the classic 1-2-3 pattern of adenopathy.

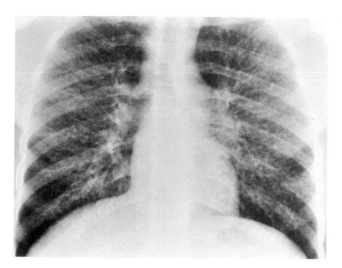

FIGURE 12-8 Sarcoidosis. Diffuse coarse interstitial pattern.

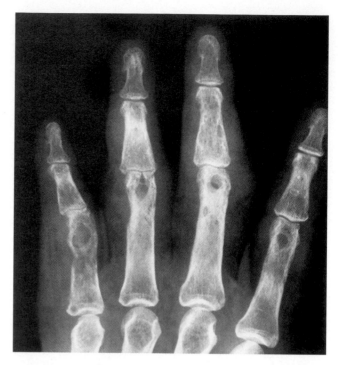

FIGURE 12-9 Sarcoidosis. Multiple osteolytic lesions throughout the phalanges produce the typical punched-out appearance. The apparent air density in the soft tissues is a photographic artifact.

subtle lymphadenopathy and parenchymal disease (ground-glass attenuation). The anterior mediastinal and left paratracheal nodes, which are obscured on the chest radiograph, are well visualized on HRCT.

Diffuse pulmonary disease develops in most patients with sarcoidosis. Although hilar and mediastinal adenopathy are often involved, there tends to be an inverse relationship between the degree of adenopathy and the extent of parenchymal disease, with the latter increasing while the adenopathy regresses. The most common appearance is a diffuse interstitial pattern that is widely distributed throughout both lungs (Figure 12-8). The alveolar pattern appears as ill-defined densities that may be discrete or may coalesce into large areas of consolidation. This pattern resembles an acute inflammatory process and may contain an air bronchogram. Infrequently, large, dense, round lesions may simulate metastatic malignancy.

The skeletal lesions in sarcoidosis involve primarily the small bones of the hands and feet. Granulomatous infiltration can cause destruction of the fine trabeculae, producing a mottled to lacelike, coarsely trabeculated pattern. Lytic destruction can produce sharply circumscribed, punched-out areas of lucency (Figure 12-9). About 10% of patients with sarcoidosis have elevated levels of serum calcium, which may lead to nephrocalcinosis. Sarcoid involvement of the stomach can produce discrete masses or generalized luminal narrowing that predominantly involves the antrum.

Treatment
Although the pulmonary lesions usually regress spontaneously or after steroid therapy, irreversible pulmonary changes develop in up to 20% of the cases.

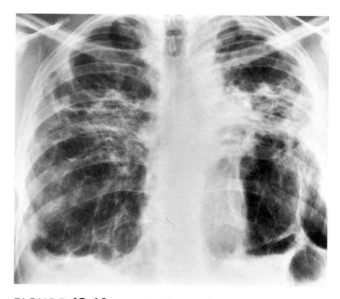

FIGURE 12-10 Sarcoidosis. In end-stage disease, there is severe fibrous scarring, bleb formation, and emphysema.

Coarse scarring is seen as irregular linear strands extending outward from the hilum toward the periphery, often associated with bulla formation (Figure 12-10). Severe fibrosis and emphysema can cause pulmonary hypertension and right-sided heart failure.

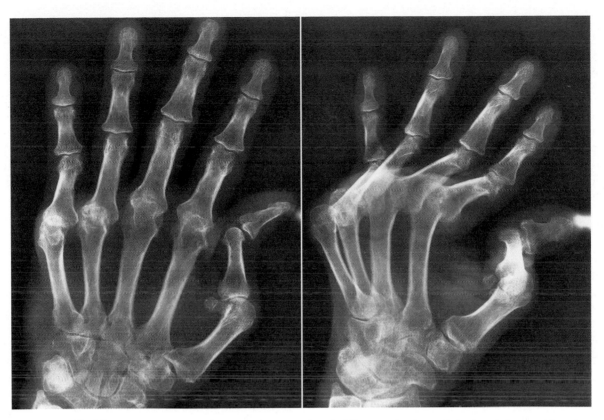

FIGURE 12-11 Systemic lupus erythematosus. Frontal and oblique projections of the hand show subluxation of the phalanges at the metacarpal articulations and hyperextension deformities of the proximal interphalangeal joints. Note the absence of erosive changes.

Systemic Lupus Erythematosus

Systemic lupus erythematosus is a connective tissue disorder that involves primarily young or middle-aged women and most likely represents an immune-complex disease. The cell activation is thought to be connected to genetic, environmental, and hormonal factors. The presentation and course of the disease are highly variable from limited skin involvement to tragic systemic disease. Characteristic findings include a butterfly-shaped rash over the nose and cheeks and extreme sensitivity of the skin to sunlight.

Radiographic Appearance
Pain in multiple muscles and joints is the most frequent clinical complaint in patients with systemic lupus erythematosus. A characteristic finding is subluxations and malalignment of joints in the absence of erosions (Figure 12-11). Cardiopulmonary abnormalities also frequently develop. Pleural effusions, usually bilateral and small but occasionally massive, occur in about half of the patients (Figure 12-12). Enlargement of the cardiac silhouette is generally the result of pericarditis and pericardial effusion.

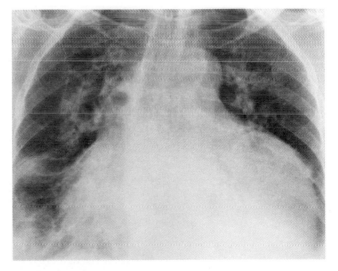

FIGURE 12-12 Systemic lupus erythematosus. Bilateral pleural effusions, more pronounced on the right, with some streaks of basilar atelectasis. Massive cardiomegaly is attributable to a combination of pericarditis and pericardial effusion.

Although kidney involvement (often leading to renal failure) is one of the most serious manifestations of systemic lupus erythematosus, no specific urographic findings are seen. Enlargement of the liver, spleen, and lymph nodes occurs in about one fourth of patients. In the gastrointestinal system, a necrotizing inflammation of blood vessels can result in massive bleeding, multiple infarctions, and bowel perforation.

Many of the radiographic manifestations of systemic lupus erythematosus tend to disappear during spontaneous remissions or after steroid therapy.

Treatment

Antiinflammatory drugs are used to treat pain in the muscles and joints. Systemic corticosteroids help prevent pathologic conditions involving the renal and central nervous system. If skin lesions occur, antimalarial drugs are prescribed.

Melanoma

Melanoma is an extremely malignant skin cancer that metastasizes widely throughout the body. The tumor develops from a benign mole (nevus), which changes size and color and becomes itchy and sore. The incidence of melanoma is rising, having increased in the United States approximately 2000% since 1930. Globally, cancer statistics from 2002 show that incidences in Australia and New Zealand are approximately six times higher in males and two times higher in females. Even though melanoma represents only 4% of all skin cancers, the mortality rate is greater than 70%.

Radiographic Appearance

Metastases from malignant melanoma frequently involve the gastrointestinal tract, usually sparing the large bowel. They are typically well-circumscribed, round, or oval nodules that may develop central necrosis and ulceration; in a barium study, this results in a dense, barium-filled central crater surrounded by a sharply marginated nodular mass (bull's-eye, or target, lesion) (Figure 12-13). Gastrointestinal metastases can be the first clinical manifestation of metastatic melanoma; at times it can be impossible to identify the primary tumor site.

Metastatic melanoma can also produce multiple nodules in the lung and destructive bone lesions with neither new bone formation nor reactive sclerosis.

Treatment

Carefully watching for changes in moles or in the skin and having a biopsy to assess the lesion is the best prevention and is highly recommended. Also, continuous protection from the sun may reduce the development of these lesions. Surgical excision of the tumor and surrounding tissue may be all that is required. A lymph node biopsy determines whether chemotherapy is required for metastases. The prognosis depends on the size of the lesion and the results of the lymph node biopsy.

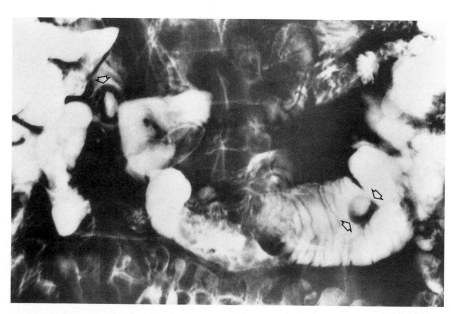

FIGURE 12-13 Metastatic melanoma. Large central ulcerations in two sharply defined filling defects in the small bowel *(arrows)*.

Muscular Dystrophy

Muscular dystrophy refers to a group of chronic inherited conditions in which fat replaces muscle; this leads to generalized weakness and eventually death caused by respiratory muscle failure or pneumonia. Males are more commonly affected because of the X-linked inheritance pattern. Of the many types, the most common is Duchenne's muscular dystrophy (DMD), which has been identified on the DMD gene as the Xp21 band. A milder form is Becker's muscular dystrophy.

Radiographic Appearance

On radiographs of the extremities, the extensive accumulation of fat within the remaining muscle bundles produces a fine striated, or striped, appearance (Figure 12-14). Because most of the muscle tissue is replaced by fat, the fascial sheath bounding the muscles may stand out as a thin shadow or as increased density as it is visualized on edge. Decreased muscular tone can lead to osteoporosis, bone atrophy with cortical thinning, scoliosis, and joint contractures.

An abnormal swallowing mechanism in muscular dystrophy can result in the failure to clear barium adequately from the pharynx; this may lead to tracheal aspiration and nasal regurgitation of contrast material (or other ingested substances).

Treatment

No curative therapy is known. Gene and cell therapy are currently under investigation as possible treatments. Currently, drug therapy is used to protect muscle mass and function. A regimen of nonstrenuous

SUMMARY of FINDINGS for Miscellaneous Disorders

disorder	cause	radiographic appearance	treatment
Lead poisoning	Ingestion of lead-containing materials	Classic lead lines (dense transverse bands extending across the metaphyses of long bones)	Eliminate source Chelation therapy to aid in elimination
Sarcoidosis	Nonspecific or unknown cause of multisystem granulomatous disease	Chest—bilateral hilar lymph node enlargement with or without diffuse parenchymal disease HRCT—demonstrates subtle lymphadenopathy in the anterior mediastinal and left paratracheal nodes and parenchymal disease as ground-glass attenuation	No treatment if spontaneous recovery Steroid therapy
Systemic lupus erythematosus	Immune-complex disease (a connective tissue disorder)	Skeletal—subluxations and malalignment of joints Chest—pleural effusions, small and bilateral; cardiac enlargement	Antiinflammatory drugs for muscle and joint pain Systemic corticosteroids help prevent renal and central nervous system pathology Antimalarial drugs for skin lesion
Melanoma	Widely metastasizing malignant skin cancer	Metastatic involvement of the GI tract; round or oval nodules with necrosis and ulceration	Prevention—watch for changes in skin and reduce sun exposure Surgical excision of lesion and surrounding tissue, biopsy needed to determine if chemotherapy is necessary
Muscular dystrophy	Replacement of muscle by fat	Extremities—fine striated (striped) appearance of remaining muscle bundles	Nonstrenuous exercise to maintain mobility and function Drug therapy is used to protect muscle mass and function

GI, Gastrointestinal.

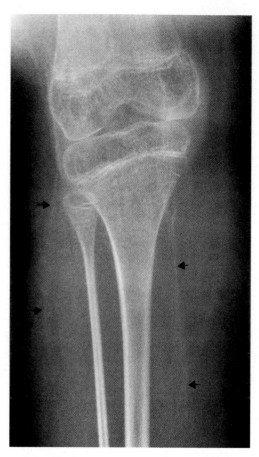

FIGURE 12-14 Muscular dystrophy. Thin, demineralized bones of the lower leg. Increased lucency, representing fatty infiltration in muscle bundles, makes fascial sheaths appear as thin shadows of increased density *(arrows)* surrounded by fat.

exercise is recommended to maintain mobility and function for as long as possible.

Hereditary Diseases

Chromosomal Aberrations

The chromosomes may mutate in many different ways and cause a multitude of disease processes. The following discussion of chromosomal aberrations includes two trisomy disorders (Down syndrome and Klinefelter's syndrome), a monosomy disorder (Turner's syndrome) and an autosomal dominant disorder (Marfan's syndrome). A **syndrome** indicates the presence of a combination of symptoms that commonly occur together and are related to a single cause.

Down Syndrome (Mongolism)

Down syndrome, the most common of the trisomy disorders (trisomy 21), is caused by an extraautosomal chromosome that results in an individual having three

strands of chromosome 21 instead of the normal two. Down syndrome is usually diagnosed at birth because of the characteristic clinical appearance: mental deficiency, short stature, poor muscle tone, short neck, and a straight skin crease that extends across the palm of the hand. The typical facial appearance includes widely set eyes, a short and flat nose, and a coarse tongue that often protrudes through a partially open mouth.

Congenital heart disease, especially septal defects, occurs in about 40% of patients with Down syndrome. There is also a greater-than-normal incidence of duodenal obstruction (duodenal atresia or annular pancreas) and Hirschsprung's disease and a substantially increased likelihood of developing leukemia.

Lab tests [chorionic villus sampling (CVS), amniocentesis, and percutaneous umbilical blood sampling (PUBS)] and the age of the mother are used to determine the risk of Down syndrome for prospective parents. Ultrasound can provide additional information. Even using these sophisticated tests, false-positive results may occur, and an accurate diagnosis can only be made after birth.

Radiographic Appearance

The major skeletal abnormality in infancy is in the pelvis, where there is a decrease in the acetabular and iliac angles with hypoplasia and noticeable lateral flaring of the iliac wings (Figure 12-15). Other common skeletal abnormalities include shortening of the middle phalanx of the fifth finger, squaring of the vertebral bodies (superoinferior length becoming equal to or greater than the anteroposterior measurement), hypoplasia of the nasal sinuses, and delayed closure of the cranial sutures.

Treatment

The many different anomalies require various treatments, which generally provide a better quality of life for the afflicted person. Experimental dietary supplements (dimethyl sulfoxide [DMSO]–amino acid formula) are believed by some to slow the retardation process, but the Food and Drug Administration has not approved these drugs.

Klinefelter's Syndrome

Klinefelter's syndrome (**testicular dysgenesis**) is a disorder characterized by small testes that fail to mature or produce sperm and testosterone. The fundamental defect is the presence in a male of two or more X chromosomes, indicating that this disorder is another sex chromosome trisomy. The pituitary sends a signal for the body to produce testosterone, but the testes do not respond. At puberty, the breasts

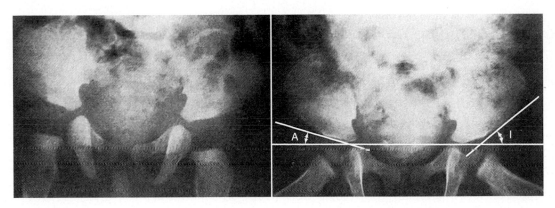

FIGURE 12-15 Down syndrome. Two examples of a typical pelvis in Down syndrome show flared iliac wings and diminished acetabular *(A)* and iliac *(I)* angles.

enlarge, and a female distribution of hair develops. The affected individual is tall, mentally deficient (often with language impairment), and sterile.

Radiographic Appearance

Radiographically, the skeletal changes are both less common and less pronounced than in patients with Turner's syndrome, its female counterpart. A positive metacarpal sign is present in fewer than 25% of the patients. Hypogonadism may lead to delayed epiphyseal fusion and retarded bone maturation.

Treatment

Hormonal therapy provides treatment of the symptoms of Klinefelter's syndrome. When young men enter puberty, testosterone therapy assists the body in developing normal male attributes (male distribution of hair growth and muscular body type).

Turner's Syndrome

Turner's syndrome (**gonadal dysgenesis**), a sex chromosome monosomy disorder, is characterized by primary amenorrhea (no ovulation or menstruation), sexual infantilism, short stature, and bilateral tiny gonads. Although the patient appears to be female, she has only one X chromosome as a result of faulty cellular division.

Various urinary tract anomalies, especially horseshoe kidney and other types of malrotation, are often seen in patients with gonadal dysgenesis. Coarctation of the aorta is the most common cardiovascular anomaly. Because coarctation of the aorta most often affects men, its appearance in a woman should indicate the possibility of underlying gonadal dysgenesis.

Radiographic Appearance

A characteristic, but nonspecific, skeletal abnormality is shortening of the fourth metacarpal and sometimes also the fifth metacarpal (Figure 12-16). This produces

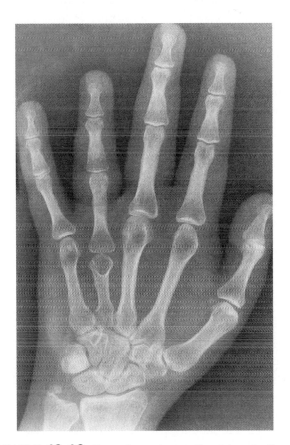

FIGURE 12-16 Turner's syndrome. Frontal projection of hand shows the short fourth metacarpal.

a positive metacarpal sign, in which a line drawn tangentially to the distal ends of the heads of the fourth and fifth metacarpals passes through the head of the third metacarpal (indicating the disproportionate shortening of the fourth and fifth metacarpals), rather than extending distally to the head of the third metacarpal as in an unaffected person. Skeletal surveys performed serially at specified intervals during adolescence demonstrate changes in bone growth.

SUMMARY *of* **FINDINGS** *for* **Hereditary Diseases**

disorder	cause	radiographic appearance	treatment
Down syndrome	Extra autosomal chromosome—trisomy 21	Pelvis—decreased acetabular and iliac angles with hypoplasia and lateral flaring of iliac wings	Various treatments to provide a better quality of life
Klinefelter's syndrome (testicular dysgenesis)	Sex chromosome trisomy disorder—male with two or more X chromosomes	Possible delayed epiphyseal fusion and retarded bone maturation	Hormonal therapy
Turner's syndrome (gonadal dysgenesis)	Sex chromosome trisomy disorder—female with one X chromosome	Shortening of the 4th and 5th metacarpals	Growth hormones for stature Hormonal therapy for gonadal dysfunction
Marfan's syndrome	Autosomal dominant disorder of connective tissue	Elongation and thinning of tubular bones (hands and feet), arachnodactyly	No cure

Treatment

Patients with Turner's syndrome can receive treatment for their short stature and for gonadal dysfunction. Human growth hormones have been available since 1994. Hormone replacement therapy of progesterone and/or estrogen may be prescribed to treat gonadal dysfunction (lack of ovulation) and to control female physical attributes (hair distribution and breast growth).

Marfan's Syndrome

Marfan's syndrome is an inherited generalized disorder of connective tissue with ocular, skeletal, and cardiovascular manifestations. Most patients with this autosomal dominant disorder are tall and slender, appearing emaciated because of the decrease in subcutaneous fat. A typical feature of Marfan's syndrome is bilateral dislocation of the lens of the eye caused by weakness of its supporting tissues. A laxity of ligaments about the joints leads to loose jointedness (or double jointedness), recurrent dislocations, and flat feet.

Almost all patients with Marfan's syndrome have abnormalities of the cardiovascular system. Necrosis of the medial portion of the aortic wall causes a progressive dilatation of the ascending aorta that produces a bulging of the upper right portion of the cardiac silhouette (Figure 12-17) and an unusual prominence of the pulmonary outflow tract as it is displaced by the dilated aorta. Dissecting aneurysm, a serious complication, may kill the patient in early life.

Radiographic Appearance

The major radiographic abnormality is elongation and thinning of the tubular bones (Figure 12-18), most pronounced in the hands and feet and seen

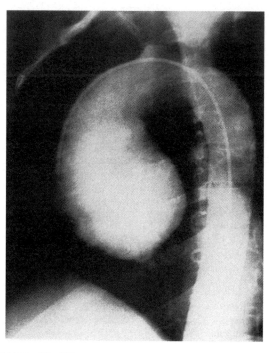

FIGURE 12-17 Marfan's syndrome. Arteriogram shows the enormous dilatation of the aneurysmal ascending aorta.

clinically as **arachnodactyly** (spiderlike digits). Patients may exhibit **pectus excavatum** (concave sternum) on a lateral chest radiograph (Figure 12-19).

Treatment

Currently, no cure exists for Marfan's syndrome. The laxity of the joints makes these patients susceptible to scoliosis; monitoring the spine and treating any curvature early help prevent spinal deformities. These patients are

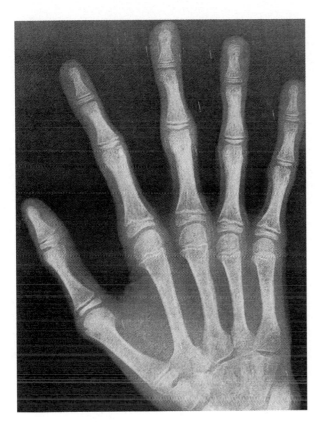

FIGURE **12-18** Arachnodactyly in Marfan's syndrome. Metacarpals and phalanges are unusually long and slender.

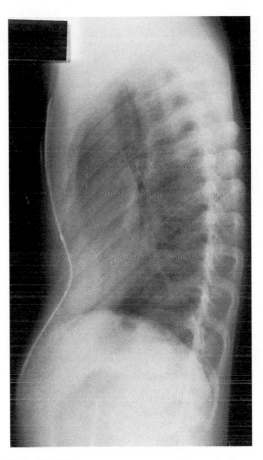

FIGURE **12-19** Pectus excavatum. Lateral chest radiograph demonstrates a concave sternum.

vulnerable to endocarditis resulting from dental procedures and commonly receive prophylactic antibiotics.

Genetic Amino Acid Disorders

The genetic amino acid disorders result from the absence of an enzyme required to produce a biochemical reaction that the body requires for normal growth and physiologic function. This genetic defect causes a decrease or an interruption in amino acid metabolism.

Homocystinuria

Homocystinuria, an inborn error of the metabolism of the amino acid methionine, causes a defect in the structure of collagen or elastin. The absence of the enzyme cystathionine B-synthase causes an elevation in the level of methionine by not allowing the metabolic cycle to complete its process. Homocystinuria occurs only if both parents carry the gene (i.e., it is an autosomal recessive trait). Patients with homocystinuria have a tendency to develop arterial and venous thrombosis, and premature occlusive vascular disease is the major cause of death. Other common signs are similar to those of Marfan's syndrome (long limbs, arachnodactyly, and scoliosis). Additional symptoms

include myopia (nearsightedness), dislocation of the lens of the eye, and mental retardation.

Radiographic Appearance

The most common and striking radiographic feature of homocystinuria is osteoporosis of the spine, which is often associated with biconcave deformities of the vertebral bodies (Figure 12-20).

Treatment

Because no cure has been found, treatment available consists of a low-methionine diet and increased doses of vitamin B$_6$ and folic acid or cysteine supplements. Not all patients have found this treatment effective.

Phenylketonuria

Phenylketonuria (PKU) is an inborn error of metabolism in which an enzyme deficiency results in the impaired conversion of phenylalanine to tyrosine. Fortunately, routine screening enables diagnosis of this disease at birth. If the condition is not diagnosed and treated early, the excessive phenylalanine in the blood usually causes the patient to suffer profound retardation (**microcephaly**), hyperactivity,

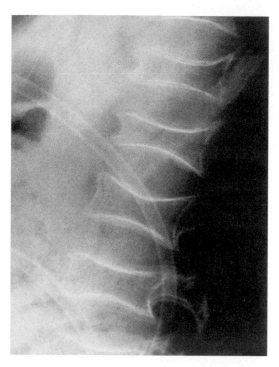

FIGURE 12-20 Homocystinuria. Striking osteoporosis of the spine is associated with biconcave deformities of the vertebral bodies.

and seizures, all related to brain atrophy. Because of an inadequate amount of tyrosine, there is impaired production of the pigment melanin, and the patient is very light in color.

Radiographic Appearance
The brain atrophy appears as dilatation of the ventricles and sulci on CT scans or magnetic resonance (MR) images.

Treatment
Treatment includes a diet low in phenylalanine and protein. Dietary measures can prevent the disease process from progressing if the treatment begins before age 1 year. Treatment instituted later in life will not improve any destructive damage that has already occurred.

Alkaptonuria and Ochronosis
Alkaptonuria is a rare inborn error of metabolism in which an enzyme deficiency leads to an abnormal accumulation of homogentisic acid in the blood and urine. The urine is either very dark on voiding or becomes black after standing or being alkalinized. The disorder often goes unrecognized until middle age, when deposition of the black pigment of oxidized homogentisic acid in cartilage and other connective tissue produces a distinctive form of degenerative arthritis (ochronosis).

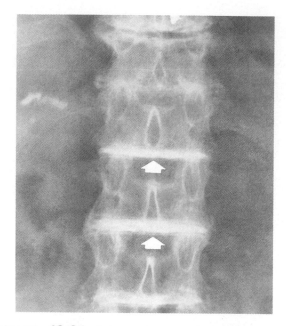

FIGURE 12-21 Ochronosis. Frontal projection of the lumbar spine shows the dense laminated calcification of multiple intervertebral disks (*arrows*).

Radiographic Appearance
The pathognomonic radiographic finding is dense, laminated calcification in multiple intervertebral disks (Figure 12-21); the calcification begins in the lumbar spine and may extend to involve the dorsal and cervical regions.

Treatment
Medical therapy can inhibit the rate of pigment deposit. A low-protein diet and added vitamin C may retard the accumulation of homogentisic acid in older children and adults.

Cystinuria
Cystinuria is an inborn error of amino acid transport characterized by impaired tubular absorption and excessive urinary excretion of several amino acids. Large amounts of cystine in the urine predispose to the formation of renal, ureteral, and bladder stones. It is common to see multiple and bilateral stones, even large staghorn calculi.

Radiographic Appearance
Pure cystine stones are not radiopaque and can be demonstrated only on excretory urography, where they appear as filling defects in the urinary tract. Stones containing the calcium salts of cystine appear radiopaque and can be detected on plain abdominal radiographs. Abdominal CT may define the filling defect better than intravenous urography.

SUMMARY of FINDINGS for Genetic Amino Acid Disorders

disorder	cause	radiographic appearance	treatment
Homocystinuria	Absence of cystathionine B-synthase	Osteoporosis of the spine—biconcave deformities of vertebral bodies	Low methionine diet; increase vitamin B_6 and folic acid or cysteine supplements
Phenylketonuria	Enzyme deficiency leading to excessive phenylalanine	CT or MRI—brain atrophy with dilatation of ventricles and sulci	Low phenylalanine and protein diet to control progression
Alkaptonuria/ochronosis	Enzyme deficiency leading to excessive homogentisic acid	Dense laminated calcification of multiple intervertebral disks	Therapy to inhibit rate of deposit
Cystinuria	Error of amino acid transport	CT—defines cystine stones in the urinary tract	No cure—increase water intake to help prevent stone formation. Thiol drugs—to aid in dissolving the cystine
Gaucher's disease	Abnormal accumulation of complex lipids	Extremity—loss of bone density, with expansion and cortical thickening of long bones	Treatment to inhibit the accumulation of complex lipids. Enzyme replacement to reverse extraskeletal symptoms

Treatment

Currently there is no cure for cystinuria. However, therapy is available to provide relief from symptoms and to prevent new stones from developing. One approach is to increase water intake to six to eight glasses a day to dilute the increased excretion of cystine in the urine. Thiol drugs may be of value in dissolving the cystine for excretion.

Glycogen Storage Diseases

The glycogen storage diseases are a group of genetic disorders that involve the pathways for the storage of carbohydrates as glycogen (in the liver) and for its use in maintaining blood glucose and providing energy. Normal or abnormal glycogen in an excess amount infiltrates and enlarges multiple organs, especially the heart and liver (Figure 12-22).

Gaucher's Disease

Gaucher's disease is an inborn error of metabolism characterized by the accumulation of abnormal quantities of complex lipids in the reticuloendothelial cells of the spleen, liver, and bone marrow. The adult (chronic) form of Gaucher's disease is most common; some cases arise in children or infants.

Aseptic necrosis (especially involving the femoral heads) is a common complication. The spleen is usually greatly enlarged, and hepatomegaly is common.

Radiographic Appearance

The most striking changes occur in the skeletal system. Infiltration of the bone marrow with abnormal lipid-containing cells causes a loss of bone density with expansion and cortical thickening of the long bones, especially the femur. Marrow infiltration of the distal femur causes abnormal modeling, flaring, and the characteristic (but nonspecific) Erlenmeyer flask deformity (Figure 12-23).

Treatment

In the past, the traditional treatment for Gaucher's was splenectomy. Today new experimental treatments are used in an attempt to inhibit the accumulation of complex lipids. Enzyme replacement is still

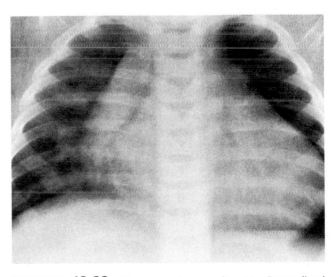

FIGURE 12-22 Glycogen storage disease. Generalized globular cardiac enlargement with left ventricular prominence.

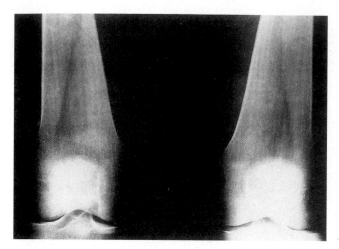

FIGURE 12-23 Gaucher's disease. The distal ends of the femurs show typical underconstriction and cortical thinning.

under investigation, though initial trials have demonstrated reversal of extraskeletal symptoms.

Internal Devices

Endotracheal Tube

A chest radiograph should always be obtained immediately after endotracheal intubation to ensure proper positioning because clinical evaluation (bilateral breath sounds, symmetric thoracic expansion, and palpation of the tube in the sternal notch) does not allow detection of the majority of malpositioned tubes. Daily radiographs are usually taken to ensure that the tube has not been inadvertently displaced by the weight of the respiratory apparatus, by the patient's coughing, or by other unforeseen events. In addition, this permits prompt detection of complications of intubation and barotrauma (positive-pressure breathing), such as pneumothorax and pneumomediastinum.

The relationship between the tip of the tube and the carina (tracheal bifurcation) must be carefully assessed. When the head and neck are in a neutral position, the endotracheal tube tip ideally should be about 5 to 7 cm above the carina (Figure 12-24). With flexion and extension of the neck, the tip of the tube will move about 2 cm caudally and cranially, respectively.

About 10% to 20% of endotracheal tubes require repositioning after insertion. A tube positioned too low usually extends into the right mainstem bronchus, where it eventually leads to atelectasis of the left lung (see Figure 3-64). A tube positioned excessively high or in the esophagus causes the inspired air to enter the stomach, causing severe gastric dilatation and a high likelihood of regurgitation of gastric contents and aspiration pneumonia.

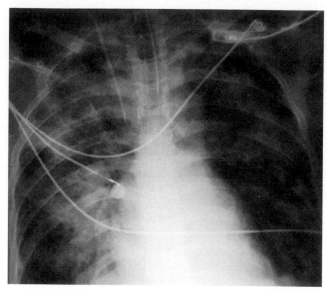

FIGURE 12-24 Proper position of the endotracheal tube.

Central Venous Catheters

Central venous catheters inserted into the subclavian vein or a more peripheral vein in the upper extremity are extremely useful for measurement of the central venous pressure (CVP) and for providing a conduit for the rapid infusion of fluid or chronic hyperalimentation. So that the CVP may be correctly measured, the catheter must be located within the true central venous system, beyond all the valves, which interfere with direct transmission of right atrial pressure to the catheter. The optimal location is where the brachiocephalic veins join to form the superior vena cava (medial to the anterior border of the first rib on chest radiographs) or within the superior vena cava itself.

Because up to one third of CVP catheters are initially inserted incorrectly, the position of the catheter should be confirmed by a chest radiograph. The most common aberrant location of a CVP catheter is the internal jugular vein (Figure 12-25). CVP catheters that extend to the right atrium are associated with an increased risk of cardiac arrhythmias and even perforation. Extension of the catheter into the hepatic veins may result in the infusion of potentially toxic substances (some antibiotics and hypertonic alimentation solutions) directly into the liver. Also, after successful placement, CVP catheters may change position as a result of patient motion or medical manipulation; therefore periodic radiographic confirmation of the catheter position is often recommended.

The anatomy of the subclavian region may lead to complications when a central catheter is introduced via the subclavian vein. Because the pleura

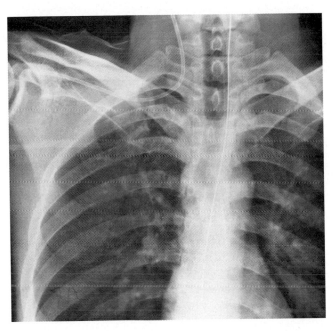

FIGURE 12-25 CVP catheter in the right internal jugular vein.

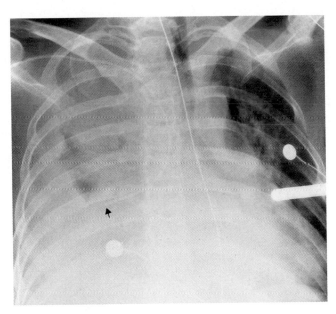

FIGURE 12-26 CVP catheter with its tip in the pleural space. A right subclavian catheter, which was introduced for total parenteral nutrition, perforated the superior vena cava and eroded into the right pleural space. Note the tip of the catheter projecting beyond the right border of the mediastinum *(arrow)*. The direct infusion of parenteral fluid into the pleural space has led to a large right hydrothorax.

covering the apex of the lung lies just deep to the subclavian vein, a pneumothorax may develop. Because this may be difficult to detect clinically, a chest radiograph (if possible with the patient in an upright position and in expiration) should be obtained whenever insertion of a subclavian catheter has been attempted. Another complication is perivascular CVP catheter placement, which may result in ectopic infusion of fluid into the mediastinum or pleural space. This diagnosis should be suggested if there is rapid development of mediastinal widening or pleural effusion after CVP catheter insertion (Figure 12-26). Other complications include inadvertent puncture of the subclavian artery, air embolism, and injury to the phrenic nerve.

The peripherally inserted central catheter (PICC) has become the long-term venous access device used for home therapy and chemotherapy patients.

Catheter breakage and embolization can result from laceration of the catheter by the needle used to insert it, fracture at a point of stress, or detachment of the catheter from its hub. The catheter fragment may lodge in the vena cava, in the right side of the heart, or in branches of the pulmonary artery (Figure 12-27), and the result may be thrombosis, infection, or perforation.

Swan-Ganz Catheters

The flow-directed Swan-Ganz catheter consists of a central channel for measuring pulmonary capillary wedge (PCW) pressure and a second, smaller channel

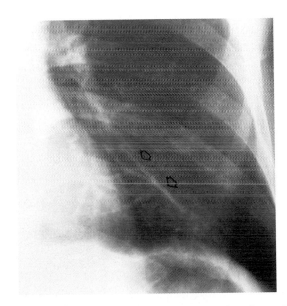

FIGURE 12-27 Broken CVP catheter. The sheared-off portion of the catheter *(arrow)* is located in the left lower lobe.

connected to an inflatable balloon at the catheter tip. Cardiac output and CVP can also be measured by use of this catheter. It can be inserted at the bedside and floated to the pulmonary artery without the need for fluoroscopic monitoring.

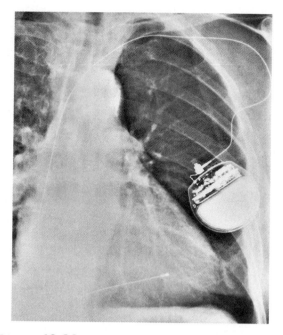

FIGURE 12-28 Pacemaker tip in coronary sinus. On the frontal projection, the tip of the electrode is angled slightly superiorly, traversing the heart in a higher plane than when it is located in the right ventricle.

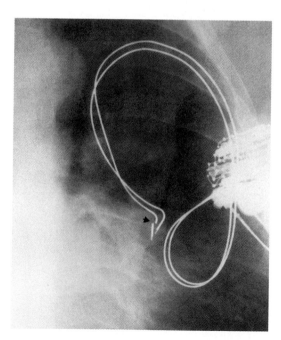

FIGURE 12-29 Fracture of a cardiac pacemaker wire *(arrow)*.

Ideally the catheter is positioned so that it lies within the right or left main pulmonary artery. Inflating the balloon causes the catheter to float downstream into a wedge position; deflating the balloon permits the catheter to recoil into the central pulmonary artery. Unlike standard intravenous catheters, the Swan-Ganz catheter has a radiopaque strip down its center.

The most common complication associated with the use of a Swan-Ganz catheter is pulmonary infarction distal to the catheter tip. Infarction may result from occlusion of a pulmonary artery by the catheter itself (if it is wedged in a too peripheral vessel) or from clot formation in or about the catheter. The pulmonary infarction appears as a patchy air-space consolidation involving the area of the lung supplied by the pulmonary artery in which the catheter lies. The appropriate treatment is simply removal of the Swan-Ganz catheter; systemic heparinization is not required once this source of emboli or obstruction has been removed.

Transvenous Cardiac Pacemakers

Transvenous endocardiac pacing is the method of choice for maintaining cardiac rhythm in patients with heart block or bradyarrhythmias. Radiographic evaluation plays an important role in the initial placement of a pacemaker and in the detection of any subsequent complications. An overexposed film can demonstrate both the generator (for permanent pacemakers) and the course of the electrodes.

Ideally the tip of the pacemaker should be positioned at the apex of the right ventricle. One common aberrant location is the coronary sinus. On a frontal radiograph, the tip often appears to be well positioned. A lateral projection is required to show that the tip is directly posterior in the coronary sinus, rather than in its proper position anterior in the right ventricle.

Although electrode fractures have become less common because of the development of new alloys, they are still a significant cause of pacing failure (Figure 12-28). The usual sites of fracture are near the pulse generator, at sharp bends in the wires, and at the point where the electrodes are inserted into the epicardium. Although most electrode fractures are easily detected on routine chest radiographs, some subtle fractures may be demonstrated only on oblique views or at fluoroscopy.

Perforation of the myocardium by an intravenous electrode usually occurs at the time of insertion or during the first few days thereafter. Perforation should be suspected when the pacemaker fails to sense or elicit a ventricular response. Plain radiographs show the electrode tip lying outside the right ventricular cavity (Figure 12-29).

SUMMARY of FINDINGS for Internal Devices

internal device	correct placement*	complications
Endotracheal tube	Tip of tube 5-7 cm above the carina	Low placement—atelectasis High placement—air entering the stomach
Central venous pressure catheters	Tip of catheter just beyond the joining of the brachiocephalic veins to form the superior vena cava	Internal jugular vein placement Right atrium—possible arrhythmias or perforation Pneumothorax with placement Infusion of fluid into mediastinum or pleural space
Swan-Ganz catheters	Right or left main pulmonary artery	Pulmonary infarction
Transvenous cardiac pacemakers	Overexpose to demonstrate the tip of the electrode at the apex of the right ventricle	Coronary sinus placement—needs a lateral chest film to distinguish Perforation at initial insertion

*Placement determined by chest radiograph.

REVIEW QUESTIONS

1. A vitamin C deficiency that years ago was common among sailors because of their lack of fresh fruit and vegetables is termed _____.

2. _____ is a vitamin deficiency disease that occurs primarily in countries in which polished rice is the main staple.

3. A deficiency of niacin, characterized by reddening and scaling of exposed skin, vomiting, diarrhea, and nervous and mental disorders is termed _____.

4. A bone disease of young children who have been deprived of adequate vitamin D is termed _____.

5. Vitamin _____ is necessary in the blood clotting mechanism.

6. A lack of vitamin _____ can result in night blindness.

7. When caloric intake consistently exceeds the amount needed for the body to function, _____ occurs.

8. A granulomatous disease of unknown origin that usually affects women more than men and African-Americans more than whites, and whose presence is most often identified on screening chest radiographs, is _____.

9. A disease of young to middle-aged women that is most likely an immune-complex disease, that can affect several systems of the body, and that is characterized by a butterfly-shaped rash across the nose and cheeks is _____.

10. A very malignant form of skin cancer, capable of metastasizing throughout the body, is _____.

11. An inherited muscular disease characterized by severe weakness and eventual death from respiratory muscle failure or pneumonia is _____.

12. The radiographer should be very alert to the possibility of _____ in patients with muscular dystrophy who lack normal swallowing ability.

13. Name three trisomy disorders: _____, _____, and _____.

14. The _____ syndrome occurs when a female has only one X chromosome.

15. Arachnodactyly, spiderlike digits, occurs in which two hereditary disorders?

16. Two common complications of intubation and barotrauma are _____ and _____.

17. A common catheter used to measure cardiac output and central venous pressure is the _____.

18. The optimal location for a central venous catheter is where the brachiocephalic veins join to form the _____.

19. An overexposed radiograph is often requested for visualizing transvenous endocardiac pacemakers to demonstrate both the _____ and the _____.

20. The most common complication associated with the Swan-Ganz catheter is _____ distal to the catheter tip.

21. Briefly describe why a lateral chest radiograph is very important for determining the correct position of the tip of the electrode of a transvenous cardiac pacemaker.

BIBLIOGRAPHY

Beers MH, Berkow R, editors : *The Merck manual of diagnosis and therapy,* ed 17, Rahway, NJ, 1999, Merck.

Goodman LR, Putman C: *Critical care imaging,* Philadelphia, 1991, Saunders.

Juhl JH, Crummy AB: *Essentials of radiologic imaging,* Philadelphia, 1987, Lippincott.

Kirks DR, McCormick VD, Greenspan RH: Pulmonary sarcoidosis, *AJR Am J Roentgenol* 117:777-786, 1973.

Lubowitz R, Schumacher HR: Articular manifestations of systemic lupus erythematosus, *Ann Intern Med* 74:911-921, 1974.

ANSWERS TO REVIEW QUESTIONS

Chapter 1

1. edema
2. phagocytosis
3. keloid
4. suppurative
5. ischemia
6. infarct
7. hematoma
8. atrophy
9. neoplasia
10. adenoma

Chapter 2

1. D
2. B
3. A
4. A
5. C
6. A
7. A
8. C
9. C
10. C

Chapter 3

1. hyaline membrane disease
2. cystic fibrosis
3. lung abscess
4. bronchography
5. emphysema
6. silicosis, asbestosis, anthracosis
7. pulmonary arteriovenous fistula
8. tension pneumothorax
9. empyema
10. pneumonia
11. histoplasmosis, coccidioidomycosis
12. coughing, droplets
13. pneumothorax
14. emphysema
15. pneumoconiosis
16. mesothelioma
17. septic embolism
18. atelectasis
19. larger and more vertical mainstem bronchi
20. subcutaneous emphysema
21. C
22. mediastinal emphysema
    (pneumomediastinum)
23. C

Chapter 4

1. B
2. A
3. D
4. D
5. B
6. B
7. A
8. B
9. C
10. A
11. D
12. B
13. D
14. C
15. B
16. C
17. B
18. D
19. B
20. C
21. A
22. C
23. D
24. B
25. B

Chapter 5

1. B
2. C
3. A
4. B
5. C
6. A
7. B
8. D
9. C
10. C
11. C
12. B
13. B
14. D
15. D
16. A
17. B
18. A
19. D
20. C
21. B
22. B

23. D
24. B
25. C
26. A

Chapter 6

1. D
2. D
3. B
4. A
5. C
6. D
7. C
8. A
9. C
10. A

Chapter 7

1. D
2. A
3. B
4. D
5. D
6. C
7. B
8. D
9. A
10. A
11. C
12. C
13. A
14. B
15. A
16. C
17. B
18. C
19. B
20. B
21. B
22. B
23. D
24. D

Chapter 8

1. C
2. C
3. B
4. D
5. D
6. B

7. A
8. C
9. B
10. C
11. CT
12. CT, MRI
13. transient ischemic attack
14. MRI
15. epilepsy
16. Alzheimer's disease
17. Parkinson's disease
18. horizontal, erect
19. hydrocephalus
20. cross-table lateral, horizontal

Chapter 9

1. C
2. A
3. C
4. B
5. B
6. C
7. C
8. C
9. A
10. C
11. B
12. B

Chapter 10

1. C
2. C
3. A
4. B
5. B
6. C
7. B
8. B
9. C
10. B
11. D
12. B
13. C
14. B
15. B
16. B
17. B
18. A
19. C
20. B
21. D

Chapter 11

1. nonionizing imaging source, high frequency sound waves
2. hysterosalpingography, mammography
3. spermatogenesis
4. testosterone
5. vasectomy
6. cancer of the prostate
7. ultrasound
8. True
9. ivory vertebra
10. ultrasound
11. testicular torsion
12. testicular, lymphatic
13. ovulation
14. ectopic
15. hysterosalpingography
16. syphilis
17. dermoid/teratoma
18. fibroids
19. breast
20. carcinoma of the cervix

Chapter 12

1. scurvy
2. beriberi
3. pellagra

4. rickets
5. K
6. A
7. obesity
8. sarcoidosis
9. systemic lupus erythematosus
10. melanoma
11. muscular dystrophy
12. aspiration
13. Down syndrome, Turner's syndrome, Klinefelter's syndrome
14. Turner's syndrome
15. Marfan syndrome, homocystinuria
16. pneumothorax, pneumomediastinum
17. Swan-Ganz
18. superior vena cava
19. generator, electrodes
20. infarction
21. In AP and PA radiographs, the tip may *appear* to be in the proper position, but a lateral view is needed to ensure that the tip is in the anterior portion of the right ventricle—the correct position.

ILLUSTRATION CREDITS

Chapter 1

Figure 1-3 courtesy Sonja Bonney, RT, (R), Phoenix, AZ.

Figure 1-6 from Bryk D et al: Kaposi's sarcoma of the intestinal tract: roentgen manifestations, *Gastrointest Radiol* 3:425, 1978.

Chapter 2

Figure 2-10 courtesy Richard Fuccillo, RT, (R), Albany, OR.

Figures 2-15, 2-16, and 2-17 courtesy Bartram J. Pierce, RT, (R)(MR), Good Samaritan Medical Center, Corvallis, OR.

Unnumbered Figures 2-1 through 2-4 from Bushong SC: *Radiologic science for technologists: physics, biology and protection,* ed 8, St Louis, 2004, Mosby.

Unnumbered Figure 2-5 from Kremkau FW: *Diagnostic ultrasound: principles and instruments,* ed 7, St Louis, 2006, Saunders.

Chapter 3

Figure 3-1 from Swischuk LE: *Radiology of the newborn and young infant,* Baltimore, 1980, Williams & Wilkins.

Figure 3-5 from Podgore JK, Bass JW: *J Pediatr* 88:154-155, 1976.

Figures 3-9, 3-26, and 3-70 from Eisenberg R: *Atlas of signs in radiology,* Philadelphia, 1984, Lippincott.

Figure 3-25 courtesy Karen Brown, RT, (R)(M), St. Joseph's Hospital and Medical Center, Phoenix, AZ.

Figures 3-32 and 3-56 from Fraser RG, Paré JAP: *Diagnosis of diseases of the chest,* Philadelphia, 1979, Saunders.

Figure 3-36 from Sargent EN, Jacobson G, Gordonson JS: *Semin Roentgenol* 12:287-297, 1977.

Figure 3-50 from Lee JKT, Sagel SS, Stanley RJ, editors: *Computed body tomography,* New York, 1989, Raven Press.

Figure 3-68 from Cappitanio MA et al: *Radiology* 103:460-461, 1972.

Figure 3-78 from Vix VA: *Semin Roentgenol* 12:277-286, 1977.

Figure 3-79 from Eisenberg RL: *Diagnostic imaging in surgery,* New York, 1987, McGraw-Hill.

Unnumbered Figure 3-1 from Thibodeau GA, Patton KT: *Anatomy and physiology,* ed 2, St Louis, 1993, Mosby.

Chapter 4

Figure 4-13 from Brown JC, Forrester DM: Arthritis. In Eisenberg RL, Amberg JR, editors: *Critical diagnostic pathways in radiology,* Philadelphia, 1981, Lippincott.

Figure 4-26 from Forrester DM, Brown JC, Nesson JW: *The radiology of joint disease,* Philadelphia, 1978, Saunders.

Figures 4-28, 4-32, and 4-34 from Rumack C, Wilson S, Charborneau JW, editors: *Diagnostic ultrasound,* ed 2, St Louis, 1998, Mosby.

Figure 4-30 from Greenspan A: *Orthopedic radiology,* Philadelphia, 1988, Lippincott.

Figures 4-31, 4-33, 4-69, and 4-83, *A* from Stark DD, Bradley WG Jr: *Magnetic resonance imaging,* ed 2, St Louis, 1991, Mosby.

Figures 4-44 and 4-104 courtesy Eric Bowlus, RT, (R), Phoenix, AZ.

Figure 4-68 from deSantos LA, Bernardino ME, Murray JA: Computed tomography in the evaluation of osteosarcoma: experience with 25 cases. *AJR Am J Roentgenol* 132:535-540, 1979.

Figures 4-84 and 4-116 from Eisenberg R: *Diagnostic imaging in surgery,* New York, 1987, McGraw-Hill.

Figure 4-91 from Dorne HL, Lander PH: Spontaneous stress fractures of the femoral neck. *AJR Am J Roentgenol* 144:343-347, 1985.

Figure 4-92 from Sty JR, Starshak RJ: The role of bone scintigraphy in the evaluation of the suspected abused child, *Radiology* 146:369-375, 1983.

Figure 4-95 from Silverman FN: *Caffey's pediatric x-ray imaging,* St Louis, 1985, Mosby.

Figure 4-103 from Bassett LW, Gold RH, Epstein HC: Anterior hip dislocation: atypical superolateral displacement of the femoral head, *AJR Am J Roentgenol* 141:385-386, 1983.

Figure 4-108 from Osborn AG: Head trauma. In Eisenberg RL, Amberg JR, editors: *Critical diagnostic pathways in radiology,* Philadelphia, 1981, Lippincott.

Figure 4-118 courtesy Bartram J. Pierce, RT, (R)(MR), Good Samaritan Regional Medical Center, Corvallis, OR.

Unnumbered Figure 4-1 from Thibodeau GA, Patton KT: *Anatomy and physiology,* ed 2, St Louis 1993, Mosby.

Chapter 5

Figures 5-14, 5-15, 5-16, 5-20, 5-21, and 5-86 from Eisenberg RL: *Gastrointestinal radiology: a pattern approach,* Philadelphia, 1990, Lippincott.

Figure 5-30 from Margulis AR, Burhenne JH, editors: *Alimentary tract radiology,* ed 4, St Louis, 1989, Mosby.

Figure 5-46 from Jeffrey RB: *CT and sonography of the acute abdomen,* New York, 1989, Raven Press.

Figure 5-55 from Rice RP et al: *Radiographics* 4:393-409, 1984.

Figure 5-56 courtesy Carol Krebs, RT, Shreveport, LA.

Figure 5-67 from Caroline DF, Evers K: Colitis: radiographic features and differentiation of idiopathic inflammatory bowel disease, *Radiol Clin North Am* 25:47-66, 1987.

Figure 5-68 from Lichtenstein JE: Radiologic-pathologic correlation of inflammatory bowel disease, *Radiol Clin North Am* 25:3-23, 1987.

Figure 5-73 from Butch RJ: In Taveras JM, Ferruci JT, editors: *Radiology: diagnosis, imaging, intervention,* Philadelphia, 1987, Lippincott.

Figure 5-81 courtesy Stephen R. Baker, New York.

Figure 5-93 from Jeffrey RB, Federle MP, Laing FC: Computed tomography of mesenteric involvement in fulminant pancreatitis, *Radiology* 147:185-192, 1983.

Figure 5-101 from Federle MP, Goldberg HL: In Moss AA, Gamsu G, Genant HK, editors: *Computed tomography of the body,* Philadelphia, 1992, Saunders.

Figure 5-108 from Koehler RE: Spleen. In Lee JKT, Sagel SS, Stanley RJ, editors: *Computed body tomography,* New York, 1983, Raven Press.

Unnumbered Figure 5-1 from Thibodeau GA, Patton KT: *Anatomy and physiology,* ed 2, St Louis, 1993, Mosby.

Chapter 6

Figure 6-9 from Friedland GW et al: *Clin Radiol* 27:367-373, 1976.

Figures 6-13 and 6-14 from Tonkin AK, Witten DM: Genitourinary tuberculosis. *Semin Roentgenol* 14:305-318, 1979.

Figure 6-20 from Eisenberg R: *Gastrointestinal radiology: a pattern approach,* Philadelphia, 1990, Lippincott.

Figure 6-34 from Bosniak MA, Ambos MA: Polycystic kidney disease, *Semin Roentgenol* 10:133-143, 1975.

Figure 6-39 from Bosniak MA, Faegenburg D: *Radiology* 84:692-698, 1965.

Figure 6-42 from McClennan BL, Lee JKT: Kidney. In Lee JKT, Sagel SS, Stanley RJ, editors: *Computed body tomography,* New York, 1983, Raven Press.

Figures 6-44 and 6-49 from Friedland GW et al, editors: *Uroradiology: an integrated approach,* New York, 1983, Churchill Livingstone.

Figure 6-47 from Merten DE, Kirks DR: In Eisenberg RL, editor: *Diagnostic imaging: an algorithmic approach,* Philadelphia, 1988, Lippincott.

Figure 6-51 from Cohn LH et al: The treatment of bilateral renal vein thrombosis and nephrotic syndrome, *Surgery* 64:387-396, 1968.

Unnumbered Figure 6-1 from Thibodeau GA, Patton KT: *Anatomy and physiology,* ed 2, St Louis, 1993, Mosby.

Chapter 7

Figures 7-2, 7-3, and 7-4 from Cooley RN, Schreiber MH: *Radiology of the heart and great vessels,* Baltimore, 1978, Williams & Wilkins.

Figure 7-5 from Rumack et al: *Diagnostic ultrasound,* ed 3, vol 2, St Louis, 2005, Mosby.

Figure 7-7 from Swischuk LE: *Plain film interpretation in congenital heart disease,* Baltimore, 1979, Williams & Wilkins.

Figure 7-10 from Stark DD, Bradley WG, editors: *Magnetic resonance imaging,* St Louis, 1988, Mosby.

Figure 7-13 from Fischell TA, Block PC: *Cardiovasc Reviews Reports* 6:89-99, 1985.

Figure 7-18 from Fraser RG, Paré JAP: *Diagnosis of diseases of the chest,* Philadelphia, 1979, Saunders.

Figure 7-22 from Burko H et al: In Eisenberg RL, Amberg JR, editors: *Critical diagnostic pathways in radiology: an algorithmic approach,* Philadelphia, 1981, Lippincott.

Figure 7-24 from Waltman AC: In Athanasoulis CA et al, editors: *Interventional radiology,* Philadelphia, 1982, Saunders.

Figure 7-27 from Eisenberg R: *Gastrointestinal radiology: a pattern approach,* Philadelphia, 1990, Lippincott.

Figure 7-29 from Thoeni RF, Margulis AR: In Eisenberg RL, editor: *Diagnostic imaging: an algorithmic approach,* Philadelphia, 1988, Lippincott.

Figure 7-31 from Fisher RG, Hadlock FP, Ben-Menachem Y: *Radiol Clin North Am* 19:91-112, 1981.

Figure 7-32 from Woodring JH, Pulmano CM, Stevens RK: The right paratracheal stripe in blunt chest trauma. *Radiology* 143:605-608, 1982.

Figure 7-35 from Ovenfors CO, Godwin JD: In Eisenberg RL, editor: *Diagnostic imaging: an algorithmic approach,* Philadelphia, 1988, Lippincott.

Figure 7-39 from Waltman AC: In Athanasoulis CA et al, editors: *Interventional radiology,* Philadelphia, 1982, Saunders.

Figure 7-41 from Katzen BT, van Breda A: Low dose streptokinase in the treatment of arterial occlusions, *AJR Am J Roentgenol* 136:1171-1178, 1981.

Figure 7-44 from Vickers SCW et al: *Radiology* 72:569-575, 1959.

Figure 7-53 from Miller SW et al: Cardiac magnetic resonance imaging: the Massachusetts General Hospital experience, *Radiol Clin North Am* 23:745-764, 1985.

Figure 7-54 From Miller SW, Gillian LD: In Eisenberg RL, editor: *Diagnostic imaging: an algorithmic approach,* Philadelphia, 1988, Lippincott.

Figure 7-55 From Holden RW, Mail JT, Becker GJ: In Eisenberg RL, editor: *Diagnostic imaging: an algorithmic approach,* Philadelphia, 1988, Lippincott.

Unnumbered Figure 7-1 from Thibodeau GA, Patton KT: *Anatomy and physiology,* ed 2, St Louis, 1993, Mosby.

Chapter 8

Figure 8-1 from Ross MR, Davis DO, Mark AS: *MRI Decisions* 4:24-33, 1990.

Figure 8-2 from Edelman RR, Hesselink JR, editors: *Clinical magnetic resonance imaging,* Philadelphia, 1990, Saunders.

Figures 8-4, 8-5, and 8-71 from Stark DD, Bradley WG: *Magnetic resonance imaging,* ed 2, St Louis, 1991, Mosby.

Figures 8-7, 8-16, 8-23, and 8-73 from Eisenberg RL: *Clinical imaging: an atlas of differential diagnosis,* Gaithersburg, Md, 1992, Aspen.

Figures 8-10 and 8-60, *B* and *C* courtesy Bartram J. Pierce, RT, (R)(MR), Good Samaritan Regional Medical Center, Corvallis, OR.

Figures 8-17 and 8-21 from Williams AL, Haughton VM: *Cranial computed tomography,* St Louis, 1985, Mosby.

Figure 8-25, *B* from Levine HL, Kleefield J, Rao KCVG: In Lee SH, Rao KCVG, editors: *Cranial computed tomography,* New York, 1983, McGraw-Hill.

Figure 8-26 from Bilaniuk LT: Adult infratentorial tumors, *Semin Roentgenol* 25:155-173, 1990.

Figures 8-31, *A* and 8-36 from Pressman BD: In Eisenberg RL, editor: *Diagnostic imaging: an algorithmic approach,* Philadelphia, 1988, Lippincott.

Figure 8-38 from Eisenberg RL: *Diagnostic imaging in surgery,* New York, 1987, McGraw-Hill.

Figure 8-41 courtesy Kenneth D. Dolan, Iowa City, IA.

Figures 8-43 and 8-45 from Dolan K, Jacoby C, Smoker W: *Radiographics* 4:576-663, 1984.

Figure 8-44 from Rogers LF: *Radiology of skeletal trauma,* New York, 1982, Churchill Livingstone.

Figure 8-54 from Drayer BP: Neuroradiology. In Rosenberg RN, Heinz ER, editors: *The clinical neurosciences,* New York, 1984, Churchill Livingstone.

Figure 8-61 from Bronen RA: Epilepsy: the role of MR imaging, *AJR Am J Roentgenol* 159:1165-1174, 1992.

Figure 8-69 from Johnson CE, Zimmerman RD: *MRI Decisions* 3:2-16, 1989.

Unnumbered Figure 8-1 from Thibodeau GA, Patton KT: *Anatomy and physiology,* ed 2, St Louis, 1993, Mosby.

Chapter 9

Figure 9-3 from Leight TF: *Radiol Clin North Am* 1:377-393, 1963.

Figure 9-6 from Moseley JE: *Semin Roentgenol* 9:169-184, 1984.

Figure 9-22 from Stoker DJ, Murray RO: Skeletal changes in hemophilia and other bleeding disorders, *Semin Roentgenol* 9:185-193, 1974.

Unnumbered Figure 9-1 from Thibodeau GA, Patton KT: *Anatomy and physiology,* ed 2, St Louis, 1993, Mosby.

Chapter 10

Figure 10-2 from Lee JKT, Sagel SS, Stanley RJ, editors: *Computed body tomography,* New York, 1983, Raven Press.

Figures 10-4 and 10-5 from Karstaedt N et al: Computed tomography of the adrenal gland, *Radiology* 129:723-730, 1978.

Figure 10-7 courtesy Nolan Karstaedt and Neil Wolfman, Winston-Salem, N.C.

Figures 10-8 and 10-13 from Stark DD, Bradley WG: *Magnetic resonance imaging,* ed 2, St Louis, 1991, Mosby.

Figure 10-12 from Welch TJ et al: Pheochromocytoma: value of computed tomography, *Radiology* 148:501-503, 1983.

Figure 10-14 from Eisenberg RL: *Diagnostic imaging in surgery,* New York, 1987, McGraw-Hill.

Figure 10-16 from Friedland GW et al: *Uroradiology: an integrated approach,* New York, 1983, Churchill Livingstone.

Figure 10-23 from Palmer EL, Scott JA, Strauss HW: *Practical nuclear medicine,* Philadelphia, 1992, Saunders.

Figure 10-42 from Stark DD et al: Parathyroid scanning by computed tomography, *Radiology* 148:297-303, 1983.

Unnumbered Figure 10-1 from Thibodeau GA, Patton KT: *Anatomy and physiology,* ed 2, St Louis, 1993, Mosby.

Chapter 11

Figure 11-5 from Russinovich NA et al: Balloon dilatation of urethral strictures, *Urol Radiol* 2:33-37, 1980.

Figure 11-8 from McCarthy S, Fritzsche PJ: In Stark DD, Bradley WG, editors: *Magnetic resonance imaging,* St Louis, 1988, Mosby.

Figure 11-12 from Thoeni RF: In Moss AA, Gamsu G, Genant HK, editors: *Computed tomography of the body,* Philadelphia, 1983, Saunders.

Figure 11-15 from Jeffrey RB: In Moss AA, Gamsu G, Genant HK, editors: *Computed tomography of the body*, Philadelphia, 1983, Saunders.

Figure 11-16 from Fritzsche PJ et al: Undescended testis: value of MR imaging, *Radiology* 164:169-173, 1987.

Figures 11-22, 11-23, 11-44, 11-47, 11-64, 11-65, 11-67, *A*, 11-70, and 11-72 from Rumack CM, Wilson SR, Charborneau JW: *Diagnostic ultrasound*, St Louis, 1998, Mosby.

Figure 11-24 from Baker LL et al: MR imaging of the scrotum: pathologic conditions, *Radiology* 163:93-98, 1987.

Figures 11-28, 11-42, 11-49, 11-51, and 11-73 from Callen PW, editor: *Ultrasonography in obstetrics and gynecology*, Philadelphia, 1983, Saunders.

Figure 11-29 from Yune HY et al: Hysterosalpingography in infertility, *Am J Roentgenol Radium Ther Nucl Med* 122:642-651, 1974.

Figure 11-32 from Eisenberg RL: *Diagnostic imaging in surgery*, New York, 1987, McGraw-Hill.

Figure 11-35 from Lee JKT, Sagel SS, Stanley RJ, editors: *Computed body tomography*, New York, 1983, Raven Press.

Figure 11-38 from Eisenberg R: *Atlas of signs in radiology*, Philadelphia, 1984, Lippincott.

Figures 11-46, 11-52, and 11-53 from Lupetin AR: In Stark DD, Bradley WG, editors: *Magnetic resonance imaging*, St Louis, 1988, Mosby.

Figure 11-48 from Gedgaudas RK et al: The value of the preoperative barium-enema examination in the assessment of pelvic masses, *Radiology* 146:609-616, 1983.

Figure 11-50 from Gross BH et al: Computed tomography of gynecologic diseases, *AJR Am J Roentgenol* 141:765-773, 1983.

Figure 11-59 from Hagen-Ansert S: *Textbook of diagnostic ultrasound*, St Louis, 2001, Mosby.

Figure 11-69 From Pasto ME, Kurtz AM: *Semin Ultrasound CT MR* 5:170-193, 1984.

Unnumbered Figure 11-1 from Thibodeau GA, Patton KT: *Anatomy and physiology*, ed 2, St Louis, 1993, Mosby.

Chapter 12

Figures 12-2 and 12-7 from Eisenberg R: *Atlas of signs in radiology*, Philadelphia, 1984, Lippincott.

Figures 12-5, 12-26, 12-27, and 12-29 from Eisenberg RL: *Diagnostic imaging in internal medicine*, New York, 1985, McGraw-Hill.

Figure 12-6 from Eisenberg RL: *Gastrointestinal radiology: a pattern approach*, Philadelphia, 1990, Lippincott.

Figure 12-11 from Brown JC, Forrester DM: In Eisenberg RL, Amberg JR, editors: *Critical diagnostic pathways in radiology: an algorithmic approach*, Philadelphia, 1981, Lippincott.

Figure 12-15 from James AE Jr et al: Radiological features of the most common autosomal disorders: trisomy 21-22 (mongolism or Down's syndrome), trisomy 18, trisomy 13-15, and the cri du chat syndrome, *Clin Radiol* 22:417-433, 1971.

Figure 12-17 from Ovenfors CO, Godwin JD: In Eisenberg RL, Amberg JR, editors: Critical diagnostic pathways in radiology: an algorithmic approach, Philadelphia, 1981, Lippincott.

Figure 12-20 from Thomas PS, Carson NA: Homocystinuria. The evolution of skeletal changes in relation to treatment, *Ann Radiol* 21:95-104, 1978.

Figure 12-23 from Levin B: *AJR Am J Roentgenol* 85:685-696, 1961.

Figures 12-25 and 12-28 from Dunbar RD: Radiologic appearance of compromised thoracic catheters, tubes, and wires, *Radiol Clin North Am* 22:699-722, 1984.

Unnumbered Figure 12-1 from Thibodeau GA, Patton KT: *Anatomy and physiology*, ed 2, St Louis, 1993, Mosby.

PREFIXES/SUFFIXES/ROOTS

Prefix/Suffix/Root	Meaning	Example
a-, ab-	away from	abduction
a-, an-	without, not	asymmetric, anencephalic
ad-	toward	adduction
-algia	pain	arthralgia
ana-	up, back again	anaplastic
ante-	before, in front of	antecubital
anti-, ant-	against antibody,	antitoxin
auto-	self	autoimmune
bi-	two	bilateral, bidirectional
-blast	budding	osteoblast
cardi-	heart	cardiology, cardiac, pericardium
caudal	tail	caudal
cephal-	head	cephalic, hydrocephaly
chondro-	cartilage	chondroma, chondrosarcoma
-clast	destroyer, breaker	osteoclast
contra-	opposite	contralateral
crani-	skull	cranium, cranial
cyano-	dark blue	cyanotic
cyto-	cell	cytoplasm, erythrocyte, leukocyte
-dactyl-	finger, toe	polydactyly, arachnodactyly
deci-	tenth	decimal
derm-	skin	dermatology, epidermis
dys-	bad, difficult	dysplasia, dysuria
ecto-	outside of	ectoderm, ectopic
endo-, ento-	within	endoderm, endometrium
erythr-	red	erythrocyte
gastr-	stomach	gastric
-genic	causing	carcinogenic, pathogenic
gyn-, gyneco-	woman	gynecology
hem-, haem-	blood	hemorrhage, hemolytic
hemi-	half	hemisphere, hemidiaphragm
hetero-	different	heterogeneous
homo-	same	homogeneous
hyper-	over, excessive	hyperthyroidism, hypertension, hyperintense
hypo-	under, too little	hypothyroidism, hypotension, hypointense
iatro-	healer, healing	iatrogenic, psychiatry
infra-	below	infratemporal
intra-	within	intramural, intradermal
ipsi-	same	ipsilateral
iso-	equal	isointense
-itis	inflammation	appendicitis, diverticulitis
juxta-	near, next to	juxtaarticular
kilo-	thousand	kilogram
leuko-, leuco-	white	leukocyte, leukemia
lipo-	fat	lipoma, liposarcoma
-lysis, -lytic	dissolve	lytic, osteolytic
macro-	large	macroadenoma
magn-	great, large	magnify, magnum (foramen)

Prefix/Suffix/Root	Meaning	Example
mal-	bad, ill	malunion, malalignment
mega-, megalo-	large	megadose
melan-	black	melanoma, melanin
micro-	small	microscope, microadenoma, microcirculation
milli-	thousandth	milligram, milliliter
mono-	one	monostotic, monoclonal
multi-	many	multilocular, multifaceted
myelo-	marrow	myelogram, osteomyelitis
myo-	muscle	myoma, myositis
necro-	dead	necrosis
neo-	new	neovascularity, neoplasm
non-	not	nonunion, nonviable
ocul-	eye	ocular, oculomotor (nerve)
oligo-	few	oligemia
-ology	study of	radiology, pathology
onco	tumor	oncology
ophthalm-	eye	ophthalmology
-osis	condition of	diverticulosis
osteo-	bone	osteomyelitis, osteosarcoma
pan-	all	pansinusitis, pancytopenia
par-, para-	beside	paraaortic, paravertebral
patho-	disease	pathology, adenopathy
peri-	around	periarticular, periventricular, pericardium
plasm-, plast-	shape, form	neoplasm, anaplastic
pleur-	rib, side	pleural, pleurisy
pneumo-	air, breath	pneumothorax, pneumonia
poly-	many	polycystic, polyostotic
post-	after, later, behind	posttraumatic, postsurgical, postoperative
pre-	before, in front of	premenstrual, prepontine
pseudo-	false	pseudotumor, pseudopolyp
psych-	mind, spirit	psychiatry, psychology
re-	again, anew	reoperate, recalcify
retro-	backward, behind	retroperitoneum
-rrhea	flow, gush	diarrhea
schizo-	split	schizophrenia
sclero-	hard	sclerotic, atherosclerosis
semi-	half	semicircular
sub-	under, below	suborbital, subphrenic, subhepatic
super-, supra-	above, more than	suprarenal, supraorbital
syn-, sym-	with, together	synthesis, symmetric
tachy-	fast	tachycardia
techn-	art, skill	technology, technique
terti-	third	tertiary
tetra-	four	tetralogy (of Fallot)
thermo-	heat	thermometer
tomo-, -tome	cut	tomography, microtome
trans-	across	transverse (colon), transvenous (pacemaker)
tri-	three	trimalleolar, trisomy
ultra-	beyond	ultrasound
uni-	one	unilateral

LABORATORY VALUES AND THEIR SIGNIFICANCE

Laboratory Values	Significance of Laboratory Values
↑ Acid phosphatase	Prostate cancer, metastatic to bone
↑ Alkaline phosphatase	Liver disease; Paget's disease; bone tumor
↑ Amylase	Pancreatitis
↑ Bilirubin	Liver disease
↑ Blood urea nitrogen (BUN)	Kidney disease
↑ Calcium	Hyperparathyroidism; bone destruction
↑ Cholesterol	Tendency toward atherosclerosis
↑ Creatinine	Kidney disease
↑ Creatine phosphokinase (CPK)	Myocardial infarction; pulmonary infarction
↑ Glucose	Diabetes mellitus; Cushing's syndrome; glucagon-secreting pancreatic tumor
↑ Lactic dehydrogenase (LDH)	Myocardial infarction; pulmonary infarction; liver disease
↑ Serum glutamic-oxaloacetic transaminase (SGOT)	Liver disease
↑ Serum glutamic-pyruvic transaminase (SGPT)	Myocardial infarction; liver disease
↑ Total protein	Dehydration; immunoglobulinopathy
↑ Uric acid	Gout; antidiuretic therapy
↓ Calcium	Hypoparathyroidism; malabsorption; osteomalacia/rickets
↓ Cholesterol	Malnutrition; liver disease
↓ Glucose	Insulin-secreting pancreatic tumor; liver disease; hypopituitarism
↓ Total protein	Chronic liver disease; malnutrition; nephrotic syndrome

GLOSSARY

aberration: Deviation from normal

abscess: Encapsulated collection of pus

achalasia: Failure of the lower esophageal sphincter to relax because of absence or destruction of cells in the myenteric nerve plexus, which results in difficulty swallowing

acid-base balance: Stable concentration in body fluids

acinus: Cluster of alveoli

acquired immunodeficiency syndrome (AIDS): Impairment of cellular immunity

acromegaly: Gradual marked enlargement and thickening of the bones of the face and jaw

active immunity: A person forms antibodies to counteract an antigen in the form of a vaccine or a toxoid

acute pancreatitis: Active inflammation of the pancreas

adenocarcinoma: Malignancy of glandular tissue

adenoma: Benign epithelial neoplasm that grows in a glandlike structure

adenopathy: Enlargement of the lymphatic glands

adnexal: Pertaining to the uterine appendages (ovaries, fallopian tubes, and ligaments)

adult respiratory distress syndrome (ARDS): Severe pulmonary congestion due to diffuse injury to the alveolar-capillary membrane

afferent: To carry toward the center

agenesis: Absence of an organ

alcoholic gastritis: Inflammation of the stomach lining caused by alcohol

alveolar, or air-space, pneumonia: Inflammatory exudates that replace air and cause the affected lung to become solid

amorphous: Without shape or definite form

anaphylactic: Reactions are characterized by hypotension and vascular collapse (shock) with urticaria (hives), bronchiolar spasm, and laryngeal edema

anaplastic: Without form

anasarca: Pronounced swelling of subcutaneous tissues throughout the body

androgens: Any steroid hormone that increases male characteristics

anechoic: Not producing internal echoes (on ultrasound)

anemia: Decreased hemoglobin in the blood below normal levels

aneurysmal bone cyst: Consists of numerous blood-filled arteriovenous communications

angioma: Tumor composed of blood vessels

angulation: Indicates an angular deformity between the axes of the major fracture fragments

ankylosis: Immobility and consolidation of a joint caused by disease, injury, or surgical procedure

annihilation: Interaction produces two high-energy photons (gamma rays) in opposite directions (separated by 180 degrees)

antibodies: Body's counteraction to control antigens

anticoagulant: Substance that suppresses or delays coagulation of the blood

antigens: Body's ability to recognize foreign substances

aortic valve: Valve between the left ventricle and aorta

aplasia: Lack of normal development resulting in a small size or developmental failure resulting in the absence of an organ or tissue

appositional growth: Flat bones grow in size by the addition of osseous tissue to their outer surfaces

arachnodactyly: Congenital condition of long, thin spiderlike fingers and toes

arachnoid membrane: Middle meningeal covering

arachnoid villa: Projections of fibrous tissue from the arachnoid membrane

arteriovenous malformation: Abnormal communication between an artery and a vein

ascites: Accumulation of fluid in the abdominal cavity

aseptic necrosis: Cystic and sclerotic degeneration caused by injury, not infection

asthma: Widespread narrowing of the airways as a result of exposure to stimuli

astrocytoma: Primary tumor of the brain composed of astrocytes

atresia: Congenital absence or closure of a normal body orifice or tubular organ

atrial septal defect: Congenital anomaly resulting in an opening between the atria

atrophy: Diminished size as a result of wasting away

autonomic nervous system: Regulates involuntary body functions

autosomes: All chromosomes except gender

avulsion fracture: Small fragments torn from bony prominences

bacteremia: Bacteria spread through the circulatory system

bacterial (phlegmonous) gastritis: Inflammation of the stomach lining caused by a bacterial infection

bacterial meningitis: Infection of the membranes covering the brain and spinal cord caused by bacteria

basal ganglia: Islands of gray matter, which is largely composed of cell bodies

basophil: Granulocyte white blood cell

Bence Jones protein: Abnormal protein typically found in the blood of patients with multiple myeloma

benign: Tumors that closely resemble their cells of origin in structure and function and remain localized

blowout fracture: Break in the floor of the orbit

bone islands: Solitary, sharply demarcated areas of dense compact bone

bougienage: Passage of an instrument through a tubular structure to increase its caliber (as in the treatment of a stricture of the esophagus)

Bowman's capsule: Cup-shaped end of renal tubule

bowing fracture: Plastic deformation caused by a stress

boxer's fracture: Fracture of the neck of the 5th metatarsal with a dorsal angulation

bronchial adenomas: Neoplastic growth of glandular structures in the bronchi

bronchiectasis: Chronic dilatation of the bronchi or bronchioles

bronchiolar (alveolar cell) carcinoma: Malignant neoplastic growth of the bronchioli spreading into the alveolar surface

bronchioloalveolar carcinoma: Adenocarcinoma of epithelial cells projecting into the alveolar spaces

bronchogenic carcinoma: Primary malignancy arising from the mucosa of the bronchial tree

bullae: Large air-containing space

butterfly fragment: Elongated triangular fragment of cortical bone generally detached from two other larger fragments of bone

cachexia: Ill health and malnutrition marked by weakness and emaciation that is usually associated with severe disease processes

callus: New bone tissue that reunites the parts of a fracture

cancellous bone: Spongy bone of the medullary cavity and bony trabeculae

cancer: Collectively, malignant tumors

carcinoma: Malignant neoplasm of epithelial cell origins

caseation: Form of necrosis in which the tissue is changed into a dry, amorphous mass resembling cheese

catamenial: Pertaining to menstruation

cavitation: Formation of cavities, as in pulmonary tuberculosis or neoplasm

centesis: Puncture and aspiration

central nervous system (CNS): Consisting of the brain and spinal cord

cerebellum: Posterior portion of the brain located behind the brainstem

cerebrovascular disease: Any process that is caused by an abnormality of the blood vessels or blood supply to the brain

cerebrum: Left and right larger superior portion of the brain

cervical rib: An extra rib that articulates with a cervical vertebra

chest physiotherapy: Chest percussions (tapping) to keep lung secretions moving

chondroblastic: Forming cartilaginous tissue

chondrosarcoma: Malignant tumor of cartilaginous origin

chordae tendineae: Thin cords that connect each cusp of the two atrioventricular valves to papillary muscles in the heart ventricles

chorion: Important fetal membrane for exchange of nutrients

choroid plexus: Tangled mass of fine blood vessels within the ventricles producing cerebrospinal fluid

chromophobe adenomas: Pituitary tumor of nonstaining cells (acid or basic dyes)

chronic atrophic gastritis: Severe mucosal wasting that causes thinning and a relative absence of mucosal folds in the stomach

chronic bronchitis: Excessive tracheobronchial mucus production leading to the obstruction of small airways

chyme: Gastric contents that have become mixed with hydrochloric acid and the proteolytic enzyme pepsin, resulting in a milky white product

closed fracture: Fracture that does not disrupt the skin

coagulation factors: Responsible for the process of blood clotting

coalesce: To merge into a single mass

coeur en sabot: Appearance resembling the curved-toe portion of a wooden shoe

colic: Intermittent abdominal pain whose fluctuation corresponds to smooth muscle peristalsis

collaterals: Blood vessels that develop or enlarge to provide an alternative route around an obstruction

collecting tubule: Funnels urine into the papillary ducts in the renal pelvis

Colles' fracture: Transverse fracture of the distal radial metaphysis proximal to the wrist with a dorsal displacement of the distal fragment

collimator: Containing multiple parallel channels to allow the rays to pass

communicating hydrocephalus: Increased cerebrospinal fluid involving the entire ventricular system and subarchnoid space

comminuted fracture: Composed of more than two fragments

community acquired: Infected by exposure in the public domain

compact bone: Outer layer that to the naked eye appears dense and structureless

complete fracture: Discontinuity between two or more fragments

compound fracture: Overlying skin is disrupted with tissue destruction

compression fracture: Compaction of bone trabeculae and results in decreased bone length or width

computed tomography: Produces cross-sectional tomographic images by first scanning a slice of tissue from multiple angles with a narrow x-ray beam

congenital: Existing at birth

conjunctivitis: Inflammation of the delicate membrane that lines the eyelids and covers the exposed surface of the sclera (white part) of the eye

constipation: Extra water is absorbed from the fecal mass to produce a hardened stool

contracture: Shortening or shrinkage of a muscle or tendon resulting in persistent flexion or distortion at a joint

corpus callosum: Mass of white matter connecting the two cerebral hemispheres

corpus luteum: Anatomic structure on the ovary surface

corrosive gastritis: Inflammation of the stomach caused by corrosive agents

cortex: Outer portion of a bone or internal organ (kidney, adrenal gland, brain)

crossed ectopic: Ectopic kidney located on the same side as the normal kidney

CT number: Attenuation of a specific tissue relative to that of water

curvilinear: Having a curved configuration

cyst: Saclike structure usually filled with fluid

cystadenoma: Benign tumor forming a large cystic mass

cytology: Microscopic examination to determine cell structure

deglutition: Swallowing

demarcate: To set or mark the limits of

de novo: From the beginning; anew

depressed skull fracture: Comminuted fracture in which fragments are driven inward

diaphysis: Shaft of a long bone

diarrhea: Results from increased motility of the small bowel, which floods the colon with an excessive amount of water that cannot be completely absorbed

diastatic fracture: Linear fracture intersecting a suture and coursing along it to cause sutural separation

diastole: Heart relaxation phase when blood enters the heart

diencephalon: Lies between the cerebrum and the midbrain and consists of the third ventricle, thalamus, and hypothalamus

diffusion imaging: Relies on the movement of molecules and random thermal motion

dilation and curettage: Dilation of the cervix to allow the scraping of the uterine wall

diploic space: Loose osseous tissue between the two tables of the skull

direct fusion: Equipment designed to image two modalities simultaneously and integrate the images

dislocation: Displacement of a bone no longer in contact with its normal articulation

displacement: Separation of bone fragments

dissection: Separation of layers

dominant: Genes that always produce an effect

dura mater: Tough outermost meningeal covering

dysphagia: Difficulty swallowing

dysplasia: Disordered growth or faulty development of various tissues or body parts

dyspnea: Shortness of breath

echogenic: Producing a relatively strong reflection in ultrasound

ectopic: Abnormally positioned

ectopic pacemaker: Initiates abnormal heartbeats

ectopic pregnancy: Implantation occurring in the fallopian tube or pelvic cavity

edema: Accumulation of abnormal amounts of fluid in the intercellular tissue spaces or body cavities

effaced: Wiped out or obliterated

efferent: To carry away from the center or part

effusion: Accumulation of fluid

Eisenmenger's syndrome: Ventricular septal defect associated with pulmonary hypertension and cyanosis resulting from right-to-left shunting

electrolyte: Element or compound that dissociates into ions in fluid

electrolyte balance: Equilibrium of electrolytes in the body

elephantiasis: Localized edema

embolus: Any foreign matter, such as a blood clot or an air bubble, carried in the bloodstream

emphysema: Pathologic accumulation of air in tissues or organs (especially as applied to a disease of the lungs)

empyema: Accumulation of pus in a cavity

emulsifier: Substance that acts like soap by dispersing the fat into very small droplets that permit it to mix with water

endemic: Present in a particular country, nation, or region

endogenous: Originating from within the body

endosteum: Inner membrane lining the medullary cavity of a bone

en face: Face to face, looking at

engorgement: Congestion of a blood vessel or tissue with blood or other fluid

eosinophils: Granulocytic bilobed leukocyte

ependymoma: Tumor arising from the wall of the 4th ventricle, especially in children, and the lateral ventricles in adults

epididymis: Tightly coiled tube enclosed in a fibrous casing where final maturation of the sperm occurs

epiphrenic diverticula: Outpouching found in the distal 10 cm of the esophagus

epiphyseal cartilage: Cartilaginous plate separating the epiphysis from the diaphysis

epiphysis: End of a long bone that at first is separated from the main part by cartilage, but later fuses with it by ossification

erythropoietin: Protein serving as the humoral regulator of red blood cell formation

estrogen: Hormonal steroid compound that promotes secondary sex characteristics in female development

etiology: The study of disease causes (*not* a synonym for *cause*)

eventration: Diaphragmatic—elevation of the diaphragm; abdominal—protrusion of the bowel or removal of abdominal viscera

exacerbation: Increase in the severity of a disease or any of its symptoms

exenteration: Removal of all organs to debulk a tumor

exogenous: Arising from outside the body

exophthalmos: Abnormal protrusion of the eyeball

external fixation: Accomplished by the use of casts and splints

external reduction: Fracture is manipulated without surgical incision

extramedullary hematopoiesis: Formation of red blood cells outside the bone marrow

extrinsic asthma: Environmental allergens

exudate: Material (fluid, cells, or cellular debris) that has escaped from blood vessels and has been deposited in tissues or on tissue surfaces, usually as a result of inflammation

fat-soluble vitamins: Vitamins stored in the body (A, D, E and K)

fat-suppressed images: Requires saturation or full magnetization on the T1 sequence to ensure a large contrast difference between fat and water

fecalith: Intestinal stone formed around a center of fecal material

fibrin: Essential portion of a blood clot

fibrinolysis: Breaking up of a blood clot

fibromuscular dysplasia (FMD): Arterial disorder characterized by intramural folds of fibrous endothelial tissue

fissures: Deep grooves that divide each cerebral hemisphere into lobes

fistula: Abnormal connection, usually between two internal organs or from an internal organ to the surface of the body

focal: Localized

follicular carcinoma: Neoplasm with a follicular arrangement of cells

functional MR (fMR): Allows the localization of specific regions of the brain that correspond to various functions

fundoplication: Taking tucks in the fundus of the stomach and distal esophagus

fusiform: Spindle shaped

Galeazzi's fracture: Combination fracture of the shaft of the radius with a posterior dislocation of the ulna

gamma camera: A sodium iodide crystal detects the ionizing radiation emitted from the patient

gastrinoma: Tumor found in the pancreas and duodenum that is associated with peptic ulcers

giant cell tumor (osteoclastoma): Frequently occurring of the end of a long bone as a mass surrounded by a thin shell of new periosteal bone

gigantism: Excessive size and stature

glioblastomas: Neoplasm consisting of embryonic epithelial cells developing around the neural tube, transforming to supportive connective tissue of the nerve cells or ventricle lining

gliomas: Largest group of primary brain tumors, composed of malignant glial cells

glomerulus: Tuft or cluster

glucocorticoid: Regulates carbohydrate metabolism and is regulated by the adrenocorticotropic hormone

glycogen: Stored excess glucose

gonadal dysgenesis: Variety of conditions related to abnormal development of the gonads

grading: Assessment of a tumor to determine the degree of aggressiveness or malignancy

Gram's method: Technique for staining microorganisms

grand mal seizure: Epileptic seizure characterized by generalized involuntary muscular contractions and cessation of respiration that precedes tonic and clonic spasms of the muscles

granulation tissue: Combination of young developing capillaries and actively proliferating fibroblasts producing connective tissue fibers

granuloma: Tumorlike mass of tissue caused by a chronic inflammatory process

greenstick fracture: Incomplete fracture of one cortex

gyri: Winding convolutions of the cerebral hemispheres

hangman's fracture: Fracture of the arch of C2 anterior to the inferior facet; associated with anterior subluxation of C2 and C3

Heberden's nodes: Small, hard nodules at the distal interphalangeal joints of the fingers produced by calcific spurs of the articular cartilage and associated with osteoarthritis

helical: Spiral continuous motion

hematogenous: Spread by means of the bloodstream

hematoma: Hemorrhage trapped in body tissues

hemodynamic: Pertaining to the movements involved in the circulation of the blood

hemoglobin: Complex protein-iron compound in the blood that carries oxygen

hemoptysis: Coughing up blood or bloodstained sputum

hemorrhage: Bleeding or abnormal blood flow from a vessel into tissue

hepatitis: Inflammatory disease of the liver

hereditary: Transmitted to offspring through genes

heterogeneous: Composed of materials that have different structures or qualities

histology: Microscopic examination to determine tissue structure

homogeneous: Composed of material of similar or identical structure or quality

horseshoe kidney: Fusion of the lower poles of the kidneys

hydrocephalus: Enlargement of the head resulting from an abnormal increase in fluid within the ventricular system

hydronephrosis: Distention of the pelvis and calyces of the kidney

hydrosalpinx: Fallopian tube cystically enlarged with clear fluid

hydroureter: Dilatation of the ureter

hyperactive: Increased activity

hyperglycemia: Greater amount of glucose than normal in the blood

hyperlucency: Overly black appearance on a radiograph

hypernephroma: Most common renal cell carcinoma

hyperparathyroidism: Excessive secretion of parathormone leading to elevated serum levels of calcium and phosphate

hyperplasia: Abnormal increase in the number of cells composing a tissue or organ

hypertension: High blood pressure

hypoactive: Decreased activity

hypocalciuria: Abnormally low calcium in the urine

hypoparathyroidism: Insufficient secretion of parathormone causing sustained muscular contraction

hypoplastic kidney: Underdeveloped kidney

hypotension: Low blood pressure

hypothalamus: Activates, controls, and integrates peripheral autonomic nervous system, endocrine system, and somatic functions

hypoxia: Deficiency (lack) of oxygen

iatrogenic: Resulting from the activity of diagnosis or treatment by medical personnel

idiopathic: Having an unknown cause for underlying disease

immune: Reaction of the body provides a powerful defense against invading organisms

incomplete fracture: Opposite cortex is intact

incontinence: Loss of urinary bladder control

indolent: Causing little or no pain; slow to heal

infarction: Death of tissue because of interruption of the normal blood supply

infectious gastritis: Inflammation of the stomach lining caused by a microorganism

infiltrating: Spreading into surrounding tissue

inflammation: Initial response of body tissue to local injury

infundibulum: Funnel-shaped organ or passage

inguinal: Pertaining to the groin

insidious: Developing in a slow or unapparent manner; more dangerous than seems evident (e.g., an insidious disease)

in situ: Confined to the site of origin

insufficiency: Less than the normal amount

insulinoma: Hormone-secreting neoplasm most frequently in the tail of the pancreas, usually benign

integrated imaging: Requires software to fuse to imaging modalities

internal fixation: Surgically placed metal plates and screws, wires, rods, or nails to maintain reduction

interstitial pneumonia: Inflammatory process predominantly involving the walls and lining of the alveoli, its septa, and interstitial supporting structures

intima: Innermost layer of an organ or blood vessel

intraluminal: Within the empty space (lumen) of a hollow viscus

intramembranous ossification: Bone formation from connective tissue

intramural: Within the wall of an organ

intrathoracic kidney: Kidney located in the thoracic cavity

intrinsic: Belonging to the real nature of a thing

intrinsic asthma: Reaction to exercise, heat or cold exposure, and emotional upset

intrinsic rhythm: Specialized pacemaker cells in the sinoatrial node that initiate impulses at regular intervals

ipsilateral: Relating to the same side (antonym: contralateral)

irritable bowel syndrome: Refers to several conditions that have an alteration in intestinal motility

ischemia: Lack of blood supply in an organ or tissue

islands of Langerhans: Another name for islets of Langerhans

isoechoic: Structures that have the same echogenicity

Jefferson's fracture: Comminuted fracture of the ring of the atlas involving both the anterior and posterior arches

Jones fracture: Transverse fracture at the base of the 5th metatarsal

juxtaarticular: Adjacent to a joint

kyphosis: Anterior convexity in the curvature of the thoracic spine, sacrum, and coccyx, as viewed from the side

left-to-right shunt: Diversion of blood from the left side of the heart to the right through a septal defect

leukocytosis: Abnormal amount of white blood cells in the blood

linear skull fracture: Jagged or irregular sharp lucent line

lipoma: Tumor composed of fat

localized ileus: Isolated distended loop of small or large bowel

loop of Henle: U-shaped portion of the renal tubule

lordosis: Anterior concavity in the curvature of the lumbar and cervical spine, as viewed from the side

lymphangitic: Spread by means of the lymphatic system

lymphatic leukemia: Malignancy of the lymph nodes in which the lymphocytes are the only white blood cells to increase

lymphatic spread: Malignant cells carried through the lymphatic system

lymphoma: Neoplastic disorder of lymphoid tissue

lytic: Destructive

magnetic resonance imaging (MRI): A strong magnet producing radiofrequencies at specified intervals and receiving a return signal to produce an image

malabsorption disorder: Multitude of conditions in which there is defective absorption in the small bowel

malaise: Vague feeling of physical discomfort or uneasiness, as early in an illness

Mallory-Weiss syndrome: Subsequent inflammation of the distal esophagus due to a laceration associated with bleeding and mediastinal penetration caused by severe retching and vomiting

marrow: Hollow, tubelike structure within the diaphysis

mast cell: Connective tissue containing large basophilic granules that contain heparin, serotonin, bradykinin, and histamine, which are released in response to injury or infection

mastication: Chewing

matrix: Basic material from which a substance (such as tissue) develops

medulla: Inner substance of a bone (bone marrow) or an internal organ (kidney, adrenal gland)

medullary carcinoma: Soft malignant neoplasm of the epithelium that contains little or no fibrous tissue

medullary cavity: Hollow, tubelike structure within the diaphysis

medulloblastoma: Poorly differentiated malignancy consisting of tightly packed spongioblastic and neuroblastic cells

megahertz (MHz): One million waves per second

menarche: Commencement of the cyclic menstrual function

meninges: Three membranes covering the brain and spinal cord

meningitis: Inflammation of the coverings of the brain and spinal cord

meningocele: Protrusion of the meninges through the skin

menopause: Cessation of the menstrual cycle

menstrual phase: Menstruation occurs, the final phase of the three

mesentery: Peritoneal folds that attach the small and large bowel to the back wall of the peritoneal cavity

mesothelioma: Tumor that develops from the surface of the pleura, pericardium, or peritoneum

metaphysis: Wider part at the end of the shaft of a long bone, adjacent to the epiphyseal plate; located between the epiphysis and the diaphysis

metastasis: Spread of disease to another organ or tissue in the body

microcephaly: Abnormally small head in relation to the body with associated underdevelopment of the brain

micturate: Act of urinating

midbrain: Major portion of the brainstem between the forebrain and hindbrain

mineralocorticoids: Regulate salt and water balance by controlling sodium retention and potassium excretion by the kidneys

mitral valve: Bicuspid valve situated between the left atrium and ventricle

monoclonal immunoglobulin: Antibodies that are formed against a specific cell type

monocytes: Large mononuclear leukocytes

Monteggia's fracture: Isolated fracture of the shaft of the ulna associated with anterior dislocation of the radius at the elbow

Morgagni's hernia: Protrusion of abdominal contents into the anterior and lateral aspects of the thoracic cavity

morphologic: Pertaining to the form and structure of an organ

multilocular: Having many cells or compartments

multiple myeloma: Bone marrow malignancy

mural thrombosis: Thrombus originating in the vessel or cavity wall

mutations: Alterations in the DNA structure that may become permanent hereditary changes

mycoplasma: Colloquial usage for any of a genus of tiny microorganisms, smaller than bacteria but larger than viruses, that appear to be the causative agents of many diseases

mycosis: Fungal infection

myelin sheath: Insulated by a fatty covering (as a nerve)

myelocytic leukemia: Unregulated production of leukocytes

myelomeningocele: Herniation of the spinal cord and meninges through the skin

myocardial infarction (MI): Infarction of the heart muscle

myxedema: Puffy thickening of the skin with slowing down of physical and mental activity caused by failure of the thyroid gland

necrosis: Death of tissue

necrotic: Dead or decayed

neoplasia: Any new and abnormal growth, especially when the growth is uncontrolled and progressive

neoplasm: Product of neoplasia

nephrocalcinosis: Calcium deposits within the substance of the kidney

neurogenic: Originating in the nervous system

neuron: Basic nerve cell

neutrophils: Polymorphonuclear granular leukocyte

nidus: Focal point, especially of a stone or an inflammatory process

noncommunicating (obstructive) hydrocephalus: Obstruction of cerebrospinal fluid flow in the ventricular system causing enlarged ventricles

normal-pressure hydrocephalus: Defective resorption of cerebrospinal fluid or an overproduction of cerebrospinal fluid causing ventricular enlargement

nosocomial: Incidences of infections being developed at the acute care facility

nuclear medicine: Using radiopharmaceuticals to produce ionizing radiation, which is detected by a gamma camera to produce an image

nutritional deficiency: Lack of nutrients or their absorption

oblique fracture: Runs a course of approximately 45 degrees to the long axis of the bone

octreotide: Radioactive peptide tracer; a long-acting analog of the hormone somatostatin

oligemia: Decreased blood volume

oligodendrocytoma: Slow-growing glioma, usually arising in the cerebrum

oligohydramnios: Very small volume of amniotic fluid

oncology: The study of neoplasms

open fracture: Overlying skin is disrupted

open reduction: Surgical procedure using direct or indirect manipulation of the fracture

ossification: Bone formation

osteoblastic: Forming bony tissue

osteoclastic: Bone resorption

osteogenic sarcoma: Malignant tumor composed of osteoblasts that produce osteoids and spicules of calcified bone

osteolytic: Destroying bone

osteomalacia: Insufficient mineralization of the adult skeleton

osteomas: Tumor composed of bone tissue

ovulation: Release of the ovum from the ovary

palpitations: Rapid or fluttering beating of the heart, of which one is aware

papillary carcinoma: Slow-growing cystic thyroid carcinoma

paradoxical: Seeming to contradict the known facts

parathormone (PTH): Secreted by the parathyroids; regulates the blood levels of calcium and phosphate

parenchyma: Essential tissue of an organ

patent ductus arteriosus: Abnormal connection between the pulmonary artery and aorta caused by lack of the fetal ductus arteriosus

pathognomonic: Especially distinctive or characteristic of a disease or pathologic condition

pathologic fracture: Occurs when the bone weakens as a result of another process, such as a tumor, infection, or metabolic disease

pectus excavatum: Funnel chest: depressed sternum

pedunculated: Having a stalk (pedicle)

Pelken spur: Marginal spur formation

pelvic kidney: Kidney located in the pelvis

pericardium: Membrane surrounding the heart

periosteum: Fibrous membrane covering the outer surface

peripheral: Outside or away from the central portion of a structure

peripheral nervous system (PNS): Nerves outside the central nervous system; motor and sensory nerves

peristalsis: Wormlike movement by which the alimentary canal or other tubular organ propels its contents

permeable: Membrane allowing fluids to pass through

permeative: Diffusely spreading through or penetrating a substance, tissue, or organ, as by a disease process, such as cancer

pernicious anemia: Progressive megaloblastic anemia that results from lack of intrinsic factor that is required for absorption of vitamin B_{12}

petit mal seizure: Characterized by sudden, momentary loss of consciousness

pia mater: Innermost meningeal covering

pinna: Cartilaginous portion of the external ear

pituitary adenomas: Tumor composed of glandular tissue of the pituitary gland

platelets: Smallest blood cell; contains hemoglobin

Pneumococcus: Genus of gram-positive bacteria

pneumoperitoneum: Presence of free gas in the peritoneal cavity

polyhydramnios: Excessive accumulation of amniotic fluid

polypoid: Resembling a polyp

pons: Part of the brain stem containing centers for some reflexes

positron emission tomography (PET): Imaging technique using a radiopharmaceutical that emits a positron and is detected by a moving gamma camera

postmenstrual phase: Follows the menstruation phase in the menstrual cycle

postpartum: After childbirth

Pott's disease: Tuberculosis of the spine

primary stage: Initial phase of a disease process

progesterone: Hormone secreted by the corpus luteum to help regulate menstrual cycle and fertilization

proliferate: To multiply rapidly, increase profusely

prostate gland: Produces fluid that makes up the semen

proximal convoluted tubule: Second part of the nephron, first part of the renal tubule

psoriatic arthritis: Rheumatoid-like destructive process involving the peripheral joints in patients with psoriasis

pulmonary mycosis: Fungal infection of the lung

pulmonary valve: Three semilunar cusps between the right ventricle and the pulmonary trunk

punctate: Marked with dots or tiny spots

purpura: Spontaneous hemorrhages in the skin or mucous membrane

pyogenic: Bacteria that lead to the production of a thick, yellow fluid called pus

pyosalpinx: Fallopian tube filled with pus

radiofrequency pulse (RF): Refers to that portion of the electromagnetic spectrum in which electromagnetic waves can be generated by alternating current—commonly in the 1- to 100-MHz range, and their effect upon a body is potential heating of tissues in MRI

radiopharmaceutical: A drug that is tagged to emit ionizing radiation

recessive: Genes that manifest themselves only when the person is homozygous for the trait

reflex arc: Simple neurologic unit to carry impulses to the central nervous system and impulses to the peripheral nervous system

resection: Partial surgical removal of an organ or bone

resorption: Bone destruction by osteoclasts

retrovirus: Any of a family of ribonucleic acid viruses containing the enzyme reverse transcriptase

right-to-left shunting: Ventricular septal defect and overriding aorta causes unoxygenated blood into the left ventricle

rudimentary: Imperfectly developed

saccular: Resembling a pouch-like sac

sarcoma: Highly malignant tumors arising from connective tissues

sclerosis: Conversion of a portion of bone into an ivory-like, densely opaque mass; an abnormal hardening of body tissues or parts, especially of the walls of arteries

secondary stage: Progression of the disease process into the phase that follows the initial stage

secretory, or postovulatory, phase: Occurs between ovulation and the onset of the menses

segmental fracture: Consists of a segment of the shaft isolated by proximal and distal lines of fracture

seminal vesicles: Paired saclike gland that secretes a thick liquid that is rich in fructose for sperm motility

sequestrum: Piece of dead bone that has become separated from the surrounding healthy bone

serosa: Outer layer of a viscus (especially in the alimentary tract)

serpiginous: Having a wavy border

shock: Acute peripheral circulatory failure

sickle cell anemia: Anemia characterized by crescentic red blood cells that contain abnormal hemoglobin molecules and are susceptible to rupture

signs: Measurable manifestations of a disorder; objective manifestations

silhouette (cardiac): Outer border of the heart, seen against the radiolucent lungs

simple bone cyst (unicameral): True fluid-filled cyst with a wall of fibrous tissue

single-photon emission computed tomography (SPECT): Gamma camera moves around the patient and detects the gamma rays produced by the radiopharmaceutical

small cell (oat cell) carcinomas: Specific type of malignant bronchogenic epithelial neoplasm

somatic nervous system: Supplies the striated skeletal muscles

spermatogenesis: Formation of sperm

spherocytosis: Anemia due to erythrocytes that have a circular rather than a biconcave shape, making them fragile and susceptible to rupture

spina bifida occulta: Mild form in which there is a splitting of the bony neural canal but no clinical symptoms

spin-echo (SE): Most common pulse sequence used in MRI using 90° radiofrequency pulses to excite the magnetization and one or more 180° pulses to refocus the spins to generate signal echoes

spiral fracture: Encircles the shaft of a long bone

spirochete: Spiral type of bacterium of the genus *Spirochaeta*

spirometry: Measure of lung capacity using a spirometer

spondylolisthesis: Spondylolysis with displacement of vertebral alignment

spondylolysis: Cleft in the pars interarticularis situated between the superior and inferior articular processes of the vertebra without displacement

squamous cell carcinoma: Cancer in which tumor cells resemble stratified squamous epithelium

stable: Resistant to change

staghorn calculus: Renal calculi filling the entire renal pelvis of the kidney

staging: Determination of the amount of spread of a neoplasm, necessary to select appropriate therapy and to predict the future course of a disease

stasis: Stagnation of some fluid in the body (as of blood in veins); reduced peristalsis of the intestines resulting in the retention of feces

stenosis: Narrowing

stress, or fatigue, fracture: Fracture caused by repetitive stresses applied to the bone

stroke: Cerebrovascular accident; denotes a sudden and dramatic focal neurologic deficit

stroma: Supporting tissue of the matrix of an organ

subarachnoid space: Space beneath the arachnoid and above the pia mater, which contains cerebrospinal fluid

subchondral: Just beneath the articular margin

subluxation: Incomplete or partial dislocation

sulci: Shallow depressions on the surface of an organ

supernumerary kidney: An extra kidney

surfactant: Agent that lowers the surface tension

symptoms: Subjective manifestations; the patient feels

synapse: Point of contact between two neurons for impulses to flow

syndrome: Indicates the presence of a combination of symptoms that commonly occur together and are related to a single cause

systemic circulation: High-pressure system that carries blood to the organs and extremities

systole: Phase in which the heart contracts

T1-weighted image: Equilibrium—high-energy protons return to the low-energy state

T2-weighted image: Image relies upon local dephasing of spins

telangiectasia: Vascular lesion formed by dilation of a group of small blood vessels

teratoma: Neoplasm composed of various kinds of embryonic tissue

tertiary: Third in rank or order

testicular dysgenesis: Characterized by small testes that fail to mature or produce sperm and testosterone

testosterone: Stimulates the development and activity of the male accessory sex organs

thalamus: Portion of the brain that receives and processes sensory information and relays it to the cerebral cortex

thalassemia: Hemolytic anemia due to a defect in hemoglobin formation

thrombus: Blood clot in the vascular system

thymoma: Tumor originating from the thymus gland

thyroxine: Hormone influencing metabolic rate

tortuous: Full of twists, turns, or curves

torus (buckle) fracture: One cortex is intact, with buckling or compaction of the opposite cortex

toxoid: Chemically altered toxin

trabeculae: Supporting or anchoring strands of connective tissue within body structures

traction: Process of placing tension between two structures

transitional vertebra: Vertebra with characteristics of another spinal region

transverse fracture: Runs at a right angle to the long axis of a bone

tricuspid valve: Valve between the right atrium and right ventricle that has three cusps

trigone: Triangular area of the posterior bladder, between the openings for the ureters and urethra

tripod fracture: Fractures of the zygomatic arch and the orbital floor or rim combined with separation of the zygomaticofrontal suture

triradiate: Radiating in three directions

trisomy: Presence of an additional (third) chromosome

trophoblastic: Relating to the layer by which the fertilized ovum is attached to the uterine wall and from which the developing embryo receives its nourishment

tuberculous arthritis: Chronic indolent infection with a slow progressive course caused by tuberculosis

ulceration: Destruction of tissue creating an opening within a structure

ulcerogenic islet cell tumors (gastrinomas): Tumor found in the pancreas and duodenum that is associated with peptic ulcers

ultrasound: Images produced by high-frequency sound waves emitted from the transducer that are echoed back to produce an image

undifferentiated: Without form

undisplaced fracture: The bone is without angulation or separation

unilateral renal agenesis: Absence of a kidney

unstable: As a result of a fracture, alignment is uncertain

urate: Salt of uric acid

uremia: Presence of excessive amounts of urea and nitrogen in the blood

vaccine: Low dose of dead or deactivated bacteria or virus

valvulae conniventes: Circular folds of the small bowel

vasculitis: Inflammation of a vessel

vas deferens: Muscular tube that passes through the inguinal canal as part of the spermatic cord connecting the epididymis and seminal vesicle to form the ejaculatory duct

vasectomy: Severing of the vas deferens

vegetations: Abnormal growth of tissue around a heart valve

ventricular septal defect: Opening between the left and right ventricles allowing blood to flow back into the right ventricle instead of entering the systemic circulation

vermis: Structure resembling a worm

villi: Fingerlike projections of the small bowel to increase the inner surface area

viral meningitis: Inflammation of the meninges caused by virus

virus: One of a group of minute infectious agents characterized by a lack of independent metabolism and by the ability to reproduce only within living host cells

viscous: Thick, sticky

viscus: Any large internal organ, especially in the abdomen

vitamins: Organic compounds essential for normal physiologic and metabolic function

volume-rendered imaging: Technique that takes all the raw CT data density information and uses them to simulate three-dimensional images

water-soluble vitamins: Vitamins B and C, which cannot be stored and therefore must be included in the daily diet

Wimberger's sign of scurvy: Epiphyseal ossification centers are demineralized and surrounded by dense, sharply demarcated rings of calcification

Zenker's diverticula: Outpouching that arises from the posterior wall of the upper esophagus

INDEX

A

Abdomen
  computed tomography of,
    21f, 25f
  magnetic resonance imaging
    of, 26f
  ultrasound of, 18f-19f
Abdominal aortic aneurysm,
  285f-286f
Abdominal radiographs, 164
Abscess
  bone, 110
  brain. *See* Brain abscess
  definition of, 5
  lung, 48-49, 49f-50f, 49t
  paravertebral soft tissue, 112
  pericolic, 198, 199f
  subphrenic, 87
  tubo-ovarian, 427f
Achalasia, 175-176, 176f-177f,
  178t
Achondroplasia, 99-100, 100f,
  101t
Acoustic neuroma, 323, 323f, 329t
Acquired immunodeficiency
    syndrome
  characteristics of, 12
  gastrointestinal manifestations
    of, 12
  Kaposi's sarcoma in, 12, 13f
  magnetic resonance imaging
    of, 13, 14f
  neurologic manifestations of,
    12-13, 14f
  personal protective
    equipment, 3
  Pneumocystis carinii pneumonia
    associated with, 12-13, 13f
  treatment of, 13
Acromegaly, 323, 391-392, 392f
Active immunity, 11-12
Acute appendicitis, 196-197,
  197f-198f, 208t
Acute cholecystitis, 212-213,
  213t, 214f
Acute idiopathic
    thrombocytopenic purpura,
    376

Acute inflammation, 5
Acute lymphocytic leukemia, 368
Acute myelocytic leukemia, 368
Acute pancreatitis, 218-220, 220f,
  222, 223t
Acute renal failure, 262-263, 264t
Acute sinusitis, 356, 356f
Acyclovir, 312
Addison's disease, 383
Adenocarcinoma. *See also* Cancer;
    Carcinoma
  description of, 8
  of lungs, 65
Adenoma
  bronchial, 64-65, 67, 67f, 69t
  cystadenoma, 429, 430f
  definition of, 8
  parathyroid, 402, 404f
  pituitary, 323-324, 324f, 329t,
    392f
  thyroid, 398, 398f, 400t
Adrenal carcinoma, 383-384,
  384f, 385t
Adrenal cortex
  description of, 380
  hyperplasia of, 7
Adrenal glands, 380-390
Adrenal insufficiency, 383, 383f
Adrenal medulla, 381, 386-390
Adrenal venography, 381
Adrenalectomy, 385
Adrenocorticotropic hormone
  description of, 7
  glucocorticoid release
    regulated by, 381
  islet cell production of, 223
Adrenogenital syndrome, 383,
  383f, 385t
Adult respiratory distress
    syndrome, 77-78, 78f, 80t
Adynamic ileus, 190-191, 192f,
  193t
Aging, 349, 353t
Air bronchogram, 65-66
Air-bronchogram sign, 47f
Air-space pneumonia, 46
Alanine, 320
Alcoholic gastritis, 179, 185t

Alcoholism
  acute pancreatitis caused by,
    219
  cirrhosis caused by, 215
Aldosterone, 380
Aldosteronism, 382-383, 385t
Aldosteronoma, 382f
Alkaptonuria, 468, 469t
Alveolar pneumonia, 46, 46f
Alzheimer's disease, 349-350,
  351f, 353t
Amino acid disorders, 467-470
  alkaptonuria, 468, 469t
  cystinuria, 468-469, 469t
  Gaucher's disease, 469-470,
    470f
  glycogen storage diseases, 469,
    469f
  homocystinuria, 467, 468f, 469t
  ochronosis, 468, 468f, 469t
  phenylketonuria, 467-468,
    469t
Amyotrophic lateral sclerosis,
  353t, 353-354
Anaphylactic reactions, 12
Anaplastic tumor, 8
Anasarca, 5
Androgens, 381
Anechoic tissue, 18-19
Anemia
  aplastic, 366
  definition of, 361
  description of, 361-366
  hemolytic, 362, 364, 367t
  iron deficiency, 362
  megaloblastic, 364, 366, 366f,
    367t
  myelophthisic, 366
  pernicious, 364
  sickle cell. *See* Sickle cell
    anemia
Anencephaly, 447f
Aneurysm
  abdominal aortic, 285f, 286f
  aortic, 286f
  berry, 342-344, 345f
  definition of, 283
  fusiform, 285

Note: Page numbers followed by "f" refer to illustrations; page numbers followed by "t" refer to tables; page numbers followed by "b" refer to boxes.

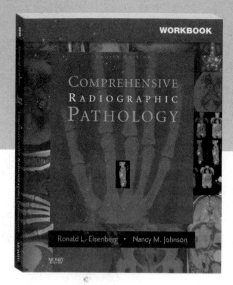
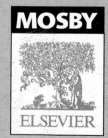